Empathy in Health Professions Education and Patient Care

Mohammadreza Hojat

Empathy in Health Professions Education and Patient Care

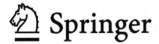

Mohammadreza Hojat
Sidney Kimmel Medical College
Thomas Jefferson University
Philadelphia, PA, USA

"Empathy in Health Professions Education and Patient Care" is an expanded and updated version of Empathy in Patient Care: Antecedents, Development, Measurement, and Outcomes published in by Springer in 2007.

ISBN 978-3-319-27624-3   ISBN 978-3-319-27625-0   (eBook)
DOI 10.1007/978-3-319-27625-0

Library of Congress Control Number: 2015960933

Springer Cham Heidelberg New York Dordrecht London

Printed on acid-free paper

Springer International Publishing AG Switzerland is part of Springer Science+Business Media (www.springer.com)

*In dedication to those who devote
their professional lives to understanding
human suffering, eliminating pain,
eradicating disease and infirmity,
curing human illnesses, and improving
the physical, mental, and social well-being
of their fellow human beings.*

Foreword to the Original Edition

Empathy for me has always been a feeling "almost magical" in medical practice, one that brings passion with it, more than vaunted equanimity. Empathy is the projection of feelings that turn *I and* you into *I am* you, or at least *I might be* you. Empathy grows with living and experience. More than a neurobiological response, it brings feelings with it. Empathy helps us to know who we are and keeps us physicians from sterile learned responses. Originally, the emotion generated by an image, empathy began as an aesthetic concept, one that should have meaning for medical practices now becoming so visual.

Empathy comes in many different guises. Empathy can be looking out on the world from the same perspective as that of the patient: to understand your patients better, sit down beside them, and look out at the world from their perspective. But empathy can be far more, therapeutic even, when physicians try to help their sick patients.

As a gastroenterologist, I have always been interested in what people feel, more than in what their gut looks like. When the flexible endoscopes began to change our vision in the 1960s, I gave up doing "procedures." Taking care of patients with dyspepsia or diarrhea up to that time had been a cognitive task: We deduced what might be seen from what our patients told us. Fortunately for our confidence, few instruments tested the truth of what we thought. The endoscopes I disdained proved forerunners of more discerning apparatus that now makes it easy for physicians to "see" an abnormality they can equate with the diagnosis. Gastroenterologists no longer trust what they hear—but only what they can see.

"Imaging," as X-ray studies have been renamed, has vastly improved medical practice. In the twenty-first century, surgeons are more likely to take out an inflamed appendix than they were in the twentieth century, thanks to the ubiquitous CAT scans that depict the offending organs. Cancer of the pancreas once was allowed to grow unchallenged in the belly when physicians had only a "barium meal" to hint at a malign process, but now they can see it at a much earlier stage. Paradoxically, such prowess makes the patients' story more important than ever: CAT scans uncover so many harmless anatomical abnormalities that, more than ever, the physician must be sure that what is to be removed from the patient will prove to be the origin of his or her complaints.

"Imaging," so seductive to the physician, sometimes stands in the way of the empathy that this book is all about. One of my favorite aphorisms, of untraceable provenance, holds that *"The eye is for accuracy, but the ear is for truth."* It is easy to see a cancer of the pancreas in a CAT scan as you jog by the view box, but it takes far longer to listen to the anguish of the patients at the diagnosis which encapsulates their abdominal pain. And modern physicians have so little time.

Moreover, this enhanced ability to see what is amiss has turned many minor symptoms into diseases, in a frenzy of reification. "Heartburn," which patients once talked about, has now been renamed "GERD," gastroesophageal reflux *disease*, which doctors must see to recognize. That once innocuous complaint, which boasted the badge of duty but could be banished by a little baking soda, has become a disease requiring treatment, not just a change of heart or mind. And it has become almost universal, thanks to the media hype magnifying attention to every little qualm of digestion.

The triumphs of medical instrumentation have led some medical students to worry that the physicians they will become may have little to do for patients as the twenty-first century moves on. They point to the "Turing experiment": Talking to someone behind a curtain, can you detect whether the answers come from a living person or a computer? Sooner or later, they fear, patients will talk to a computer with about as much idea of what or who is responding as Dorothy before the Wizard of Oz. How will tomorrow's physicians compete with the all-knowing and all-seeing "Doc in the Box!"

I hope they will learn that the sick need the right hand of friendship; for neither robots nor computers can compete with humans when it comes to empathy, sympathy, or even love for those in trouble or despair. Empathy is a crucial component of being truly human and an essential characteristic of the good physician. Yet critics assert that modern physicians lack empathy. If that is true, the selection process may be at fault: Physicians are winnowed by victories, from the competition to get into college and then the struggle to get into medical school. Having clambered up the greasy pole, students may have little feeling left for the defeated, the humble, those who have not made it to the top. Once in medical school, they don white coats—unwisely I think—helping to see themselves separate from their patients and the world. As they learn to be experts fixing what is damaged, they learn the primacy of the eye over the ear.

Sadly, current medical school education squeezes empathy out of the students who learn the body and forget the spirit/mind, while their teachers inculcate more detachment from the "still sad music of humanity." Later, the experience of postgraduate hospital training quenches the embers of empathy, as they see young lives cut too short by disease and old lives suffering too long. They learn to talk about the case rather than the person, medical writing is objective and impersonal, and imperturbability becomes their watchword. Medical students, as so many studies have shown repeatedly, lose their empathy as they go through medical school training that "clinical medicine" has been relabeled "cynical medicine."

That is what this book is intended to counter, just as the program it depicts has changed medical education at Jefferson. In *Empathy in Patient Care*, Dr. Mohammedreza Hojat expands on what we physicians do not see, but can only imagine. **The Jefferson**

Longitudinal Study of Medical Education, which he has headed for so long, provides the bedrock for this volume. He and his colleagues have studied how empathy begins—how medical students develop—and how empathy affects "outcomes"—how patients fare. We humans are social beings who need to live with others and who depend on interpersonal relationships for support. That need for human relationship, Hojat finds essential to the patient–physician dyad, as much as to the work of the ministry. Basing his conclusions on data obtained by the research instruments he has utilized and perfected, Dr. Hojat does not just talk about empathy, he measures it.

A Ph.D. psychologist of estimable attainment, Dr. Hojat has been drawn to viewing empathy as integral to the practice of medicine. The whole aim of this longitudinal study is to select medical students who will be empathic practitioners and to keep them empathic throughout life. "Attainment" and "success" provide the benchmarks of this long-term comprehensive psychosocial study of what makes for successful medical students and turns them into good physicians.

Teachers must find paths to refresh students' feelings for the human condition early; for that, the humanities loom so important. Beginning in college, premedical students—at least those who are not committed to a career in research—should focus less on the hard sciences and far more on the social sciences and literary fields. Liberal studies should make it easier for them to fold real human emotions into the care they give and—just as important—into their character. The humanities are not forgotten in this book, which recommends more experience with poetry and literature to nurture an empathic attitude in medical students.

It may be easier to recognize the absence of empathy than its presence. Knowing that it had its first openings in the Nazi concentration camp at Theresienstadt (Terezin), I cannot watch the play *Brundibar* without anguish. Its children/actors sing a song of defiance and survival on stage, but they know, Maurice Sendak its illustrator avers, that at its end they will be shipped to Auschwitz, to burn in the ovens of the death camps. Where was the empathy that makes us human in the German guards and officials of that place? In other concentration camps, it is said, prisoners who were musicians were ordered to play chamber music for the guards and officials who, afterwards, would send them off to be gassed. Not much empathy there. Pleasure in music, but no humanity.

Empathy is both rational *and* emotional, for many physicians. Dr. Hojat devotes attention to how much empathy comes from thinking—what the trade calls cognition—and how much from emotion. When we reason, he asks, do we also have emotions appropriate to our thoughts? Surely the answer must depend on what we are thinking about, but here I yield to his appraisal of the data.

Physicians may find his distinction between empathy as a cognitive act and sympathy as an emotional attribute to be more daring, since for us sympathy involves compassion. We physicians, licensed by the state and more knowledgeable than our patients because of experience, try to feel what they experience. Can we feel too much? Get too involved? Can doctors take care of friends? Is it possible for a physician to manage the medical problems of a spouse or children? Are people better off being taken care of by a friend who treats them as patient than by a stranger? Such questions arise from reflecting on his studies.

Dr. Hojat's strong views on human connections are echoed by the phrase "A *friend* a day keeps the doctor away!" Friends, marriage, and all social arrangements help; falling sick, illness, and disease test those relationships. Aging tests them too, especially in the loss of friends, so few left for the funeral. Dr. Hojat attends to some optimistic psychological studies from California claiming that emotional support for women with breast cancer improves their longevity—but, I must caution, most of the time, prognosis depends more on the presence of metastases in lymph nodes than on the circuits of the brain, or even on the spirit.

Hojat finds the roots of empathy nourished by the mother–child relationship, even as he elucidates the nature–nurture conflict. Emotional support in childhood must be enormously fruitful, and the nurturing of infants crucial in establishing a model. Culture must have equal influence, along with the central role of genetic endowment.

Hospital chaplains understand the importance of connections when they talk about "being there" with the patient; no need for talk, just being there, actively present. Dr. Hojat traces the physiological path of that clinical mystery, as he puts it, a gift to the patient. Or is it our duty?

His words on brain imaging bring everything into balance, as up to date as possible. Nevertheless, I wonder whether psychiatry as talk therapy will survive the burgeoning skills of computers. Neurobiology seems to suggest that the mind is like a secretion from the brain, like insulin from the pancreas, that the tide of neurotropic drugs can sweep clean. I prefer to dream that the mind arises from the brain more like smoke from a burning log, to obey quite different physical laws. Just as smoke flies free from its earth-bound roots, so from our protoplasm springs poetry, from the circuits of the brain our hope for a Creator. Yet Leibnitz wisely asked, if we could stroll through a brain as through a room, where would we find charity, love, or ambition? A Creator may have fashioned the channels, but will we ever locate them in that gray matter of the brain? Much depends on culture and environment, as the author so wisely points out.

Empathy is crucial to clinical practice, to treatment especially, though not all physicians agree. Some time ago, an essay *"What is empathy and can it be taught?"* was quickly rejected by a well-known journal of opinion, its editor observing that "Empathy has no place in medical practice." After the essay appeared in a less austere journal, however, many supportive letters and comments encouraged a book on that topic, one that welcomed the return of emotion to medicine.

Hojat sees empathy as largely cognitive, but some will think of empathy as present at birth, innate, waiting to be developed but unlikely to be created by any act of will. That could be too much like play-acting, for if the physician–patient relationship is as central to practice as I believe, there are mystical relationships not yet pictured by our models.

Psychologists will find much of interest in the chapters on techniques and testing. A remarkable collection of abstracts from the Jefferson Longitudinal Study, published in 2005, supports the conclusions in this book. One hundred and fifty-five of those abstracts eventuated in papers published elsewhere provide the outcome data that has changed much at Jefferson. Some, unfamiliar with such studies, will wonder about psychometrics, and how often answers can be "socially desirable," as

Dr. Hojat puts it. They remember that to test how well a subject bears pain in a labo-ratory setting cannot replicate the state of mind of a patient lying in a bed despairing of unfamiliar abdominal pain and wondering what will happen next. Knowing that an experimenter is causing your pain makes it a lot easier to bear than when you are in the dark. Psychometrics is a complicated science.

The "wounded healer" represents a model. Something good has to be said for the narcissistic satisfaction that comes from patient–physician relationships: working with patients, caring for them, and sharing their emotional life but respecting bound-aries. That can be therapeutic for physicians. The physician who has been sick is more likely to be empathic in future practice. Physicians who have had their own troubles have confessed that they have found surcease in talking with patients. Physicians who "burn out" or are bored are often, I imagine, those who regard their tasks as purely medical and technical. Countertransference can play a dynamic ther-apeutic role for physicians, at times.

The social revolutions of the late twentieth century brought the physician–patient relationship from the distant "professional" ideal of William Osler to one that encourages an intimacy that must vary with cultural norms. Physicians of the twenty-first century in America ask about sexual habits and proclivities, questions which once were taboo. With the fading of parentalism, we are far more frank about the uncertainties of our practices. Prudently, Dr. Hojat has studied the influence of culture and environment, the expectations that mold our behavior. As educators, we might wish to have had empathy poured into our students before they come to medi-cal school, but, as the Jesuits knew, for that we would have to train them from early childhood. The habits and norms of physicians vary with the passage of time; the ideal of what is proper for a physician to do or say also has varied remarkably: Sometimes touching the patient is appropriate and comforting, and sometimes it is misunderstood and inappropriate.

Empathy varies with age and experience. Am I more empathic now than 40 years ago because I have experienced so much more? Does empathy develop? Or does it atrophy or weaken? In recognizing the differences between men and women, Hojat comes down firmly on the side of women as more empathic than men, at least in Western culture. Women are new in medicine, at least in America still finding their way; and the data may change with the "maturation" of their medical practices.

Not all physicians need empathy, for patient–physician encounters comprise many different relationships. Chameleon-like, physicians have to vary with circum-stances. Treating a patient with pneumonia is quite different from evaluating some-one with abdominal pain of uncertain origin. Their faith in the efficiency of computers has convinced some physicians that empathy is an unnecessary addition to their character. Time is at such a premium; family care doctors complain that they do not get paid for being nice to patients. They have to see more patients ever more briefly just to pay expenses. That must be why fewer graduates are choosing pri-mary care or even internal medicine.

Analysis of videotaped interviews must be a good way to refresh and recover the empathy that students bring to medical school. They can relearn empathy in discussing why patients have asked certain questions, and what answers are most fitting, and what comfortable phrases may make patients feel better. Rita Charon and others have gotten medical students to write about diseases from their patients' perspective, a very appropriate stimulus to empathy and understanding, the "narrative competence" that Hojat praises.

That also requires the reading of stories and novels, and the discussion of narratives, and it certainly requires more collegiality than trainees tell about in the beginning of the twenty-first century. Empathy can be strengthened through stories. I have no wish to add to what others have written about the medical school curriculum, but I am convinced that rhetoric—the equivalent of persuasion—needs a rebirth in medical practice. We physicians are more than conduits of pills and procedures; we need to build bridges between our medical practice and the world of suffering around us. Conversation is essential, continuing discussions about patient–doctor relationships, about human relationships in general. We can fan the passion of empathy in medicine by both science and poetry, reason and intuition; we can provide more than the robots and computers, for only men and women are capable of empathy.

Team medicine, now looming so large, may supply that remedy through some other member of the group. A nurse or medical student, someone other than a doctor, can readily ask questions and provide the comfort that the physicians on the team do not always find the time to give. Now that hospitalists go from one desperately sick patient to the next, medical practice in the hospital has become too complex for any one person, and the emotional burdens of hospital care cannot be any less trying.

As technology takes over the physicians' task of making diagnoses, empathy will need more attention than equanimity. What physicians can do in the twenty-first century is vastly more effective than before. But physicians no longer find the time to talk to each other, let alone their patients. Conversation helps to develop empathy, empathy overcomes our isolation, and in empathy we rediscover ourselves.

Dr. Hojat wisely provides an agenda for future research ranging from selecting prospective medical students for their empathy to evaluating the neurobiological components of empathy and compassion. He and his coworkers are keen to provide measurements that will predict clinical competence and clinical empathy to help in the selection of medical students. But it may be a long time before the personal qualities of prospective medical students will trump their scientific know-how or their desirably high scores in the MCAT. Gentleness does not loom as captivating as high science grades to most deans of admission. Hojat's utopia wisely provides goals which medical practitioners and teachers can ponder and try to reach for in their daily activities. We are in his debt.

Howard Spiro, M.D.
Emeritus Professor of Medicine
Yale University School of Medicine
New Haven, CT
1924–2012

Foreword to the Expanded Edition

It was in a 1964 decision (Jacobellis vs. State of Ohio) in which he was trying to define obscenity, that Supreme Court justice Potter Stewart famously said, "I shall not today attempt further to define the kinds of [obscene] material I understand to be embraced ... *but I know it when I see it.*" Much the same can be said for defining and researching empathy, especially in the context of health professions education and patient care. For example, between The Oxford English Dictionary (Compact Edition) and Wikipedia I recently found no fewer than 14 different definitions of empathy some of which conflicted with, and even contradicted, one another.

For a concept with so many different definitions, empathy's history is surprisingly brief, the word having entered the lexicon in the late nineteenth and early twentieth centuries. This is not to say that caring, concern, and compassion for patients, all mentioned in various definitions of empathy, didn't exist prior to 1900. On the contrary, one can trace the philosophy and practice of these skills to ancient Greek physicians as Plato showed (Prangle, 1988). Nor does a literal translation of the word, derived from the Ancient Greek (*empatheia*), "physical affection, passion, partiality" which, in turn, derives from (*pathos*) "passion" or "suffering," help explain why empathy has been the subject of such wide-ranging thought. The answer lies in the fact that the English term "empathy" is actually a translation of the German word, "Einfühlung" (roughly translated as "to feel into"), that first appeared in an 1873 doctoral thesis entitled, *On the Optical Sense of Form: A Contribution to Aesthetics* (Vischer et al., 1994). The thesis focused on the philosophy of idealism and its application to appreciating architectural forms. In its original form, empathy had nothing to do with the connection of human beings to one another and their suffering. The term was translated and reintroduced as "empathy" in 1909 by a British-born psychologist, Edward B. Titchener, who used it in *his* theory of introspection and the problem of intersubjectivity, that is, how it is possible to know others' minds and experiences (Titchener, 1909). Given its intellectual history, it is not that surprising, even today, that there is so little agreement about what empathy is and the canons of evidence that surround it.

The history of an incomplete translation from one language and disciple to another, plus the current lack of precision in meaning and use, has led to the same sort of definitional quagmire that faced Justice Stewart half a century ago. Few researchers have attempted, and even fewer have succeeded, in operationalizing empathy in a comprehensive theoretical framework and measuring it in valid and reliable ways. The good news is that this is exactly what Dr. Hojat has done in the expanded and updated edition of *Empathy in Health Professions Education and Patient Care*. Building on his closely reasoned view of empathy and the extant literature in 2007, when the original edition appeared, this expanded edition provides the reader with updates to the field including exciting developments in the neuroscience of empathy, physiological correlates and heritability, psychodynamics, communication, gender, and the relationship of empathy to personal characteristics such as career choice, knowledge acquisition, and clinical competence. Included in the expanded edition are also updated chapters on the development and use of the Jefferson Scale of Empathy (JSE) as well as results from a worldwide network of scholars who have used it in their research. In short, this book is a treasure trove of information and practical wisdom about studying empathy that is unparalleled in depth, breadth, and scholarship.

It was Thomas Kuhn, in his book, *The Structure of Scientific Revolutions* (Kuhn, 1963), who described the evolution of paradigmatic thought in science, thought that normally develops through the accretion of evidence over time and is sometimes disrupted or revolutionized by new ways of thinking. Darwin and Wallace's work on the origin of species through natural selection, Einstein's theory of relativity, and Crick and Watson's discovery of DNA are a few examples of such paradigmatic shifts that have occurred in the modern scientific era. While these paradigm shifts are spectacular and often bring about rapid change, the slow evolution of paradigms in science is more normative. Each paradigm shift brings with it opportunities to add new knowledge as a field matures.

Applying Kuhn's notion of paradigm development in the social and behavioral sciences, Inui and Carter (Inui et al., 1983; Carter et al., 1982) surveyed the field of doctor-patient communication in the early 1980s and concluded that it was slowly evolving from a phase of descriptive work to a more advanced stage in which specific communication behaviors in doctor-patient encounters could be linked to both biomedical and functional outcomes of care. For example, in a series of outcome-based studies, Greenfield, Kaplan, and Ware found that a simple 20-min communication coaching intervention designed to enable patients to ask more questions produced measurably better outcomes in hypertension, diabetes, and ulcer disease (Greenfield et al., 1985). Likewise, in pediatrics, Starfield and her colleagues (1981) showed that patient-practitioner agreement on the nature of a child's problem and the proposed solution had a direct and positive effect on outcomes of care. Given the diversity in scholarship in and around empathy, it has been difficult, until recently, to imagine a similar movement toward outcome-based studies. And yet, if the gold standard of clinical research is the ability to connect specific qualities, characteristics, and behavior outcomes of care, Dr. Hojat's recent research on the role of empathy in diabetes stands out as a telling example of the scientific maturation of research on empathy and the movement from descriptive studies to predictive models (Hojat et al., 2011). The same can be said for his work in medical education and his finding that there is a decided decrease in empathy in the third year of medical school (Hojat et al., 2009), a finding that is both significant and actionable. In addition to these studies, the reader will find in the expanded edition of *Empathy in Health Professions Education and Patient Care* chapters on the evidence supporting empathy training in health professions education, its effect(s) on patient outcomes, and a road map for future research in the field.

I grew up professionally as a health services researcher and educator in an academic division of general internal medicine where we trained primary care physicians to diagnose and treat 80 % of office-based patient problems and to know when to refer the rest. To succeed in this environment one must be flexible, adaptable, and like solving lots of different kinds of problems. I recall attending a grand rounds presented by a well-known basic scientist who was working at the time on the human genome project. In introducing him it was noted that he had spent the majority of his career working on sequencing the DNA of a single insect, the common fruit fly (*Drosophila melanogaster*)! I was blown away by the investment of time and energy this researcher had put into a single problem, which might or might not produce meaningful results, and might ultimately fail. As it turned out, the investment was worth it and the combined efforts of many basic scientists paid off when the human genome was successfully sequenced in 2013. The point is that single mindedness, persistence, and focus in scientific research, while risky, often lead to significant advances in the field.

The expanded edition of *Empathy in Health Professions Education and Patient Care* is the latest installment in one researcher's lifelong commitment and focus to defining, measuring, and disseminating research on the role of empathy in medical education and practice. It is learned, lucid, and accessible to those who have a passing interest in this area as well as established researchers and medical educators tasked with training future physicians and other health care professionals who hope to realize the promise of medicine to heal as well as cure. It was Sir Isaac Newton, in a letter to a rival, who wrote, "What Descartes did was a good step. You have added much in several ways [but] … *If I have seen further it is by standing on the shoulders of Giants*" (Turnbull, 1959). Indeed, with the publication of this expanded edition of *Empathy in Health Professions Education and Patient Care*, we can see more clearly what lies just over the horizon for research, education, and practice on the role of empathy in health professions education and patient care. As a communication researcher, educator, and sometimes patient, I am especially grateful to Dr. Hojat for his long-standing interest and focus on this topic and for the path he has blazed in bringing clarity and precision to the science and practice of empathy.

Richard M. Frankel, Ph.D.
Professor of Medicine and Geriatrics
Indiana University School of Medicine
Indianapolis, IN

References

Carter, W.B., Inui, T.S., Kukull, W.A., & Haigh, V.H. (1982). Outcome-based doctor-patient inter-action analysis: II. Identifying effective provider and patient behavior. *Medical Care, 20*, 550–566.

Greenfield, S., Kaplan, S., & Ware, Jr., J.E. (1985). Expanding patient involvement in care: Effects on patient outcomes. *Annals of Internal Medicine, 102*, 520–528.

Hojat, M., Louis, D.Z., Markham, F.W., Wender, R., Rabinowitz, C., & Gonnella, J.S. (2011). Physicians' empathy and clinical outcomes in diabetic patients. *Academic Medicine, 86*, 359–364.

Hojat, M., Vergare, M., Maxwell, K., Brainard, G., Herrine, S.K., Isenberg, G.A., …, Gonnella, J.S. (2009). The devil is in the third year: A longitudinal study of erosion of empathy in medical school. *Academic Medicine, 84*, 1182–1191.

Inui, T.S., Carter, W.B., Kukull, W.A., & Haigh, V.H. (1982). Outcome-based doctor-patient inter-action analysis 1: Comparisons of techniques. *Medical Care, 20*, 535–549.

Kuhn, T. (1963). *The structure of scientific revolutions*. Chicago, IL: The University of Chicago Press.

Prangle, T.L. (1988). *The laws of Plato*. Chicago, IL: The University of Chicago Press.

Starfield, B., Wary, C., Hess, W., Gross, R., Birk, P.S., & D'Lugoff, B.C. (1981). The influence of patient-practitioner agreement on outcome of care. *American Journal of Public Health, 71*, 127–131.

Titchener, E.B. (1909). *Lectures on the experimental psychology of the thought-processes*. New York, NY: Macmillan.

Turnbull, H.W. (Ed.). (1959). *The correspondence of Isaac Newton: 1661–1675*. Volume I. London: The Royal Society at the University Press.

Vischer, R., Mallgrave, H. F., & Ikonomou, E. (1994). *Empathy, form, and space: Problems in German aesthetics, 1873–1893*. Santa Monica, CA: Getty Center for the History of Art and the Humanities.

From Preface to the Original Edition

All human beings are in truth akin,
all in creation share one origin.
When fate allots a member pangs and pain,
no ease for other members then remains.
If, unperturbed, another's grief canst scan,
thou are not worthy of the name of human.

—Saadi (classic Persian poet, 1210–1290 AD)

Although the primary intention of this book is to describe the antecedents, development, measurement, and consequences of empathy in the context of health professions education and patient care, some of the material presented goes beyond that purpose. For the sake of a more comprehensive analysis, one cannot isolate such a complex and dynamic entity as empathy in health professions education and patient care from a string of determining factors (e.g., its evolutionary, genetic, developmental, and psychodynamic aspects) and multiple consequences (e.g., physical, mental, and social well-being). Thus, to achieve a broader understanding of empathy in health professions education and patient care, I discuss the issue in the wider context of a dynamic system, the function of which rests on the following six premises:

- Human beings are social creatures.
- The human need for affiliation and social support has survival value.
- Interpersonal relationships can fulfill the human need for affiliation and social support.
- The interpersonal relationship between clinician and patient is a special case of a "mini" social support system that can fulfill the need for affiliation and support.
- Empathy in patient care contributes to the fulfillment of the need for affiliation and support.
- An empathic clinician–patient relationship can improve the physical, mental, and social well-being of the patient as well as the clinician.

Human beings are designed by evolution to form meaningful interpersonal relationships through verbal and nonverbal communication. Human beings possess a system of needs for social affiliation—for bonding and attachment, forming a social network, feeling felt, for understanding and being understood. The grand principle is the same whether the individual is an infant, a child, an adolescent, or an adult, or

xvii

whether the individual is male or female, healthy or ill: *Being connected is beneficial to the human's physical, mental, and social well-being; it has survival value.*

The aforementioned principle is indeed the theme underlying all chapters of this book. In some chapters, it may seem that I take my eyes off the intended target of health professions education and patient care, but I always return to the underlying theme to link the discussion to the clinician–patient relationship. When appropriate, I frequently use the terms "clinician" and "client," rather than "doctor," "physician," or "patient," to make the discussion more general and thus applicable to all health care disciplines and professions, not to medicine and physicians alone.

Empathy is viewed in this book from a multidisciplinary perspective that includes evolution; neurology; clinical, social, developmental, and educational psychology; sociology; medicine; and other health professions. Some theoretical aspects of antecedents, development, and outcomes of empathy are discussed, and relevant experimental studies and empirical findings are presented in support of the theoretical discussion. The book is based on my years of experiences in medical education research, and in particular on our research in empathy in physicians-in-training and in-practice at Jefferson (currently Sidney Kimmel) Medical College at Thomas Jefferson University. This research resulted in the development and validation of the Jefferson Scale of Empathy, a psychometrically sound instrument that has been used by many researchers in the USA and in other countries.

The book is written for a broad audience that includes physicians, residents, medical students, and students and practitioners of all other health professions including the disciplines of nursing, dentistry, pharmacy, psychology, and clinical social work, and other health professions students and practitioners who are involved in patient care. In particular, faculty involved in the education and training of health professionals can use the book as a reference in their courses in the art (and science) of patient care.

Because the book is intended to serve as a reference source on the topic of empathy in patient care, on many occasions I have cited multiple references for critical issues for those who need to further review the issues in more detail beyond what I have presented in this book. Although a critical review of the literature was not among the intended purposes of the book, occasionally when appropriate I reported additional information such as measuring instruments used, and described the sample used in the cited research to help readers judge the merit of the findings.

It is my hope that this book can help to improve our understanding of empathy in the context of health professions education and patient care. A problem that is well understood is a problem that is half solved. The more that health professions teachers and practitioners understand the importance of empathy in patient care, the better the public is served.

Mohammadreza Hojat, Ph.D.
Philadelphia, PA
September, 2006

Preface to the Expanded Edition

The original edition of this book, "*Empathy in Patient Care: Antecedents, Development, Measurement, and Outcomes*," was published in 2007. The book contributed to a surge of interest in empathy research in medical and other health profession disciplines, based on the feedback from national and international readers, researchers, and scholars. In addition to the attention to the book by educators and practitioners in the health professions disciplines, the following three factors prompted me to embark on this journey to expand and update the original edition of my book. First and foremost, empathy as an important element of professionalism in health care, and as a pillar of the art of patient care, has received increased attention in recent years by leaders, administrators, and educators in academic health centers, by practitioners of patient care, by students and researchers in health professions education, and by the public media. This shift of attention has contributed to a new wave of research on empathy in the context of health professions education and patient care that needed to be included in the expanded edition of the book.

Second, another major advancement in empathy research has been the increasing volume of published research in health profession students and practitioners in the USA and abroad in which the *Jefferson Scale of Empathy* has been used. Indeed, this wave of national and international research imparts great pleasure to me and my research team to witness the impact of our work in the advancement of empirical research on empathy in health professions education and patient care. I have included findings of some of this accumulating volume of national and international research in the annotated bibliography in this expanded edition of the book (see Appendix A).

Third, since the publication of the original edition, a major development ensued in empathy research. An increasing number of studies in the emerging field of social cognitive neuroscience have been published in which brain imaging techniques have been used to explore neurological activities involved in empathy. These advances are important to be reported in an independent chapter which is included to this expanded edition of the book (Chap. 13).

The book is divided into two parts. The first part consists of Chaps. 1 through 5, in which empathy is discussed from a broader perspective in the general context of human relationships. This part lays the foundation for the second one, without which the discussion of empathy in the second part would look like a structure without supporting pillars.

In the second part, consisting of Chaps. 6 through 14, the focus shifts more specifically to empathy in the context of health professions education and patient care. The two parts are closely interrelated, evident by frequently referring readers to different chapters in the book to avoid redundancies. Each chapter begins with a preamble (an Abstract) presenting the major highlights of the text and ends with a recapitulatory paragraph that provides a brief global view of the chapter.

Chapter 1 presents a historical background about the concept of empathy and discusses the ambiguity associated with the definitions and conceptualization of empathy. The long-standing confusion between empathy and sympathy is discussed and specific features of each construct are listed to distinguish the two. In addition, distinctions are made between cognition and emotion and between understanding and feeling, as specific features of empathy and sympathy, respectively. Finally, the implications of such distinctions are outlined to clarify their different consequences in the context of patient care.

Chapter 2 is based on the assumption that human beings are evolved to connect together for survival. Thus, the importance of making and breaking human connections in health and illness is emphasized. The beneficial effects of a social support system on health and the detrimental effects of isolation, loneliness, and disconnection are presented to underscore the nature, mechanisms, and consequences of interpersonal relationships. The chapter concludes with a notion that the positive relationship between clinician and patient is formed by the drive for human connectedness and serves as a special kind of social support system with all its beneficial healing power.

In Chapter 3, empathy is viewed from an evolutionary perspective, and the psycho-socio-physiological function of empathic engagement is described. In addition, the chapter discusses the genetic studies of empathy. The chapter ends with the notion that the foundation of the capacity for empathy developed during the evolution of the human species; thus, empathy is likely to be a hard-wired human attribute.

Chapter 4 discusses the psychodynamics of empathy by emphasizing the importance of prenatal, perinatal, and postnatal factors in the development of prosocial and altruistic behaviors. In particular, the effects of the early rearing environment, especially the mother's availability and loving responsiveness, in the development of internal working models that provide a framework for later interpersonal relationships are described. Experimental studies are presented to show that early relationships with a primary caregiver influence the regulation of emotions that becomes an important factor in interpersonal relationships in general, and in empathic engagements in particular.

Chapter 5 briefly describes several instruments that researchers have used most often to measure empathy in children and adults. The contents of the items in these instruments indicate that these instruments are useful for measuring empathy in the general population; thus their content relevance (or face and content validities) in the context of health professions education and patient care is limited. The chapter concludes with the notion that a psychometrically sound instrument, developed specifically to measure empathy in the context of health professions education and patient care, was required to satisfy an urgent need to measure empathy among students and practitioners of the health care professions.

In Chapter 6, empathy in patient care is discussed in relation to the World Health Organization's definition of health and the triangular bio-psycho-social paradigm of illness. In that context, empathy in patient care is defined, and four key features in the definition are emphasized: cognition, understanding, communication, and intention to help. The chapter concludes with the point that the patient's recognition of the clinician's empathy through verbal and nonverbal communication plays an important role in the outcome of empathic engagement.

Chapter 7 describes in detail the developmental phases and psychometric properties of the Jefferson Scale of Empathy (JSE), which was developed specifically to measure empathy among students and practitioners in the medical and other health professions. A large volume of empirical evidence is presented from our research team and from other national and international researchers in support of the validity and reliability of the three versions of the JSE. The chapter ends with the thought that the accumulating research evidence from the USA and abroad in support of the JSE's validity and reliability should instill confidence in those who are searching for a psychometrically sound instrument that can be used in empirical research on empathy among health professions students and practitioners.

Chapter 8 discusses the interpersonal dynamics involved in an empathic relationship between clinician and patient, and proposes that both can benefit from empathic engagement. The chapter presents several experimental studies that describe how role expectations, the tendency to bind with others for survival, uncritical acceptance of and compliance with authority figures, the effects of the clinical environment, and bystanders' empathy can influence clinicians' and patients' behavior in clinical encounters. In addition, the chapter argues that such psychological mechanisms as identification, transference, and countertransference, plus placebo effects, and cultural factors, personal space, and boundaries make clinician–patient encounters unique. The chapter ends with a notion that for achieving a better empathic engagement, the clinician should learn to listen with the "third ear" and to see with the "mind's eye."

Chapter 9 describes the link between empathy, psychological, and social variables, clinical performance, career interest, and choice of specialty. The chapter reports a number of desirable personality attributes, conducive to relationship building, that are positively correlated with empathy, and a number of undesirable personal qualities, detrimental to positive interpersonal relationships, that are negatively correlated with it. Data reported in this chapter suggest that high empathy scores are associated with greater clinical competence, and more interest in people-oriented specialties as opposed to technology- or procedure-oriented specialties.

In Chapter 10, gender differences in favor of women observed in a large number of studies of students and practitioners in the health professions are discussed. While the contribution of social learning in gender differences cannot be ignored, I propose that other factors can provide plausible explanations for gender differences in social skills and capacity for empathy. The ancestral history in mate selection, parental investment, division of labor, and hormonal and physiological factors has endowed women with a greater propensity for social skills and empathic engagement. It is argued that women may be endowed at an early age with a greater sensitivity to social stimuli and a better understanding of emotional signals that can result in a greater capacity for empathic engagement. This argument is reflected in studies reporting gender differences in the practice styles of male and female health professionals.

Chapter 11 reports the theoretical link between empathy and positive patient outcomes and provides evidence concerning the quality of clinician–patient relationships that can lead to more trusting relationships between clinician and patient, which in turn could lead to more accurate diagnoses, and to patients' greater satisfaction with their health care providers, better compliance with clinicians' advice, firmer commitment to treatment plans, and a reduced tendency to file malpractice litigations. Based on the reported empirical studies, and particularly recent findings that showed significant associations between physician's level of empathy and tangible clinical outcomes in diabetic patients, it is concluded that empathy should be considered as an important component of the overall clinicians' competence.

Chapter 12 describes obstacles to the enhancement of empathy in health professions education and practice—the cynicism that students develop during their professional education, the changes evolving in the health care system, and the current overreliance on biotechnology. The chapter also presents some empirical evidence suggesting that empathy is amenable to change by targeted educational programs and describes a variety of approaches used in psychological and health education research to enhance empathy. In particular, ten approaches used for enhancing empathy in the context of patient care were described including interpersonal skill training, perspective taking, role playing, exposure to role models, imagining, exposure of students to activities resembling patients' experiences while hospitalized or during encounters with health care providers, the study of literature and the arts, development of narrative skills and reflective writing, and the Balint approach to training physicians. The chapter presents an overall view that empathy can be taught through targeted educational programs, but the challenge is to retain the improvement.

Chapter 13 describes a new wave of research in social cognitive neuroscience, in exploring the neurological underpinnings of empathy. Recent findings from neuroimaging studies and a new line of research on the mirror neuron system hold promise of helping to understand the neurological underpinnings of empathy. Relying on the conceptualization of empathy (Chaps. 1 and 6), and findings from neuroimaging research and neurological impairment linked to deficiencies in empathy, it can be assumed that particular cortical regions of the brain may be implicated in empathic responses. The importance of making a clear distinction between empathy (predominantly a cognitive attribute) and sympathy (predominantly an affective reaction) in exploring the neurological underpinnings of empathy is discussed. However, challenges exist in developing a research paradigm to evoke empathic responses in one occasion and sympathetic reactions in another to examine similarities and differences in brain activities in the two situations. It is argued that exploring neurological underpinnings of empathy as opposed to sympathy is important for finding ways to maximize empathy and regulate sympathy in patient care.

In Chapter 14, the final chapter, empathy in the context of health professions education and patient care is viewed from the broad perspective of the systems theory. I suggested that a systemic paradigm of empathy in patient care includes the following subsets that interactively operate in the system: the clinician related, non-clinician related, social learning, and educational subsets. The elements within each subset and the interactions of the elements within and between subsets during clinical encounters that lead to functional (positive) or dysfunctional (negative) patient outcomes are discussed. Finally, an outline of an agenda for future research on several topics involving empathy in patient care is presented. The chapter concludes that the implementation of remedies for enhancement of empathy is a mandate that must be acted upon and that any attempt to enhance empathic understanding among people is a step toward building a better civilization.

It is my hope that the instruments we developed—Jefferson Scale of Empathy—and our research in empathy in health professions education and in patient care can continue to generate greater motivation and inspire researchers to undertake more inquest on the topic, and hopefully help to improve our understanding of the concerns, pain, and suffering of our fellow human beings in general, and to enhance health professionals' empathic engagement in patient care, in particular. As indicated in the entire text of this book, empathic understanding can not only enhance the quality of patient-clinician relationships and improve outcomes of patient care, but also serve as a binding means for achieving global peace and harmony in all humans, everywhere, regardless of any so-called divisive factors.

Mohammadreza Hojat, Ph.D.
Philadelphia, PA
August, 2015

A Personal Odyssey

Life is full of surprises!

—(A popular cliché)

A mother and her young daughter sat in the examination room, waiting for the doctor to show up. They looked anxiously at the closed door, expecting a stranger in a white coat to open it at any moment. Time seems to stand still when a patient is waiting for a doctor to come. It is interesting that patients always view a doctor as the most trusted of all strangers unless an adverse event occurs, usually during the first encounter.

At the recommendation of the pediatrician, the mother brought her teenaged daughter to this pediatric cardiologist to be examined for heart palpitations. The pediatrician had indicated that, at that age, occasional palpitations were not necessarily a serious cause for concern: They could be a result of too much caffeine for a coffee-lover like that young girl, a sign of test-taking anxiety at school, or a sign of a transitory emotional state. However, to eliminate the possibility of a serious heart condition, the pediatrician referred the girl to an expert in cardiology.

Here they were waiting for the expert to deliver the final verdict—either a clean bill of health or a long-term treatment that eventually could involve surgical procedures. The fear of the unknown that always haunts human beings was escalating with the passage of time. Finally, the doctor entered the room shadowed by a young woman also wearing a white coat. He pointed to her and said, "This is my resident." No greetings were exchanged, and the doctor seemed indifferent and in a rush. The encounter was cold. Without looking at the mother or the girl, he opened the medical chart the pediatrician had sent him and announced that additional tests were needed. The test he suggested was a heart monitor the girl would wear 24 hours a day, seven days a week, for at least a month. After each abnormal heartbeat, the device would transmit the recorded signals to a monitoring center via a telephone line connected to the monitor.

When the anxious mother asked the doctor how her daughter could be hooked up to a heart monitor for a month without missing her classes, the cardiologist said the monitor was light and could be attached to a belt around her waist and connected to a watch-like device on her wrist. The only additional information he offered was that the monitor could be rented for a month and that the expense might not be covered by insurance. He seemed to be more concerned about how the monitor would be paid for than about the mother's and daughter's need for comforting comments.

The doctor informed the mother that the next appointment would be in a month or so, after the heart monitor test was completed. The anxious mother expected, to no avail, more information about her young daughter's condition, some sign from the doctor that would make her daughter, who was looking hopelessly into the doctor's emotionless eyes, feel a little hopeful at least. As the doctor and his resident were leaving the examination room (where no examination had been performed), the mother, with a despairing look, asked the doctor: "Is my daughter's

> heart condition really serious enough to need constant monitoring for a month? Couldn't her
> condition be transitory?" The doctor looked at his resident and mumbled, "We've got another
> doctor in here," and the two left the room, leaving mother and daughter feeling desperate and
> confused. The mother did not trust the expert, never rented the monitor, and the heart palpita-
> tion stopped abruptly when the daughter stopped drinking coffee. However, memories of cold
> encounters can last forever.

It is interesting that an adverse event occurring when a person is in a heightened
state of emotional arousal tends to leave a deeper scar in the sufferer's mind than it
would otherwise. Or it may be that a lack of empathic understanding has a more
lasting effect than the presence of expressing concerns. It is true that negative experiences have a more lasting trace than positive ones. Is it any wonder that many
patients hate to go to a doctor's office? (By the way, that mother happened to be my
wife and the young patient was my daughter.)

It is interesting to note the gift of presence of a lovingly responsive and empathic
human being can become a panacea to other's pain and suffering. Here is a personal
observation:

> The baby startled first at the touch of the immunization needle in her tiny thigh, then came
> bursts of cries. The mother anxiously rushed to her baby's side, held her tight in her arms,
> gently put the baby on her chest, while patting her back started to talk in a calm motherly voice:
> "Oh my little girl … don't cry baby, it's over …" The little girl gazed at her mother's eyes,
> stopped crying, cuddling in the security of her mother's arms as if her pain had gone away to
> the sky …

I accompanied my wife and my daughter that day to the pediatrician's office,
observed this event, and wondered: What is in the mother's tender loving care that
soothes her baby's pain? Could it be a miraculous outcome of an empathic
understanding?

The aforementioned events, plus my long-standing curiosity about and fascination with the two opposing poles of human connectedness versus lack of connectedness—namely interpersonal relationship versus loneliness—compelled me to
embark on a journey that would lead to a better understanding of why empathy is so
important in patient care.

Since my college years, I have been curious about why people behave as they do
in making or breaking human connections. What are the foundations on which
human beings build, or fail to build, the capacity to form meaningful interpersonal
relationships? Has human evolution included development of the ability to form
interpersonal connections? What roles do genetic predisposition, rearing environment, personal qualities, educational experiences, and social learning play in
achieving personal and professional success, in clinician–patient encounters, or in
student–teacher relationships, or even in achieving likeability or attaining the qualities of professional, educational, or political leadership?

While earning my master's degree at the University of Tehran, I attempted to
satisfy my curiosity about the personal attributes leading to popularity and success
by examining the qualities of popular students using a sociometric methodology. I
found that the human attribute of likeability, or popularity, was rooted in the early
rearing environment and was also linked to positive personality traits, such as
sociability and self-esteem. Furthermore, academic and professional success is the

end result of these social skills. This research culminated in my master's thesis, *An Empirical Study of Popularity*.

While earning my doctoral degree at the University of Pennsylvania several years later, I continued to pursue my research interests, which eventually resulted in my doctoral dissertation, *Loneliness as a Function of Selected Personality, Psychosocial and Demographic Variables*. During this period, I studied factors contributing to loneliness, an indication of an inability to form meaningful interpersonal relationships. The findings showed that a set of personality factors, early experiences in the family environment, perceptions of the early relationship with a primary caregiver, early relationships with peers, and later living environment could predict experiences of loneliness in adulthood.

From the results of both studies, I learned that a common set of psychosocial attributes can contribute to the development of a capacity (or incapacity) to make (or break) human connections. These psychosocial attributes that are conducive to making human connections are similar to the elements of "emotional intelligence," such as social competency and the ability to understand the views, feelings, and emotions of others: that is, the capacity for empathic understanding.

As a psychologist by academic training, I entered a new territory of medical education research more than three decades ago. At the beginning, I was not sure whether my interests, knowledge, skills, and academic background in psychology could serve the purpose of medical education research. However, I soon discovered that the field of medical education research was a rich and challenging territory at the crossroad of several disciplines, including psychology, education, and sociology as well as medicine. As a result of learning more about the field, I became convinced that both the art of medicine and the alleviation of human suffering would flourish by incorporating ideas from the behavioral and social sciences into the education of physicians.

I started my career in medical education research at a great academic medical center, Jefferson (currently Sidney Kimmel) Medical College of Thomas Jefferson University, where I was charged with administrative and research responsibilities for the Jefferson Longitudinal Study of Medical Education. This now well-known longitudinal study retrieves data about Jefferson's medical students and graduates from the most comprehensive, extensive, and uninterrupted longitudinal database of medical education maintained in a single medical school. The Jefferson Longitudinal Study was initiated under the supervision of Joseph S. Gonnella, M.D., a decade before I joined the faculty. Joe was then the Director of the Office of Medical Education. Joe initiated the study because he had a vision concerning the need to empirically assess the outcomes of medical education at a time when most medical faculty and leaders in academia did not believe in the value of such an extensive (and expensive) study and thus were unwilling to devote resources to it.

My involvement with the Jefferson Longitudinal Study not only opened up a new window of opportunity for me but also proved to be an extremely interesting beginning to my professional life. I enjoyed the freedom bestowed on me to add new dimensions (e.g., personality and psychosocial measures) to the longitudinal database to address psychosocial aspects of academic success in medical school. Given my academic background in psychology, to me, that green light which allowed me to include personality and psychosocial measures in the longitudinal study was analogous to offering a cool glass of water to a thirsty man in the heat of a desert! The job provided me with a golden opportunity to incorporate my ideas about psychosocial attributes into research on the contribution of those attributes to the academic attainment and professional development of medical students, to the professional success of physicians, and to clinical outcome which is the ultimate goal of health professions education. So far, this highly productive research enterprise has resulted in more than 200 publications in peer-reviewed journals.

Meanwhile, my long-term interest in why people behave as they do in making or breaking human connections shifted to a more specific interest in empathy in health professions education and patient care. Then the question became the following: Why are some health professionals more capable than others of forming empathic relationships with their patients? More important, how can empathy be conceptualized and quantified in the context of health professions education and patient care? How does the capacity for empathy develop? How can it be measured? And what are the antecedents and consequences of empathy in the context of patient care?

Approximately 15 years ago, in pursuit of answers to these questions, we began to develop an instrument for physicians to measure empathy in patient care (see Chap. 7). During that time, I was fortunate to benefit from the intellectual input and instrumental support of a group of medical education scholars and practicing physicians making up the team of physician empathy project at the Jefferson (currently Sidney Kimmel) Medical College (see "Acknowledgments").

All the elements in this interrelated chain of events brought me to the uncharted terrain of empathy in health professions education and patient care. Interestingly, empathy has proved to be an extremely rich area of research requiring a multidisciplinary approach that links views, concepts, theories, and data from diverse disciplines, such as evolutionary psychiatry; ethology; developmental, clinical, and social psychology; psychoanalysis; sociology; neuroscience; philosophy; art; and literature. What prompted me to embark on a search for the answers to my questions about how empathy develops and what its antecedents and outcomes are in the health professions was fascination with the richness of this uncharted territory, in combination with my long-time interest in the mysteries of interpersonal relationships, my academic background in the behavioral and social sciences, and my professional experience in medical education research.

If a fortune-teller had told me at the beginning of my college years that I would end up with a career as a researcher in medical education, I would have laughed uproariously in disbelief! And that wise fortune-teller probably would have responded by saying, "Well, young man! Life is full of surprises." It is indeed!

Acknowledgments

I am indebted to many for their influence on my thoughts, for inspiring me to pursue this line of research, and for their encouraging and supporting my research ideas and activities. Because of space constraints, I cannot name them all.

There is a popular saying in the Persian language: "Forever remain my masters those from whom I have learned." Following this piece of advice, I must begin with my mother—that angel from whom I heard before taking my first breath, who taught me to say my first word, who is engraved vividly in my mind as the foremost symbol of love, care, and empathic understanding.

Then there are others: among them, those who are the most valuable of all human resources, the teachers. There are many of them, but I would like to mention two of my undergraduate psychology teachers, Professor Reza Shapurian, Ph.D. (who joined the eternity after publication of the original edition of this book), and Professor Amir Hooshang Mehryar, Ph.D.; both of them not only opened up a window for me to the study of human behavior but also instilled self-confidence in me by asking me, when I was a novice undergraduate student, to write a critical review of their book for publication.

There are others who trained me on the job and encouraged me in my professional development, particularly in medical education research. Among them are Joseph S. Gonnella, M.D., and Carter Zeleznik, Ph.D. Joe Gonnella is one of the best and brightest role models of an exemplary clinician-academician, teacher, leader, scholar, and researcher in medical education, whom I consider my mentor in medical education research. His great advice to me that "perfectionism is an obstacle to progress" has made my research career productive. Carter Zeleznik often said, humorously I hope, that his worst mistake was to hire me at Jefferson! His ideas, kind heart, and sense of humor made medical education research fun for me. (Carter joined the eternity after publication of the original edition of this book.) Joe has continued to be a source of inspiration to me, and unceasingly providing me with his intellectual input and instrumental support to pursue my research on empathy in medical education and patient care. I must confess that it was indeed his idea to empirically study patient outcomes of physician empathy (and to use diabetes as the disease of choice, since it has well-defined criteria for patient improvement) that led to the publication of our two key studies on linking physician empathy to clinical outcomes, which enjoyed broad media coverage (these studies are cited in Chap. 11).

Enormous appreciation is due to colleagues at Sidney Kimmel Medical College who contributed to the inception and development of the Jefferson physician empathy project. This book is an offshoot of that project. Those colleagues are (in alphabetical order) Clara A. Callahan, M.D., the Lillian H. Brent Dean of Students and Admissions, and Director of the Center for Research in Medical Education and Health Care, Sidney Kimmel Medical College; James B. Erdmann, Ph.D., Emeritus Dean of Jefferson College of Health Professions; Joseph S. Gonnella, M.D., Emeritus Dean of then Jefferson Medical College, Distinguished Professor of Medicine, and Founder and Emerirus Director of the Center for Research in Medical Education and Health, Sidney Kimmel Medical College at Thomas Jefferson University; Daniel Z. Louis, M.S., Research Associate Professor of Family and Community Medicine, Managing Director, Center for Research in Medical Education and Health Care; Thomas J. Nasca, M.D., former Anthony and Gertrude DePalma Dean of then Jefferson Medical College, and current President and Chief Executive Officer of the Accreditation Council for Graduate Medical Education (ACGME) and ACGME International; Salvatore Mangione, M.D., Associate Professor of Medicine, Course Director for Physical Diagnosis, Sidney Kimmel Medical College; and Jon Veloski, M.S., Director of the Medical Education Research Division, Center for Research in Medical Education and Health Care, Sidney Kimmel Medical College. Throughout the book, I have frequently used the plural pronoun "we," rather than the singular "I." Such phrases as "our research findings," rather than "my research findings," reflect my acknowledgment of the contributions of these colleagues.

There are others whom I would like to thank; among them are Mark Tykocinski, M.D., Provost and Executive Vice President for Academic Affairs, Thomas Jefferson University, and Anthony F. and Gertrude M. De Palma Dean and Professor of Pathology, Sidney Kimmel Medical College at Thomas Jefferson University; Michael Vergare, M.D., Chair, Department of Psychiatry and Human Behavior; and of course Joe Gonnella for encouraging me to pursue the idea of expanding and updating my book. All of them provided me with the opportunity to do so by graciously approving my sabbatical leave.

The Jefferson physician empathy project was supported in part for a few years at its inception by a grant from the Pfizer Medical Humanities Initiative, Pfizer Inc., New York. Mike Magee, M.D., who at that time was Director of the Pfizer Medical Humanities Initiative and a member of the Jefferson physician empathy project, provided me with continued support, and encouragement in my pursuit of this line of research. At the beginning, I could not imagine that a modest financial support could lead to such an important project. Also, I would like to acknowledge funding provided by Dr. Yoshihisa Asano, founder and chairman emetirus of Noguchi Medical Research Institute in Japan to partially support our continuous research on empathy in health professions education and patient care.

Several colleagues reviewed different chapters of this book and made valuable suggestions for improvement. Joe Gonnella was kind enough to review all the chapters and his valuable feedback has been incorporated in the text. Herbert Adler, M.D., Ph.D., Clinical Professor of Psychiatry and Human Behavior, Sidney Kimmel Medical College, reviewed Chaps. 8 and 13; Marianna LaNoue, Ph.D., Assistant Professor of Family and Community Medicine, and Director of the Greenfield Research Center, Sidney Kimmel Medical College, and Jon Veloski, M.S., Director of Medical Education Research, Center for Research in Medical Education and Health Care, Sidney Kimmel Medical College, reviewed Chap. 7. Alice Eagly, Ph.D., Distinguished Professor of Psychology, Northwestern University, and Judith A. Hall, Ph.D., University Distinguished Professor, Northeastern University, reviewed Chap. 10; and Nuno Sousa, M.D., Ph.D. Professor of Neuroscience at University of Minho, Portugal, reviewed Chap. 13. All of these colleagues made valuable comments to improve the chapters they reviewed, but I take full responsibility for any possible shortcomings in the text.

Kaye Maxwell has played a major role in the development of computerized testing services and compiling the User's Guide for the Jefferson Scale of Empathy (see Chap. 7), and preparing computerized reports for the scale. I am also grateful to Dorissa Bolinski for her valuable help in editorial polishing of the text. Shira Carroll helped me in proofreading, checking for consistencies in citations in the text and reference list and for stylistic corrections to conform with the APA publication guidelines.

I chose Springer Science + Business Media over other book publishers, not only because of its reputation as a publisher of scholarly books, but also because of the professional manner in which Janice Stern, the acquisitions editor, responded to my original book proposal. I was pleased and impressed by her initial and encouraging feedback—she would seek an expert to endorse the value of the book, rather than offering the standard response that the book's merit must first be judged by the publisher's reviewers. She also encouraged me to pursue the idea of expanding and updating the text for this new edition of the book. Scholarly publishers would do well with more editors like she—those who empathically understand the strong bond that exists between authors and their intellectual property.

My children, Arian, Anahita, and Roxana, filled me with additional joy and energy by repeatedly asking "Dad! How is your book going?" when I was writing the original and this edition of the book. They are my inspiring source of joy and energy. A recent addition to my family, my first grandchild, Alexander Bijan, who has become a new joyful energizing attraction, is a reminder of the notion that in a broader context, we all somehow contribute to the eternity of the garden of life by our surviving DNA, or by leaving traces of our thoughts, intellectual products, or creations. Last, but certainly not the least, I would like to thank my charming wife, Mimi, who provided me with all I needed to work in an atmosphere full of peace and love at home during my sabbaticals to write the original as well as this edition of the book.

Contents

Part I
Empathy in Human Relationships

Chapter 1
Descriptions and Conceptualization

To be one in heart is enchanting,
more than to be one in tongue.

—Rumi (Persian mystical poet and philosopher, 1207–1273 AD)

Abstract

- Empathy, a translation of the German word *Einfühlung*, has been described as an elusive and slippery concept with a long history marked by ambiguity and controversy.
- There has been an ongoing debate about the construct of empathy, described sometimes as a cognitive attribute featuring understanding of experiences of others (cognitive empathy); at other times, as an emotional state of the mind featuring sharing of feelings (emotional empathy); and at still other times as a concept involving both cognition and emotion.
- Distinctions are made in this chapter between cognition and emotion and also between their corresponding underlying mechanisms of understanding and feeling.
- The unsettled issue of the differences between empathy and sympathy in the context of patient care is addressed by viewing empathy in patient care as a predominantly cognitive attribute featuring understanding of others' concerns (cognitive empathy, or clinical empathy) that has a positive and linear relationship with patient outcomes and by viewing sympathy (synonymous to emotional empathy) as a primarily emotional concept featured by sharing emotions and feelings that has a curvilinear relationship (an inverted U shape) with patient outcomes.
- Distinctions between cognition and emotion, understanding and feeling, and empathy and sympathy are utterly important because of their implications not only for relevant conceptualization and valid measurement of empathy in patient care but for their different consequences in patient outcomes as well.

© Springer International Publishing Switzerland 2016

M. Hojat, *Empathy in Health Professions Education and Patient Care*,

DOI 10.1007/978-3-319-27625-0_1

Introduction

The concept of empathy has received a lot of attention in the past few decades in public media, academia, national and international politics, arts, ethics, health professions education and patient care (Coplan, 2014). Despite the popularity of the concept, there is no consensus on the definition of empathy among researchers (Matravers, 2014). The notion of "empathy" has a long history marked by ambiguity, discrepancy, disputation, and controversy among philosophers and behavioral, social, and medical scholars (Aring, 1958; Basch, 1983; Preston & deWaal, 2002; Wispe, 1978, 1986). Because of conceptual ambiguity, empathy has been described as an "elusive" concept (Basch, 1983)—one that is difficult to define and hard to measure (Kestenbaum, Farber, & Sroufe, 1989). Eisenberg and Strayer (1987a, p. 3) described empathy as a "slippery concept ... that has provoked considerable speculation, excitement, and confusion." Also, because of the ambiguity associated with the concept of empathy, Pigman (1995) suggested that empathy has come to mean so much that it means nothing! More than half a century ago, Theodore Reik (1948, p. 357), the prominent psychoanalyst, made a similar comment: "The word empathy sometimes means one thing, sometimes another, until now it does not mean anything at all."

Because of the conceptual ambiguity, Wispe (1986) suggested that the outcomes of empathy research might not be valid because empathy means different things to different investigators, who may believe they are studying the same thing but actually are referring to different things! As a result, Lane (1986) suggested that empathy might not even exist in reality after all. Later, Levy (1997) proposed that the term should be eliminated and replaced by a less ambiguous one.

Despite the conceptual ambiguity, it is interesting to note that empathy is among the most frequently mentioned humanistic dimensions of patient care (Linn, DiMatteo, Cope, & Robbins, 1987). Many successful clinicians know intuitively what empathy is without being able to define it. In that respect, empathy may be analogous to love, which many of us have experienced without being able to define it! Thus, while we all have a positive image of the concept of empathy and a preconceived idea about its positive outcomes in interpersonal relationships in general and in patient care in particular, we wonder how to define it operationally. Needless to say, no concept can be subject to scientific scrutiny without an operational definition.

The Origin and History of the Term *Empathy*

The concept of empathy (not the English term) was first discussed in 1873 by Robert Vischer, a German art historian and philosopher who used the word *Einfühlung* to address an observer's feelings elicited by works of art (Hunsdahl, 1967; Jackson, 1992). According to Pigman (1995), the word was used to describe the projection of human feelings onto the natural world and inanimate objects.

However, the German term was originally used not to describe an interpersonal attribute but to portray the individual's feelings when appreciating a work of art, specifically when those feelings blurred the distinction between the observer's self and the art object (Wispe, 1986).

In 1897, the German psychologist-philosopher Theodore Lipps brought the word *Einfühlung* from aesthetics to psychology. In describing personal experiences associated with the concept of *Einfühlung*, Lipps indicated that "when I observe a circus performer on a hanging wire, I feel I am inside him" (cited in Carr, Iacoboni, Dubeau, Mazziotta, & Lenzi, 2003, p. 5502). In 1903, Wilhelm Wundt, the father of experimental psychology, who established the first laboratory of experimental psychology in 1879 at the University of Leipzig in Germany, used *Einfühlung* for the first time in the context of human relationships (Hunsdahl, 1967). In 1905, Sigmund Freud (1960) used *Einfühlung* to describe the psychodynamics of putting oneself in another person's position (Pigman, 1995).

The English term "empathy" is a neologism coined by psychologist Edward Bradner Titchener (1909) as an English equivalent or the translation of the meaning of *Einfühlung*. The term empathy derives from the Greek word *empatheia*, which means appreciation of another person's feelings (Astin, 1967; Wispe, 1986). Although Titchener (1915) used the term empathy to convey "understanding" of other human beings, Southard (1918) was the first to describe the significance of empathy in the relationship between a clinician and a patient for facilitating diagnostic outcomes. Thereafter, American social and behavioral scientists have often used the concept of empathy in relation to the psychotherapeutic or counseling relationship and in the discussion of prosocial behavior and altruism (Batson & Coke, 1981; Carkhuff, 1969; Davis, 1994; Eisenberg & Strayer, 1987b; Feshbach, 1989; Feudtner, Christakis, & Christakis, 1994; Hoffman, 1981; Ickes, 1997; Stotland, Mathews, Sherman, Hansson, & Richardson, 1978). Empathy also has been discussed frequently in the psychoanalytic literature (Jackson, 1992) and in social psychology, counseling, and clinical psychiatry and psychology (Berger, 1987; Davis, 1994; Eisenberg & Strayer, 1987b; Ickes, 1997).

Definitions, Descriptions, and Features

A review of the literature indicates that more disagreement than agreement exists among researchers about the definition of empathy. Presenting a long list of definitions and descriptions of empathy would take us far beyond the intended scope of the book and space constraints do not allow such an extensive review. I have deliberately chosen a few definitions and descriptions that seem to be most relevant to health professions education and can also provide a framework for the conceptualization and definition of empathy in the context of patient care that will be presented in Chap. 6.

Carl Rogers (1959, p. 210), the founder of client-centered therapy, suggested the following often-cited definition of empathy as an ability "to perceive the internal frame of reference of another with accuracy *as if* one were the other person but without ever losing the "as if" condition" (emphasis added). In addition, Rogers (1975) described the experience of empathy as entering into the private perceptual world of another person and becoming thoroughly at home in it. Similarly, in one of the first psychoanalytic studies of empathy, Theodore Schroeder (1925, p. 159) suggested that "empathic insight implies seeing *as if* from within the person who is being observed" (emphasis added).

George Herbert Mead (1934, p. 27) suggested the following definition of empathy more than eight decades ago: "The capacity to take the role of another person and adopt alternative perspectives." More than half a century ago, Charles Aring (1958) described empathy as the *act* or *capacity* of appreciating another person's feelings *without* joining those feelings. Robert Hogan (1969, p. 308) defined empathy as "the intellectual or imaginative apprehension of another's condition or state of mind *without* actually experiencing that person's feelings" (emphasis added). Clark (1980, p. 187) defined empathy as "the unique capacity of the human being to feel the experience, needs, aspirations, frustrations, sorrows, joys, anxieties, hurt, or hunger of others *as if* they were his or her own" (emphasis added). These definitions by Hogan and Clark are in line with Rogers's (1959) "as if" condition in describing empathy and with Aring's (1958) "without joining" feature of empathy described earlier. I will assert later in this chapter that the "as if" condition is a key feature that distinguishes empathy from sympathy.

Wispe (1986, p. 318) described empathy as "the attempt by one self-aware self to comprehend nonjudgmentally the positive and negative experiences of another self." Baron-Cohen and Wheelwright (2004) described empathy as the "glue" of the social world that draws people to help one another and stops them from hurting others. Levasseur and Vance (1993, p. 83) described empathy as follows: "Empathy is not a psychological or emotional experience, nor a psychic leap into the mind of another person, but an openness to, and respect for, the personhood of another." Similarly, Shamasundar (1999) described empathy as related to open-mindedness and tolerance for ambiguity and complexity.

Mead (1934) described empathy as an element of social intelligence. This description resembles the notion of emotional intelligence introduced originally by Salovey and Mayer (1990) and later by Goleman (1995) who proposed that empathy, as an ability to recognize emotions in others, is one domain of emotional intelligence. The proposition that empathy has a significant overlap with measures of emotional intelligence and social skills has been supported (Schutte et al., 2001).

Greif and Hogan (1973) described empathic development as a parallel function of moral maturity. Schafer (1959, p. 343) defined empathy as "the inner experience of sharing and comprehending the momentary psychological state of another person." Stefano Bolognini (1997, p. 279) described empathy as "a state of complementary conscious-preconscious contact based on separateness and sharing." William Ickes (1997, p. 183) defined empathy as "a state of our mind upon which we reflect." Bellet and Maloney (1991, p. 183) defined empathy as "the capacity to understand what the other person is experiencing from within the other person's frame of reference, i.e., the capacity to place oneself in another's shoes." Hamilton (1984, p. 217) defined empathy as a "vehicle for understanding one another in a meaningful way."

Levasseur and Vance (1993, p. 82) described empathy as "a mode of caring," adding that "Empathy is not for those who are flourishing or happy. … Empathy is for those who need help or are suffering or struggling in some way." Similarly, Shamasundar (1999) suggested that the intensity of empathic resonance is deeper for negative states, such as sadness, anger, and hostility. These descriptions portray the importance of empathy in situations where others are suffering or are sad. Thus, the importance of empathic relationships in patient encounters is apparent.

Recently, empathy has been described as the neural matching mechanism constituted of a mirror neuron system in the brain that enables us to place ourselves in the "mental shoes" of others (Gallese, 2001, 2003). Briefly, mirror neurons are brain cells (not visual cells) that are activated when we observe another person who is performing a goal-directed action as if we are performing that act (Carr et al., 2003; Gallese, 2001; Iacoboni et al., 1999). Brain imaging studies have shown that watching on a television screen a needle prick a specific hand muscle influences the same hand muscle in the observer (Singer & Frith, 2005). These new studies suggest the possibility that, in the future, empathy may be defined in neurological terms and be measured by physiological indicators (see Chap. 13 for a more detailed discussion).

Empathy Viewed from the Cognitive and Emotional Perspectives

In general, empathy has been described as a cognitive or an emotional (or affective) attribute or a combination of both. Cognition requires mental activities involved in acquiring and processing information for better understanding, and emotion is sharing of the affect manifested in subjectively experienced feelings (Colman, 2001). Two types of empathy, cognitive empathy and emotional empathy, fit these descriptions of cognition and emotions, respectively. I believe that emotional empathy is conceptually synonymous to sympathy and vicarious empathy, which will be addressed later.

Cognitive Perspective

Rosalind Dymond (1949) viewed empathy as a cognitive ability to assume the role of another person. Heins Kohut (1971, p. 300) described empathy as "a mode of *cognition* that is specifically attuned to the perception of a complex psychological configuration" (emphasis added). Basch (1983) also described empathy as a complex cognitive process involving cognitive functions, such as judgment and reality testing. MacKay, Hughes, and Carver (1990, p. 155) described empathy as "the ability to understand someone's situation without making it one's own."

Cognitive activities, such as perspective taking and role taking, are among the features some authors have presented in their definition of empathy. For example, Dymond (1949, p. 127) defined empathy as "the imaginative transposing of oneself into the thinking, feeling, and acting of another, and so structuring the world as he does." Blackman, Smith, Brokman, and Stern (1958) defined empathy as an ability to step into another person's shoes and to step back as easily into one's own shoes again when needed. Similarly, Decety and Jackson (2004) described empathy as subjective experience of similarity between feelings experienced by self and others without losing sight of whose feelings belong to whom. Those who advocate the cognitive view of empathy, place more emphasis on understanding and social insight than on emotional involvement (Rogers, 1975).

Emotional Perspective

Some authors have defined empathy as an emotional response by generating identical feelings and sharing emotions between people. For example, Batson and Coke (1981, p. 169) defined empathy as "an emotional response elicited by and congruent with the perceived welfare of someone else." Rushton (1981, p. 260) defined empathy as "experiencing the emotional state of another." Eisenberg (1989) described it as "an emotional response that stems from the apprehension of another's emotional state or condition and is congruent with the other's emotional state or condition" (p. 108). Halpern (2001, p. xv) described empathy as "a form of emotional reasoning with risks of error that such reasoning involves." Katz (1963, p. 26) defined it as "the inner experience of feeling oneself to be similar to, or nearly identical with the other person." Kalisch (1973, p. 1548) defined it as "the ability to enter into the life of another person, to accurately perceive his current feelings and their meaning"; and Hoffman (1981, p. 41) defined it as "a vicarious affective response to someone else's situation rather than one's own." However, Underwood and Moore (1982) suggested that an emotional perspective is not a sufficient condition to define empathy. I will describe later that emotional empathy is analogous to sympathy.

A number of researchers, however, believe that empathy involves both cognition and emotion (Baron-Cohen & Wheelwright, 2004; Davis, 1994). For example, Bennett (2001, p. 7) defined empathy as "a mode of relating in which one person comes to know the mental content of another, both *affectively* and *cognitively*, at a particular moment in time and as a product of the relationship that exists between them." Mark Davis (1994) believes that cognitive and affective facets of empathy interact in his organizational model of empathy. He defined empathy as "a set of constructs having to do with the responses of one individual to the experiences of another. These constructs specifically include the process taking place within the observer and the affective and non-affective outcomes which results from those processes" (Davis, 1994, p. 12). Hodges and Wegner (1997, p. 313) suggested that "empathy can have either an emotional component … or a cognitive component, or both."

Cognition and Emotion

Silvan Tomkins (1962, 1963) viewed cognition and emotion as two separate systems working side by side to process incoming data. The processing of cognitive information often involves specific mental activities, such as reasoning and appraisal (Tausch, 1988). In contrast, emotional mental processing often entails an affective response experienced spontaneously without involvement of the higher mental processes that are activated in reasoning (Basch, 1996). Therefore, *reasoning* and *appraisal* are the features of cognitive responses, and *spontaneity* and *arousal* are the hallmarks of emotional responses (Tucker et al., 2005). Solomon's (1976) description of the wisdom of "reason" against the treachery of the "passions" is somewhat analogous to the nature of a cognitive response as opposed to an emotional one.

Basic emotions and their expressions, as Charles Darwin (1965) was first to note, are universally similar regardless of cultural factors, personal background, or educational experiences. On the contrary, the processing of cognitive information is not culture free and is heavily dependent on personal background, learning, and educational experiences. Thus, the contribution of learning is more significant in a cognitive response (e.g., empathy) than it is in an emotional reaction (e.g., sympathy). Manifestation of cognitive behaviors is more *effortful*, and its behavioral roots are more *advanced* (Schulte-Ruther, Markowitsch, Fink, & Piefke, 2007). The same is true of empathy. Expression of emotion is *effortless*, and its behavioral roots are more *primitive*. The same is true of sympathy. An emotional response is colored more by subjective judgments, leading to a less accurate interpretation than would result from a cognitive response.

At the neuroanatomical level, different brain mechanisms appear to be involved in the processing of cognitive and emotional input (Nathanson, 1996). Cognitive mental processing is primarily an *advanced intellectual process* that often involves social perception, analysis of information, and generation of appropriate responses based on one's understanding of another person and the situation. Emotional responses consist primarily of more *primitive* mental processes, wherein the person responds, through a process of contagion, with emotions similar to the emotions of others who are present (Mehrabian, Young, & Sato, 1988). Thus, emotion often is contagious in interpersonal exchanges, but cognition is not (Doherty, 1997).

Despite these differences between cognition and emotion, some authors do not make such distinctions and assign equal weight to both cognition and emotion in the construct of empathy (Bennett, 2001). Freud (1958a, 1958b), for example, emphasized the intellectual or cognitive component while recognizing emotion as another important aspect of empathy in forming empathic relationships between clinician and patient.

It is indeed virtually impossible to treat emotion and cognition as two completely independent entities because one cannot fully exist without the other. For practical reasons, however, the distinction between the two is important, particularly in the context of patient care, to avoid confusion between the concepts of understanding and feeling (and thus between empathy and sympathy). I will discuss this further in the following sections.

Understanding and Feeling

The distinction between cognition and emotion provides a context for distinguishing between the two other corresponding interrelated concepts of understanding and feeling, which are often used interchangeably. In the context of interpersonal relationships, however, it is useful to define understanding as the awareness of meaning (Sims, 1988) and to define feeling as the perception of emotions. All meaningful social relationships are based on both mutual understanding of one another and feeling of emotions.

Understanding is often based on *tangibility* and *objectivity*, whereas feeling is more a product of *subjectivity* and thus can be subject to *prejudice. Accuracy in judgment* is more likely to emerge from effortful mental activities associated with understanding than from spontaneous and effortless emotional arousal. Understanding is more likely to be based on learning and requires active efforts, whereas feeling is more likely to be *innate* and *effortless* (Wispe, 1986). A higher mental processing is involved when attempting to understand another person's concerns, whereas a primitive mental processing is involved in feeling another person's emotions. Empathy is associated more with cognitive response and understanding, whereas sympathy is associated more with emotions and affects. To be empathic, according to Bellet and Maloney (1991, p. 1831) "the physician does not have to experience the intense feelings or emotions that grip the patient … but only to understand these feelings and relate to them while maintaining a sense of self." According to Shamasundar (1999), the less empathy between individuals, the more difficult it is to reach a mutual understanding of each other regardless of the use of a larger and more precise vocabulary.

Empathy and Sympathy

Both empathy and sympathy are important components of interpersonal relationships. Sympathy derives from the Greek *sym* (being with) and *pathos* (suffering, pain) (Black, 2004). The two distinct concepts of empathy and sympathy are often mistakenly tossed into the same terminological basket in empathy research—a mistake that has created conceptual confusion and debates for years but has never been settled (Black, 2004; Chismar, 1988; Gruen & Mendelsohn, 1986; Wispe, 1986; Zhou, Valiente, & Eisenberg, 2003). The two constructs of empathy and sympathy reflect different human qualities that have different measurable influences on clinicians' professional behavior, utilization of resources, and clinical outcomes (Nightingale, Yarnold, & Greenberg, 1991; Yarnold, Greenberg, & Nightingale, 1991).

We showed in an empirical study that it is possible to differentiate and quantify empathic and sympathetic responses to patient care (Hojat, Spandorfer, Louis, & Gonnella, 2011). In that study, we asked medical students to respond to clinical

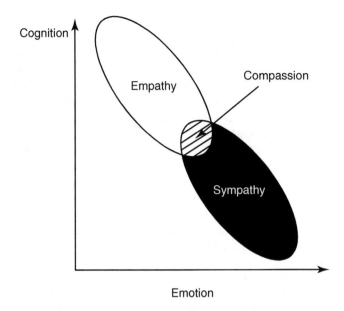

Fig. 1.1 Empathy and sympathy as related to cognition and emotion

scenarios by using one scale pertaining to empathic engagement (for measuring a student's inclination toward *understanding* the patient's pain and suffering); and using another scale pertaining to sympathetic response (to measure the student's tendency to *feel* a patient's pain and suffering). Findings indicated that inclination toward empathic engagement was significantly correlated with a validated measure of cognitive empathy (Jefferson Scale of Empathy, Hojat et al., 2002c, see Chap. 7), and sympathetic responses were significantly associated with measure of emotional empathy measured from scales of the Interpersonal Reactivity Index (Davis, 1983, 1994, see Chap. 7).

According to Decety and Jackson (2004, p. 85) "an essential aspect of empathy is to recognize the other person as like self while maintaining a clear separation between self and other." The key feature of empathy is the preponderance of *cognitive* information processing that distinguishes it from the predominantly *emotional* mental processing involved in sympathy (Brock & Salinsky, 1993; Streit-Forest, 1982; Wolf, 1980). Although one cannot claim that empathy and sympathy are fully independent from cognition and emotion, but one can argue that the degree of cognitive and emotional involvement is different in the two concepts of empathy and sympathy. Figure 1.1 is a graphic presentation showing the relative contribution of cognition and emotion in empathy and sympathy and the overlap between them. (My colleague Jon Veloski conceived the idea for this graphic presentation.) As it is shown in the figure, empathy is in the area of higher cognition than emotion. Conversely, sympathy is in the area of higher emotion than cognition. Compassion, I propose, resides in the area of the overlap between empathy and sympathy, where both of these attributes are expressed in a moderate amount.

Empathy is an *intellectual* attribute, whereas sympathy is an *emotional* state of mind (Gruen & Mendelsohn, 1986). Empathy refers to one person's attempt to comprehend nonjudgmentally another person's experiences (Wispe, 1986). Self-awareness is augmented in empathy, but it is reduced in sympathy. Whereas the aim of empathy is to *understand* another person's pain, suffering, and concerns better, the aim of sympathy is to *feel* another person's pain, suffering, and emotions better. The empathic relationship implies a *convergence* of understanding between two people, and the sympathetic relationship implies a *parallelism* in the feelings between the two (Buchheimer, 1963). According to Kohut (1984), empathy is a "value-neutral" mode of observation. Similarly, Olinick (1984) believed that empathy is an affect-free phenomenon, whereas sympathy involves an affect-laden perception.

The underlying behavioral motivation in empathy is likely to be altruistic, but it is more likely to be egoistic in sympathy. The ultimate goal of altruistically motivated helping behavior is to reduce another person's distress without any expectation of reward, whereas the primary goal in egoistically motivated helping behavior is to reduce one's own level of stress, to avoid adverse feelings, or to receive rewards (Coke, Batson, & McDavis, 1978). A genuine attempt to understand the experiences of another person—or *empathic understanding*—increases the likelihood of altruistic helping behavior. However, feeling the emotions of others, or sympathetic sharing of emotions, leads to physiological arousal, thus increasing the likelihood of egoistic behavior to reduce emotional arousal and avoid aversive experiences.

In clinical encounters, empathy involves an effort to *understand* the patient's experiences without joining them, whereas sympathy involves an effortless feeling of *sharing* or joining the patient's pain and suffering (Aring, 1958). Olinick (1984) suggested that empathy entails separateness and sympathy entails closeness; empathy "feels into" and sympathy "feels with." Titchener (1915), who first coined the term empathy, distinguished empathy from sympathy by describing empathy as a tendency to perceive another person's experiences and by describing sympathy as "feeling together" with another person. McKellar (1957, pp. 220–221) suggested that "One can, however, empathize without necessarily experiencing sympathy for the other person; empathy involves understanding rather than 'siding with.'" Wilmer (1968) described empathy as entering into the sufferer's mind and understanding his pain from within as if the pain were ours but remains his own. In contrast, sympathy, according to Wilmer, is sharing feelings together with the patient as if the pain was ours and remains so.

Hinshelwood (1989) wrote that empathy, in contrast to sympathy, involves a sophisticated mental operation in which two interacting people are clearly separated, but one conceives of the other person's mental landscape without losing sight of reality and his or her own identity. Similarly, Black (2004) believes that empathy is a sophisticated and conscious act and that sympathy is an involuntary propensity that makes affective attunement possible.

Understanding the *kind* and *quality* of the patient's experiences is the territory of empathy, whereas feeling the *degree* and *quantity* of the patient's pain and suffering falls within the terrain of sympathy. A patient will feel felt if the clinician understands the kind and quality, not the degree and quantity, of the patient's experiences

(Greenson, 1960). Whereas empathy is an internal cognitive process that should be communicated, sympathy seems to be more transparent. Benjamin Disraeli described the transparency of feelings in the following statement: "Never apologize for showing feelings. When you do so, you apologize for the truth" (retrieved March 2015 from http://www.quotationspage.com/quote/2563.html).

Empathy has been described as the art of understanding (Agosta, 1984; Starcevic & Piontek, 1997). This notion of empathic understanding is reflected in different features attributed to empathy, such as perspective taking, role-playing, standing in another person's shoes, tolerance, openness, uncritical judgment, and unconditional acceptance. The difference between empathy and sympathy is more than a semantic one because each involves different mental activities during information processing (Gruen & Mendelsohn, 1986). The predominantly cognitive nature of empathy and the primarily emotional nature of sympathy imply additional differences between the two terms that go beyond semantics. A cognitive response (in empathy) is more likely to be nonspontaneous because it is influenced by the regulatory process of *appraisal.* An affective reaction (in sympathy) is more likely to be spontaneous because it is influenced by the psychological regulatory process of *arousal* (Siegel, 1999).

Also, empathy as a cognitive response is characterized by an *inhibitory* energy-conserving state in the *parasympathetic* branch of the neurological regulatory process. However, sympathy as an emotional reaction is characterized by an *excitatory* energy-consuming state related to the *sympathetic* neurological regulatory process (Siegel, 1999). Despite the differences between empathy and sympathy, they cannot be completely independent from one another. For example, in one of our studies (Hojat, Mangione, Kane, & Gonnella, 2005), we found a moderate correlation ($r=0.48$, $p<0.01$) between cognitive empathy (measured by the Jefferson Scale of Empathy) and emotional empathy (which is synonymous to sympathy) measured by scores on the Empathic Concern scale of the Interpersonal Reactivity Index (Davis, 1983, 1994, see Chap. 7). A correlation of this magnitude indicates that the overlap between the two concepts is approximately 23 % (coefficient of determination: $r^2=0.48^2=23$ %). More empirical research is needed to examine the degree of overlap between measures of empathy and sympathy. Similar patterns of relationships between empathy and sympathy were observed in an earlier study (Hojat et al., 2001b).

Empathy and Sympathy in the Context of Patient Care

The distinction between sympathy (also known as emotional empathy, or vicarious empathy) and empathy (also known as cognitive empathy, or clinical empathy in the context of patient care) has important implications for the clinician–patient relationship because joining the patient's emotions, a key feature of sympathy, can impede clinical outcomes. A clinician should sense the patient's feelings only to a limited extent to improve objectivity in his or her understanding of the patient without impeding professional judgment (Starcevic & Piontek, 1997). When experiencing empathy, individuals are able to disentangle themselves from others, whereas individuals experiencing sympathy have difficulty maintaining a sense of whose feelings belong to whom (Decety & Jackson, 2006).

Ehrlich and Jaffe (2002) indicated that empathy must be distinguished from sympathy and sentimentalism because neither of the latter two concepts is desirable in the context of patient care. Starcevic and Piontek (1997) argued that because a clinician, as a separate human being, can never fully share the patient's feelings, perfect sympathy can never be achieved. Furthermore, as Truax and Carkhuff (1967) suggested, it would be undesirable for the clinician to feel the patient's emotions too strongly. Black (2004) points out that sympathy is a concept that psychoanalysts avoid, in contrast to empathy, which they use with pride. Wilmer (1968, p. 246) compared the outcomes of pity, sympathy, and empathy in the patient care context and concluded that "pity rarely helps, sympathy commonly helps, empathy always helps."

Because of the emotional nature of sympathy, its overabundance can be overwhelming and therefore can impede the clinician's performance. This notion about the restraints in sympathetic clinician–patient relationships and clinical outcomes implies that the relationship between sympathy and a clinician's performance is likely to be *curvilinear*—an inverted U function similar to that between anxiety and performance on achievement tests. Although a certain amount of anxiety can improve performance, too much anxiety can hinder it by disrupting cognitive functioning. Thus, to a certain degree, sympathy can be beneficial in clinician–patient encounters—beyond that, however, it can interfere with clinical objectivity and professional effectiveness. The relationship between empathy and a clinician's performance, however, is considered to be *linear*. That is, the more empathic the relationship, the better the clinical outcomes. Therefore, the general conclusion is that sympathy must be restrained or regulated in clinical situations, whereas empathy needs no restraining boundary.

The differences in features between empathy and sympathy are summarized in Table 1.1. I already described some of these differences when discussing the notions of cognition and emotions, and of understanding and feelings that correspond to empathy and sympathy, respectively.

In the context of patient care, when expressed in abundance, empathy would be an "enabling" factor, whereas sympathy in excess would be a "disabling" factor. Thus, it seems desirable to maximize empathy, and regulate (or optimize) sympathy in patient care for optimal patient outcomes. As I indicated previously, the two concepts of empathy and sympathy have mistakenly been used interchangeably as if one can replace the other without any serious consequences. However, in the context of patient care, the two terms must be used in their proper context because of their different consequences in patient outcomes. It is my hope that the differences described in Table 1.1 can help to settle the longstanding debate about empathy and sympathy. I will return again to the issues of empathy's definition and the differences between empathy and sympathy in the context of patient care in Chap. 6.

Table 1.1 Specific features of empathy and sympathy

Feature	Empathy	Sympathy
Contribution of learning	More significant	Less significant
Contribution of cognition	More significant	Less significant
Contribution of affects	Less significant	More significant
Contribution of innate or genetic factors	Less innate	More innate
Objectivity vs. subjectivity	More objective	More subjective
Likelihood of accuracy	More accurate	Less accurate
Behavioral roots	Advanced	Primitive
Required efforts	More effortful	More effortless
Relation to clinician's performance	Linear	Inverted U shape
Reaction time	Nonspontaneous	Spontaneous
Patient's emotions	Appreciated without joining	Perceived by joining
Feeling felt	The kind and quality of the patient's feelings	The degree and quantity of the feelings
Brain processing area	Predominantly neocortex	Predominantly limbic system
Psychological regulatory process	Appraisal	Arousal
Neurological regulatory process	Parasympathetic (inhibitory)	Sympathetic (excitatory)
Psycho-physiological state	Energy conserving	Energy consuming
Behavioral motivation	Altruistic	Egoistic
State of mind	Intellectual	Emotional
Effect of caregiver	Personal growth, satisfaction	Exhaustion, burnout, fatigue
Typical expression to patient	I understand your suffering	I feel your pain
Key mental-processing mechanism	Cognitive/intellectual/understanding	Affective/emotional/feeling

Recapitulation

Empathy is a vague concept that has been described sometimes as a cognitive attribute, sometimes as an emotional state of mind, and sometimes as a combination of both. The ambiguity associated with the definition of empathy obstructs our view to clearly see what we intend to study, and hinders our ability of how to measure it in the context of patient care. Also, we should realize that the fundamental differences that exist between cognition and emotion, between understanding and feeling, and between empathy and sympathy have important implications not only for the conceptualization and measurement of empathy in patient care but also for the assessment of patient outcomes as well as for the development of proper research design, and accurate interpretation of research outcomes (see Chap. 13). Research findings on empathy will continue to be subject to serious challenges if differentiations between concepts of cognition and emotion, and between mechanisms of understanding and feeling, and between empathy and sympathy remain unsettled.

Chapter 2
Human Connection in Health and Illness

Hear the reed's complaining wail!
Hear it tell its mourning tale!
Torn from spot it loved so well,
Its grief, its sighs our tears compel.

—Rumi (Persian mystical poet and philosopher, 1207–1273 A.D.)

It is not good for the man to be alone.

—(Genesis 2:18)

Abstract

- Humans are evolved to connect together for survival. Among the factors that fulfill the human need for affiliation and connectedness are social institutions, such as marriage, family, and the social support network, including clinician–patient empathic relationships.
- Human connection serves to promote health and prevent illness. Conversely, an absence of satisfactory human connection, experienced as loneliness, is detrimental to physical, mental, and social well-being.
- The mechanisms involved in linking the quality of human connection to health or illness are not well understood. However, opportunities for empathic engagement and involvement of a multisystem of psychoneuroimmunology may provide some explanations for the beneficial effects of human connections.
- The clinician–patient relationship is formed in part by the drive for connectedness which increases with illness. The empathic connection between clinician and patient can serve as a special kind of social support system with all of its beneficial effects.

© Springer International Publishing Switzerland 2016   17
M. Hojat, *Empathy in Health Professions Education and Patient Care*,
DOI 10.1007/978-3-319-27625-0_2

Introduction

Human beings are evolved to be social. We are, according to Larson (1993) "pre-wired" to be connected by evolutionary design for the sake of survival. Our survival depends on our ability to understand others and the skills to communicate our understanding. Social relationships provide opportunities for empathic engagement, which in turn reinforces human connections, a cycle that has always been in motion in the evolution of humankind. In the often-cited list of basic needs proposed by psychologist Henry Murray (1938), the need for "affiliation" as well as the needs for "understanding" and "succorance" (to be gratified by being understood; seeking empathy, affection, and support) are included among the human being's basic psychosocial needs. Without fulfillment of those needs, Murray said, self-actualization cannot be fully achieved. In this chapter, I describe the importance of human ties in health and illness and discuss the consequences of making and breaking human connections on one's physical, mental, and social well-being. Also, I will attest that the human factors involved in clinician–patient empathic engagement make it the epitome of human connection.

The Need for Connectedness

The need for affiliation is a powerful motivator that guides human interactions in health and illness (Lieberman, 2007). Human connection is the bedrock of empathic growth. The urge for connectedness arises from the human need for affiliation. That basic need prompts us to fall in love, marry and establish a family, raise children, associate with other people, enjoy the company of others, and develop interpersonal relationships. The need for affiliation has survival advantages and is deeply rooted in the evolutionary history of humankind.

   Human connection leads not only to psychological pleasure but also to biophysiological changes and activities in the endocrine system (Uchino, Cacioppo, & Kiecolt-Glaser, 1996). For example, female students living together in university dormitories noticed that their menstrual cycles had become synchronized, and this hormonal synchronization occurred not only among roommates but among networks of close friends as well (McClintock, 1971).

   People interacting with one another often show behavioral synchronization, usually unconsciously, that is reflected in such nonverbal clues as facial mimicry, imitation, and the motor mirroring reaction (see Chaps. 3 and 13). These signals are not necessarily learned; they seem to be the outcomes of a pre-wired built-in behavioral repertoire that facilitates interpersonal exchanges (see Chap. 8).

The Making of Connections

It is now widely recognized that making connections has a powerful effect on the maintenance of health and that breaking connections can lead to the development of illness (Cohen, 1988). This recognition is not new, however. Early research by the French sociologist Emile Durkheim on factors contributing to suicide found that erosion of the capacity for social integration and human connection was the triggering factor for social miseries, including people's attempt to end their lives (Durkheim, 1951).

In their widely cited epidemiological research conducted more than four decades ago, Berkman and Syme (1979) showed that the absence of human connections was significantly linked to an increase in disease and mortality. So much evidence has been accumulating that it is now beyond doubt that being connected and feelings acknowledged are beneficial to physical, mental, and social well-being—the three pillars of health defined by the constitution of the World Health Organization (WHO, 1948) (see Chap. 6). Social connections in epidemiological research are typically defined in terms of marital status, family, friends and peer relationships, and membership in social or religious groups (Cacioppo et al., 2002). In this context, marriage, family, peer relations, and belonging to social or religious groups as well as clinician–patient empathic engagement have a common denominator: They connect people together and serve as social support systems.

Marriage and the Family

Traditionally, the family is built on the covenant of marriage for the purpose of bringing couples together, to make a commitment to share their concerns, feelings, and experiences in health and illness and in happiness and sadness "till death do us part." Thus, marriage and the family are important social support systems that can fulfill the human needs for affiliation, intimacy, and connectedness.

The social support system originates in the family, which is regarded as a secure base for the development of the capacity for human connection from cradle to grave. The relationships inside the family between parents and children, spouses, and among other family members become a prototypical working model, or a representational model of human connections outside the family, extending to friends, peers, colleagues, and others (see Chap. 4).

Consistent with the notion that fulfillment of the need for affiliation promotes health, research has shown that the mortality rate of death for medical causes is significantly lower for married couples than it is for single, separated, divorced, and widowed individuals (Goodwin, Hunt, Key, & Samet, 1987; Ortmeyer, 1974; Wiklund, Oden, & Sanne, 1988). In addition, married people are the healthiest group, with the lowest rates of chronic disease and disabilities, followed by single, widowed, divorced, and separated people in that order (Verbrugge, 1979).

The proportion of elderly people living in an assisted living or nursing home facility was highest among those who were single or divorced and lowest among married elderly people (Verbrugge, 1979). Research also indicates that married patients with cancer live longer than their single counterparts (Goodwin et al., 1987).

Numerous studies indicate that spouses, children, other family members, and a network of friends play important roles in prevention of disease and maintenance of health. Among patients who underwent coronary angiography and had at least one blocked coronary artery, those who were not married or lacked a companion to talk to regularly were significantly more likely to die within 5 years after the procedure (Williams et al., 1992).

It has been suggested that a stable marriage and close family relationships can free a person from becoming entrapped in serious psychopathology (Valliant, 1977). Consistent with this finding, empirical data from a longitudinal study conducted in Sweden found that single people and those living alone had an elevated risk of dementia compared with married people living with their spouses (Fratiglioni, Wang, Ericsson, Maytan, & Winblad, 2000). In summarizing his family studies, Lewis (1998) pointed out that marriage and family have beneficial effects because couples often express their affects openly to one another and family members frequently communicate empathically, in particular.

It is interesting to note that although making a connection through marriage is beneficial for both men and women, men benefit more from marriage than women do. In addition, although breaking the marital connection is harmful for both men and women, men seem to suffer more than women from separation, divorce, and spousal death (Glynn, Christenfeld, & Gerin, 1999). Gender differences in sociability, interpersonal skills, social behavior, and empathic capacity (see Chap. 10) can provide plausible explanation for the differential effects of making and breaking human connections in men and women.

It also should be noted that because breakdown of human connections resulting from disruption of marriage, separation, and divorce is detrimental to physical, mental, and social well-being (Bloom, Asher, & White, 1978; Verbrugge, 1979), fragmentation of this important social institution raises a red flag for public health in society at large. Such a trend toward the breakdown of the family places additional responsibility on health care providers to fill the gap and serve as part of a social support system. Having a supportive clinician who listens empathically to the patient's personal illness narrative with a "third ear" and sees patient's concerns with the "mind's eye" helps the patient sort out those experiences and is, in itself, therapeutic.

Social Support

Social support is defined as a multidimensional construct of social relationships that enhances well-being (Rodriguez & Cohen, 1998). It also has been described as the interpersonal resource people use to share understanding and emotions and to develop a sense of belonging (Wellman, 1998). A social support system provides psychological and material resources that benefit an individual's ability to cope with stress (Blumenthal et al., 1987; Cohen, 2004). A social support network of peers and friends is important for the well-being of both children and adults (Cohen, 2004; Hartup & Stevens, 1999). A substantial volume of accumulated evidence indicates the extent to which supportive social relationships are related to individuals' physical, mental, and social well-being (Berkman, 1995). The positive effect of social support on increasing longevity is as strong as the negative effects of obesity, cigarette smoking, and hypertension on life expectancy (Sapolsky, 2004). It has been reported that Vietnam veterans who benefitted from social support were significantly less likely to develop posttraumatic stress disorders (PTSD) than those with low level of support systems (Boscarino, 1995). Because of the benefits of a social support system in promoting health and well-being, Berkman (1995) suggested that social support networks, such as family, friends, and community, should be incorporated into treatment interventions. A review of 81 studies showed that social support was significantly associated with health beneficial effects on cardiovascular, endocrine, and immune systems (Uchino et al., 1996). According to Morgan (2002), a functional social support system requires empathy for more optimal health benefits.

Beneficial Outcomes of Making Connections

The association between social connection and health outcomes is fairly well established in epidemiological research (Glynn et al., 1999). Dean Ornish (1998) described the healing power of intimacy and social relationships in coronary artery disease, beyond drugs and surgery, as follows: "Our heart *is* a pump that needs to be addressed on a physical level, but our hearts are more than just pumps. A true physician is more than just a plumber, technician, or mechanic. We also have an emotional heart, a psychological heart, and a spiritual heart. Our language reflects that understanding." (p. 11).

Cohen (1988) reported that when research participants were exposed to the common cold virus, the perceived social connections served as a protective factor against the virus. Sociability and social activity were found to predict longer survival among women with breast cancer (Hislop, Waxler, Coldman, Elwood, & Kan, 1987), and it is widely recognized that one factor that contributes to improving the health of patients with cancer is social connection (Holland, 2001). The aforementioned studies support the notion that meaningful social relationships, manifested in empathic engagement, can enhance human immunocompetence to a miraculous degree.

Although the well-known Framingham Heart Study has concentrated primarily on physiological and lifestyle factors in heart disease (Levy, 1999); however, this and several other large-scale epidemiological studies provide strong support for the proposition that human connection is beneficial to health and a lack of it is an independent risk factor leading to illness. For example, in a study of the mortality rate caused by heart disease among Italian American residents in two adjacent towns in eastern

Pennsylvania, the researchers found that the death rate among the residents of Roseto was higher than it was among the residents of Bangor (Egolf et al., 1992; Wolf, 1992). The researchers attributed this difference in mortality rates to changes in the social support system and to lower family and community cohesiveness among Italian-Americans in Roseto as a result of becoming a more "Americanized" community.

Remarkable recoveries from life-threatening diseases have been linked to the power of social connections, such as an enduring marriage, family relationships, and friendships (Hirshberg & Barasch, 1995). In a study of Japanese people who emigrated to the USA, Marmot and Syme (1976) found that the immigrants who maintained their traditional family ties had a low prevalence of heart disease similar to their counterparts living in Japan, but the immigrants who became acculturated by adopting the Western lifestyle were 3–5 times more likely to suffer from heart problems.

Another epidemiological study, conducted in Alameda County near San Francisco, found that perception of a lack of social network (family, friends, religious and other group affiliations) significantly increased the mortality rate during the 9-year follow-up period (Berkman, 1995; Berkman, Leo-Summers, & Horwitz, 1992; Berkman, Glass, Brissette, & Seeman, 2000; Berkman et al., 2000, 1992; Berkman & Syme, 1979). Using residents of the same county, researchers found that during their 5-year study, the mortality rate for breast cancer was twice as high among the women who lacked a strong social connection (Raynolds, Boyd, & Blacklow, 1994).

Investigators in the Tecumseh Community Health Study conducted in Michigan found that during a period of 10–12 years, the morbidity rates for stroke, other cardiac problems, cancer, arthritis, and lung disease increased 2–3 times during the study period as a result of participants' weakening of social support systems (House, Robbins, & Metzner, 1982). Blazer (1982) found that people who expressed dissatisfaction with their social support system were more than three times as likely as their satisfied counterparts to die sooner of disease.

These and other epidemiological studies indicate that the risk of a physical illness doubles, at least, when a person's social connections become weak or fragmented (Kaplan, Salonem, & Cohen, 1988; Orth-Gomer & Johnson, 1987; Schoenbach, Kaplan, Fredman, & Kleinbaum, 1986; Seeman, Berkman, & Kohout, 1993). On the basis of the findings just described, it appears that vigilance, inquiries, and advice about patients' social connections not only can help clinicians find remedies that will improve their patients' health status but also can confirm the importance of empathic connection between clinician and patient as a prototype of a support system that in itself is therapeutic.

Pennebaker (1990) suggested that a social support system has a potent benefit because it serves as an outlet for people to talk about their concerns and feelings. Similarly, the healing power of "opening up" during consultations with a health care provider is facilitated by the provider's active listening and empathic interpersonal connection with the patient (see Chap. 8). Pennebaker, Kiecolt-Glaser, and Glaser (1988) reported that self-disclosure during a clinician–patient encounter can have beneficial effects on the patient's immune system. The clinician's empathic understanding can strengthen the clinician–patient connection that leads the patient to self-disclose at deeper levels, which in turn results in a more positive health outcome. In support of this notion, Greenberg, Watson, Elliot, and Bohart (2001) suggested that an empathic relationship can help strengthen the self and free a person from isolation and loneliness.

The precise mechanisms that promote health as an outcome of human connection are not well understood. However, research suggests that some neurobiological (e.g., endocrine and immune functions) as well as psychological mechanisms (e.g., stress-buffering effects, emotional support) are involved (Uchino et al., 1996). Berkman (1995) also confirmed that the immune and neuroendocrine systems are involved in the linkage of social connection and health outcomes. In a review article, Cohen (1988) concluded that health-promoting effects of social ties reflected in social integration (e.g., marriage, network of family and friends, group activities, and religious affiliation) are the combined outcomes of psychosocial factors (e.g., regulation of emotions, cognitive processes, lifestyle, and health behaviors) as well as biophysiological functions (e.g., neuroendocrine, immune, and cardiovascular systems).

Social connections are protective because of the satisfaction that results from human relationships—an important health-promoting factor. For example, Berkman (2000) emphasized that satisfaction with one's spouse, children, relatives, and friends is more important than the frequency of contact with them. In other words, the perceived *quality* of one's social connections is more important than the *quantity* of such connections in maintaining health. Similarly, Seeman and Syme (1987) showed that the size of one's social network is less important than the quality of the interpersonal relationships within that network in lowering the risk of coronary artery disease. Evidence has been accumulating that social support serves as a protective "buffer" against fear and anxiety associated with stress (Cohen, 1988; LaRocco, House, & French, 1980), which in turn could prolong the lives of patients with breast cancer (Spiegel, Bloom, Kraemer, & Gottheil, 1989).

The health-promoting aspects of human connection could be a consequence of certain patterns of psychophysiological response involving the relaxing effect of affiliation, decreased sympathoadrenal activity, and hormonal and metabolic activities associated with human contact (Uvnas-Moberg, 1997). It appears that perceptions of interpersonal connection affect the nervous, endocrine, and immune systems (collectively called psychoneuroimmunology) and that the combined effects of the interactions of these systems contribute to either health (when connections are satisfactory) or illness (when connections, such as negative or stressful relationships are dissatisfactory).

According to the aforementioned studies, the risk of illness should be lower among people who have strong social connections in several domains, including the perception of support from their health care providers. This is important for health care providers to know, because Berkman (2000) suggested that one type of satisfactory social relationship can fill the gap for another. Thus, empathic engagement in clinician–patient encounters can serve as a substitute for, or an additional source of human connection, with all its beneficial outcomes.

Detrimental Outcomes of Breaking Connections

Making and breaking human connections obviously will have opposite consequences for health. An inadequate social network is associated with a high degree
of loneliness experiences (Seeman & Syme, 1987). Lonely people obviously are
deprived of the protective effects of human connections. According to House,
Landis, and Umberson (1988), social isolation is a significant risk factor for morbidity and mortality comparable to obesity, sedentary lifestyle, and even smoking.
A detailed discussion of loneliness and its corrosive effects on human well-being is
beyond the intended scope of this book. However, because loneliness reduces the
likelihood of empathic engagement, I will briefly discuss its detrimental outcomes
as well as its link to empathy.

Loneliness, defined as the perception that one lacks meaningful connections with
others, is a complex phenomenon that is an outcome of many factors, including the
early rearing environment, insecure attachment relationships in childhood, a dysfunctional social network, a nonfacilitative living environment, social forces, and
the lack of interpersonal skills (Hojat & Crandall, 1989). These same factors also
contribute to a deficient capacity for empathy (see Chap. 4).

Loneliness not only impedes psychosocial well-being but also has a negative
effect on physical health through the pathway of the immune system (Kennedy,
Kiecolt-Glaser, & Glaser, 1988). It has been shown that human disconnectedness,
experienced as loneliness, leads to a compromised immune system and thus
increases a person's vulnerability to infection and disease. For example, medical
students who were lonely had poor immune function, as measured by decreases in
the proportions of T-helper lymphocytes and in the number and function of natural
killer cells (Kiecolt-Glaser et al., 1984).

Disconnected people lack social skills and are similar to people with deficient
empathic capacity. For example, in one of our recent studies with medical students
(Hojat, Mangione, Kane, & Gonnella, 2005), we found that scores on the Jefferson
Scale of Empathy (see Chap. 7) were negatively correlated with scores on the
UCLA Loneliness Scale (Russell, Peplau, & Cutrona, 1980) but were positively
correlated with sociability scores on the Extraversion subscale of the Zuckerman–
Kuhlman Personality Questionnaire (Zuckerman, 2002).

Research shows that lonely people are likely to score low on measures of positive aspects of personality that are conducive to relationship building (e.g., self-
esteem, extraversion) (Hojat, 1982a, 1982b, 1983; Shapurian & Hojat, 1985).
Conversely, lonely people are likely to score high on negative aspects of personality
that are detrimental to interpersonal relationships (e.g., depression, anxiety, neuroticism, tough-mindedness) (Hojat, 1982a, 1982b, 1983; Hojat & Shapurian, 1986;
Hojat, Shapurian & Mehryar, 1986; Shapurian & Hojat, 1985). Disconnected people are less likely to trust others, as is indicated by a significant correlation between
scores on the UCLA Loneliness Scale and scores on a scale measuring misanthropy
or faith-in-people (Hojat, 1982a). The findings that lonely people lack the skills
required to achieve interpersonal connections and tend not to trust others suggest

that loneliness is not conducive to forming empathic relationships. In a recent study (Hojat, Michalec et al., 2015), we found that medical students who were recognized by their classmates as positive influencers, compared to others, scored significantly lower on the UCLA Loneliness Scale, but scored higher on the JSE. In a study by Papadakis and colleagues (2005), it was found that impaired peer relationships during medical school could predict later disciplinary action by medical boards against physicians. Thus, capacity to connect can have a lasting effect on physicians' professional behavior.

In his intriguing book with the telling title *The Broken Hearts: The Medical Consequences of Loneliness*, James Lynch (1977, p. 181) proposed that "the lack of human companionship, the sudden loss of love, and chronic human loneliness are significant contributors to serious disease (including cardiovascular disease) and premature death." For example, being surrounded by family or friends reduced the likelihood of premature death by half among elderly patients compared to the rate of death among those who were lonely (Penninx, van Tilburg, & Kriegsman, 1997).

Another study found that living alone was an independent risk factor in recurrent major cardiac events (Case, Moss, Case, McDermott, & Eberly, 1992). However, it is reported that feeling alone is more detrimental to health than living alone (Berkman, 2000; Hojat, 1992). A growing body of evidence in epidemiologic and psychosomatic medicine suggests that disconnectedness is a significant stressor that can be a causative element in the onset or exacerbation of a large and diverse number of medical illnesses, including asthma, cancer, congestive heart failure, diabetes mellitus, infectious hepatitis, leukemia, peptic ulcer, hypertension, hyperthyroidism, and rheumatoid arthritis and in the onset of medical catastrophes, such as sudden death after bereavement (for a review, see Hojat & Vogel, 1989). The perceived distress emerging from dissatisfaction with the social network adversely affects the psychoneuroimmune system, which leads to the progression of illness and deterioration of health (Keller, Shiflett, Schleifer, & Bartlett, 1994).

A number of studies have documented that patients who are lonely, single, or lack a confidant have a higher mortality rate after a myocardial infarction (Berkman, Leo-Summers, & Horwitz, 1992; Case et al., 1992). Low levels of social resources were identified as important risk factors, independent of important medical prognostic factors, in patients medically treated for coronary artery disease (Williams et al., 1992). The harmful outcomes associated with the lack of interpersonal connections result in a reduced ability to adapt to environmental changes, which can inflict damage on the cardiovascular, metabolic, and immune systems (McEwen, 1998).

A recent report indicates that myocardial stunning was an outcome of emotional stress resulting from the death of a family member or close friend in 47 % of the patients with stress-related cardiomyopathy (Wittstein et al., 2005). The authors suggest that exaggerated sympathetic stimulation (or "broken heart" syndrome) as a result of overwhelming emotional stress after loss of a loved one might be central to the myocardial stunning.

Windholz, Marmar, and Horowitz (1985) reported that bereaved spouses were at greater risk for deteriorating health and had a higher mortality rate. In a longitudinal study of volunteers of mammography, Fox, Harper, Hyner, and Lyle (1994) found that experiencing the death of a spouse or another close family member within the previous 2 years significantly increased the risk of breast cancer. To summarize, misery will knock on the door when human connection is broken by death of a loved one, divorce, separation, or loneliness. Empathic engagement can overhaul the misery of human disconnectedness.

Human Connections in Therapy

Human connection can generate an interpersonal dynamic that has a healing effect. For example, group therapy is a method of therapy conducted with a group of patients who often have similar problems. Support groups composed of patients or former patients who get together to discuss illness related experiences represent another therapeutic approach. The unique elements of these types of therapies are interpersonal connection, mutual understanding, and sharing of experiences and concerns, all of which are elements of empathic engagement as well. Shamasundar (1999) postulated that participants in such groups, experience relief from anxiety and distress through the process of diluting emotional states during empathic engagement that occurs while sharing of experiences with others. Spiegel (1990, 1994), Spiegel and Bloom (1983), Spiegel, Bloom, and Yalom (1981) demonstrated that as a means of providing members with social support, group therapy and support groups lead to longevity for patients with cancer. In a series of articles, Spiegel (1993, 1994, 2004) and Spiegel et al. (1989) demonstrated that the perception of belongingness associated with group membership could significantly increase the longevity of patients with metastatic breast cancer.

In one clinical study, patients with metastatic breast cancer were encouraged to express their feelings about their illness in a group (Spiegel et al., 1989). On the average, those patients lived approximately 18 months longer than did members of a control group. The researchers concluded that group support and expression of feelings can mobilize patients' vital resources more effectively. A similar phenomenon occurs during empathic clinician–patient engagement.

In a meta-analytic study, Bohart, Elliot, Greenberg, and Watson (2002) confirmed that group therapy led to slightly better patient outcomes than did individual therapy. A study with addicted physicians found that a peer-led self-help program similar to Alcoholics Anonymous (AA) was successful in treating the physicians' addiction (Galanter, Talbott, Gallegos, & Rubenstone, 1990). The authors identified three factors that contributed to the program's positive outcomes—shared beliefs, group cohesiveness, and mutual understanding—all of which are elements of empathic engagement. Development of an empathic understanding among participants in group therapy or support groups as a result of sharing common goals and experiences could be a contributing factor to changes that occur in group behavior (Shamasundar, 1999). Feelings of being understood generate connectedness that diminishes patients' feelings of loneliness and perceptions of alienation that lead to the therapeutic alliance (Book, 1991).

The phenomenon known as mass psychogenic illness often occurs at a group level among members of a network consisting of family members, friends, coworkers, and classmates who share similar experiences and concerns (Colligan & Murphy, 1982). The empathic relationship has been identified as a factor that contributes to the contagion of group psychogenic illness (Colligan & Murphy, 1982). Also, contagious yawning triggered by seeing or imagining another person's yawning has been linked to the ability to empathize with others (Platek, Critton, Myers, & Gallup, 2003; Platek, Mohamed, & Gallup, 2005). For example, after-dinner yawning that triggers others at the dinner table to yawn may be akin to mass psychogenic behavior that is analogous to interpersonal mimicry or synchronized posture elicited by empathic engagement (Boruch, 1982). According to Newberg and Waldman (2010), yawning evokes neural activities in the brain that are involved in social awareness and empathy. Platek and colleagues (2005) proposed that contagious yawning is an expression of cognitive processes involved in awareness of self and others and may be driven by the so-called mirror neuron system (see Chap. 13).

The Gift of Being Present in Patient Care

The human drive for connectedness increases during times of illness-related distress because illness often makes patients feel disconnected (Platt & Keller, 1994). Therefore, the availability of social support for patients is crucially important. As Morgan (2002) indicated, social support is somewhat synonymous with treatment in the context of health care. Being present when a person is in need of help is, in itself, a social support factor and is a therapeutic remedy described as the "gift of presence" (Nicholas, 2002). The clinician's presence is especially supportive when an empathic relationship is formed between clinician and patient.

The presence of a supportive ally, such as an empathic health care provider, serves as a buffer against the cardiovascular stress response (Christenfeld & Gerin, 2000). In particular, the presence of a woman who provides social support has been found to be more significant than the social support provided by a man (Christenfeld & Gerin, 2000). In an experiment on the influence of social support provided by men and women, study participants were assigned to deliver a short speech on euthanasia (Glynn et al., 1999). The researchers found that when the support was provided by women, who were in the audience and nodding in agreement, the magnitude of the systolic blood pressure was reduced in both male and female speakers. However, a cardiovascular effect of that magnitude was not observed in the speakers when men in the audience nodded in agreement. From the results of this experiment, the researchers concluded that the gift of the presence of supportive individuals, especially supportive women, would probably lead to fewer heart conditions (Glynn et al., 1999). (See Chap. 10 for a discussion of gender differences in medical practice.) These findings also suggest the important role that nurses (most of whom have traditionally been women) often play in providing care and support to the patients (e.g., the concept of caring versus curing described in Chap. 8).

The Empathic Clinician–Patient Relationship as the Epitome of Human Connection

The term "social support" applies to a broad range of conceptualizations of social network structures and their health-promoting functions (Blumenthal et al., 1987; Cohen & Matthews, 1987). In that regard, the clinician–patient relationship can be conceptualized as a special kind of social support system. Cohen (2004) suggested that social support can provide the following three types of resources: (a) instrumental, involving the provision of material aids; (b) emotional, involving the expression of empathy, caring, and reassurance; and (c) informational, involving the provision of relevant information to help the individual understand the problem better and cope with difficulties. An empathic clinician–patient relationship provides all of the aforementioned resources because research shows that empathic understanding of pain and suffering enhances cooperative relationships (Goubert et al., 2005).

The patient's perception of the clinician's support is a complex phenomenon that is a function of the nature of the patient's help-seeking behavior, desire for affiliation, and the clinician's feedback loop through empathic communication. When a trusting relationship is established and is further reinforced by empathic engagement, constraints in the relationship will diminish and a heart-to-heart human communication will prevail (see Chap. 11). This kind of human connection, characterized by full trust, can be formed between lovers as well as between clinicians and their patients.

The relevance and importance of the notion of social support in clinician–patient relationships becomes more evident, considering that patients exhibit an increased desire for affiliation that is naturally expected when people are in distress (Taylor, Klein, Gruenewald, Gurung, & Fernandes-Taylor, 2003). In his experiment, Stanley Schachter (1959) demonstrated that stress increases our desire to affiliate. In the experiment, participants in the high-stress condition (they were told they would receive painful shocks) were twice as likely as other participants to wait in the company of others than to wait alone to participate in the experiment. It has been shown that the presence of others can reduce the experience of pain and suffering (Romano, Jensen, Turner, Good, & Hops, 2000).

One plausible explanation is that human connectedness has a fear-reducing effect that contributes to positive health outcomes (House et al., 1988). Accordingly, it has been suggested that a positive encounter between a clinician and a patient, in itself, has a potential healing power (Novack, 1987; Spiro, 1986). Because of this powerful impact, Balint (1957) described clinicians as the most frequently used therapeutic agents in the history of medicine.

The positive influence of clinician–patient encounters on patient outcomes has been called "Factor X", an unknown factor in healing human suffering (White, 1991). The patient's social support system in general and the nature and quality of the clinician–patient relationship in particular are among the components of the human factor in health and illness. In the process of interpersonal connection, empathy has a mediating role in improving the strength of the connections by increasing a sense of common identity, and reducing prejudice (Stephan & Finlay, 1999). Thus, empathy paves the road to the interpersonal connection between clinicians and patients which is a special kind of social support system, with all of its beneficial healing powers.

Recapitulation

The human tendency to seek connections has an evolutionary root and a survival advantage. Abundant evidence indicates that satisfying the need for affiliation and human connectedness through marriage, family, peers, friends, community, and other social support networks leads to physical, mental, and social well-being. Conversely, breaking social connections leads to loneliness and its detrimental health outcomes. The opportunity for empathic engagement is one underlying reason for the health-promoting outcomes of human connections. Because the drive for human connection increases during times of distress and illness, the presence of an empathic clinician is a gift for the patient that epitomizes the human connection, with all of its beneficial effects.

Chapter 3
An Evolutionary Perspective, Sociophysiology, and Heritability

Empathy can lead to the evolution of fairness.

—(Karen Page & Martin Novak, 2002, p. 1101)

Abstract

- For a better grasp of empathy, we need to understand its evolutionary roots and its sociophysiological functions.
- During the course of evolution, human beings have been endowed with an innate capacity to express and understand emotions from nonverbal cues, which contributed to survival and is conceptualized as primitive empathy.
- Evidence showing infant's reactive crying, facial mimicry, physiological synchronicity in interpersonal interactions, and universal expression of emotions indicates that aspects of interpersonal behaviors cannot be attributed to social learning.
- Twin studies suggest that heritability is also a significant component of empathy more often when a measure of emotional empathy (rather than cognitive empathy) is used.

Introduction

In Chap. 2, I described human beings as social creatures that evolved to be connected with other human beings because social groupings provided increased defense against predators (Plutchik, 1987). Empathic engagement, particularly at the time of distress, was viewed in that chapter as a special kind of social support system. In this chapter, I discuss empathy as having an evolutionary root with a sociophysiological function and a heritability component. Long before they developed the capacity for verbal communication and invented language, our ancestors could relay their feelings, intentions, and expectations by nonverbal means, such as facial expressions, imitation, motor mimicry, and bodily postures. Nonverbal empathic communication has a longer history in the course of human evolution than

© Springer International Publishing Switzerland 2016   31
M. Hojat, *Empathy in Health Professions Education and Patient Care*,
DOI 10.1007/978-3-319-27625-0_3

does verbal communication. Thus, if the brain has areas for verbal communication and language (e.g., Broca's and Wernicke's areas), it must have areas for nonverbal communication and understanding of emotions. Because empathy implies understanding of feelings, emotions, and inner experiences, any means of communicating these concepts would be relevant to studies on the capacity for empathy.

Empathic exchanges, according to Buck and Ginsburg (1997a, p. 481), involve "a genetically based, spontaneous communication process that is fundamental to all living things and that includes innate sending and receiving mechanisms (visual, auditory, or chemical displays, and pre-attunements to such displays); empathy involves communicative genes." If one assumes that empathy is based on an *innate* mechanism and involves "communicative genes," then it must have an evolutionary root, a neuroanatomical structure, and a sociophysiological function.

An Evolutionary Perspective

Evolution lays out the historical path along which humankind has traveled to reach the present point. To understand human behavior, we must understand its evolution. According to the notion of evolution espoused by Charles Darwin (1965, 1981) human beings have evolved during a long evolutionary history of struggle for existence that resulted in the survival of the fittest. During that long history, emotions and their expressions and social cognition evolved for their adaptive advantages in dealing with the fundamental task of survival (Ekman, 1992).

Allport (1924) suggested that the expression of emotion originated from experiences *common* to all human beings. Similarly, Ekman (1992) proposed that our cognitive appraisal of situations that evoke emotions (e.g., those that threaten our survival) is primarily determined by our ancestral past. Carl Gustav Jung (1964) proposed the notion of "collective unconscious" as a transpersonal residue of experiences inherited from one generation to the next. These views imply the existence of a common evolutionary root in the expression of emotion and in cognitive appraisal that are vehicles of empathic communication.

In her thought-provoking article on the biological perspective of empathy, Leslie Brothers (1989) proposed that the capacity for empathy improves fitness for survival. The capacities our ancestors developed to read emotions from nonverbal clues (e.g., facial expression, bodily movement, tone of voice) provided a means of distinguishing foes from friends and danger from safety. The ability to understand social signals conveyed by facial expressions and bodily movements provides a competitive advantage over adversaries and protects against being deceived by them (Brothers, 1989).

Obviously, people who were armed with the capacity to understand other people's states of mind could escape danger more easily than others who lacked that skill; thus, they were more fit for survival. People who failed to develop the capacity for empathy because of genetic predisposition, inappropriate psychosocial experiences, a nonfacilitative rearing environment, or arrested neurological development were less likely to survive. Natural selection, therefore, favored empathy (Humphrey, 1983; Ridley & Dawkins, 1981). Parallel to sensitivity in detecting social signals, human beings developed the skills of deception and manipulation to conceal their emotions and intentions from predators. Studying these evolutionary adapted skills can enhance our understanding of empathy in interpersonal exchanges.

Evolutionary adaptation is linked not only to the physiological activities but also to such social behaviors as mate selection (Buss, 2003), reproductive strategies (Buss, 1995; Buss & Schmitt, 1993), parental investment (Trivers, 1972) (see Chap. 10 for more detailed descriptions of these notions), and prosocial behavior, altruism, and empathy (Buck & Ginsburg, 1997a; Ridley & Dawkins, 1981). During the history of human evolution, capacities have gradually evolved to achieve the ultimate purpose of life—survival or preservation of genes. Dawkins (1999) proposed that the engine of the survival machine is driven by the "selfish gene," which determines whether to protect, fight, or flee to increase the probability of survival. All of these actions require understanding of others' intentions. However, Buck and Ginsburg (1997b, p. 19) argued that "some genes are selfish, and function to support the survival of the individual organism, but other genes are social functioning to support the survival of species."

Buck and Ginsburg's notion was supported by Hamilton (1964) who, in discussing the evolutionary concept of exclusive fitness, proposed that human beings are not programmed exclusively and egoistically to protect their own individual genes but are programmed inclusively and altruistically to protect the survival of others who share similar characteristics. The capacity for empathy evolved to serve that purpose.

In support of this notion, de Quervain and colleagues (2004) used positron emission tomography (PET) to study the neural basis of *the social brain* with regard to intrinsic rewards for prosocial behaviors (e.g., cooperation and observing social norms) and punishment for violating them. The researchers found that people derive intrinsic satisfaction from punishing norm violators, which suggests that such altruistic punishment for the sake of the group's survival has been a decisive force in the evolution of human social behavior. A reward-related region of the brain, the dorsal striatum, has been implicated in the processing of rewards that accrue for socially desirable behavior (de Quervain et al., 2004), including inclination for empathic engagement.

The idea of a "non-selfish" gene that protects the survival of the group suggests that the unit of observation for the purpose of survival may be the group of individuals with common characteristics, rather than the individual. Perhaps this is a reason why empathic engagement becomes stronger with similar rather than dissimilar individuals. The chance of group survival increases with prosocial and altruistically motivated behaviors. The evolutionary basis of empathy, according to Hoffman (1978), can be linked to altruistic behavior in helping others to survive, sometimes even at a cost to the self.

Altruistic behaviors have puzzled evolutionary scholars who believe that the purpose of the struggle for existence is preservation of the individual's genes. However, the notion of a "non-selfish" gene can explain the underlying motivation for altruism.

For example, sacrificing one's own life for the good of the country (patriotic behavior) was dramatically illustrated by Japan's kamikaze pilots during World War II. Political suicidal missions can also be explained by the concept of a "non-selfish" gene aiming at group rather than individual survival. Empathy may have a role in such self-sacrificing behaviors, rooted in the understanding of pain and suffering of others who share some common features.

The issue of whether unconscious (or conscious) efforts to survive are selfishly and egoistically directed toward the preservation of individual genes or are selflessly and altruistically directed toward maintaining the group's genes has been hotly debated by evolutionary scholars. Although the details of such a debate are beyond the intended scope of this book, we should always remember that we are the product of millions of years of evolutionary adaptation for the purpose of either individual or group survival. Empathy is a by-product of this evolutionary adaptation.

Nonverbal Means of Empathic Communication

Through the process of evolution, the human brain has evolved to send and receive messages through nonverbal cues, such as facial expressions, motor mimicry, bodily gestures, change of facial skin color, sweating, and trembling as well as through vocal sounds, such as voice pitch, crying, and laughter, so that happiness, friendliness, and well-intended behaviors could be distinguished from sadness, disagreement, and hostile intent (Adolphs, Tranel, Damasio, & Damasio, 1994; Siegel, 1999). As a result of this evolutionary process, according to Darwin (1965), basic affects, such as happiness, sadness, anger, fear, and disgust, and the nonverbal means of expressing them can be understood and communicated easily regardless of language or cultural barriers.

The ability to send and receive communicative signals in interpersonal encounters is a means of survival. In interpersonal behavior, described by Westerman (2005, p. 22) as "a person's contributions to doing something with other people," expression of emotions plays a major role. The ability to understand other people's emotions from external signals, such as facial expressions and bodily gestures, also is a core ingredient in inferring other's inner feelings and intentions, thus facilitating to form an empathic relationship (Ekman & Friesen, 1974; Zahn-Waxler, Robinson, & Emde, 1992). Empathy can be conveyed through lexical as well as kinetic means of communication (Mayerson, 1976). It has been suggested that behavioral or nonverbal cues, because of difficulty to conceal them, may be even more effective in conveying emotional messages than lexical or verbal communication which can be easily faked (Bayes, 1972). Nonverbal means of communication, according to Mehrabian (1972), include observable actions such as facial expressions; emotional expressions; hand and arm gestures; postures; bodily positions; various movements of the body, head, hand, and legs; eye contact and gaze aversion; as well as subtle aspects of speech such as speech errors, slip of the tongue, pauses, long silence, speech rate, and deliberate choice of words. Better understanding of these nonverbal cues in interpersonal or clinical encounters can enhance empathic engagement.

Facial Expression, Mimicry, Imitation, and Bodily Posture

The human face presents fascinating and meaningful clues about a person's physical and mental status. The facial muscles, controlled by the central nervous system, have the unique ability to produce a wide variety of expressions (Dawson, 1994; Siegel, 1999). Because facial expressions and bodily postures are the external manifestation of the internal world, they facilitate empathic communication, especially in clinician–patient encounters. For example, the degree of rapport between clinician and patient, according to Goldstein and Michaels (1985, p. 107), is correlated with the occurrence of "shared posture." Observing facial expression unconsciously triggers similar expression (and muscle tone measured by electromyography) in the observer (Dimberg, Thunberg, & Elmehed, 2000).

Experimental evidence suggests that the human brain is designed to be attentive to emotional signals emitted via facial expressions. For example, using the "still-face" procedure, Tronick, Als, Adamson, Wise, and Brazelton (1978) found that young children become distressed and withdrawn when their mothers assume an emotionless face, rather than revealing their emotions (see Chap. 4). Evidence also indicates that infants can imitate human facial gestures, such as sticking out the tongue, protruding the lips, and opening the mouth (Meltzoff & Moore, 1977, 1983). Also, emotional expressions can be mimicked (Field, Woodson, Greenberg, & Cohen, 1982; Kugiumutzakis, 1998). Thus, mimicry is a nonverbal means of communicating experiences, which occurs when one observes another person's expression and responds with a similar motor representation (Hess, Blairy, & Phillippot, 1999). For example, we all tend to assume the postural strains of athletes or dancers during moments when we are absorbed in observing their actions (Davis, 1985). Furthermore, most of us have either experienced or observed that while spoon-feeding their infants, mothers often open their own mouth *as if* they are spoon-feeding themselves! These examples suggest that mimicry is a nondeliberate imitation that serves the function of communication (Schaflen, 1964).

Mimicry and the ability to imitate facial gestures and to understand facial expressions have been conceptualized as a type of primitive empathy, rooted in the history of human evolution (Bavelas, Black, Lemery, & Mullett, 1986). Mimicry and imitation behaviors can be explained by the principle of ideomotor action postulated by William James (1890) and the perception-action coupling proposed by Preston and deWaal (2002) (see Chap. 13), suggesting that observing another person's behavior increases a tendency in the observer to behave similarly.

Because mimicry and its associated somatosensory outcomes can help us to understand another person's experiences (Wicker et al., 2003), its relevance to empathy is evident (Chartrand & Bargh, 1999). According to Davis (1985), appraising the concept of mimicry is important when analyzing the component of empathy. Mimicry and facial expression generate changes in the autonomic nervous system associated with feelings that correspond to the facial expression (Decety & Jackson, 2004). Basch (1983) proposed that unconscious, automatic imitation of another person's facial expressions (facial mimicry) and bodily gestures (motor mimicry) generates an automatic and synchronized response in the observer that leads to better understanding of experiences identical to those experienced by the observed individual.

Carr, Iacoboni, Dubeau, Mazziotta, and Lenzi (2003) proposed that individuals with a high degree of empathy compared with others exhibit more unconscious mimicry of other people's facial expressions and bodily postures. Chartrand and Bargh (1999) described this phenomenon as the "chameleon effect"—the mere perception of another person's behavior can automatically increase the likelihood of imitating the perceived behavior. Lakin, Jefferis, Cheng, and Chartland (2003) reported that chameleon effect is a kind of social glue that represents the evolutionary significance of nonconscious mimicry, and serves to foster interpersonal relationships. Chartrand and Bargh suggested that the chameleon effect is the mechanism behind motor mimicry that satisfies the human need for connection and affiliation. Furthermore, they reported that individuals with high empathy scores on the Interpersonal Reactivity Index (Davis, 1983) (see Chap. 5) exhibited the chameleon effect to a greater degree than others with low empathy scores. Chartrand and Bargh (1999) report that a number of researchers have conceptualized mimicry in terms of empathy.

Imitation of another person's behavior is a different type of mimicry that generates a tendency to repeat an observed action (Meltzoff & Prinz, 2002). Imitation of an action implies striving to achieve the goal of that action (Baldwin & Baird, 2001). This indicates that in observing a behavior, either positive or negative, the underlying intention is also inferred which is perhaps more important in prompting imitative behavior. This explains why role models in health professions education and practice are important motivators of professional behavior. In his theory of violence, Berkowitz (1984) postulated that violence shown in public media contributes to imitating aggressive and criminal behaviors which can be explained by the principle of ideomotor action (James, 1890), and the perception-action model (Preston & de Waal, 2002) (see Chap. 13).

One indicator of recognizing emotions early in life is the observation that newly born infants will cry in response to the sound of another infant's cry (Sagi & Hoffman, 1976; Simner, 1971). This reactive crying does not occur in response to either a loud sound or a vocal sound that lacks the affective components of the other infant's cry, or even to the recorded crying of the newborn infant itself. According to Hoffman (1978), the human infant's reactive crying is based on a built-in mechanism that is an early precursor of empathic understanding.

Sociophysiology

The link between human physiology and social interaction has attracted the attention of scholars for a long time. For example, more than half a century ago, Boyd and DiMascio (1957) studied the concept of the "sociophysiology" of social behavior and found a relationship between emotions expressed in clinical interviews and autonomic physiologic responses, such as heart rate, skin resistance, and facial temperature. The notion of "interpersonal physiology" in clinician–patient interactions was first introduced in a study by DiMascio, Boyd, and Greenblatt (1957), who found that patients' and therapists' heart rates and skin temperatures were synchronized during clinical interviews. Goldstein and Michaels (1985, p. 68) reported that synchronization typically occurs between individuals who have "good rapport" with one another. Accuracy in perception of negative emotions was found to be a function of physiological synchrony between the perceiver and the target person (Levenson & Ruef, 1992). It is suggested that empathy can emerge as a result of the autonomic nervous system, which tends to simulate another person's physiological state (Ax, 1964). In other words, an empathic engagement reflected in good interpersonal rapport facilitates physiological synchronization during clinical interviews.

In another early experiment, investigators noticed that the physiological responses of healthy young soldiers were different when interacting with an officer (who was a psychiatrist) compared with a person who was an enlisted man (Reiser, Reeves, & Armington, 1955). The researchers concluded that the sociophysiology of the relationship in clinician–patient encounters could be a function of the client's view regarding the care provider's prestige or status (Reiser et al., 1955). In their study, Chartrand and Bargh (1999) found that greater time in contact with elderly people was associated with poorer memory, and more forgetfulness, indicating that even mental status of others can be adapted by frequent observations.

In a review article, Adler (2002) proposed that the experience of an empathic relationship in clinical encounters reduces the secretion of stress hormones and concluded that "the immediate effect of a caring relationship flows from the physiologic consequences of feeling cared about, because the neurobiology of such a relationship promotes an endocrine response pattern that favors homeostasis and is the antithesis of the fight–flight response" (p. 878).

A physiological feedback loop is set in motion during clinical interviews that is a reflection of mutual understanding. Observing emotion in another person has been reported to result in a similar display of emotion in the observer (Lanzetta & Englis, 1989). Similarly, emotional distress in one person can automatically trigger similar distress in another person when the two are interacting (Eisenberg, 1989). A study of physiological changes, such as heart rate, during interpersonal interactions revealed that a clinician's interpersonal style (e.g., praising or criticizing) can influence the patient's physiological reaction (Malno, Boag, & Smith, 1957). For example, these investigators observed that patients' heart rates rose significantly when the clinician had had a "bad" day. The results of a study indicate that physiological synchronicity (e.g., in heart rate and muscle activity) between people can lead to more accurate perceptions of their feelings (Decety & Jackson, 2006).

Maurer and Tindall (1983) observed that patients' perceptions of the therapist's empathic understanding increased when therapist's arm and leg positions were congruent (mirror image) of the patients. Mimicry, imitation, and body posture synchronization serve as an adaptive function to facilitate interpersonal interaction (Chartrand & Bargh, 1999). Schaflen (1964) observed that the more people in group share similar viewpoints, the more they tend to mimic one another's postures. It is also reported that patients perceive more empathic engagement when the clinicians mimicked their body posture; and the effect is reciprocal if the clinician and client are acquainted with each other (La France, 1979). It has also been observed that students' ratings of their teacher's involvement in class activities improved when there is more postural synchronicity between students and their teacher (La France, 1982).

Kaplan and Bloom (1960, p. 133) proposed the idea that the empathic process involves not only placing oneself in another person's "psychological" shoes but also placing oneself in that person's "physiological" shoes as well. However, Szalita (1976, p. 145) suggested that in empathic engagement with patients, "it is good to be able to put yourself into someone else's shoes, but you have to remember that you don't wear them." In a study of couples examined by using functional magnetic resonance imaging (fMRI), Singer and colleagues (2004) found that couples who scored higher on the Empathy Scale (Hogan, 1969) (see Chap. 5) and the Empathic Concern Scale of the Interpersonal Reactivity Index (Davis, 1983) (see Chap. 5) showed more intense brain activity when they observed their partner experiencing pain.

These findings suggest that empathic resonance involves shared physiological–neurological activities between people who are interacting. The notion of shared physiology between interacting people is intriguing (Ax, 1964; Kaplan & Bloom, 1960; Levenson & Ruef, 1992), and it opens up a window for studying the "physiological dance" that takes place in empathic engagement. More research is needed to investigate the underlying mechanisms involved in the psycho-socio-physiology of social behavior and the relevance of shared physiologic responses to empathic understanding and sympathetic feelings (see Chap. 13 on neurological underpinnings of empathy).

Heritability

Mumford (1967) regarded empathy as a genetically determined quality that can be enhanced or inhibited by positive or negative life experiences, respectively (cited in Szalita, 1976). A standard approach to research on heritability is the "twin study." In this research design, genetically identical or monozygotic (MZ) twins (who share 100 % common genes) are compared with fraternal or dizygotic (DZ) twins (who share approximately 50 % of their genes). Heritability can be determined with regard to a particular trait when MZ twins are more highly correlated than DZ twins on the trait, assuming a similar rearing environment. In a sample of 278 MZ and 378 DZ twins, strong genetic influences were found in 78 % of the twins younger than 11 years of age and in 66 % of those aged 11 years or older concerning the heritability of social cognitive skills relevant to empathy (Scourfield, Martin, Lewis, & McGuffin, 1999).

In a study involving 114 MZ and 116 DZ twins, the researchers found a significant heritability component of 72 % on a derived index of empathic concern (Matthews, Batson, Horn, & Rosenman, 1981). In yet another study involving 94 MZ and 90 DZ twins, the investigators found modest evidence of heritability in empathy (Zahn-Waxler et al., 1992). In another study of 573 adult twin pairs of both sexes, empathy, as measured by the Emotional Empathy Scale (Mehrabian & Epstein, 1972) (see Chap. 5), had a relatively broad heritability estimate of 68 % (Rushton et al., 1986). In a study of 174 pairs of MZ twins, and 148 pairs of DZ twins, it was found that 42 % of prosocial behavior was due to the twins' genes, 23 % to twins' shared environment, and the remaining to the twins' non-shared environment (Rushton, 2004).

Knafo, Zahn-Waxler, Van Hule, Robinson, and Rhee (2008) studied the genetic and environmental influences on empathy among 409 young twins and noticed increased contribution of genes, but decreased effects of environment with age. The results of another study (Davis, Luce, & Kraus, 1994) using the Interpersonal Reactivity Index (Davis, 1983) (see Chap. 5) showed evidence of significant heritability for the scales of Empathic Concern and Personal Distress (indicators of emotional empathy of the Interpersonal Reactivity Index, Davis, 1983) but not for the Perspective Taking Scale (an indicator of cognitive empathy of the Interpersonal Reactivity Index). These findings generally suggest that indicators of the so-called emotional empathy, which is more akin to sympathy, are more likely to have a higher heritability component than the cognitive indicators of empathy.

Recapitulation

In this chapter, I presented an evolutionary perspective on precursors of empathy through nonverbal behavior such as facial mimicry, imitation, and body posture. Data from twin studies were also presented to suggest that the capacity for empathy could be heritable to some extent. Research findings on the sociophysiology of interpersonal behavior, linking empathy to unconscious mimicry, imitation, and postural synchronicity, were discussed to show that empathic relationship in general, and empathic engagement in patient care in particular, resembles a synchronized dance between the involved parties which is orchestrated by sociophysiological factors to harmonize the dynamic exchanges and optimize interpersonal communication.

Chapter 4
Psychodynamics and Development

Love, and lack of it, changes the young brain forever.

—(Thomas Lewis, Fari Amini, & Richard Lannon, 2000, p. 89)

The key to the heaven is under mother's footsteps.

—(A popular Persian saying)

The hand that rocks the cradle rules the world.

—(A popular cliché)

Abstract

- Empathy is nurtured in a facilitative early rearing environment, particularly in relation to the quality of child's relationship with the mother or a primary caregiver.
- Evidence regarding the newborn's preference for its mother's voice; maternal investment in child rearing, lactation and breast-feeding; and attachment relationships suggest that nature has endowed the mother with the innate ability to be the most important participant in the development of a child's capacity for empathy.
- Experimental findings obtained by using the "still-face" and "visual cliff" paradigms indicate that infants can understand and react to their primary caregiver's emotional state.
- The foundation for a child's mental representation (internal working models) of the world is the early relationship with the mother that becomes an influential force in the regulation of emotions and empathic behavior throughout life.
- Associations between empathy and facial imitation and mimicry in childhood, and theory of mind are discussed.

© Springer International Publishing Switzerland 2016

M. Hojat, *Empathy in Health Professions Education and Patient Care*,

DOI 10.1007/978-3-319-27625-0_4

Introduction

The search for the roots of the capacity for empathy is of paramount importance in understanding the course of its optimal development or the arrest of its development. In this chapter, I describe some of the factors that contribute to the nourishment of empathy. The central notion emphasized throughout the chapter is that empathy is nurtured in the early rearing environment in relation to the quality of the early attachment relationship with a primary caregiver (Henderson, 1974; Schaflen, 1964).

The Nature–Nurture Debate

The issue of whether nature or nurturing contributes more to prosocial behavior has been debated for a long time. Proponents of nature place great emphasis on the notion that genetic makeup has an undeniable role in the development of human behavior. Recent developments in the Human Genome Project have provided more fuel in support of their argument (Collins, 1999).

However, proponents of nurture use Watsonian and Skinnerian approaches to classical conditioning and operant learning as evidence that human behavior can be molded according to the principles of behavior modification, and they believe that environmental and experiential factors have a more prominent role than genes do in the development of prosocial or antisocial behavior. The often-cited statement made by John Brutus Watson (1924, p. 82), the founder of the school of behaviorism in psychology, supports the nurture notion:

> Give me a dozen healthy infants, well formed, and my own special world to bring them up, and I will guarantee to take any one at random and train him to become any type of specialist I might select—doctor, lawyer, artist, merchant-chief, and yes, even beggar and thief, regardless of his talents, penchants, tendencies, abilities, vocations, and race of his ancestors.

Although some experts still believe that nurturing matters more than nature does in determining human behavior (Hoover, 2000), most scholars nowadays are of the opinion that it is the interaction of nature and nurturing that contributes to the development of social behavior. Human beings are born with a potential for "engageability," which is triggered to a certain degree by, and will develop to a certain extent depending on, environmental and experiential factors (Neubauer & Neubauer, 1990).

Although many genetics-oriented scientists were excited about the discoveries of the Human Genome Project (Collins, 1999), determining the basis of human behavior proved to be a more complicated matter than simply mapping the human genome. For example, findings in a study of 44,788 sets of twins indicated that environmental and lifestyle factors as well as inherited genes make significant contributions in the development of different types of cancers (Lichtenstein et al., 2000). Abundant research evidence has accumulated in support of the proposition that the family environment and parental care play an important role in the development of adults' prosocial behavior, including the propensity for empathic relationships.

The Family Environment

The family is the oldest and the most important social institution in the history of human civilization. It is "the seedbed of commitment, love, character, and social as well as personal responsibility" (Ashcroft & Straus, 1993, p. 1). The United Nations Convention on the Rights of the Child, adopted unanimously by the General Assembly, recognized that for full and harmonious development, children must grow up in a facilitative family environment in an atmosphere of happiness and love provided by their parents (Grant, 1991; Hojat, 1993, 1997). The calming experience of feeling felt and the echoes of love spring to life in the family first, then expand to embrace a broader social network, even the entire human race (Eibel-Eibesfeldt, 1979).

The family environment early in life not only shapes the quality of later interpersonal relationships (Fonagy, 2001) but also sows the seed for the growth of the capacity for empathic engagement. The way we are brought up in the early periods of our lives influences "all our later relationships, all our later days" (Neubauer & Neubauer, 1990, p. 81). The child whose emotional needs are unmet or denied in the family will not develop a sense of trust, a problem that will have a lasting negative influence on later social relationships (Rempel, Holmes, & Zanna, 1985). The capacity for empathy also can be negatively influenced by unmet emotional needs in the family (Eisenberg & Strayer, 1987b; Perry et al., 2001) because, as Guzzetta (1976) proposed, empathy springs from interpersonal relationships within the family. Development of empathy, according to Barnett (1987), occurs in a family environment in which parental warmth and responsiveness satisfy the child's emotional needs and provide opportunities for the child to observe and experience warm interpersonal responses in a variety of situations.

It is the family's importance in the development of the capacity for empathy that has led to health care researchers' apt description of the clinician's family of origin as the bedrock for the development of interpersonal skills in patient care (Farber, Novack, & O'Brien, 1997; Mengel, 1987).

The Parents

Empathy has a rich and complex developmental history (Shapiro, 1974). It arises from early sensory and tactile communication between mother and child (Schwaber, 1981). In a review of the literature on parental behavior that contributes to the development of empathy in children, Mehrabian, Young, and Sato (1988) concluded that the parents of children with a strong capacity for empathy were more verbally explicit about their feelings, offered more emotional support, and were more tolerant. Early interactions with parents, according to Roe (1957), determine the child's future vocational choice in people-oriented versus other occupations.

Human beings differ from all other animals in the length of their dependency on a caregiver for survival and protection. This period of dependency is crucial for neurological development (e.g., the process of myelination) (Davison & Peters, 1970) and social growth. The critical period of susceptibility opens a window of opportunity during which activation of specific brain functions are essential for ongoing development of different areas of the brain related to social behavior (Siegel, 1999). That window will close after a certain period of time.

The importance of the critical period of neurological development was first noticed by Hubel and Wiesel who found that suturing one eye closed in kittens during the first few weeks after birth caused a sharp decline in the number of cells in the visual cortex (Hubel, 1967; Hubel & Wiesel, 1963). The investigators found that up to 5 years after the eye was opened, only a minimal amount of the visual cortex had recovered (Hubel & Wiesel, 1970). Hubel (1967) noticed that when kittens were not exposed to horizontal lines during a certain critical period of development, their visual cortex was unable to process horizontal input later in life.

Abundant evidence supports the existence of a sensitive period of neurological development. For example, baby chimpanzees reared in darkness during that period will be blind for the rest of their lives (Chow, Riesen, & Newell, 1957). MacLean (1967) found that if certain neural circuits were not formed during a crucially receptive period in the brain's development, the circuits were unlikely to ever be fully developed. The assumption is that the repeated activation of specific neuronal pathways as a result of early experiences reinforces the strength of connections between groups of neurons. The neurons that create interconnections through early experiences, according to Hebbian neuron cell assembly theory (Hebb, 1946; Keysers & Perrett, 2004), fire together later in life, so to speak, because "neurons that fire together wire together" (see Chap. 13).

In addition to physical stimulation, emotionally rich interactions in early life contribute to neurological development. One early experiment on the importance of early life experiences to human survival was conducted in the thirteenth century by Emperor Frederick II who wanted to know what language children would speak if no one talked to them. Thus, "he bade foster mothers and nurses to suckle the children, to bathe and wash them, but in no way to prattle with them. ... But he labored in vain, because the children died" (Ross & McLaughlin, 1949, pp. 366–367).

Supportive parenting fosters capacity for empathy (Soenens, Duriez, Vansteenkiste, & Goossens, 2007) because in addition to genetic predisposition, supportive parents serve as the model of empathic understanding for their children (Chase-Lansdale, Wakschlag, & Brooks-Gunn, 1995; Krevans & Gibbs, 1996). Parental warmth has been hypothesized to promote children's capacity for empathy and prosocial behavior (Hoffman, 1982; Janssens & Gerris, 1992). Children of empathic parents reacted vicariously to others' negative emotions (Robinson, Zahn-Waxler, & Emde, 1994; Trommsdorff, 1995). Cross-sectional and longitudinal research, using structural equation modeling, has confirmed that parents' (particularly mothers') expression of positive emotions is the mechanism that mediates a causal relationship between parental warmth and children's empathic capacity (Zhou et al., 2002). On the contrary, Zahn-Waxler and Radke-Yarrow (1990) suggested that family risk factors such as parental depression, marital discord, and parental maltreatment, particularly in the first two years of life could contribute to the arrest of empathy development in children and can be manifested in the adults' deficit in interpersonal relationships.

The Hand that Sows the Seeds

Parents usually provide the love and affection their children need for healthy development. Research has shown that a supportive relationship with both parents is predictive of high empathy scores as well as social sensitivity in children (Adams, Jones, Schvaneveldt, & Jenson, 1982). However, although both parents must share childcare responsibilities for their children to achieve ideal social development, some findings suggest that the mother's role may be more crucial than that of any other caregiver, including the father.

For example, in a study of Harvard University graduates who were followed up for 35 years, Russek and Schwartz (1997) found that 91 % of the graduates who retrospectively perceived the lack of a warm and friendly relationship with their mother had serious health problems in midlife (e.g., coronary artery disease, high blood pressure, alcoholism) compared with 45 % of the graduates who retrospectively perceived their relationship with their mother as having been warm and friendly. The corresponding figures for their perceived relationship with their father were 82 % and 50 %, respectively. Consistent with these findings, we found that medical students who perceived a satisfactory childhood relationship with their mother rated their general health more positively and reported more resilience in appraising stressful life events (Hojat, 1996).

Individuals' perceptions of their early relationships with parents generally are positively associated with personality attributes that are conducive to interpersonal relationships (Hojat, Borenstein, & Shapurian, 1990). In our study of 422 medical students, we examined the differential effects of satisfactory early relationships with the mother and father and found that higher scores on the Jefferson Scale of Empathy (see Chap. 7) were significantly associated with students' retrospective reports concerning the level of satisfaction with the early relationship with their mother (Hojat et al., 2005). Such an association was not found regarding the students' perceived relationship with their father.

These findings are consistent with those in another study in which undergraduates reported that their mothers, more than fathers, spent more time with them, were more affectionate with them, and expressed more empathy toward them (Barnett, Howard, King, & Dino, 1980). The undergraduates' scores on Mehrabian and Epstein's Emotional Empathy Scale (1972) (see Chap. 5) showed stronger association with their interactions with their mothers than with their fathers.

In another study, medical students' retrospective perceptions of a satisfactory relationship with the mother were significantly associated with a positive personality profile, such as higher self-esteem and more satisfactory relationships with peers

(Hojat, 1998). In the same study, perceptions of satisfactory relationships with the mother were inversely associated with personality attributes that are detrimental to interpersonal relationships, such as depression, anxiety, and loneliness. Such patterns of significant associations were not observed for students' perceptions of their early relationships with the father. Also, the students' perceptions of the availability of the mother in childhood were significantly associated with higher scores on self-esteem and lower scores on depression and loneliness (Hojat, 1996).

In a study with kindergarten children and their mothers, a substantial correlation was observed in the empathy between mother and child (Trommsdorff, 1991). One explanation is that empathic mothers are likely to engage in empathic exchanges with their children, and empirical research supports this speculation. For example, Wiesenfeld, Whitman, and Malatesta (1984) observed that the mothers' scores on Mehrabian and Epstein's Emotional Empathy Scale predicted their emotional responses to their infant's emotional distress and their desire to pick up the baby when baby was in distress. Other researchers found that mothers with high scores on the Emotional Empathy Scale were less disturbed by their infant's cry and rated the crying as less irritating than low-empathy mothers (Lounsburg & Bates, 1982). Conversely, a link was reported between mothers' low levels of empathy and maternal child abuse. For example, Letourneau (1981) reported that scores on Hogan's Empathy Scale and Mehrabian and Epstein's Emotional Empathy Scale could differentiate abusive and nonabusive mothers better than a measure of stressful life events. In a study of 177 adolescents and their mothers, Soenens et al. (2007) found that maternal support served as a mediator of the intergenerational transmission of empathy and quality of friendship. A child who never developed the capacity for empathy will become an ineffective parent (Tucker, Luu, & Derryberry, 2005).

Why do mothers have a more crucial role in the development of their children's prosocial and empathic behavior? Nature has bestowed them with some unique privileges that enable them to perform their caregiving role. Some of these privileges are described here.

The Infant's Preference for the Mother's Voice and Face

Under normal circumstances, the voice the developing fetus hears most often is the voice of the expectant mother, who talks, may sing, shouts, laughs, and cries. Thus, the onset of interpersonal connection is with the mother's voice. Although the fetus is unable to respond, it is able to hear the mother's voice again, again, and again. Her voice is different from the low-frequency rhythmic sound of her heartbeat, which probably has a calming effect.

Because the mother's voice is the most intense acoustical signal in the amniotic environment of the uterus, the newborn infant shows a clear preference for the sound of her voice within the first 3 days after birth (DeCasper & Fifer, 1980; Fifer & Moon, 1994). Fifer and Moon (1994) suggested that early experiences with mother's voice have an enduring influence on the development of the infant's brain.

In addition, the specific tone and range of pitch that mothers use to get the attention of preverbal infants have been described as the universal "maternal melodies" that serve as a potent mediator of affective communication (Papousek, Papousek, & Symmes, 1991).

By using a non-nutritive nipple attached to an electronic recorder that monitored the rate and amplitude of the infant's sucking pattern, DeCasper and Fifer (1980) found that newborn infants changed their sucking pattern when they heard a recording of their own mother's voice, but no such change was recorded for other female voices. Their sucking pattern also did not change when they heard a recording of their own father's voice (DeCasper & Prescott, 1984). DeCasper and Fifer (1980) suggested that the infant's preference for its mother's voice is important for initiating bonding with the mother. Thus, it appears that the biological mother has a unique advantage that is not shared by any other caregiver—the ability to establish the early attachment relationship with her newborn infant through the newborn's recognition of her voice. The onset of empathy can be traced back to this kind of early exchange between mother and child (Burlingham, 1967).

Preference for the maternal voice can lead the child to prefer the mother's face. Indeed, empirical data suggest that neonates quickly learn to recognize their mother's face. The infant not only shows a preference for her voice but pays particular attention to her varying facial expressions as well. Pascalis, DeSchonen, Morton, Deruella, and Fabre-Grenet (1995) reported that the 4-day-old neonate looks longer at its mother's face than at a stranger's face.

The Mother's Investment in Child Rearing

Trivers (1972) pointed out that in all mammalian species, the mother is usually more involved in child-rearing than any other caregiver, including the father. The following factors contribute to greater investment on the mother's part: scarcity of gametes and maternal certainty, the psychology of pregnancy, the neurochemistry of motherhood, lactation and breast-feeding, and the mother–child attachment.

The Scarcity of Gametes and Maternal Certainty

Evolutionary scholars have proposed two reasons for more maternal than paternal investment in child care. First, women have far fewer gametes than men do—usually one ovum every 4 weeks during the limited period of fertility versus millions of sperm per ejaculation. This scarcity of gametes leads to the mother's greater protection of offspring and consequently to her greater investment in their care (Bjorklund & Kipp, 1996; Buss & Schmitt, 1993). Second, because of internal gestation and childbirth, maternal certainty (the mother's confidence that she is the biological mother) has historically been much greater than paternal certainty (the father's confidence that he is the biological father), which has resulted in greater maternal investment in preserving one's own genes (Bjorklund & Kipp, 1996; Buss, 2003; Buss & Schmitt, 1993; Trivers, 1972).

The Psychology of Pregnancy and the Neurochemistry of Motherhood

The psychology of internal gestation leads to a fundamentally unique maternal experience of bringing new life into the world (Ballou, 1978). Early in her pregnancy, the mother perceives the child as a developing part of herself. The initial attachment begins to develop at this stage. Nine months of carrying the fetus, the subsequent experience of childbirth, and a long period of breastfeeding and nourishing the infant, provide a sense of emotional investment that is a unique experience for the expectant mother and no one else.

The neurochemistry of motherhood, including hormonal changes during pregnancy, after birth, and during lactation, is unique to the biological mother. For example, levels of oxytocin increase drastically in human mothers around the time of childbirth. These high concentrations of oxytocin are believed to serve as the thread that weaves the ties between mother and child (Lewis et al., 2000), ties that Freud (1964, p. 188) described as "unique, without parallel, established unalterably for a whole lifetime as the first and the strongest love-object and as the prototype of all later love relations—for both sexes."

Oxytocin can influence the activation of dopamine-producing neurons (Insel, 2000; Oliver, 1939), which makes motherhood more pleasurable under normal circumstances. Studies have shown that increased oxytocin can induce maternal behavior in nonpregnant rats (Pedersen & Prange, 1979; Pedersen, Ascher, Monroe, & Prange, 1982). Conversely, other studies have shown that reduced binding of oxytocin in the brain inhibits the onset of maternal behavior (Fahrbach, Morrell, & Pfaff, 1985; Insel, 2000).

Lactation and Breast-Feeding

Oxytocin prepares the biological mother to feed her newborn by stimulating the release of prolactin and thus lactation (Mori, Vigh, Miayata, & Yoshihara, 1990). Breast-feeding is another physiological privilege that nature has bestowed only on the biological mother. In addition to the nutritious quality of mother's milk, which contributes to the enhancement of the infant's immunocompetence and neurological development, breast-feeding is the first human interactive experience that satisfies the newborn's physiological and psychological needs. Winnicott (1987, p. 79) described the infant's breast-feeding experience as a means of communication that "sings a song without words." It paves the road to empathy.

The sequence of breast-feeding activities, such as proximity seeking toward the nipple; rhythmic movement of the head, mouth, and tongue; sucking that stimulates secretion of milk; ingestion of milk; and withdrawal and disengagement from the nipple, provides a unique opportunity for the behavioral and physiological regulation that develops in the mother–infant dyad (Smotherman & Robinson, 1994). Nursing at the breast is physiologically pleasurable for both mother and infant. The female physiological responses during coitus and lactation have been reported to be similar. For example, uterine contractions, nipple erection, and ejection of milk can occur during both sexual intercourse and breast-feeding (Newton & Newton, 1967). Breast-feeding not only has a calming effect on the human infant, mediated by activation of the opioid system (Smotherman & Robinson, 1994) but also serves as a thermoregulatory mechanism for the exchange of body warmth between mother and infant. During sucking, uterine contractions and increased skin temperature occur that are pleasurable to the lactating mother (Newton, Feeler, & Rawlins, 1968). The gratifying sensation mothers experience when breast-feeding their infants serves as a positive reinforcement of mother–child bonding. The seeds of empathy grow in the ecstasy of such loving interactions.

The universal synchronicity observed between mother and infant during breast-feeding (e.g., the holding position, visual gazes, and vocal exchanges) is, in itself, a unique model of human communication. According to Schore (1996), empathy is rooted in this early psychobiological attunement between mother and child. Isabella and Belsky (1991) reported that synchronous interactions between mother and infant open the highway to a secure attachment between them. All these early experiences affect the infant's growing brain by altering the strength of the synaptic connections that contribute to affective and cognitive behavior later in life.

It is these early physiological and psychological exchanges between the newborn child and the lactating mother that can alter the trajectories of neural development and later interpersonal behavior. The attachment between mother and child that is strengthened by these exchanges between the two can be viewed as a prototypical example of an empathic engagement.

The Attachment Relationship

The bonding between a mother and her child strengthens at the moment of birth during skin-to-skin contact between the mother and her newborn baby (Klaus & Kennell, 1970; Klaus et al., 1972). John Bowlby (1973, 1980, 1982) elegantly described the dynamics and consequences involved in the infant's repeated encounters with the primary caregiver in his attachment theory, which he systematically formulated, advanced, and elaborated in the widely cited trilogy of books. The theory not only was conceived as a general theory of psychosocial development but also was viewed specifically as a framework for later interpersonal and social relationships. According to the tenets of the theory, a lovingly responsive mother serves as a secure base that allows the child to explore the world comfortably.

The mother's presence (or absence), her attentiveness and loving responses (or her inattentiveness or lack of responses) to her baby's signals, and her provision (or lack of provision) of physical and emotional nourishment gradually become a fact of life for the growing child. The formation of a secure mother–child attachment is most likely to occur in the presence of a lovingly responsive mother, whereas the opposite (an insecure attachment) is likely to occur if the mother is physically or emotionally unavailable (Bowlby, 1988). (For a review, see Hojat, 1995, 1996, 1998.) A strong mother–child attachment is a major antecedent of early interest in others and is a necessary condition for the development of the capacity for empathy (Mussen & Eisenberg-Berg, 1977).

The quality of the mother–child attachment relationship is assessed by the Strange Situation Procedures, a frequently used test developed by Ainsworth, Blehar, Waters, and Wall (1978). Individual differences among infants and toddlers concerning the quality of attachment with their primary caregiver can be measured with this controlled laboratory procedure, which takes approximately 20 min and includes the following seven episodes, each lasting 3 min or less: (1) an infant or a toddler (usually aged 12–18 months) and its mother are brought into a laboratory room containing some toys; (2) a stranger (usually a woman) enters the room, sits down, and talks to the mother and child; (3) the mother then leaves the room while the stranger stays in the room; (4) the mother then returns and the stranger leaves the room; (5) again, the mother leaves the room, leaving the child alone; (6) the stranger returns; (7) finally the mother returns.

According to Ainsworth and her colleagues, the reaction of the child, particularly in the two episodes of mother–child reunion in this procedure (Episodes 4 and 7) reflected the nature and quality of the mother–child attachment. Originally, the researchers identified three types of mother–child attachment. Briefly, if the child explored and played with the toys when the mother was present, expressed less interest in the toys when she left the room, and sought to be near her and initiate positive expression with her when she returned, the attachment was classified as a *secure* attachment (Ainsworth, 1985b). However, if the child continued to explore the toys during all seven episodes, exhibited no distress when the mother left the room, and avoided her when she returned, the child's attachment was classified as *avoidant*. Finally, if the child tended to be wary of the stranger, became intensely upset when the mother left, and exhibited ambivalent behavior when she returned (wanting to approach her and simultaneously being angry and avoiding being near her, thus difficult to soothe), attachment was classified as *ambivalent*. Main and Solomon (1990) introduced a new category of attachment, the "disorganized attachment," in an attempt to explain the situation when none of the other three patterns of attachment applied.

The type of attachment developed in early childhood is likely to endure throughout life (Ainsworth, 1985a, 1985b). Research has shown that securely attached children develop a sense of trust with caregivers who respond to them empathically and therefore develop the capacity to respond sensitively and empathically toward others in later relationships (Kestenbaum, Farber, & Sroufe, 1989). Furthermore, research has shown that the lack of a secure attachment with the mother can result in aggressive and noncompliant behaviors in later years that are not conducive to empathic engagement (Belsky, 1988; Karen, 1994) (for a review, see Hojat, 1995).

In a study of preschool children, Kestenbaum et al. (1989) observed a continuity between the quality of a child's early relationship with the primary caregiver and the child's capacity to respond empathically later. This observation confirmed the notion that "it is with the aid of modified mother–child signals that we establish and maintain friendly contact with our fellow men" (Eibel-Eibesfeldt, 1979, p. 230). Severe abnormalities in interpersonal relationships have been observed in infants, such as Romanian orphans, who have been deprived of maternal love (Konner, 2004). The abnormality in connecting to others known as "reactive attachment disorder" is another testimony to the importance of the quality of early attachment to later empathic behavior or the lack thereof.

According to Bowlby (1988, p. 82), the need for a secure attachment remains "from cradle to grave." More important, as Bowlby pointed out, the quality of the child's early relationship with the mother will lead to the development of cognitive schemata regarding the world that reside deep in the child's mind and "tend to persist and are so taken for granted that they come to operate at an unconscious level" (p. 130). In other words, the prototypical model of the world as friendly and caring or as hostile and uncaring becomes an influential property of the child's cognitive structure, serving primarily as an unconscious motivational force that significantly influences the adult's interpersonal relationships and the capacity for empathic engagement (Ainsworth, 1985a, 1985b).

The nature and quality of the child's early interpersonal experiences with the primary caregiver and the positive or negative outcomes engrave relatively permanent cognitive images on the mind that attachment scholars describe as "internal working models" (Bretherton, 1987). This mental representation of the world, or the psychological "script," becomes a major motivational factor in empathic relationships later in life (Nathanson, 1996; Tomkins, 1987). The assertion that attachment relationships in childhood can influence interpersonal behavior across the life span has broad implications for developmental, social, and clinical psychology.

Also, it has been reported that relationships with family members, peers, and others are influenced by early attachment experiences (Bartholomew & Horowitz, 1991). Shaver and Hazan (1989) reported that adult love relationships share similarities with, and are rooted in the early attachment experiences with a primary caregiver. It has also been reported that attachment history can predict medical students' specialty preferences. For example, students with a secure attachment history are more likely to choose specialties that require more interaction with patients (Ciechanowski, Russo, Katon, & Walker, 2004). Early attachment experiences also can influence the style of clinical practice. For example, clinical psychologists with an insecure attachment history who reported less empathic parental responses, were more in need of support, and were more vulnerable to work stress (Leiper & Casares, 2000).

The child's attachment behavior in all cultures becomes extremely strong in the second year of life, when major pathways of the limbic system become encased in myelin. According to Konner (2004), the aforementioned phenomenon improves the function of the subcortical circuits that process emotions and social behavior.

Therefore, the quality of the mother–child attachment exerts a lasting influence on the development of the brain and prosocial behavior as well.

Because the capacity for empathy is deeply rooted in the early attachment relationship with a primary caregiver, a number of empirical studies have addressed the link between empathy and relationships with one's parents. The outcomes of these studies generally confirm a significant relationship between scores on empathy and the nature and quality of the early relationship with the primary caregiver and the rearing environment.

Kestenbaum et al. (1989) reported that children aged 12–18 months with a secure attachment to their mothers grew up to be more empathic to others and exhibited more prosocial behavior. Zahn-Waxler, Radke-Yarrow, and King (1979) reported that empathic caregiving (determined by whether mothers responded promptly to their child's call for help, anticipated dangers, and provided nurturing caregiving) was significantly associated with greater prosocial and altruistic behavior in the children. The aforementioned theoretical perspectives and empirical findings suggest that the seeds of empathy are sowed by the same hand that rocks the cradle. Because of the importance of the mother–child relationship in the development of children's capacity for empathy, Goldstein and Michaels (1985) proposed a series of training programs to enhance empathic communication between mothers and their children.

There are resemblances between the mother–child attachment and the clinician–patient relationship. The child needs the mother's help and protection to survive, and the attachment behavior (e.g., proximity seeking) intensifies when the child is in distress or pain. Similarly, patients have a natural tendency to bond with a caring figure (the clinician) to maintain their health during a time of pain and suffering. Therefore, clinician–patient bonding is associated, though unconsciously, with the early attachment relationship. One can speculate that people with a history of a secure attachment are more likely to form stronger empathic relationships quickly than are those with a history of ambivalent or avoidant attachment. This behavioral tendency also should be true for both clinician and patient.

Other Paths to the Development of Empathy in Childhood

The following factors feed the development of empathy and social behavior in children.

Facial Imitation and Motor Mimicry

Nature has bestowed human infants with the gift of an imitative brain, which allows them not only to understand others' affective state of mind but to learn from the emotions of others as well. As was mentioned in Chap. 3, Meltzoff and Moore

(1977, 1983) found that infants only 12–21 days old could imitate human facial gestures, such as protruding their tongue or lips and opening their mouth—an ability conceptualized as a type of primitive empathy (Bavelas et al., 1986; Bavelas, Black, Lemery, & Mullett, 1986). Early in life, the infant pays attention to expressions of emotion on the human face. The infant's attention to facial expressions and its apparent responses are described as "telepathic" exchanges that lay the foundation for empathic communications (Burlingham, 1967). Understanding one's own emotions and those of others emerges from these exchanges (Ickes, 1997). According to Decety and Jackson (2004), one adaptive advantage of mimicry is that it connects people together and fosters empathy.

Motor mimicry (e.g., wincing when a person or an animal is injured, mimicking a facial expression similar to the expression of another person who is in pain) is indeed a nonverbal mode of communication based on observing another person's affect. This phenomenon, which has been observed in children and adults alike, supports the notion that individuals are intricately and visibly connected in their interpersonal interactions (Bavelas et al., 1986). According to Decety and Jackson (2006), people can "catch" the emotional states of others as a result of motor mimicry. Bush, Barr, McHugo, and Lanzetta (1989) suggested that an observer's mimetic facial responses may play an important role in the development of empathic responses.

The Theory of Mind

The capacity to represent the mental states of others is described in the theory of mind (Fonagy & Target, 1996; Wellman, 1991) as part of the human being's cognitive-emotional development. Empathy is linked to the theory of mind, because both are involved with the capacity to stand in another person's *mental shoes* (Gallese, 2001). Perspective taking ability, a major feature of empathy, according to Eslinger (1998), is also a feature of the theory of mind. In contrast to Jean Piaget's proposition (1967) that children between the ages of 2 and 7 years are primarily egocentric and unable to stand in another person's shoes, subsequent research demonstrated that young children are aware of other people's emotions and therefore are capable of responding empathically to other people's feelings (Borke, 1971). Research in the theory of mind found that children often in the fourth year of life develop the ability to understand the other's mental states (Lieberman, 2007). The mechanisms involved in the human neonate's ability to understand and imitate facial gestures provide the foundation for understanding other people which is precursor to the theory of mind, a key ingredient in the conceptualization of empathy (see Chap. 1).

The theory describes meta-cognitive abilities that make a distinction between thoughts, desires, and intentions of self and others which are among the ingredients of interpersonal relationships. Mentalization is a feature of the theory of mind which refers to the process of making inferences of other's mental states. It has been demonstrated that in the mentalization process, brain activities in the medial prefrontal cortex are involved (Lieberman, 2007). The same brain area is also implicated in empathic responses (see Chap. 13).

The "Still-Face" Experiments

Additional evidence supporting the infant's capacity to understand other people's emotions is provided by the "still-face" procedure developed by Tronick, Als, Adamson, Wise, and Brazelton (1978). In this procedure, the mother is instructed to distort her affective feedback to her infant by assuming an expressionless face (a still face) after a period of normal playful exchanges with her child. The child first becomes unpleasantly surprised to observe the mother's emotionless expression; the child then attempts to get her attention in an effort to restore affect to her emotionally blank face. When these efforts fail, the child becomes overtly uncomfortable, distressed, and anxious. Finally, when the mother's face does not change, the child becomes indifferent, detached, and apathetic. Most infants react physiologically to the mother's still face with an increased heart rate, which Weinberg and Tronik (1996) attributed to disruption of the infant's goal of relating to others. The still-face experiments with infants indicate that although the infant has not developed language to facilitate verbal communication, the face-to-face interactions between a mother and her child is a goal-directed, reciprocal system of communication that serves as a regulator of emotions in social relationships and a primary step toward the development of empathic capacity.

The "Visual Cliff" Experiments

Young children's understanding of others' emotions was also demonstrated in experiments involving the "visual cliff" apparatus (Gibson & Walk, 1960). This apparatus consisted of a sheet of heavy glass supported approximately one foot off the floor by a table-like frame. Patterned material in the open space under the glass looked to the infant like a bottomless crevasse. The baby was placed on one side of the frame and the mother stood on the other side and encouraged the child to come to her by crawling over the glass. Human infants can recognize depth as soon as they are old enough to crawl; the infants refused to crawl over the glass.

Sorce, Emde, Campos, and Klinnert (1985) demonstrated that by 12 months of age, children were more likely to feel confident enough to cross over the visual abyss when their mothers looked joyful or assumed a positive facial expression. However, when the mother adopted a negative facial expression, such as fear or anger, the children hesitated to cross over the glass. These findings suggest that young children not only can recognize the mother's emotional expressions but also can be encouraged by her positive look to risk crossing the cliff. The relevance of these findings to empathy was described by Campos and Sternberg (1981), who suggested that one developmental root of empathic understanding is a form of emotional communication known as "social referencing," through which children attempt to infer emotional information from interactions with others to adjust their own behavior accordingly.

Infants' ability to imitate facial expressions and mimic motor activities and to understand emotions indicates that infants possess a remarkable innate ability to establish social connections in the early days of life. Nurturing this ability lays the foundation for the development of a capacity to understand other people's positive and negative emotional states (Stern, 1985). Such understanding is the royal road to empathy.

Regulation of Emotions

According to Marx, Heidt, and Gold (2005), regulation of emotions is defined as the process that enables individuals to control the quality, frequency, intensity, or duration of their emotional responses. It is reported that regulation of emotion is positively linked to an important aspect of empathy: namely, being concerned for others (Decety & Jackson, 2004). One mechanism for linking caregivers' behavior to the development of empathy in children can be explained by the process of regulation of emotions, which plays an important role in organizing, motivating, and sustaining social behavior and attributing meaning to experiences (Nathanson, 1996). Human infants are well-equipped for socialization because they are endowed with a system of affect that can be regulated and therefore lays the foundation for a key ingredient in the development of interpersonal relationships.

Some developmental scholars have proposed that regulation of emotions begins extremely early—from the face-to-face interactions with the primary caregiver (as attested to by infants' reactions in the "still-face" and "visual cliff" experiments) and from the quality of the mother–child attachment (as attested to by the experiments regarding secure and insecure attachment).

Regulation of emotions develops as a result of emotional attunement between mother and child (Black, 2004) and involves a process in which people recognize and express their emotions (Archer, 2004). Regulation of emotions is a necessary condition for demonstrating prosocial behavior, and it functions as a mechanism to achieve an internal state that is optimal for social relationships. Regulation of emotion plays an important role in maintaining a boundary between the self and others (Decety & Jackson, 2006) which is an important aspect of empathic engagement in patient care.

Although emotions play an important role in social behavior, their regulation also is believed to play an essential role in empathic relationships (Demos, 1988). The infant's emotional response depends on his or her regulatory capacities and the regulatory scaffolding provided by the mother (Weinberg, Tronick, & Cohn, 1999). Thus, the mother is the most important first regulator of emotions because she provides a supplementary context for the development of her infant's social behavior (Lott, 1998). The self-regulated behavior is a function of the quality of interactions with a primary caregiver during the formative period of brain development (Nathanson, 1996). Together, the mother and infant are a regulatory unit, and the mother's role in the regulatory exchanges is influenced by her own early attachment relationships (Mays, Carter, Eggar, & Pajer, 1991).

The nature and quality of the neonate, infant, or young child's interaction with the mother sets the stage for the development of a psychological script (Nathanson, 1996; Tomkins, 1962, 1963), an internal working model (Ainsworth, 1985a, 1985b; Bretherton, 1987), and an emotional regulatory system (Lott, 1998; Weinberg et al., 1999) that will serve as a guiding force for empathic behavior during the rest of one's life. The implicit memories of the early warm relationship with the primary caregiver lead to the development of an enduring neural structure that influences self-regulatory behavior reflected in interpersonal relationships (Amini et al., 1996). The emotional arousal generated by feelings of other people's pain and suffering needs regulation and control for empathic understanding (Decety & Jackson, 2004). According to Watson (2002), a propensity to regulate emotions in clinical encounters can enhance empathic engagement and improve patient outcomes.

Recapitulation

Evidence suggests that infants are endowed with a capacity to understand and respond to emotions. Empathy is nurtured in a facilitative family environment where opportunities are provided for forming secure attachment relationships with a primary caregiver (usually the mother). The motivation for prosocial behavior and the capacity for empathic relationships are the outcomes of early social–emotional exchanges that lead to the development of an internal working model, a mental script, and an emotional regulatory system that guide interpersonal responses from the cradle to the grave.

Chapter 5
Measurement of Empathy in the General Population

If you cannot measure it, you cannot improve it.

(Lord William Thompson Kelvin, 1824–1907)

Abstract

- Some of the instruments that have been developed to measure empathy in children and adults, and used by researchers other than their own authors, are briefly described.
- The three that have been used most often in medical education and health care research are Hogan's Empathy Scale, Mehrabian and Epstein's Emotional Empathy Scale, and Davis's Interpersonal Reactivity Index. These instruments were developed for administration to the general population; therefore their relevance to the context of health professions education and patient care is limited for two reasons. First, as the content of the items in the three instruments implies, none is framed in the context of physician-patient (clinician-client) relationships. Thus, the validity of their use in that context is questionable. Second, the three instruments were not developed specifically to address the cognitively defined concept of empathy, a conceptualization that is more relevant and desirable in the context of patient care.
- The biotechnological advancements in functional brain imaging and the recent discovery of the mirror neuron system have opened up a new window for assessing empathy that is extremely promising.
- Given the findings that empathy tends to erode during medical and other health professions education, and in an era of changes in the health care system that hamper the clinician-patient relationship, a psychometrically sound instrument for measuring empathy in the context of health professions education and patient care is in high demand.

Introduction

In Chap. 1, I indicated that one reason for the dearth of empirical research on empathy in the health professions was the lack of a psychometrically sound instrument that can be used to measure the concept in health professions education and patient care. This chapter briefly describes some of the instruments that have been used most often to measure empathy in the general population and presents sample items enabling us to judge their *face validity* in the context of patient care. Although a detailed analysis of the psychometric properties of these scales can be informative, such a technical discussion is beyond the scope of this book. However, in Chap. 7, I will describe in detail the step-by-step development and psychometric properties of the Jefferson Scale of Empathy, which was specifically designed to measure empathy in medical and other health professions students, practicing physicians, and other health professionals.

In general, an instrument serves not only as a device for measurement but also as the basis of a common language that researchers use to communicate their empirical findings. Therefore, familiarity with the instruments and the scores they generate is necessary to comprehend and compare the results of research. For that purpose, I have selected a few research instruments designed to measure empathy in child and adult populations that are described in the following sections.

Measurement of Empathy in Children and Adolescents

Reflexive or Reactive Crying

Simner (1971) systematically investigated newborn infants' reactive crying and reported that newborns who heard another newborn crying cried significantly more often in response (reflexive crying) than they did to any other nonstartling noise. These findings were later replicated in other studies (Martin & Clark, 1982; Sagi & Hoffman, 1976). It is interesting to note that the newborns did not respond to their own cries (Martin & Clark, 1982) suggesting that infants are capable of distinguishing between self and others early in life (Decety & Jackson, 2004). The reaction of one infant to another infant's crying has been used as an indicator of empathy in infants based on the assumption that an infant crying in response to another infant's distress is a reflection of an empathic response (Eisenberg & Lennon, 1983). Eisenberg (1989) suggested that the capacity to respond to cues of another person's distress in childhood is a primitive precursor of more mature empathic sensibilities that develop later. However, the assumption that reflexive crying in infants is an indicator of empathy needs to be verified empirically in longitudinal studies.

According to Eisenberg and Lennon (1983), no convincing evidence is available to confirm that reflexive crying necessarily implies an empathic response. Martin and Clark (1982) reported that children of both sexes cried more in response to a male newborn's crying than to a female newborn's crying. These reports raise questions about the validity of reflexive crying as an indicator of empathic capacity.

The Picture or Story Methods

One popular method of measuring empathy in young children, developed by Eisenberg and Lennon (1983), has been to expose children to another person's distress by showing them pictures or telling them stories depicting hypothetical situations. The children are subsequently asked to describe their own feelings about the story's protagonist either verbally or by choosing an image from a set of pictures representing a variety of faces exhibiting various expressions, such as a happy or sad face. A match between the child's feelings and the protagonist's feelings is considered to be an indication of empathic understanding. The difficulty of differentiating empathy from sympathy when using picture or story methods of assessment raised concern about the validity of this method. Also, the predictive validity of this method awaits empirical verification.

The Feshbach Affective Situations Test of Empathy

The Feshbach Affective Situations Test of Empathy (FASTE), published by Feshbach and Roe (1968), is a widely used variation of the picture or story method of measuring empathy in children. Children (usually aged 6 or 7 years) are shown cartoons on a series of slides accompanied by hypothetical stories depicting children in different affectively charged conditions (happiness, sadness, fear, and anger). The children are then asked to describe their own feelings and emotions about the picture or story either verbally or by choosing a response from a set of facial expressions depicting different emotions. For example, a theme for happiness is a picture of a birthday party, a theme for sadness is a lost dog, a theme for fear is a frightening dog, and a theme for anger is a false accusation. The child's capacity for empathy is determined by a match between the child's expressed feeling and the theme depicted in the picture or story. The FASTE has been modified to accommodate studies by different researchers (Zhou, Valiente, & Eisenberg, 2003).

Some have criticized the FASTE because of its weak psychometric support, its suggestive test instructions (e.g., instructions designed in a way that elicits the desired behavior), and a lack of clarity in scoring (Eisenberg-Berg & Lennon, 1980; Eisenberg & Lennon, 1983; Hoffman, 1982; Zhou et al., 2003). Concern also has been raised about the confounding effect of the "demand characteristic" in children's responses (Goldstein & Michaels, 1985). This phenomenon makes the respondents modify their responses to what they believe the testing situation demands. The demand characteristic (e.g., a tendency to respond in a certain way that can undermine the validity of the results) is inherent in children's self-reports when an adult constantly asks them about their feelings. Another concern is the confounding effect of the experimenter's gender on the results of the FASTE because research indicated that when the experimenter was a woman, girls scored higher than boys did (Levine & Hoffman, 1975; Roe, 1977).

The Index of Empathy

The self-report Index of Empathy, developed by Bryant (1982), consists of 22 items designed to measure empathy in children and adolescents. The measure is comparable to Mehrabian and Epstein's Emotional Empathy Scale, which was developed to measure empathy in the adult population (this scale will be described later in this chapter). The author of the Index of Empathy indicated that these comparable instruments can be useful for exploring changes in empathy at different ages. A sample item is "I really like to watch people open presents, even when I don't get a present myself." The internal consistency reliability coefficients of this measure were reported to be 0.54 for first graders, 0.68 for fourth graders, and 0.79 for seventh graders (Bryant, 1982; Zhou et al., 2003).

Although the abovementioned methods of measuring empathy in children and adolescents seem to be useful for measuring reactions to affective situations, no convincing evidence is available in support of the instrument's predictive validity as indicators of the capacity for empathy.

Measurement of Empathy in Adults

The Most Frequently Used Instruments

The first three self-report measures of empathy discussed in this section—Hogan's Empathy Scale, Mehrabian and Epstein's Emotional Empathy Scale, and Davis's Interpersonal Reactivity Index—have been the most frequently used instruments in empathy research. Although they were developed for use in the general population, rather than with health professions students and practitioners, they have been used frequently in health care research. These measures are briefly described in the order in which they were originally published. Although other instruments have been designed to measure empathy, they have not received widespread attention. Some of them will be briefly described later in this chapter.

The Empathy Scale

Published by Robert Hogan (1969) and based on his doctoral dissertation at the University of California at Berkeley, the Empathy Scale includes 64 true–false items adopted from the California Psychological Inventory (CPI), the Minnesota Multiphasic Personality Inventory (MMPI), and other tests used at the Institute of Personality Assessment and Research. The scale was developed within the framework of the theory of moral development. A typical item is "I have seen some things so sad that I almost felt like crying."

Evidence in support of the scale's validity was provided by showing that high scorers were more likely than low scorers to be socially acute and sensitive to nuances in interpersonal relationships, and low scorers were more likely to be hostile, cold, and insensitive to the feelings of others (Hogan, 1969). Also, in a group of medical students, Hogan found a significant and positive correlation between scores on this scale and a criterion measure of sociability on the CPI ($r = 0.58$) and a significant negative correlation with social introversion on the MMPI ($r = -0.65$) (Hogan, 1969). Factor analysis of the Empathy Scale across different studies resulted in an inconsistent factor structure. For example, Greif and Hogan (1973) reported the following factors: "even-tempered disposition," "social ascendancy," and "humanistic sociopolitical attitudes," and Johnson, Cheek, and Smither (1983) reported "social self-confidence," "even temperedness," "sensitivity," and "nonconformity." These inconsistent findings raised questions about the scale's construct validity. Based on the factor analytic findings, it is suggested that the entire scale may not capture the essence of empathy (Baron-Cohen & Wheelwright, 2004). The scale's reliability has also been questioned (Cross & Sharpley, 1982).

The Emotional Empathy Scale

This instrument was developed by Albert Mehrabian and Norman Epstein (1972) and includes 33 items intended to measure emotional empathy. "It makes me sad to see a lonely stranger in a group" is a typical item. The title of the measure and the contents of the items pertain to susceptibility to emotional contagion (Zhou et al., 2003), indicating that the authors used an affective conceptualization of empathy when developing the scale (Davis, 1994). This conceptualization conflicts with the definition of empathy as a primarily cognitive concept in the context of patient care that was adopted in this book (see Chap. 6).

Items are answered on a 9-point Likert-type scale (Very Strongly Agree = +4, Very Strongly Disagree = −4). The split-half reliability of this scale was reported to be 0.84, and the internal consistency reliability was 0.79 (Zhou et al., 2003). The validity of this scale was determined by using an experimental paradigm similar to Milgram's experiments (1963; 1968) in which high scorers on this scale were less likely than low scores to administer electric shocks to the experimental subjects (Mehrabian & Epstein, 1972) (see Chap. 8 for a description of Milgram's experimental paradigm). On the basis of their subjective view, Mehrabian and Epstein reported that the scale included the following components and identified the items that measured each of these components: extreme emotional responsiveness, appreciation of the feelings of unfamiliar and distant others, tendency to be moved by others' emotional experiences, and tendency to be sympathetic. A study by Dillard and Hunter (1989) failed to support the aforementioned multidimensional components.

Later, Mehrabian, Young, and Sato (1988) changed the scale's name to the Emotional Empathic Tendency Scale. More recently, Mehrabian introduced a new instrument, the Balanced Emotional Empathy Scale (BEES), to measure vicarious empathy (Mehrabian, 1996) which is similar in content to the Emotional Empathy Scale. It contains 30 items, each answered on a 9-point Likert scale (4 = Very Strongly Agree, −4 = Very Strongly Disagree). A sample item is "Unhappy movie endings haunt me for hours afterward." Information about the scale is posted on Mehrabian's personal website, and to my knowledge no empirical study has been published to specifically address psychometrics of the BEES. In a study of empathy and aggression, a Cronbach's alpha coefficient of 0.87 was reported for this scale (Mehrabian, 1997).

The Interpersonal Reactivity Index

As part of his doctoral dissertation at the University of Texas at Austin, Mark Davis developed the Interpersonal Reactivity Index (IRI) (Davis, 1983) to measure individual differences in empathy. The instrument includes 28 items tapping four components of empathy in the cognitive and emotional domains. These four components are reflected in four subscales (Perspective Taking, Empathic Concern, Fantasy, and Personal Distress), each of which includes seven items answered on a 5-point scale ranging from 0 (Does not describe me well) to 4 (Describes me very well). These components were originally determined by subjective judgment without statistical support. However, confirmatory factor analysis provided mixed results concerning the existence of the four subscales (Cliffordson, 2002; Litvack-Miller, McDougall, & Romney, 1997).

The Perspective Taking subscale measures the tendency to adopt the views of others spontaneously. "I sometimes try to understand my friends better by imagining how things look from their perspective" is a typical item. The Empathic Concern subscale measures a tendency to experience the feelings of others and to feel sympathy and compassion for unfortunate people. A typical item is "I often have tender, concerned feelings for people less fortunate than me." The Fantasy subscale measures a tendency to imagine oneself in a fictional situation. A typical item is "After seeing a play or movie, I have felt as though I were one of the characters." The Personal Distress subscale taps a tendency to experience distress in others. "When I see someone who badly needs help in an emergency, I go to pieces" is a representative item. According to Davis, the Perspective Taking subscale is more likely to measure cognitive empathy, whereas the other three subscales are more likely to measure emotional empathy.

The internal consistency reliability coefficients ranged from 0.71 to 0.77 for the four subscales, and their test–retest reliabilities ranged from 0.62 to 0.71 (Davis, 1983). The test–retest reliabilities in an adolescent sample over a 2-year period ranged from 0.50 to 0.62 (Davis & Franzoi, 1991; Zhou et al., 2003). In correlating the IRI subscale scores with scores on Hogan's Empathy Scale, the highest positive correlation was found for the Perspective Taking subscale ($r = 0.40$) and the highest negative correlation was found for the Personal Distress subscale ($r = -0.33$) (Davis, 1983). The Perspective Taking subscale of the IRI yielded the lowest correlation with the scores of Mehrabian and Epstein's Emotional Empathy Scale ($r = 0.24$), and the Fantasy and Empathic Concern subscales yielded the highest correlations (0.52 and 0.60, respectively) (Davis, 1983). This pattern of correlations confirms Davis's claim about the cognitive nature of the Perspective Taking subscale.

In 1994, Davis stated that convincing evidence existed in support of some psychometric aspects of the IRI, although no satisfactory statistical evidence has been presented to confirm the stability of the four components of the index. In a study with physicians and undergraduate psychology students, Yarnold, Bryant, Nightingale, and Martin (1996) discovered an additional component called "involvement" in their statistical analysis of the IRI. The findings that scores on the Personal Distress subscale of the IRI were negatively correlated with scores on the Perspective Taking subscale raise a serious question about the validity of scoring the IRI by summing up the scores of all its subscales, including the Personal Distress subscale. According to D'Orazio (2004), because of the negative correlation between the Personal Distress and Perspective Taking subscales and because high scores on Personal Distress are associated with dysfunctional interpersonal relationships, summing up the scores of all four subscales of the IRI would not be meaningful.

Other Instruments

Several other instruments for measuring empathy in the adult population are described here in chronological order. Kerr developed a test of empathy with the intention of measuring respondents' ability to "anticipate" certain typical reactions, feelings, and behavior of other people (Kerr, 1947). The test consists of three sections which require respondents to rank the popularity of 15 types of music, the national circulation of 15 magazines, and the prevalence of 10 types of annoyances for a particular group of people (Chlopan, McCain, Carbonell, & Hagen, 1985). The respondent's rankings are compared to the empirical data to assess the accuracy of the respondent's rankings. This test seems to be a measure of general information, rather than a measure of empathy. Nevertheless, Kerr and Speroff (1954) claimed that the test was an indicator of empathic understanding and that it could predict a person's popularity, feelings for others, leadership, and sales records.

A measure of insight and empathy was introduced by Dymond (1949, 1950). This measure was based on the conceptualization of empathy as the imaginative transposing of oneself into another person's thinking, feeling, and acting. In Dymond's Rating Test (of empathic ability), respondents rate themselves and one another on a 5-point scale on six attributes such as "superior–inferior," "friendly–unfriendly," "leader–follower," "self-confidence," "selfish–unselfish," and "sense of humor." The concordance between individual's ratings of himself or herself and the individual's predictions of how others would rate him or her was considered as a measure of empathic ability. High scorers on the Dymond's Rating Test were classified as empathizers by analyses of their responses to the Thematic Apperception Test (TAT) (Dymond, 1949). Although no satisfactory evidence is available to confirm the instrument's validity as a measure of empathy, some preliminary data on its psychometric characteristics were presented by Chlopan et al. (1985). However, those investigators raised concerns about the measure's lack of easy administration and scoring procedures.

Barrett-Lennard (1962) developed an instrument called the Relationship Inventory, which was designed to investigate changes in the clinician–client relationship in the psychotherapeutic context. The instrument can be completed by either the clinician or the client. The original inventory included 92 items. However, one revised version consists of 64 items divided into four subjectively determined subtests of interpersonal relationships: (1) Empathic Understanding, described as the extent to which one person is conscious of the awareness of another person; (2) Level of Regard, the affective aspect of one person's response to another; (3) Unconditionality of Regard, the degree of constancy of regard one person feels for another person; and (4) Congruence, the degree to which one person is functionally integrated in the context of his or her relationship with another person (Barrett-Lennard, 1986). The "Willingness To Be Known" subtest included in the original version of the Relationship Inventory was defined as the degree to which a person wants to be known as a person by another person. This subtest was dropped in the revised version because of its nonsignificant predictive validity concerning therapeutic outcomes (Barrett-Lennard, 1986). Subsequent versions of the Relationship Inventory have been developed for use in nonclinical situations involving family, friendship, coworker, and teacher–pupil relationships (Bennett, 1995).

A 16-item subtest of this instrument called Empathic Understanding contains such items as "He [clinician/client] understands me." Items are answered on a Likert-type scale ranging from −3 ("No," as strongly felt disagreement) to +3 ("Yes," as strongly felt agreement). A negligible clinician–client correlation of 0.09 was reported for the Empathic Understanding subtest (Barrett-Lennard, 1962).

Truax and Carkhuff (1967) developed the 141-item Relationship Questionnaire to measure clients' perceptions of psychologists or counselors in psychological counseling and psychotherapy. Forty-six of the 141 items of the Relationship Questionnaire form a subscale called the Accurate Empathy Scale, which consists of such items as "He sometimes completely understands me so that he knows what I am feeling even when I am hiding my feelings." A number of questions have been raised about the validity, reliability, and score stability of the Accurate Empathy Scale (Beutler, Johnson, Neville, & Workman, 1973; Blass & Hech, 1975; Chinsky & Rappaport, 1970).

Carkhuff (1969) developed the Empathic Understanding in Interpersonal Processes Scale. This single-item instrument gives clinicians an overall empathy score based on five levels of empathic behavior, as judged by observers. Clinicians who score at Level 1 are judged as unable to express any awareness of even the most obvious of a client's feelings, whereas those who score at Level 5 are judged to be fully aware of and able to respond accurately to all of the client's feelings. Because an observer rates clinicians' empathic global behavior on a single item, the validity of this instrument is questionable (LaMonica, 1981).

The Fantasy-Empathy (F-E) Scale developed by Stotland, Mathews, Sherman, Hansson, and Richardson (1978) measures the tendency to respond emotionally to situations. The scale contains three items answered on a 5-point scale: for example, "When I watch a good movie, I can very easily put myself in the place of a leading character." Some psychometric data on this brief scale have been reported (Stotland, 1978). For instance, a correlation of 0.44 was reported between scores of the F-E Scale and Mehrabian and Epstein's Emotional Empathy Scale (Williams, 1989).

Layton (1979) developed the Empathy Test, a two-part 48-item instrument, as part of a research project designed to teach empathy to nursing students. The purpose of this measure was to evaluate whether empathy can be learned by observing models of empathic behavior. Each part of the Empathy Test consists of 12 true–false items and 12 multiple-choice items. According to Layton's reports, the reliability coefficients for the measure are unacceptably low (in the 0.20s), and no significant correlations were found between this measure and the Empathic Understanding subtest of Barrett-Lennard's Relationship Inventory and Carkhuff's Empathic Understanding in Interpersonal Processes Scale (Carkhuff, 1969).

Another instrument for measuring empathy is the Empathy Construct Rating Scale developed by LaMonica (1981). The instrument consists of 84 items about the respondent's feelings or actions toward another person, answered on a 6-point Likert-type scale (−3, Extremely Unlike; +3, Extremely Like). A typical item is "Seems to understand another person's state of being." The bipolar grand factor of this scale includes the notion of "well-developed empathy" (e.g., "Shows consideration for a person's feelings and reactions") at one pole and "lack of empathy" (e.g., "Does not listen to what the other person is saying") at the opposite pole.

A 15-item unidimensional instrument (The Emotional Contagion Scale) was developed by Doherty (1997) to measure emotional empathy. Each item is answered on a 5-point Likert-type scale. A sample item is "I cry at sad movies." A Cronbach's alpha coefficient of 0.90 is reported for the scale. Higher correlation was found between scores of this scale and those of the Empathic Concern scale ($r = 0.37$) than scores of the Perspective Taking scale of the IRI ($r = 0.14$).

A measuring instrument—Empathy Quotient (EQ)—was developed in England by Baron-Cohen and Wheelwright (2004) that contains 40 empathy items plus 20 filler items to distract the participants from relentless focus on empathy (Lawrence, Shaw, Baker, Baron-Cohen, & David, 2004). Each item is answered on a 4-point Likert-type scale from Strongly Agree to Strongly Disagree. Although the authors claim that the EQ was explicitly designed to have clinical applications, the contents of most of the items do not support such an application. Sample items are "I really enjoy caring for other people" and "I tend to get emotionally involved with a friend's problems." A test–retest reliability of 0.83 is reported for the EQ. Three factors, Cognitive Empathy, Emotional Reactivity, and Social Skills, emerged from factor analyses of the EQ. With the exception of the Cognitive Empathy factor, which was not correlated with any subscales of the IRI, the EQ yielded moderate correlations with the Empathic Concern and Perspective Taking subscales of the IRI and a negligible negative correlation with the Personal Distress subscale (Lawrence et al., 2004).

Another empathy measuring instrument for the general population is the Toronto Empathy Questionnaire (TEQ) for measuring emotional empathy (Spreng, McKinnon, Mar & Levine et al, 2009). This instrument contains 16 questions. A sample item is "I become irritated when someone cries." Some psychometric data exist in support of the validity and reliability of the TEQ in a study by its authors (Spreng et al., 2009).

Mercer, Maxwell, Heaney, and Watt (2004) and Mercer, McConnachie, Maxwell, Heaney, and Watt (2005) developed the Consultation and Relational Empathy (CARE) instrument for administration to patients to assess their doctors' or health care providers' empathic engagement in clinical encounters. This instrument includes ten items; each is answered on a 5-point Likert scale (1 = Poor, 5 = Excellent). A sample item is "How was the doctor at being interested in you as a whole person." Data in support of validity of the instrument and a Cronbach's alpha coefficient of 0.92 have been reported by the test authors (Mercer, Maxwell, Heaney, and Watt (2004).

There are a few review articles about empathy measuring instruments. For example, Yu and Kirk (2009) identified 20 empathy measures used in nursing research, and concluded that none of the reviewed measures was psychometrically robust. Hemmerdinger, Stoddart, and Lilford (2007) reported that based on their systematic review of the literature, 36 empathy measuring instruments were identified, but only eight demonstrated evidence in support of their validity, internal consistency, and reliability. There are other instruments, claimed by their authors as measures of empathy; however, either no convincing evidence has been presented to support their psychometrics, or they have not been used by other researchers except their own authors.

Physiological and Neurological Indicators of Empathy

Some social psychologists have studied empathy by using physiological measures, such as heart rate, skin conductance, palmar sweating, and vasoconstriction, as indicators of understanding other people's distress (Goldstein & Michaels, 1985; Stotland et al., 1978). Although most of these physiological measures are likely to be free of a social desirability response bias, they seem to be indicative of a person's emotional reaction to another person's distress. Such physiological reactions are more likely to be akin to sympathy than to empathy. Correspondingly, they may not be appropriate for the measurement of cognitively defined empathy in patient care.

Recently, functional brain-imaging methods (e.g., fMRIs and PET scans) have been used as indicators of brain activity in individuals experiencing empathy (Carr, Iacoboni, Dubeau, Mazziotta, & Lenzi, 2003; Wicker et al., 2003). In addition to advancements in functional brain imaging, the discovery of the mirror neuron system activated by observing another person in pain or performing an act (see Chap. 13) is, I believe, the beginning of a promising approach to quantifying neurophysiological manifestations of empathy in future research (see Chap. 13 for more detailed discussion).

Relationships Among Measures of Empathy

The results of studies attempting to determine correlations among different measures of empathy have not been encouraging. For example, Jarski, Gjerde, Bratton, Brown, and Matthes (1985) tested a group of medical students and found no significant correlations among the Empathy Scale (Hogan, 1969), the Empathic Understanding subtest of the Relationship Inventory (Barrett-Lennard, 1962), or the Empathic Understanding in Interpersonal Processes Scale (Carkhuff, 1969).

Another study with registered nurses examined correlations among four measures of empathy (Layton & Wykle, 1990). The results showed that Carkhuff's Empathic Understanding in Interpersonal Processes Scale was moderately correlated ($r = 0.25$) with Layton's Empathy Test but was not correlated with the Empathic Understanding subtest of Barrett-Lennard's Relationship Inventory. In addition, LaMonica's Empathy Construct Rating Scale was not correlated with Layton's Empathy Test but was moderately correlated ($r = 0.37$) with Carkhuff's Empathic Understanding in Interpersonal Processes Scale and highly correlated ($r = 0.78$) with the Barrett-Lennard's Empathic Understanding subtest of the Relationship Inventory.

In a review article, Chlopan et al. (1985) reported the findings of studies on the validity and reliability of several measures of empathy, including Mehrabian and Epstein's Emotional Empathy Scale and Hogan's Empathy Scale. They argued that both of these scales seem to measure two different aspects of empathy. As its name indicates, the Emotional Empathy Scale is more likely to measure the affective aspects of empathy, or general emotional arousability (Mehrabian et al., 1988), whereas the Empathy Scale is more likely to measure role-taking ability, a cognitive aspect of empathy. Chlopan and colleagues also reported that the subscales of the IRI seem to tap both the emotional (e.g., Personal Distress subscale) and the cognitive (Perspective Taking subscale) aspects of empathy.

The intercorrelations among these empathy measures are often weak and inconsistent and, in most cases, nonsignificant or negligible (Bohart, Elliot, Greenberg, & Watson, 2002; Gladstein & Associates, 1987). One reason for these inconsistent findings is that different instruments tap different aspects of empathy based on different definitions of the concept. Although these instruments can have potential value in particular situations, none can be recommended as the best for all patient-care situations (Bennett, 1995). With the exception of the Perspective Taking subscale of the IRI, the contents of the other instruments described in this chapter do not reflect the cognitive conceptualization of empathy adopted in this book (see Chap. 6). Thus, their face validity (and content validity) would be questionable when empathy is conceptualized as a predominantly cognitive attribute in the context of patient care advocated in this book.

A Need for an Instrument Specifically Designed to Measure Empathy in Patient Care

A measure that assesses empathy in patient care—particularly in medical and surgical treatment—needs to be more specific than the instruments I have discussed in this chapter so far. Because of the findings on the decline of empathy during health professions education (see Appendix A), and changes evolving in the market-driven

health care systems that hamper clinician-patient relationships, the empirical study
of empathy in health care education and practice is both important and timely.
Among prerequisites to empirical research on empathy in the health professions
education and the practice of patient care are (1) an operational definition of the
concept (see Chaps. 1 and 6), and (2) a psychometrically sound instrument for quantifying the concept in the context of health professions education and patient care.
In 2000, in response to a need for a psychometrically sound instrument to measure
empathy in the context of patient care, our research team in the Center for Research
in Medical Education and Health Care at Jefferson (currently Sidney Kimmel)
Medical College developed an instrument specifically designed to measure empathy
among students and practitioners in the health care professions. This scale will be
described in detail in Chap. 7.

Recapitulation

Several instruments exist that claim to measure empathy in children and adults. The
three frequently used instruments intended to measure empathy in adults—Hogan's
Empathy Scale, Mehrabian and Epstein's Emotional Empathy Scale, and Davis's
IRI—were developed for administration to the general population. The examination
of their contents suggests that they do not tap the essence of empathy in the context
of health professions education and patient care. In other words, their face and content validities in the context of health professions education and patient care are
questionable. Recently, functional brain imaging technology that has been used to
address brain activities in interpersonal relationships has emerged as a promising
path for measuring empathic engagement. I suspect that the findings of most of the
studies in which the instruments described in this chapter were used are questionable in addressing empathy issues in the context of patient care. The reason is that
the content of the bulk of the items in the self-reported instruments, described in this
chapter, taps on feeling the pain and suffering of others (described as emotional or
affective empathy, synonymous to sympathy and arousability) rather than empathic
understanding (e.g., cognitive empathy) which has a different consequence in
patient care (see Chaps. 1 and 6). Thus, there was a need for an instrument specifically developed to measure empathy in the context of patient care which will be
described in Chap. 7.

Part II
Empathy in Health Professions Education and Patient Care

Chapter 6
A Definition and Key Features of Empathy in Patient Care

*Clinical study amounts to the study of one person by another, and
dialogue and relationship are its indispensable tools.*

—(George L. Engel, 1990, p. 15)

Abstract

- Empathy in patient care is addressed in this chapter with regard to the World Health Organization's (WHO) definition of health, consistent with the notion of a biopsychosocial paradigm of illness.
- Empathy in the context of patient care is defined as a predominantly cognitive attribute that involves an understanding of the patient's experiences, concerns, and perspectives, combined with a capacity to communicate this understanding and an intention to help. The importance of the four key features (cognition, understanding, communication, and an intention to help) used in the definition of empathy is elaborated and suggestion is made to make a distinction between cognition and emotion, between understanding and feeling, and between empathy and sympathy because of their different consequences in patient outcomes.
- Because of its cognitive nature, an abundance of cognitively defined empathic engagement is always beneficial in the context of patient care, whereas excessive sympathetic involvement (akin to emotional empathy), because of its affective nature, can be detrimental to both the clinician and the patient, leading to exhaustion and burnout.
- In the context of patient care, empathy bonds the patient and the health care provider together, whereas sympathy blinds them to objectivity and reason. Thus, efforts should be made to maximize empathy and regulate sympathy for optimal patient outcomes.
- To achieve optimal patient outcomes, communication of understanding in empathic engagement between physician and patient must be reciprocal, confirming the patient's significant role in the outcome of patient care.

Introduction

We cannot scientifically study empathy in patient care unless an agreement exists concerning its definition and unless a psychometrically sound instrument is available to measure the defined concept. The descriptions of empathy presented in Chap. 1 provide a framework for the definition and conceptualization of empathy in the context of health professions education and patient care. I begin in this chapter by describing the definition of health proposed by the WHO and briefly describe the biopsychosocial paradigm of health and illness. Then I offer a definition of empathy in patient care and elaborate on the definition's key features and their implications for patient outcomes.

The World Health Organization's Definition of Health and a Biopsychosocial Paradigm

The constitution of the WHO (1948, p. 1) defines health as "a state of complete physical, mental, and social well-being, and not merely an absence of disease or infirmity." This definition is consistent with the biopsychosocial paradigm of illness in medicine (Engel, 1977, 1990; Hojat, Samuel, & Thompson, 1995). Generally, human infirmity can be viewed from two different perspectives: biomedical and biopsychosocial.

The *biomedical* paradigm of disease, postulated by the German physician Robert Koch and the French scholar Louis Pasteur, although still valid for some diseases, presents an incomplete picture of infirmity suffered by humankind. This "microbe hunting" model of disease (DeKruif, 1926) has a more limited scope than the triangular *biopsychosocial* paradigm of illness (Engel, 1977, 1990; Hojat et al., 1995; Ray, 2004). In the biopsychosocial paradigm, the targeted treatment of an affected organ is replaced by curing the whole patient, who is viewed as a system of being, always in relation to the biological, psychological, and social elements interacting closely with one another (see Chap. 14 for a discussion of the systems theory). Because of its limited scope, the biomedical model can neither describe the underlying interpersonal reasons for the victories in overcoming human illnesses (Frenk, 1998; McKinlay & McKinlay, 1981) nor explain the health-promoting effects of human connections, including empathic physician–patient engagement in health and illness.

In addition to the importance of pathophysiological determinants of infirmity, in the biopsychosocial paradigm of health and illness, psychological, social, and interpersonal factors are taken into consideration as well (Engel, 1977, 1990). This paradigm of health and illness attests that curing occurs when the science of medicine (the biomedical and pathophysiological aspects of disease) and the art of medicine (the psychological, social, and interpersonal aspects of illness) merge into one unified holistic approach to patient care. Empathy is a key element in the holistic care system.

The art of medicine, according to Blumgart (1964), consists of skillfully apply-ing the science of medicine in the context of human relationships to maintain health and ameliorate illness. The unit of observation in the art of medicine is the indi-vidual person in relation to social and cultural factors, whereas the unit of observa-tion in the science of medicine is the affected organ or the pathophysiology of disease. Empirical evidence is available to support the art and science of medicine dichotomy (Hojat, Paskin et al., 2007).

The science of medicine in the treatment of diseases and the art of medicine in the curing of illnesses are not independent entities; they supplement one another (Peabody, 1984). As Peabody (1984, p. 814) pointed out, "Treatment of disease may be entirely impersonal, but the care of the patient must be completely per-sonal." Considering that the physician–patient relationship is an indispensable tool in clinical situations to achieve better patient outcomes (Engel, 1990), health care professionals should pay attention not only to the biomedical aspects of disease but to the psychosocial factors of illness as well (Spiro, 1992). Treating a pathophysi-ological disease may not require as much empathy as is required in curing the patient's illness (Novack, 1987; Novack, Epstein, and Paulsen 1999).

Definition and Key Features of Empathy in Patient Care

Empathy in patient care has been characterized as arising "out of a natural desire to care about others" (Baron-Cohen, 2003, p. 2). Gianakos (1996, p. 135) referred to empathy in patient care as "the ability of physicians to imagine that they are the patient who has come to them for help." Greenson (1967, p. 367) described empa-thy in patient care as follows: "I have to let a part of me become the patient, and I have to go through her experience *as if* I were the patient." (Remember the "as if" condition in Rogers's definition of empathy described in Chap. 1.)

The notion of an empathic relationship with the patient was elegantly described in a statement attributed to Sir William Osler (1932): "It is as important to know what kind of man [sic] has the disease, as it is to know what kind of disease has the man." This quotation is often attributed to Osler, as cited in White, 1991, p. 74; it also is attributed to Hippocrates, as cited by Ray, 2004, p. 30.) In any case, this statement best describes the biopsychosocial paradigm in which science and the art of medicine are complementary. To Larson and Yao (2005, p. 1105) empathy is the royal road to treatment and "a symbol of the health care profession." Engaging in empathic relationships makes physicians more effective healers and makes their careers more satisfying. Freud (1958a) suggested that empathy is not only a factor in enhancing the clinician–patient relationship; it also provides a condition for cor-rect interpretation of the patient's problems. Therefore, empathy is valuable both in making accurate diagnoses and in achieving more desirable treatment outcomes. Both the patient and the physician benefit from empathic engagement. This topic will be discussed in more detail in Chap. 8.

Definitions of the key concepts in research serve as a common language to understand the nature of the concepts under study. Although not all experts may agree on all aspects of any definition, at least some agreement should exist on the key features of a definition; otherwise, research based on a vague concept obviously will prove to be fruitless. By considering the various descriptions and features of empathy that were described in Chap. 1 and by taking into account the specific nature of empathy in the context of patient care and its implications for positive patient outcomes, our research team proposed the following definition of empathy in the context of patient care (Hojat et al., 2001b, 2002b, 2009a, 2009b; Hojat, Erdmann, & Gonnella, 2014; Hojat, Spandorfer, Louis, & Gonnella, 2011):

> Empathy is a predominantly *cognitive* (rather than an affective or emotional) attribute that involves an *understanding* (rather than feeling) of experiences, concerns and perspectives of the patient, combined with a capacity to *communicate* this understanding, and an *intention to help*.

The four key terms in this definition are printed in italics to underscore their significance in the construct of empathy in the context of patient care. We developed this definition after a comprehensive review of the literature (Hojat et al., 2001b, 2002c) and a careful consideration of the factors that contribute to positive patient outcomes. Our original intention was to present a working definition that would clarify the key ingredients we believed were conceptually relevant to empathy in the health professions education and in patient care to provide a framework for quantifying the defined concept by developing an instrument with which to measure empathy in the context of the health professions education and patient care (the instrument will be described in detail in the next chapter). Also, in our definition we intended to make a distinction between empathy and sympathy in the context of patient care. Our deliberate choice of the four key ingredients in the definition of empathy—*cognition, understanding, communication,* and *intention to help*—needs some elaboration.

Cognition

Our research team viewed empathy as a predominantly cognitive (rather than an emotional) attribute based on a belief that in patient care situations, empathy emerges as a result of mental activities described in Chap. 1 as facets of cognitive information processing. Such facets include reasoning and appraisal, which are the basis of clinical judgment. Although cognitive mental processing (a key feature of empathy) can lead to positive patient outcomes, overwhelming emotion (a key feature of sympathy, see Chap. 1) can impede the optimal outcomes by obscuring objectivity in clinical judgments.

Cognition and emotion, although seemingly related, have different qualities independent of their joint appearance (Lazarus, 1982). Experienced therapists tend to respond to patients' distress with cognitive rather than emotional feedback. For example, an analysis of the interpersonal responses between Carl Rogers and his patients showed that approximately two-thirds of his responses were referred to as cognitive as opposed to emotional reactions (Tausch, 1988).

The distinction between cognition and emotion (and correspondingly, between empathy and sympathy) may not seem as important in situations where patient care is not a primary consideration. In the context of patient care, however, such a distinction must be made because of the different implications and consequences in patient outcomes. Physicians should feel their patients' feelings only to the extent necessary to improve their understanding of the patients without impeding their professional judgment (Starcevic & Piontek, 1997). It is not essential for physicians to experience their patients' feelings, pain, and suffering to an overwhelming degree. Emotional overinvolvement is a feature of sympathy, not empathy (Olinick, 1984). However, for the purpose of more accurate diagnoses, it is essential for physicians to understand, as much as possible, their patients' feelings and concerns.

The notions of "detached concern," "compassionate detachment," "affective distance," "exhaustion," and "professional burnout" have been mistakenly used to describe the limits of empathic engagement in clinician–patient relationships (Blumgart, 1964; Halpern, 2001; Jensen, 1994; Lief et al., 1963). However, I strongly believe that linking those notions to empathy is a grave mistake. They are indeed most relevant to sympathetic involvement (not empathic engagement) in patient care, based on the definitions of empathy and sympathy (see Chap. 1).

Ayra (1993) suggested that physicians' dissociation from patients' emotions can help them to retain their mental balance. Farber, Novack, and O'Brien (1997) reported that although medicine is a profession characterized by caring and empathy, it has also been characterized throughout history as aspiring to "objective detachment." This is possible when emotional involvement in clinician–patient encounters is restrained. However, *complete* emotional detachment has its own perils in the context of patient care (Friedman, 1990). As I described in Chap. 1, emotion is acceptable to some extent, and sometimes it is difficult to distinguish when emotion ends and cognition begins in the context of patient care. The controversy about "detached concern" in clinician–patient encounters arises from confusion about the nature and meaning of empathy and sympathy. Maintaining an affective distance to avoid emotional overinvolvement (a feature of sympathy) makes the physician's clinical judgment more objective, but cognitive overindulgence (a feature of empathy) can always lead to a more accurate judgment. Objectivity when making clinical decisions can be better achieved by avoiding emotional overinvolvement, which clouds medical judgment (Koenig, 2002).

It is difficult to be highly emotional and objective at the same time (Wispe, 1986) because excessive emotion in patient care can interfere with the principle of objectivity when making diagnostic decisions and choosing treatments (Blumgart, 1964; Gladstein, 1977; Spiro, 1992). Perhaps one reason why physicians are advised not to treat close family members who have serious health problems is the notion that excessively sympathetic feelings toward close family members can impede clinical objectivity (Aring, 1958). Indeed, the professional guidelines on the treatment of immediate family members in the American Medical Association's Code of Ethics (Section E-8.19) state that "Professional objectivity may be compromised when an immediate family member of the physician is the patient; the physician's personal feelings may unduly influence his or her professional medical judgment, thereby interfering with the care being delivered."

Borgenicht (1984) suggested that in performing certain procedures, physicians must maintain a certain degree of emotional distance from the patient because overwhelming emotional involvement may prevent them from making objective decisions at times of crisis. Too much affect impedes effective communication between physician and patient, whereas an abundance of understanding facilitates it. Brody (1997) suggested that the real danger to the physician's effectiveness lies in sympathetic overengagement with the patient. Issues such as dependency, exhaustion, burnout, compassion fatigue, and vicarious traumatization (Figley, 1995; Linley & Joseph, 2007) which are often mistakenly attributed to empathic engagement in patient care are indeed the results of sympathetic overengagement which is overwhelming to the health care providers and their patients. This speculation was confirmed in a large-scale study of board-certified practicing physicians in Argentina (Gleichgerrcht & Decety, 2013) in which it was found that compassion fatigue, burnout, and secondary traumatic job-related stress were closely associated with personal distress (which is a feature of emotional empathy which is analogous to sympathy).

Lief and Fox (1963) introduced the concept of "detached concern" in the medical education literature to prevent emotional overengagement (certainly different from empathic engagement) between physicians and patients. In contrast, no one has ever expressed concern about excess in understanding (or empathic understanding). An "affective distance" between physician and patient is desirable not only to avoid an intense emotional involvement, which can jeopardize the principle of clinical neutrality, but also to maintain the physician's personal durability (Jensen, 1994). Empirical evidence suggests that physicians who had difficulty to regulate their emotions were likely to experience more exhaustion and lower sense of accomplishments (Gleichgerrcht & Decety, 2013). Because excessive emotions (different from cognition and understanding) can obscure the physician's judgment concerning the patient's predicament, Freud (1958b) proposed that to achieve better therapeutic outcomes, clinicians must put aside all of their human sympathies! (not empathies).

For practical reasons, a distinction between cognition (a major ingredient of empathy) and emotion (a major ingredient of sympathy) is important because of its implications with regard to determining the contents of the items in instruments intended to measure empathy in the context of patient care (see Chap. 7), developing educational programs to regulate sympathy, maximize empathy, and assess their consequences in clinical outcomes. The amenability to change will vary for cognitive and emotional behaviors. Cognitive attributes (e.g., empathy) are more prone to change as a result of educational programs than are emotional responses (e.g., sympathy).

Understanding

Understanding others' feelings and behaviors is central to human survival (Keysers & Perrett, 2004). Understanding is also a key ingredient of empathic engagement in the clinician–patient relationship (Levinson, 1994). Patients' perception of being understood, according to Suchman, Markakis, Beckman, and Frankel (1997), is intrinsically therapeutic because it helps to restore a sense of connectedness and support. Empathy in patient care is built on the central notion of connection and understanding (Hudson, 1993; Sutherland, 1993). Because being understood is a basic human need, the physician's understanding of the patient's physical, mental, and social needs, in itself, can fulfill that need. Accordingly, we proposed elsewhere that "when an empathic relationship is established, a basic human need is fulfilled" (Hojat, Gonnella, Mangione, Nasca, & Magee, 2003, p. 27).

According to Schneiderman (2002, p. 627), "the better we understand them [the patients], the closer we come to discovering the true state of affairs, and the more likely we will be able to diagnose and treat correctly." Understanding of the patient's perspective was considered as an essential element of physician–patient communication by a group of medical education experts in the Kalamazoo, Michigan, conference held in 1999 (Makoul, 2001). A specific feature of understanding in the physician–patient relationship is the ability to stand in a patient's shoes (knowing that the shoes belong to someone else), and to view the world from the patient's perspective without losing sight of one's own personal role and professional responsibilities. With this background in mind, we decided to consider "understanding" (rather than "feeling") as a keyword in the definition of empathy in the context of patient care.

Accuracy of understanding is another topic of discussion in empathy research. As Rogers (1975, p. 4) advised clinicians, "perhaps if we wish to become a better therapist, we should let our clients tell us whether we are understanding them accurately." In general, the accuracy of understanding depends on the strength of the empathic relationship and the feedback mechanisms. Because the accuracy of understanding is an issue that may be a subject of debate, physicians should occasionally verify the degree to which their understanding is accurate by *communicating* with the patent—another essential ingredient of empathy in patient care that will be discussed in the following section.

Communication of Understanding

Communication of understanding is indeed a behavioral aspect of empathic engagement in patient care. According to Carkhuff (1969) and Chessick (1992), the central curative aspect of clinician–patient relationships rests not only on the clinician's ability to understand the patient but also on his or her ability to communicate this understanding back to the patient. Reynolds (2000), and Diseker and Michielutte (1981) included communication of understanding as a feature of empathy in clinician–patient relationships. Carkhuff (1969, p. 315) indicated that "[empathy is] the

ability to recognize, sense, and understand the feelings that another person has associated with his (her) behavioral and verbal expressions and to accurately communicate this understanding to him or her." Similarly, Reynolds (2000, p. 13) defined
empathy as "an accurate perception of the client's world and an ability to communicate this understanding to the client."

Communication of understanding also is a key feature in LaMonica's description
of empathy: "Empathy ... involves accurate perception of the client's world by the
helper, communicating this understanding to the client, and the client's perception
of the helper's understanding" (LaMonica, 1981, p. 398). Truax and Carkhuff
(1967, p. 40) described empathy as involving the ability to sense the client's "private world" and to communicate this understanding in "a language attuned to the
client's current feelings." A physician who has an empathic understanding of the
patient but does not communicate such an understanding would not be perceived as
an empathic physician (Bylund & Makoul, 2005). According to Branch and Malik
(1993), there are windows of opportunities in clinical encounters for expressing
mutual understanding when patients describe emotional, personal, and family concerns. Physicians must capture these moments of "potential empathic opportunities" (Suchman et al., 1997) to express their understanding of patients' concerns.

An important aspect of communication in patient care is the notion of "reciprocity"
or "mutuality" (Makoul, 1998; Miller, 2002; Raudonis, 1993). Although the idea that
empathy involves mutual understanding is not widely discussed in empathy research
(Bennett, 2001), it must be regarded as an essential ingredient of empathic engagement in patient care. Mutual understanding generates a dynamic feedback loop that is
helpful not only in strengthening empathic engagement but also in making a more
accurate diagnosis and thus providing better treatment. It is important to note that
mutual understanding and reciprocal feedback during verbal and nonverbal exchanges
indicate that both clinician and patient must play an active role to enhance empathic
engagement. Without such features, empathic engagement cannot fully develop.

Physicians should let their patients know that their health problems and their psychosocial concerns are fully understood. It is also desirable for a patient to confirm
the physician's understanding. By using a coding system (Empathic Communication
Coding System), Bylund and Makoul (2005) reported that most patients do provide
physicians with potential empathic opportunities. In their coding system, physicians'
reactions to these potential opportunities were recorded on a 7-point scale (0 = physician ignores the empathic opportunity, 6 = physician makes an explicit statement to
express understanding of the patient's concerns). They found that more than 80 % of
physicians could detect the opportunities and reacted either by confirmation,
acknowledgment, or pursuing or elaborating the issues of concern. The patient's
belief concerning the physician's understanding reinforces the empathic engagement
between the two. The following statements represent some simple approaches to the
communication of empathic understanding: "I understand your feelings. You have
gone through a lot of difficulties"; "I can see how being in a cast would make you
helpless" (the expression of empathic understanding approach); "I can understand
why this problem is so difficult for you" (the validation approach); "I understand your
problem very well because I went through a similar situation" (the self-disclosure

approach); "I want to make sure that I understand your concern. Let me rephrase it this way ..." (the rephrasing approach); "It is saddening to have that kind of feeling" (sympathy); or "This reminds me of the story of ..." (the metaphorical approach) (Matthews, Suchman & Branch, 1993; Mayerson, 1976).

Mutuality generates a belief in the patient that not only enhances the empathic relationship but also has a mysterious beneficial effect on clinical outcomes (Hudson, 1993). Although the mechanism of the positive effect of mutuality in understanding is not well understood, one could speculate that the beneficial outcomes are attributable to greater satisfaction with the health care provider, to better compliance with treatment, or to such psychological factors as reduced anxiety, enhanced optimism, and perceptions of social support, which are activated in mutually understood interpersonal relationships. The reciprocal communication can help to remove the constraints of physician–patient relationships because, as a golden rule in interpersonal relationships, when constraints diminish, people begin to reveal their secrets.

Intention to Help

Intention to help is another specific feature of empathic engagement in patient care. Decety and Jackson (2006) described empathy as the capacity to understand and respond to the needs of others. Understanding in itself does not necessarily imply that the individual is compelled to help. However, readiness to respond to another person's call for help is indeed synonymous to the intention to help. Such intention in patient care often derives from altruistic motivation, making it different from the empathy of, for example, a sales agent, whose understanding of potential consumers often rests on egoistic motivation for personal gain. This feature of empathic engagement in patient care is consistent with the golden ethical principle of medical practice that the best interest of the patient must be of primary consideration.

Empathy Versus Sympathy in Patient Care

A large number of empathy researchers have failed to make a distinction between empathy and sympathy, and used the terms interchangeably. A clear distinction between these two terms, as I indicated before, is utterly important in patient care. The conceptual confusion and interchangeable use of "empathy" and "sympathy" may not cause a serious problem in social psychology, but separating the two in the context of patient care is important. In social psychology, both empathy and sympathy can lead to a similar outcome (e.g., prosocial behavior), albeit for different behavioral motivations. A prosocial behavior induced by empathic understanding is more likely to be elicited by a sense of altruism (Hojat, Spandorfer et al., 2011). A prosocial behavior prompted by sympathetic feelings, however, is more likely to be triggered by a self-serving egoistic motivation to reduce the observer's personal distress. In patient care, the two constructs must be distinguished because, in that context, they lead to different outcomes. For example, Nightingale, Yarnold, and Greenberg (1991) have shown that in simulated conditions empathic physicians, compared with their sympathetic counterparts, used resources appropriately by ordering fewer laboratory tests, had less preference for unwarranted patient intubation, and did not perform cardiopulmonary resuscitation for an excessively long time. In an empirical study we showed that it is possible to differentiate empathic and sympathetic responses to patient care and test the validity of such responses (Hojat, Spandorfer et al., 2011).

Empathy Bonds, Sympathy Blinds

Our definition of empathy in the context of patient care as a predominantly *cognitive* attribute implies that it involves understanding another person's concerns. Sympathy as an *emotional* reaction implies that it involves feeling another person's pain and suffering. Some researchers have described two types of empathy: "cognitive empathy" and "emotional empathy" (e.g., Davis, 1983). Davis (1994) used cognitive empathy as "attempts to entertain the perspective of others" (p. 17) and "the capacity for role taking" (p. 29). However; he used emotional empathy (synonymous to sympathy) as "a tendency to react emotionally to the observed experiences of others" (Davis, 1994, p.55). Others have also described emotional empathy in terms of vicarious empathy (Mehrabian & Epstein, 1972).

To understand the operational definition of a concept, researchers must not only describe specific features of the concept but also take into consideration the clinical relevance of the features (Morse & Mitcham, 1997). Our definition of empathy in the context of patient care is close to Davis's description of cognitive empathy, whereas our conceptualization of sympathy is somewhat similar to Davis's description of emotional empathy, and analogous to Mehrabian and Epstein's (1972) vicarious empathy. The distinction between cognitively defined empathy and affectively defined empathy (or sympathy) has important implications for both health professions education and health care research. As I discussed before, it can be speculated that, in the context of patient care, cognitively defined empathy almost always leads to positive clinical outcomes, whereas sympathy in excess, due to its emotional nature, can be detrimental to objectivity in clinical decision making. In addition, empathy can lead to professional growth, career satisfaction, and optimal clinical outcomes, whereas sympathy can lead to unhealthy patient-physician dependency, career burnout, compassion fatigue (Figley, 1995), exhaustion, and vicarious traumatization (Linley & Joseph, 2007). These speculations await empirical verifications.

If my assumptions (see Chap. 1) that (1) the relationship between empathy and positive clinical outcomes is linear (that is, the outcomes progressively become better as a function of an increase in empathic engagement), and (2) the relationship between sympathy and clinical outcomes resembles an inverted U shape (similar to that between anxiety and performance) are confirmed, then the following outcomes would be expected. (1) Abundance of empathy is always beneficial in patient care; (2) sympathy — to a limited extent — is beneficial, but excessive sympathy is detrimental to patient outcomes. In other words, for more optimal patient outcomes, empathy must be maximized, but sympathy must be optimized or regulated for its best effect.

Soenens, Duriez, Vansteenkiste, and Goossens (2007) have confirmed that past studies generally ignored the distinction between empathy and sympathy. I agree, and take it as a justification for my repeated reminder of differences between empathy and sympathy throughout this book which may seem redundant. However, I have deliberately placed the emphasis on this distinction in several pertinent occasions, because I believe that such differentiation is extremely important in the context of patient care, but has been benignly neglected in that context. This failure is not certainly inconsequential in the empathy research outcomes in patient care (see Chaps. 1 and 3), and particularly on exploring the neurological underpinnings of empathy as a separate entity than sympathy (see Chap. 13).

In summary, the distinction made by Solomon (1976) between the wisdom of "understanding" against the treachery of "emotion" with regard to the differences between empathic and sympathetic engagements in clinician–patient relationships can be translated into the following statement that *"empathy bonds, sympathy blinds!"*

Recapitulation

The triangular biopsychosocial paradigm of health and illness, consistent with the definition of health in the WHO's constitution, suggests that empathic engagement in clinician–patient encounters should lead to improvement in physical, mental, and social well-being. The distinction between cognition and affect and their corresponding attributes of empathy and sympathy has important implications for the health professions education, effects on patient outcomes, and explorations of their neurological roots. Empathy, due to its cognitive nature, is always beneficial to patient outcomes; thus attempts must be made to maximize empathic engagement in patient care. However, sympathy in excess, because of its emotional nature, can be detrimental to the patient and health care provider; thus, it is desirable to regulate or optimize sympathy to prevent dependency, exhaustion, and career burnout.

Chapter 7
The Jefferson Scale of Empathy

If anything exists, it exists in some amount,
If it exists in some amount, it can be measured.

—(E. L. Thorndike, 1926, p. 38)

Abstract

- On the basis of the belief that empathy-measuring instruments which were developed for the general population did not embrace the essence of empathy in the context of health professions education and patient care, we developed a new instrument to specifically measure empathy in that context.

- This chapter describes the steps taken in the development and psychometric analyses of the *Jefferson Scale of Empathy* (*JSE*). The evidence is presented in support of the JSE's validity (face, content, construct, criterion-related, convergent, and discriminant validities) and reliability (Cronbach's alpha coefficient in support of internal consistency and test–retest reliability in support of score stability).

- The significant relationships observed between JSE scores, clinical competence, and patient outcomes can boost the confidence of researchers who are searching for a psychometrically sound instrument for measuring empathy in the context of health professions education and patient care.

- The general findings on the JSE's measurement properties in samples of students and practitioners in a variety of health professions disciplines and in different cultures suggest that the instrument can serve as a sound measure of empathy among medical students (S-Version), students in the other health professions (HPS-Version), and practitioners in the health professions including physicians (HP-Version).

- Further research is needed to investigate the relationship between scores on the JSE and outcomes such as accuracy of diagnosis, patient compliance, reduced risk of malpractice claims, and patient outcomes in different settings and cultures. Furthermore, large-scale research is needed with national samples to develop national norm tables and cutoff scores for the JSE to identify low and high scorers in different populations of health professions students and practitioners.

© Springer International Publishing Switzerland 2016

M. Hojat, *Empathy in Health Professions Education and Patient Care*,
DOI 10.1007/978-3-319-27625-0_7

Introduction

Empathy has been described in the literature as the most frequently mentioned attribute of the humanistic physician (Linn, DiMatteo, Cope, & Robbins, 1987); yet empirical research on the topic is insufficient because of the ambiguity of the term (see Chap. 1) and the lack of psychometrically sound instruments to measure empathy in the context of patient care. Some researchers believe that the instruments developed for the general population do not grasp the essence of the construct of empathy in the context of patient care and are not adequate for that purpose (Evans, Stanley, & Burrows, 1993).

To the best of my knowledge, prior to the development of the JSE, no psychometrically sound instrument was available to measure empathy among students and practitioners in health professions. None of the instruments described in Chap. 5 is specific enough to capture the essence of empathy in the context of patient care. In more technical terms, none of the instruments has "face" and "content" validity in the context of health professions education and patient care.

More than a decade ago our research team at Jefferson (currently Sidney Kimmel) Medical College recognized the need for an instrument that could enable researchers to conduct empirical investigations to assess empathy in professional development of students and practitioners, to investigate the changes in empathy among them, to study group differences, and to examine correlates, antecedents, development, and outcomes of empathy in different stages of training as well as in different types of health professions disciplines and practices. In response to this need, we developed our empathy-measuring instrument. Originally designed for medical students (Hojat, Mangione, Nasca et al., 2001) and entitled the Jefferson Scale of Physician Empathy (JSPE), it was subsequently modified to be applicable to not only medical students, but also to a broader populations of practicing physicians and other health professions students and practitioners (Hojat et al., 2002b). Thus, it was renamed as the Jefferson Scale of Empathy. A brief history of JSE's development and modifications is presented in the following sections.

Development of a Framework

Review of the Literature

To construct a test, one must embark on a journey to develop a framework for understanding the concept and its related elements that one intends to measure. The journey begins with a comprehensive review of the literature to explore conceptual frameworks, theoretical views, and empirical research on the topic and to identify behaviors that are relevant to the concept in question. Accordingly, in 1999, we began to search the Medline database for all studies published beginning in 1966 (the starting date in the Medline database) that would identify contexts and contents to guide us in drafting items for the preliminary version of the instrument. Using "empathy" as a keyword in our search, we found 3541 published sources in English. Cross-searching with the terms "empathy" and "physician/physicians" resulted in 107 published entries. A review of these and other relevant references, most of which were cited in the original 107 entries, provided us with some ideas about what the contents of items in the preliminary version of the instrument should be to measure empathy among health professions students and practitioners.

Drafting Preliminary Items and Examination of Face Validity

The second step, subsequent to the review of the literature, was to draft preliminary items and examine the face validity of the drafted items. Face validity involves subjective judgments, usually by nonexperts, about the relevance of the contents of the items to the concept being measured. We drafted 90 items for the preliminary version of the JSE that appeared to be relevant to empathy in patient care and, therefore, seemed to have face validity.

The items in the preliminary version covered broad areas, such as understanding subjective experiences of the patients and their families; interpersonal relationships with the patients; attention to verbal and nonverbal signals in physician–patient communications; humor; appreciation of art, poetry, and literature; narrative skills; absorption in stories, plays, and movies; cognitive and affective sensitivities; emotional closeness and affective distance between physician and patient; objectivity in clinical decision making; clinical neutrality; clinicians' emotional expression and regulation of emotions; sentiments; imagination; tactfulness; perspective taking; role playing; and cues in verbal and nonverbal communications.

It is important to notice that during the process of examining the face validity of the items, a particular item may seem, at first glance, to be irrelevant to the topic. Consequently, including such an item must be justified. A convincing argument should support the inclusion of every item, in case a question is raised concerning the item's relevance to empathy. We used the rational scale method of theory-based item selection (Reiter-Palmon & Connelly, 2000) for that purpose. For example, we included items related to an interest in literature and the arts based on the theoretical view that studying literature and the arts can improve a person's understanding of human pain and suffering (Herman, 2000; McLellan & Husdon Jones, 1996; Montgomery Hunter et al., 1995). Therefore, such an interest would be relevant to the capacity for empathy. Another example was inclusion of an item about humor based on the assumption that a clinician's sense of humor can reduce the stress perceived by the patient, thus contributing to an improved clinician–patient relationship (Yates, 2001). According to Martin (2007, p. xv) "humor is a ubiquitous human activity that occurs is all types of social interaction." Humor generally can reduce the harmful impact of stressful experiences (Martin & Lefcourt, 1983). Additional theoretical support for this proposition is based on observations that humor can reduce the restraints in clinician–patient relationships by relieving tension and reducing inhibitions (Lief & Fox, 1963). Also, a sense of humor has been listed as an element of professionalism in medicine (Duff, 2002). According to Golden (2002), humor is a "magical force" that detaches patients from their pain and suffering through the healing power of laughter. A popular movie based on the true story of the life of doctor Patch Adams beautifully depicted the role of humor in medical care. Thus, we included an item about sense of humor in the instrument.

In addition, we made every effort to incorporate components that were consistent with our conceptualization and definition of empathy (see Chaps. 1 and 6). For example, because "understanding" is a key component of our definition, the word appears in approximately one-third of the items (seven items) in the final scale.

Examination of Content Validity

In addition to face validity, examining the content validity of a new instrument is another important step in its development. Content validity involves the systematic examination of the instrument's contents, usually by experts, to confirm the relevance and representativeness of the items in covering the domains of behavior the test intends to measure (Anastasi, 1976). We probed the instrument's content validity to ensure that the instrument included a representative sample of the behaviors expected to fit within the concept of empathy, particularly in relation to patient care situations.

To examine the content validity of the preliminary version of the JSE, we used a version of the Delphi technique (Cyphert & Gant, 1970), which is usually used to obtain systematic and independent judgments from a group of experts. We mailed the preliminary version of the instrument to 100 clinician and academic physicians. A cover letter described the purpose of our study as the development of an instrument to measure empathy among health professionals, such as physicians. The letter briefly described empathy as an "understanding" of patients' experiences, emotions, pain, and feelings as opposed to sympathy, which was described as "feeling" of patients' pain, suffering, and emotions similar to the way patients experience them.

Respondents were asked to cross out any item they considered to be irrelevant to the measurement of empathy, as described in the aforementioned brief definition. They were also asked to edit the remaining items for simplicity and clarity and to add new items they regarded as important to include in an instrument intended to measure empathy in the context of patient care. The 55 physicians who responded offered suggestions, made editorial improvements, and provided additional comments. They also made recommendations about revisions, additions, and deletions.

During this stage of the study, we excluded all items from the preliminary version that five or more physicians had crossed out. We also incorporated appropriate editorial suggestions the respondents had made. After several iterations and revisions to assure that the items reflected distinct and relevant aspects of empathy in patient care situations, 45 of the original 90 items were retained (Hoja, Mangione, Nascat et al., 2001). It was this 45-item version of the instrument that was used in the preliminary psychometric analyses.

Preliminary Psychometric Analyses

For the purpose of a preliminary psychometric study, the 45-item instrument was administered to 223 third-year students at Jefferson Medical College (193 completed the instrument, an 86 % response rate). Also, a group of 41 residents in the internal medicine program at Thomas Jefferson University Hospital and its affiliated hospitals completed the instrument.

Likert-Type Scaling

A 7-point Likert-type scale (1 = Strongly disagree, 7 = Strongly agree) was used to respond to each item in the 45-item instrument. We chose a Likert-type scale rather than a simple, dichotomous (Agree/Disagree, Yes/No) response format because Likert-type scales (Likert, 1932) provide a wider range of item scores, which allows for more variation and thus more precise discriminatory power (Oppenheim, 1992). Furthermore, a Likert scale usually yields a distribution that resembles a normal distribution (Likert, 1932) and results in numeric scores that can be treated as an interval scale of measurement. The underlying assumptions for using more powerful parametric statistical techniques would not be violated by the presence of a distribution approaching a normal distribution and an interval scale of measurement. We also chose a 7-point Likert-type scale, rather than the more common 5-point scale, because the two additional points could reduce respondents' tendency to consistently use the extreme points of the scale (Polgar & Thomas, 1988; Reynolds, 2000).

Factor Analysis to Retain the Best Items

Exploratory factor analysis (EFA) is a statistical method used to explore the underlying constructs associated with a set of items. Items that are highly correlated with one another would emerge under one factor (or a hypothetical construct). In addition, factor analysis can be used to reduce the length of an instrument by proving information to retain the items that have relatively high factor loadings (e.g., greater than |0.30|) under the important and meaningful factors (Gorsuch, 1974). Another type of factor analysis is used to test if the empirical relationships among a set of items (or variables) can be efficiently summarized by a theoretical model (a confirmatory factor analysis (CFA)).

To screen for the best items to include in the next version and thus reduce the length of the preliminary instrument, we used EFA with the data collected from 193 medical students for the 45-item instrument. We used principal component factor extraction (the most frequently used factor extraction method), followed by orthogonal varimax rotation. This type of mathematical rotation is frequently used to obtain a simpler factor structure and to produce independent (uncorrelated) factors.

The "Generic Version" of the Scale

On the basis of the results of the EFA, we retained 20 of the 45 items in the generic or original version of the instrument, the JSPE, which was later renamed the Jefferson Scale of Empathy subsequent to making some slight modifications in the content for administration of the instrument to medical as well as other health professions students, and all practicing health professionals. Those 20 items had the highest factor structure coefficients (greater than 0.40) on the first extracted factor (grand factor). The eigenvalue (latent root) of this grand factor was 10.64, which was much higher than the eigenvalue for the next factor, 3.45. Eigenvalues indicate the importance of extracted factors in terms of the proportion of variance accounted for. A relatively large eigenvalue for the first factor is indicative of the factor's importance. A sudden drop in the magnitude of the eigenvalue and no significant decrease in the eigenvalues of subsequent factors are used to retain the substantial factors and disregard the trivial ones. This guideline is known as the "scree test" (Cattle, 1966). Because the sample size of 41 residents was insufficient (e.g., the ratio of the size of the sample of medical residents to the number of variables was less than 10; Baggaley, 1983), we did not perform a factor analysis for that sample. However, an examination of the patterns of inter-item correlations showed considerable similarities between medical students and residents (Hojat, Mangione, Nasca et al., 2001).

The item with the highest factor structure coefficient on the grand factor was "I believe that empathy is an important therapeutic factor in medical and surgical treatment." This item was regarded as an "anchor" with which to evaluate the other items by examining the magnitude and direction of correlations between the anchor item and the other items. In the generic version of the scale, 17 items with positive factor structure coefficients and positive and statistically significant correlations with the "anchor" item were directly scored on the 7-point Likert-type scale (e.g., 1 = Strongly disagree; 7 = Strongly agree). The other three items, which had negative factor structure coefficients on the grand factor and also yielded negative correlations with the "anchor" item, were reverse scored (1 = Strongly agree, 7 = Strongly disagree). The descriptive statistics for the generic version of the two preliminary study samples of medical students and residents are reported in Table 7.1.

Construct Validity of the Generic Version

Construct validity refers to the extent to which a test measures the theoretical constructs of the attribute that it purports to measure (Anastasi, 1976). Factor analysis helps to determine whether the scale's dimensions (underlying factors) are consistent with the theoretical constructs of the concept one intends to measure. Therefore, using factor analysis to examine construct validity can reveal the major dimensions that characterize the test scores (Anastasi, 1976).

Table 7.1 Descriptive statistics for the generic version of the JSE

Statistics	Residents ($n=41$)	Medical students ($n=193$)
Mean	118	118
Standard deviation	12	11
Median (50th percentile)	119	117
Mode	119	112
25th percentile	110	111
75th percentile	126	126
Possible range[a]	20–140	20–140
Actual range[b]	88–140	87–139
Alpha reliability estimate	0.87	0.89

©2001 *Educational and Psychological Measurement*. Reproduced with permission (Hojat, Mangione, Nasca, et al., 2001)
[a]The minimum and maximum possible scores
[b]The lowest and highest scores obtained by the samples

To investigate the underlying structure of the generic version, data collected from the medical students were subjected to principal component factoring with orthogonal varimax rotation. Four factors emerged, each with an eigenvalue greater than 1. An eigenvalue equal to or greater than 1 known as the Kaiser's criterion (Kaiser, 1960) is often used to retain the most important factors. The four extracted factors accounted for 56 % of the total variance. Ten items had factor coefficients greater than 0.40 on the first factor (eigenvalue=7.56, accounting for 38 % of the variance). We chose the magnitude of 0.40 as the minimum salient factor loading needed to assume a meaningful relationship between the item and the relevant factor (Gorsuch, 1974).

Assigning a title to a factor in factor analytic studies is a subjective judgment made according to the contents of the items with higher factor coefficients under the corresponding factor. Based on the contents of the ten items with the highest factor coefficients, the first factor was called a construct of "the physician's view of patient's perspective" (perspective taking). Five items had a factor coefficient greater than 0.40 on the second factor, which accounted for 7 % of the variance (eigenvalue=1.30). Based on the contents of items with high factor coefficients, this factor was entitled "understanding patient's experiences" (compassionate care). Two reverse-scored items had factor coefficients greater than 0.40 on the third factor (eigenvalue=1.14, accounting for 6 % of the variance), which was entitled "ignoring emotions in patient care." (This is the opposite pole of standing in a patient's shoes.) Finally, two items had factor coefficients greater than 0.40 on the fourth factor (eigenvalue=1.01, accounting for 5 % of the variance), which was entitled "thinking like the patient." According to Velicer and Fava (1998), a minimum number of three items per factor is required for a stable factor pattern. According to this criterion, the last two factors may not be as stable as the first two.

Also, a relatively considerable change in the magnitude of the pre-rotational eigenvalue after extracting the first factor suggests that the first factor is the most salient and reliable among all other extracted factors. The factor structure of the generic version of the JSE is consistent with the multifaceted concept of empathy reported in the literature (Spiro, McCrea Curnen, Peschel, & St. James, 1993). Details regarding the factor analysis of the generic version of the JSE and a table of factor structure coefficients are reported elsewhere (Hojat, Mangione, Nasca et al., 2001).

Criterion-Related Validity of the Generic Version

Criterion-related validity involves an examination of the correlations between the test scores and selected criterion measures. One approach to criterion-related validation is to demonstrate significant correlations between scores on the scale and conceptually relevant variables (convergent validity) accompanied by nonsignificant correlations with conceptually irrelevant measures (discriminant validity). Convergent and discriminant validities are concepts derived from the method introduced by Campbell and Fiske (1959) which was initially used in their analysis of the multitrait–multimethod matrix of correlations to describe a pattern of higher relationships among conceptually more relevant variables (convergent validity) than among conceptually less relevant variables (discriminant validity) in different methods of assessment.

We included the criterion measures listed in Box 7.1 in a questionnaire to examine the criterion-related validity of the generic version of the instrument. Criterion measures 1–6 were available for both samples of medical students and residents. The remaining ten measures of personal attributes (items 7–16 in Box 7.1) were defined on the questionnaire and were answered on a 100-point scale. These criterion measures were available for the sample of students only. Respondents were asked to place a mark on the scale to identify the extent to which they perceived themselves as having each of those particular personal attributes. We also used scores of three scales (Perspective Taking, Empathic Concern, and Fantasy of the Interpersonal Reactivity Index (IRI, Davis, 1983) described in Chap. 5). We did not use the Personal Distress scale of the IRI for two reasons: We wanted to reduce the length of the questionnaire and increase the response rate, and we thought that the Personal Distress scale was less germane to patient care situations. The Pearson correlation coefficients between scores of the generic version of the instrument and all 16 criterion measures (in Box 7.1) are reported in Table 7.2. The correlations with the scores of the three scales of the IRI were statistically significant but moderate in magnitude.

Although statistically significant, the correlations between scores of the generic version and conceptually relevant variables, such as compassion, warmth, dutifulness, faith-in-people, trust, tolerance, personal growth, and communication, were not large in magnitude—possibly the result of the low reliability of the single items used as criteria. However, the fact that all these conceptually relevant criteria yielded positive and statistically significant correlations is consistent with our

Box 7.1: Criterion measures used for the validity study

1. *Empathic concern*. A scale of the IRI (Davis, 1983) (see Chap. 5).
2. *Perspective taking*. A scale of the IRI.
3. *Fantasy scale*. A scale of the IRI.
4. *Warmth*. A facet of personality (eight items) from the revised version of the NEO Personality Inventory (NEO PI-R©), a widely used instrument measuring the big five personality factors and their facets (Costa & McCrea, 1992). The inventory has been used in the USA with samples of both physicians and members of the general population. Physicians scored higher than the general population on Warmth (Hojat, Glaser, Xu, Veloski, & Christian, 1999a). Also, positive female role models in medicine scored higher than the general population on this facet of personality (Magee & Hojat, 1998).
5. *Dutifulness*. A facet of personality from the NEO PI-R © (eight items). Both male and female positive role models in medicine scored higher than the general population on this facet (Magee & Hojat, 1998).
6. *Faith-in-people scale*. This scale was developed by Rosenberg (1957, 1965) and contains five items measuring one's degree of confidence in the trustworthiness of people (Robinson, 1978). A typical item is "Most people are inclined to help others."
7. *Global empathy*. Defined as "Standing in the patient's shoes in the experience of the illness."
8. *Global sympathy*. Defined as "Developing feelings for the patient's sufferings."
9. *Global compassion*. Defined as "Sympathy for the patient combined with the intention of doing good and a desire to help."
10. *Trust*. Defined as "Belief that patients report their illness experience honestly."
11. *Tolerance*. Defined as "The ability to evaluate a patient who shows offensive and self-destructive behavior without becoming judgmental or losing interest in helping."
12. *Personal growth (through interaction with the patient)*. Defined as "Learning and gaining reward through emotionally intense (either positive or negative) interactions with patients."
13. *Communication (of the understanding)*. Defined as "The capacity to reflect patients' emotions by providing some statements which validate the patient's feelings."
14. *Self-protection*. Defined as "Protecting one's self from being overwhelmed by patients' emotions and/or suffering."
15. *Humor*. Defined as "Ability to laugh with the patients about human foibles and absurdities related to their illness and treatment, as well as to appropriate jokes and lighter topics unrelated to illness."
16. *Clinical neutrality*. Defined as "Controlling expressions of emotional reactions to patients, whether their reactions are positive or negative."

Table 7.2 Correlations of scores of the generic version of the JSE with criterion measures

Criterion measures	Residents ($n=41$)	Medical students ($n=193$)
IRI scales[a]		
Empathic concern		0.41**
Perspective taking		0.29**
Fantasy		0.24**
Self-report (7-point scale)[b]		
Compassion	0.56**	0.48**
Sympathy	0.27***	0.33**
NEO PI-R personality facets[c]		
Warmth[c]	NA	0.33**
Dutifulness[c]	NA	0.24**
Faith-in-people (misanthropy)[d]	NA	0.12***
Self-report (100-point scale)[e]		
Empathy	NA	0.45**
Compassion	NA	0.31**
Trust	NA	0.27**
Sympathy	NA	0.26**
Tolerance	NA	0.25**
Personal growth	NA	0.15*
Communication	NA	0.13***
Self protection	NA	0.11
Humor	NA	0.05
Clinical neutrality	NA	−0.05

© 2001 *Educational and Psychological Measurement*. Reproduced with permission (Hojat, Mangione, Nasca et al., 2001)
*$p<0.05$; **$p<0.01$; ***$p<0.10$
NA data were not available
[a]Scales from the Interpersonal Reactivity Index (Davis, 1983)
[b]Single items
[c]Personality facets from the NEO PI-R (Costa & McCrea, 1992)
[d]Faith-in-People Scale (Rosenberg, 1957, 1965)
[e]Self-reported personal attributes on a 100-point scale

expectations, thus providing support for the scale's "convergent" validity. Conversely, a lack of significant relationships between scores on the JSE and on personal attributes that seemed conceptually irrelevant to empathy (e.g., self-protection and clinical neutrality) supports the scale's "discriminant" validity.

Sympathy overlapped with scores of the scale to a limited degree, with correlations ranging from 0.27 to 0.33 (see Table 7.2). Self-reported empathy and compassion yielded the highest correlations with the JSPE scores, with correlations ranging from 0.31 to 0.56 (see Table 7.2). These correlations provide evidence supporting the criterion-related validity of the generic instrument. (Details of these findings are reported elsewhere; Hojat, Mangione, Nasca et al., 2001)

The moderate magnitude of the correlations with the criterion measures suggests that empathy, as measured by the original scale, can be regarded as a distinct personal attribute with a statistically significant but practically limited overlap with compassion, concern, sympathy, perspective taking, imagination, warmth, dutifulness, tolerance, personal growth, trust, and communication.

Internal Consistency Reliability of the Generic Version

The reliability of an instrument is an indication of the precision in a single testing situation (internal consistency) or score stability in multiple testing situations. We studied the internal consistency aspect of the reliability by calculating Cronbach's alpha coefficient (Cronbach, 1951). The coefficient obtained was 0.89 for the sample of medical students and 0.87 for the sample of residents (Hojat, Mangione, Nasca et al., 2001). Reliability coefficients of this magnitude are desirable for educational and psychological instruments (Anastasi, 1976).

Revisions to Develop Three Versions of the Jefferson Scale of Empathy

The generic version of the scale was originally developed to measure medical students' orientations or attitudes toward empathic relationships in the context of patient care. However, there was a demand to use the scale for administration not only to medical students, but also to physicians and other health professionals involved in patient care, and all health professions students other than medical students. Thus, we decided to slightly modify the content of the generic scale so that three versions would be available: one version for administration to medical students (the S-Version, see Appendix B); a second version for administration to physicians and other practicing health professionals (the HP-Version; see Appendix C); and the third version for administration to students in all health professions disciplines other than medicine (the HPS-Version; see Appendix D).

The HP-Version was to be geared more toward the clinician's empathic behavior in patient encounters; the S-Version and HPS-Version were to reflect students' orientation or attitudes toward empathy in patient care. The content in the three versions was very similar with only minor modifications to make the items appropriate for the target groups. For example, the item in the S-Version reading "It is difficult for a physician to view things from patients' perspectives" was modified as follows in the HP-Version: "It is difficult for me to view things from my patients' perspectives," and it was modified as follows in the HPS-Version: "It is difficult for a health care provider to view things from patients' perspectives."

Revisions to Balance Positively and Negatively Worded Items

There were only three negatively worded items (reverse scored) in the generic version of the scale. Reversed scored items are used in personality tests to disrupt aberrant responses (Paulhus, 1991; Weijters, Baumgartner, & Schillewaert, 2013) and to reduce the confounding effects of those unusual responses. The following three mechanisms often lead to invalid responses. 1) the "acquiescence response style" defined as a tendency to agree or disagree constantly with the test items (in the sociopolitical context, these individuals are called "yeasayers" or "naysayers"); 2) "careless responding" refers to random or inattentive responses to the test items regardless of their content; 3) "confirmation bias," a tendency to express beliefs that are consistent with the way in which the question is stated (Davies, 2003). For example, when question is about extraversion, respondents tend to think about situations in which they are extraverted, and when the question is about introversion, respondents tend to think about situations in which they are introverted (Weijters, Baumgartner, & Schillewaert, 2013).

In the modified version, a balance was maintained by making ten items positively worded and the other ten negatively worded. The positively worded items were directly scored according to their Likert weights (1 = Strongly disagree, 7 = Strongly agree), whereas the negatively worded items were reverse scored (1 = Strongly agree, 7 = Strongly disagree).

Revisions to Improve Clarity for an International Audience

Minor revisions also were made in the wording of a few items to improve their clarity for international audiences. For example, while researchers in Italy and Mexico were translating the instrument into Italian and Spanish, a question arose about the verbatim translation of the verb "touch" in the following item: "I do not allow myself to be touched by intense emotional relationships between my patients and their family members" (a negatively worded item). The symbolic meaning of "to be touched by" (to be affected or influenced by) was not apparent in the translated versions. Therefore, we revised this item by substituting "to be influenced" for "to be touched" to avoid confusion in translations in foreign languages.

Comparisons of the Generic (JSPE) and the Revised Versions (JSE)

To study the effects of our modifications and revisions on the JSE, we administered the generic version and the HP-Version to a group of 42 residents in internal medicine by using a crossover design so that half the residents completed the HP-Version first and then the generic version, and the other half completed the two versions in the reverse order. The correlation between scores on the two versions was 0.85 ($p<0.01$). We noticed an extremely slight nonsignificant trend toward improvement in the Cronbach's alpha coefficient reliability estimate of the HP-Version (an increase from 0.81 to 0.85). No significant change occurred in the descriptive statistics of the two versions. For example, the mean score on the generic version was 120.9 ($SD=10.1$), and it was 120.2 ($SD=10.7$) for the HP-Version. Recently collected data on medical students using the S-Version showed descriptive statistics that were similar to those reported in Table 7.1 on medical students who completed the generic version. Similar data on the HPS-Version of the JSE have also been reported in nursing students (Fields, Mahan, Hojat, Tillman, & Maxwell, 2011), and pharmacy students (Fjortoft, Van Winkle, & Hojat, 2011) (see Appendix A).

We conducted studies to examine the psychometric characteristics of different versions of the JSE. For example, in the following study, we examined the psychometric properties of the HP-Version in a relatively large sample of practicing physicians. In the second study, we investigated the psychometric properties of the S-Version using a large sample of medical students.

Psychometrics of the JSE HP-Version

To study the psychometric and other aspects of the HP-Version, we mailed the JSE to 1007 physicians in the Jefferson Health System, affiliated with Thomas Jefferson University Hospital and Jefferson Medical College in the greater Philadelphia area (postage-paid return envelopes were provided). After two follow-up reminders, 704 physicians completed and returned the questionnaire, a response rate of 70 % (Hojat et al., 2002b). A response rate of 70 % is considerably higher than the typical rate of 52 % reported for surveys mailed to physicians (Cummings, Savitz, & Konrad, 2001). However, some researchers have suggested that a response rate of at least 75 % should be achieved for surveys mailed to professionals to ensure the representativeness of the sample (Gough & Hall, 1977). A comparison of respondents and nonrespondents failed to show any significant differences between the two groups with regard to the distribution of their specialties, providing support for the representativeness of the study sample regarding their specialties (Hojat et al., 2002b).

To study the stability of scores on the HP-Version over time (test–retest reliability), 100 physicians who had completed the HP-Version were selected at random to receive a second copy of the scale plus a letter thanking them for their participation and requesting that they complete the second copy of the scale to help us establish the scale's reliability. Seventy-one physicians responded, and their scores on the two tests were correlated. The exact time interval between completion of the two tests could not be determined accurately because we did not ask physicians to specify the date on which they completed the survey. However, by examining the postmarks, we were able to reach a rough estimate of approximately 3–4 months as the testing interval. The test–retest reliability was 0.65 ($p<0.01$) (Hojat et al., 2002b).

Underlying Components (Factors) of the JSE HP-Version

We conducted an EFA to investigate the underlying components of the HP-Version. Three factors with eigenvalues greater than one emerged (4.2, 1.5, and 1.3) accounting for 21 %, 8 %, and 7 % of the total variance, respectively (Hojat et al., 2002b). The factor coefficients, the magnitudes of eigenvalues, and the proportions of variance are reported in Table 7.3. The ten positively worded items had factor coefficients of at least 0.45 on Factor 1 (shown in bold). This factor can be regarded as the grand component of the scale, as the magnitude of its eigenvalue indicates. On the basis of the contents of items with high factor coefficients, the first factor can be titled "Perspective Taking," a component of the JSE that has been described as the core cognitive ingredient of empathy (Davis, 1994; Spiro et al., 1993) and as the stepping stone in empathic engagement (Jackson, Brunet, Meltzoff, & Decety, 2006; Jackson, Rainville, & Decety, 2006). This major component is similar to the grand factor of "Physician's View of the Patient's Perspective" that emerged in the generic version.

Factor 2 included eight of the negatively worded items with factor coefficients of at least 0.37. This factor can be regarded as a construct involving "Compassionate Care" according to the contents of the items (the positive pole of the contents of the items that were negatively worded but reverse scored). Conceptually, this construct is similar to the two factors that emerged in the generic version: "emotions in patient care" and "understanding patient's experiences." Finally, Factor 3 included two other negatively worded items with high factor coefficients (≥ 0.66) that can be called "Standing in the Patient's Shoes" (the positive pole of the contents of the negatively worded but reverse-scored items). This is a trivial component that is similar to the factor "Thinking Like the Patient," which emerged in the generic version.

These findings suggest that the factor structure of the JSE is consistent with the notion of the multidimensionality of empathy (Davis, 1983, 1994; Kunyk & Olson, 2001). In addition, the stability and the similarity between the factor structure and components across different samples (medical students and physicians) and across different versions (generic and revised) provide further support for the JSE's construct validity.

Item Characteristics and the Corrected Item-Total Score Correlations of the HP-Version

The means of item scores on the HP-Version ranged from a low of 4.8 to a high of 6.5 on the 7-point scale (Hojat et al., 2002b). This finding suggests that the physicians' responses to the items tended to be skewed toward the upper tail of the scale although the distribution of their responses showed that the physicians actually used the full range of possible responses on all items. The standard deviations for the items ranged from 0.9 to 1.6 (Hojat et al., 2002b). The corrected item–total score correlations were all positive and statistically significant ($p < 0.01$), ranging from 0.30 to 0.60 with a median correlation of 0.43.

Table 7.3 Rotated factor loadings of items in the HP-Version of the JSE[a]

Items	Factors		
	1	2	3
1. An important component of the relationship with my patients is my understanding of their emotional status as well as that of their families	**0.70**	0.21	−0.08
2. I try to understand what is going on in my patients' minds by paying attention to their nonverbal cues and body language	**0.62**	0.06	0.23
3. I believe that empathy is an important therapeutic factor in medical and surgical treatment	**0.60**	0.28	−0.25
4. Empathy is a therapeutic skill without which my success in treatment would be limited	**0.58**	0.22	−0.16
5. My patients value my understanding of their feelings which is therapeutic in its own right	**0.58**	0.32	0.03
6. My patients feel better when I understand their feelings	**0.50**	−0.02	0.16
7. I consider understanding my patients' body language as important as verbal communication in caregiver–patient relationships	**0.48**	−0.18	0.30
8. I try to imagine myself in my patients' shoes when providing care to them	**0.46**	0.29	0.28
9. I have a good sense of humor that I think contributes to a better clinical outcome	**0.45**	−0.02	0.14
10. I try to think like my patients in order to render better care	**0.46**	0.20	0.25
11. Patients' illnesses can be cured only by medical treatment; therefore, affectional ties to my patients cannot have a significant influence on medical or surgical outcomes	0.17	**0.60**	−0.01
12. Attentiveness to my patients' personal experiences does not influence treatment outcomes	0.07	**0.59**	0.07
13. I try not to pay attention to my patients' emotions in history taking or asking about their physical health	0.02	**0.54**	0.02
14. I believe that emotion has no place in the treatment of medical illness	0.22	**0.50**	−0.03
15. I do not allow myself to be touched by intense emotional relationships between my patients and their family members	0.13	**0.44**	0.26
16. My understanding of how my patients and their families feel does not influence medical or surgical treatment	−0.03	**0.43**	0.14
17. I do not enjoy reading nonmedical literature or the arts	0.05	**0.37**	0.13
18. Asking patients about what is happening in their lives in not helpful in understanding their physical complaints	0.10	**0.37**	−0.12
19. It is difficult for me to view things from my patients' perspectives	0.10	0.05	**0.74**
20. Because people are different, it is difficult for me to see things from my patients' perspectives	0.17	0.20	**0.66**
Eigenvalues	4.2	1.5	1.3
Variance (%)	21	8	7

©2002. American Psychiatric Association. Reproduced with permission from the *American Journal of Psychiatry* (Hojat et al., 2002b)
Responses were based on a 7-point Likert-type scale. Responses were reverse scored on items 11–20 (strongly agree = 1, strongly disagree = 7); otherwise, items were directly scored (strongly agree = 7, strongly disagree = 1)
[a]Items are listed based on the descending order of the magnitude of the factor structure coefficients within each factor. Values greater than 0.36 are in boldface

Descriptive Statistics and Reliability of the HP-Version

The descriptive statistics and the distribution of scores for the HP-Version are reported in Table 7.4. Also, the internal consistency aspect of reliability (Cronbach's alpha coefficient) was 0.81 for the sample of physicians, and the test–retest reliability coefficient was 0.65 (Hojat et al., 2002b). The reliability coefficients indicate that the HP-Version is internally consistent and its scores are relatively stable over time (see Table 7.4).

Desirability of National Norms and Cutoff Scores

It would be desirable to develop norms based on representative national samples of physicians for comparative purposes or for evaluation of each individual physician's score (e.g., a female physician practicing family medicine) against the norm

Table 7.4 Score distributions, percentiles, and descriptive statistics for the HP-Version of the JSE ($n = 704$ physicians)

Score interval	Frequency	Cumulative frequency	Cumulative percentage
≤75	3	3	<1
76–80	3	6	1
81–85	2	8	1
86–90	3	11	2
91–95	13	24	3
96–100	21	45	6
101–105	31	76	11
106–110	57	133	19
111–115	97	230	33
116–120	111	341	48
121–125	114	455	65
126–130	126	581	83
131–135	85	666	95
136–140	38	704	100
Mean	120		
Standard deviation	11.9		
25th percentile	113		
50th percentile (median)	121		
75th percentile	128		
Possible range	20–140		
Actual range	50–140		
Alpha reliability estimate	0.81		
Test–retest reliability[a]	0.65		

©2002 American Psychiatric Association. Reproduced with permission from the *American Journal of Psychiatry* (Hojat et al., 2002b)
[a]Test–retest reliability is calculated for 71 physicians within an interval of approximately 3–4 months between testing

(e.g., percentile ranks) derived from a corresponding national sample (e.g., a national sample of female physicians in family medicine). Also, determining cutoff scores to identify those with marginal JSE scores could be helpful for assessment purposes. Obviously, the data reported in Table 7.4 cannot serve those purposes.

Psychometric Properties of the JSE S-Version

To examine the psychometrics and other measurement properties of the S-Version, we collected data from 2637 students who matriculated at Jefferson (currently Sidney Kimmel) Medical College between 2002 and 2012 and completed the JSE (S-Version) at the beginning of medical school (orientation day, before they were exposed to formal medical education). There were 1336 (51 %) women and 1301 (49 %) men in this sample, which represented 94 % of all matriculants during the 11-year study period ($n = 2802$). Frequency and percent distributions of the study sample by matriculation year and gender are reported in Table 7.5. Although the proportion of women varied from 46 % (in year 2002) to 57 % (in year 2006), no significant difference was found in gender composition in different matriculation years ($\chi^2_{(10)} = 9.8$, $p = 0.45$) (for more detailed report of this study, see Hojat & Gonnella, 2015).

Descriptive Statistics of the S-Version

Means, standard deviations, medians, score ranges, skewness, and kurtosis indices for the entire sample and for matriculants of each year are presented in Table 7.6. As shown in the table, the JSE (S-Version) mean score for the entire sample was

Table 7.5 Frequency and percent distributions of the study sample (2637 medical students) by matriculation year and gender

Matriculation year	Men, n (%)	Women, n (%)	Total, n (%)
2002	120 (54 %)	101 (46 %)	221 (100 %)
2003	105 (48 %)	113 (52 %)	218 (100 %)
2004	103 (46 %)	121 (54 %)	224 (100 %)
2005	126 (51 %)	121 (49 %)	247 (100 %)
2006	107 (43 %)	140 (57 %)	247 (100 %)
2007	132 (53 %)	116 (47 %)	248 (100 %)
2008	120 (51 %)	117 (49 %)	237 (100 %)
2009	111 (46 %)	128 (54 %)	239 (100 %)
2010	124 (49 %)	128 (51 %)	252 (100 %)
2011	125 (50 %)	127 (50 %)	252 (100 %)
2012	128 (51 %)	124 (49 %)	252 (100 %)
Total	1301 (49 %)	1336 (51 %)	2637 (100 %)

©2015 Karger. Reproduced with permission (Hojat & Gonnella, 2015)
$\chi^2_{(10)} = 9.8$, $p = 0.45$ (nonsignificant)

Table 7.6 Means, standard deviations, range, skewness and kurtosis indices, and reliability coefficients (Cronbach's α coefficient) of the JSE by matriculating classes and summary results of statistical analysis

Matriculating class	n	Mean	SD	Median	Range	Skewness	Kurtosis	Cronbach α
2002	221	114.1	9.9	114	81–137	−0.24	0.04	0.80
2003	218	113.9	10.0	115	75–140	−0.44	0.52	0.79
2004	224	115.9	9.8	117	82–140	−0.35	0.12	0.78
2005	247	114.5	9.7	116	82–133	−0.66	0.46	0.78
2006	247	114.8	9.4	115	86–135	−0.46	0.19	0.75
2007	248	114.6	10.6	114	71–136	−0.47	0.74	0.81
2008	237	113.5	12.1	114	52–140	−0.92	2.66	0.84
2009	239	113.2	11.3	113	73–140	−0.28	0.05	0.84
2010	252	113.8	10.7	114	70–140	−0.62	0.88	0.81
2011	252	114.1	10.1	116	76–140	−0.57	0.79	0.79
2012	252	114.8	10.6	116	79–140	−0.65	0.90	0.81
Total	2637	114.3	10.4	115	52–140	−0.56	0.92	0.80

©2015 Karger. Reproduced with permission (Hojat & Gonnella, 2015)
$F_{(10,2626)}=1.2$, $p=0.29$ (nonsignificant)

114.3 ($SD=10.4$), which varied from a low of 113.2 ($SD=11.3$) for matriculants of 2009 to a high of 115.9 ($SD=9.8$) for matriculants of 2004. Analysis of variance was used to test the significance of differences in mean scores of matriculants in different years. No statistically significant difference was observed ($F_{(10,2626)}=1.2$, $p=0.29$), meaning that students during the 11 years of this study period had similar empathy scores at the beginning of medical school. These descriptive statistics are somewhat similar to most of those reported for medical students in the USA by other researchers (see Appendix A).

Skewness index is a measure of symmetry in score distribution. In a perfectly normal distribution the skewness is close to zero. As shown in Table 7.6, the skewness index was negative for the entire sample (−0.56) and for each matriculating year (ranging from −0.92 for matriculants of 2008 to −0.24 for matriculants of 2002, with a median of −0.53). Negative skewness indicates that the peak of JSE score distributions tended to be to the right side of the distribution (bulk of data to the side of higher scores). However, the magnitudes of the skewness indices suggest that distributions were just moderately skewed (distributions with skewedness indices out of the −1 to +1 range are considered highly skewed).

Kurtosis is an index of the peak of score distribution. Higher values indicate a higher peak, and lower values a flatter peak. Normal distributions have a kurtosis index close to three (mesokurtic); those greater than three are high-peaked distributions (leptokurtic), and those with kurtosis less than three are flatter peaked (platykurtic). The kurtosis for the entire sample was 0.93, ranging from a low of 0.04 (for matriculants of 2002) to 2.66 (for matriculants of 2008) with a median of 0.52 (Table 7.6). These findings indicate that the distributions of the JSE scores tend to be platykurtic (Hojat & Gonnella, 2015).

Internal Consistency Reliability of the S-Version

We calculated Cronbach's α coefficient for the entire sample which was 0.80, ranging from a low of 0.75 (for matriculants of 2006) to a high of 0.84 (for matriculants of 2008 and 2009) with a median of 0.80 (Table 7.6). These reliability coefficients are in the range of most JSE studies by other national and international researchers (see Appendix A).

Score Distributions and Percentile Ranks of the S-Version

Frequency distributions of the JSE scores and percentile ranks for men, women, and the entire sample are presented in Table 7.7. As shown in the table, the mean, median, and standard deviation for the entire sample were 114.3, 115, and 10.4, respectively. Because we found significant gender difference on the JSE scores, we examined the score distributions for men and women separately (Hojat & Gonnella, 2015). Later in this chapter I will discuss how the data reported in Table 7.7 can be used as "proxy" norm and for determining "tentative" cutoff scores.

Item Statistics of the S-Version

Respondents used the full range of possible answers (1–7) for each item. Item mean scores ranged from a low of 3.6 ($SD = 1.4$) for this item: "Physicians should not allow themselves to be influenced by strong personal bonds between their patients and their family members" to a high of 6.5 ($SD = 0.8$) for this item: "Patients feel better when their physicians understand their feelings."

The corrected item-total score correlations ranged from a low of 0.13 (for the aforementioned item with the lowest mean score) to a high of 0.61 (for this item: "Physicians' understanding of the emotional status of their patients, as well as that of their families, is one important component of the physician-patient relationship"). The median item-total score correlation was 0.44. All correlations were positive and statistically significant ($p < 0.01$) which indicates that all items contributed positively and significantly to the total score of the JSE scale (for more detailed information see Hojat & LaNoue, 2014). Item-total score correlations are reported in Table 7.8.

To address the discrimination power of each item, we calculated an item discrimination effect size index. For that purpose, we divided the total sample into two groups of approximately top-third high scorers on the JSE (score > 119, $n = 835$) and bottom-third low scorers (JSE score < $111 < n = 857$). For each item, we calculated the mean score difference between the top-third and bottom-third JSE scoring groups, divided by the pooled standard deviation of the item to calculate the item discrimination effect size index, similar to the Cohen's d (item discrimination effect

Table 7.7 Frequency and percent distributions and descriptive statistics of scores on the Jefferson Scale of Empathy (S-Version) by gender

Score interval	Men (n = 1301)			Women (n = 1336)			Total (n = 2637)		
	Freq.	Cumulative freq.	Percentile ranks (%)	Freq.	Cumulative freq.	Cumulative %	Freq.	Cumulative freq.	Percentile ranks (%)
≤80	11	11	1	5	5	<1	16	16	<1
81–85	8	19	1	2	7	<1	10	26	1
86–90	22	41	2–3	1	8	1	23	49	2
91–95	48	89	4–7	21	29	2	69	118	3–4
96–100	87	176	8–13	56	85	3–6	143	261	5–10
101–105	136	312	14–24	89	174	7–13	225	486	11–18
106–110	214	526	25–40	165	339	14–25	379	865	19–33
111–115	252	778	41–60	258	597	26–45	510	1375	34–52
116–120	232	1010	61–78	279	876	46–65	511	1886	53–71
121–125	159	1169	79–90	221	1097	66–82	380	2266	72–86
126–130	91	1260	91–97	171	1268	83–95	262	2528	87–96
131–135	34	1294	98–99	56	1324	96–99	90	2618	97–99
>135	7	1301	100	12	1336	100	19	2637	100
Descriptive statistics									
Mean[a]	112.3			116.2			114.3		
Median	113			117			115		
Standard deviation	10.8			9.7			10.4		
Possible range	20–140			20–140			20–140		
Actual range	70–140			52–140			52–140		

©2015 Karger. Reproduced with permission (Hojat & Gonnella, 2015)

[a] $t_{(2635)} = 9.9$, $p < 0.0001$ for testing the null hypotheses that JSE mean scores for men and women are not different

Table 7.8 Rotated factor pattern for the Jefferson Scale of Empathy[a], item-total score correlations, and effect size estimates of item discrimination indices (n = 1380)

Items[b]	Factors			Item-total score correlation[*c]	Discrimination index effect size[c]
	Factor 1	Factor 2	Factor 3		
• Patients value a physician's understanding of their feelings which is therapeutic in its own right (10)	**0.66**	0.02	0.01	0.55	1.3
• Physicians should try to stand in their patients' shoes when providing care to them (9)	**0.64**	−0.05	0.02	0.50	1.2
• Physicians should try to think like their patients in order to render better care (17)	**0.61**	−0.16	0.00	0.37	1.0
• Physicians' understanding of the emotional status of their patients, as well as that of their families is one important component of the physician–patient relationship (16)	**0.46**	**0.29**	0.00	0.61	1.4
• I believe that empathy is an important therapeutic factor in medical treatment (20)	**0.44**	**0.26**	−0.02	0.59	1.3
• Patients feel better when their physicians understand their feelings (2)	**0.44**	0.00	0.03	0.41	0.89
• Physicians should try to understand what is going on in their patients' minds by paying attention to their nonverbal cues and body language (13)	**0.40**	0.17	0.04	0.49	1.2
• Empathy is a therapeutic skill without which the physician's success is limited (15)	**0.36**	0.20	−0.04	0.44	1.2
• Understanding body language is as important as verbal communication in physician–patient relationships (4)	**0.30**	0.09	0.08	0.35	0.88
• A physician's sense of humor contributes to a better clinical outcome (5)	**0.29**	0.03	0.00	0.26	0.79
• Patients' illnesses can be cured only by medical or surgical treatment; therefore, physicians' emotional ties with their patients do not have a significant influence in medical or surgical treatment (11)	0.03	**0.59**	0.01	0.52	1.2
• I believe that emotion has no place in the treatment of medical illness (14)	0.23	**0.54**	0.04	0.46	1.0
• Attentiveness to patients' personal experiences does not influence treatment outcomes (8)	0.01	**0.52**	0.05	0.48	1.1

(continued)

Table 7.8 (continued)

Items[b]	Factors			Item-total score correlation*[c]	Discrimination index effect size[c]
	Factor 1	Factor 2	Factor 3		
• Asking patients about what is happening in their personal lives is not helpful in understanding their physical complaints (12)	0.03	**0.49**	0.00	0.44	1.0
• Physicians' understanding of their patients' feelings and the feelings of their families do not influence medical or surgical treatment (1)	0.04	**0.49**	−0.09	0.35	0.94
• Attention to patients' emotions is not important in history taking (7)	0.01	**0.48**	0.09	0.43	1.0
• I do not enjoy reading nonmedical literature or the arts (19)	0.00	**0.25**	0.00	0.20	0.62
• Physicians should not allow themselves to be influenced by strong personal bonds between their patients and their family members (18)	−0.02	0.21	0.01	0.13	0.50
• Because people are different, it is difficult to see things from patients' perspectives (6)	−0.05	0.06	**0.75**	0.15	0.59
• It is difficult for a physician to view things from patients' perspectives (3)	0.06	−0.06	**0.68**	0.14	0.57

©2014 *International Journal of Medical Education*. Reproduced with permission (Hojat & LaNoue, 2014)

[a]Principal component factor extraction with oblique rotation was used for approximately half of the sample ($n = 1380$). CFA was performed for the other half of the sample to examine the three-factor model

[b]Items are listed by the order of magnitude of factor loadings within each extracted factor. Factor loadings equal to or greater than 0.25 are in bold. Numbers in parentheses represent the sequence of the items in the actual scale. Items were scored using a 7-point Likert-type scale. Half of the items are reverse scored

[c]These are partial correlations between score of each item and total JSE score by excluding the corresponding item score from the total score. Item-total score correlations and discrimination indices were calculated based on data for the entire sample ($n = 2612$). For calculation of the effect size estimates of discrimination indices, the item mean score for JSE high scorers (top 33 %) was subtracted from the item mean score for JSE low scorers (bottom 33 %), divided by the pooled standard deviation of the corresponding item

*$p < 0.001$ for all of the reported correlations

size index = $M_{\text{top-third}} - M_{\text{bottom-third}}$/pooled SD) (Hojat & LaNoue, 2014). The item discrimination effect size indices ranged from a low of 0.50 for the aforementioned item which showed the lowest item-total score correlation to a high of 1.4 for the abovementioned item with the highest item-total score correlation. The median effect size was 1.2 (see Table 7.8). Cohen (1987) suggests that the effect size values around 0.30 or lower are considered negligible, around 0.50 are moderate, and around 0.70 and higher are large and practically important. According to these operational definitions, the item discrimination effect size indices were all substantial, and practically (clinically) important (Hojat & Xu, 2004).

Underlying Components of the S-Version

For factor analytic studies we divided the sample into two groups: (1) matriculants between 2002 and 2007 ($n = 1380$): data from this group were used for EFA and (2) matriculants between 2008 and 2012 ($n = 1232$): data from this group were used for CFA. We used principal component factor extraction with oblique rotation in our EFA to reexamine the underlying components of the JSE. CFA was performed by using structural equation modeling (SEM), and several measures of model fit were evaluated including root mean square error of approximation (RMSEA) (Arbuckle & Wothke, 1999) to confirm the latent variable structure of the scale.

In almost all of the factor analytic studies of the JSE, orthogonal (varimax) rotation was used to obtain independent factors. In the present study, we used oblique rotation (promax) to allow correlations among the extracted factors in order to examine if previously reported factor pattern in our study of physicians for the HP-Version (Hojat et al., 2002c) would remain unchanged. We also limited the number of retained factors to three to make the findings comparable to the previously reported factor analytic study with physicians (Hojat et al., 2002c). Indeed, the scree test to determine the appropriate number of factors to retain before rotation showed that the plot of the eigenvalues leveled off after extraction of the third factor, supporting our decision to retain three factors for rotation. The Kaiser-Meyer-Olkin measure for sampling adequacy (MSA) was used prior to factor extraction which resulted in an overall index of 0.86, supporting the adequacy of data for factor analysis. Also, the Bartlett's test for sphericity showed that the intercorrelation matrix was factorable ($\chi^2_{(190)} = 5332.5$, $p < 0.0001$).

The eigenvalues for the first, second, and third retained factors were 4.7, 1.6, and 1.4, respectively. The first factor, "Perspective Taking," included ten items with relatively high factor coefficients of at least 0.28, accounting for 23 % of the total variance. A sample item (with the highest factor coefficient) is "Patients value a physician's understanding of their feelings which is therapeutic in its own right." The Cronbach's alpha coefficient for items under this factor was 0.79.

The second factor, "Compassionate Care," included seven items with relatively high factor coefficients (>0.25), accounting for 8 % of the total variance. A sample item is "Patients' illnesses can be cured only by medical or surgical treatment; therefore, physicians' emotional ties with their patients do not have a significant influence on medical or surgical treatment." This is a negatively worded item which is reverse scored. The Cronbach's alpha coefficient for items under this factor was 0.69.

The third factor, "Standing in the Patient's Shoes," included only two items with factor coefficients greater than 0.67, accounting for 7 % of the total variance. A sample item is "Because people are different, it is difficult to see things from patients' perspectives" (reverse scored). The Cronbach's alpha coefficient for items under this factor was 0.68. One item had a low factor coefficient (0.21) on Factor 2. However, this item showed a significant item discrimination effect size index and yielded a statistically significant (but low in magnitude) item-total score correlation.

Summary results of the EFA are reported in Table 7.8. The general pattern of findings is similar to that in most other studies in the USA and abroad. For example, similarities in factor pattern are observed in studies reported for the physicians (Hojat et al., 2002b) and nurses (Ward et al., 2009) in the USA and for samples of physicians in Italy (DiLillo, Cicchetti, Lo Scalzo, Taroni, & Hojat, 2009) and medical students in Iran (Shariat & Habibi, 2013); Korea (Roh, Hahm, Lee, & Suh, 2010); Japan (Kataoka, Koide, Ochi, Hojat, & Gonnella, 2009); Mexico (Alcorta-Garza, Gonzalez-Guerrero, Tavitas-Herrera, Rodrigues-Lara, & Hojat, 2005); South Africa (Vallabh, 2011); mainland China (Wen, Ma, Li, Liu, Xian, & Liu, 2013; Wen, Ma, Li, & Xian, 2013); Taiwan (Hsiao, Tsai, & Kao, 2012); Brazil (Paro, Daud-Gallotti, Tiberio, Pinto, & Martins, 2012); Austria (Preusche & Wagner-Menghin, 2013); and England (Tavakol, Dennick, & Tavakol, 2011a, 2011b). The two factors of "Perspective Taking" and "Compassionate Care" emerged in almost all factor analytic studies of the JSE.

Confirming the Latent Variable Structure of the S-Version

In CFA, all 20 items were modeled as functions of three underlying latent variables which emerged in the EFA and have been widely reported (see Appendix A). Maximum likelihood (ML) estimation was used. The regression coefficient for one item-to-latent variable path for each latent variable was set to 1.0 to scale the latent variable. Additionally, the variance of one error term (that is corresponding to item 6) was set to 0.0 to facilitate convergence of the ML estimation. Without this constraint, the model was inadmissible due to the negative error variance of item 3 (Kolenikov & Bollen, 2012).

As an exploratory analysis, we also evaluated a two-factor model, one which omitted the two items which comprise factor 3—"Standing in the Patient's Shoes." This was done because of the failure of the maximum likelihood CFA to converge without constraining one error variance, which can indicate a mis-specified model (Kolenikov & Bollen, 2012), and the other CFA studies of the scale which modeled only two factors (Tavakol et al., 2011a, 2011b; Williams, Boyle, & Earl, 2013; Williams, Brown, Boyle, & Dousek, 2013; Williams, Brown, & McKenna, 2013). We compared the fit of this two-factor model to the fit of the three-factor model (Hojat & LaNoue, 2014).

   Assessment of model fit was made through the use of several well-accepted metrics in structural equation modeling (SEM). First, the χ^2 test for the model was reviewed. In SEM, it is a measure of fit, rather than a test statistic, and desired values are small and nonsignificant. However, since χ^2 is sensitive to sample size, it is possible to obtain a large and significant value even when the fit of the model to the data is acceptable. To address this, a widely used "rule of thumb" was also evaluated—the ratio of the χ^2 to its degrees of freedom, which is suggested to reflect good fit at values <4.0 (Joreskog, 1993).

   We also evaluated the adjusted "goodness-of-fit" index (AGFI) which indexes the proportion of the observed covariance matrix that is explained by the model-implied covariance matrix (Kline, 1998). The Tucker-Lewis Index (TLI) was used to compare the fitted model to a null model. Hu and Bentler (1998) recommend values >0.95. Finally, the RMSEA for the structural model was evaluated. Hu and Bentler (1998) showed that a cutoff of 0.06 for RMSEA indicates a good model fit.

   For model comparisons, an additional fit and an incremental fit improvement metrics were used. The models were first compared to each other through the use of the χ^2 test for the significance of the difference in fit. The non-normed fit index (NNFI; also known as the TLI) was used to assess improvements in fit from model to model. The TLI normally results from SEM output as a comparison to a "null" model, but a version can be calculated for the improvement in fit between any two competing models. Hu and Bentler (1998) suggested that improvements in the TLI greater than 0.02 are of "substantive interest."

   See Fig. 7.1 for the measurement model structure of 20 variables and three correlated factors.

   The two-factor solution did not indicate a good fit (RMSEA = .07, AGFI = 0.88); however, the three-factor CFA yielded a marginally good fit to the data; RMSA = 0.05 and AGFI greater than 0.90. Both the χ^2 difference test and the TLI suggest that the three-factor model is a better fit than the two-factor model. Summary results for fit statistics are shown in Table 7.9.

   Results of CFA support the three-factor model of the JSE, and are in agreement with those reported in Iranian medical students (Shariat & Habibi, 2013), and British medical students (Tavakol et al., 2011a, 2011b). A satisfactory three-factor model fit was also achieved in Portuguese medical students after relaxing model restrictions (Magalhäes, Salgueira, Costa, & Costa, 2011). The two-factor model ("perspective taking" and "compassionate care") in Australian paramedic students (Williams, Boyle, et al., 2013; Williams, Brown, Boyle, et al., 2013; Williams, Brown, & McKenna, 2013) partly resembles findings of the present study. Although we acknowledge that these findings overall are not definitive with regard to the structure of the scale, we do not agree with suggestions made by some that a few JSE items should be excluded for a better latent variable structure model (Williams, Boyle et al., 2013; Williams, Brown, Boyle et al., 2013; Williams, Brown, & McKenna, 2013). First, deletion of items can cause an incompatibility problem in comparative research. Second, in most of the psychometric studies of the JSE (including our own study), significant item-total score correlations have been reported suggesting that each item contributes significantly to the total score of the

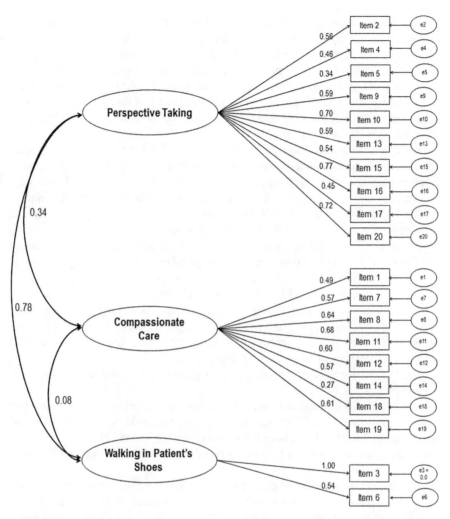

Fig. 7.1 Three-factor model (latent variable structure) of the Jefferson Scale of Empathy ($n=1232$). ©2014 *International Journal of Medical Education*. Reproduced with permission (Hojat & LaNoue, 2014)

JSE. In addition, we showed in this study that each item can discriminate substantially between high and low scorers of the JSE (Hojat & LaNoue, 2014).

As noted above, our study did not conclusively support a three-factor latent variable scale structure for the JSE. Further exploratory studies may be desirable to reexamine this issue in different samples of health profession students and practitioners. In our sample, we noticed a ceiling effect, or relatively high mean scores (>6.0) across seven items, which may have contributed to the marginal model fit (Hojat & LaNoue, 2014).

Data in our large-scale study supported the previously reported findings on the reliability (Cronbach's α coefficient), underlying constructs, and confirmation of

Table 7.9 Summary results of confirmatory factor analysis fit statistics ($n = 1232$)

Model	Parameters estimated	χ^2	df	χ^2/df	AGFI	TLI	RMSEA	AIC
Fitted three-factor model	42	887.87	168	5.28	0.93	0.89	0.05	971.87
Fitted 2-Factor Model	36	984.51	135	7.29	0.88	0.843	0.071	
Difference		205.65	33*			0.47[a]		
Null model (1 factor model)	20	6469.32	190	34.05	0.39	0.00	0.16	7468.25

©2014 *International Journal of Medical Education*. Reproduced with permission (Hojat & LaNoue, 2014)

*$p < 0.05$

[a]Calculated as recommended in Hu and Bentler (1998), this value represents a significant improvement in fit over the two-factor model

the latent variable structure of the JSE (S-Version). Similarities in factor pattern of the JSE in different samples and in different countries indicate that the underlying components of the scale are relatively stable, regardless of cultural variation. The three components of "Perspective Taking," "Compassionate Care," and "Standing in the Patient's Shoes" which emerged in our study and some other factor analytic studies of the JSE are consistent with the ingredients of empathy often reported in the literature. These underlying factors are also supportive of the pillars of empathic engagement in patient care, namely seeing with the mind's eye (e.g., Perspective Taking and Walking in Patient's Shoes) and hearing with the third ear (e.g., Compassionate Care). Based on the findings from this and other CFA studies (Magalhães et al., 2011; Shariat & Habibi, 2013; Tavakol et al., 2011a, 2011b), we suggest to retain all 20 items in the instrument not only for the goodness of the fit of the three-factor model, but also because of significant item-total score correlations and substantial item discrimination effect size indices obtained for all items (Hojat & LaNoue, 2014). Deletion of items can also lead to an incompatibility problem in comparative research. In addition, because the initial process of item generation for the JSE was not based on a preconceived idea of a specified factor structure, it is possible that sufficient number of items were not generated to address the third factor (or any additional factors) to emerge as reliable components.

The psychometric properties of an attribute, such as empathy in patient care, can be a function of several factors including sociocultural, educational, and environmental factors which necessitate a continued effort to examine psychometrics of the JSE in different sociocultural environment, populations, and translated versions of the scale to assure that the psychometric soundness of the JSE can be retained in a variety of settings. Such broad psychometric support would further add to the credibility of the JSE and raise confidence of its users wherever it is applied.

Proxy Norm Data for the S-Version

Data for a large sample of medical students ($n = 2637$) provided an opportunity for exploring the possibility of providing norm data and cutoff scores (Hojat & Gonnella, 2015). Because of the large sample from a large medical school—which is similar to other large medical schools in the USA with regard to its 4-year medical education curriculum, composition of student body, attrition rate, and career choices—the statistics reported in Table 7.7 can serve as proxy norm data for matriculating students in other US medical school under the condition that descriptive statistics and score distributions of the JSE in those medical schools are not substantially different from data reported in Table 7.7. For example, a score of 120 on the JSE obtained by a male matriculant would place him in the 78th percentile, and the same score obtained by a female matriculant would place her in the top 65th percentile of the score distributions.

The score distributions and percentile ranks reported in Table 7.7 can be used as proxy norms for the purpose of comparing individual scores and determining the relative rank for male and female medical school matriculants (assuming that the score distributions and descriptive statistics of the medical school from which the JSE score is being compared are not substantially different from data reported in Table 7.7). For example, the JSE score of a male first-year matriculant to medical school "X" who falls between 131 and 135 would place him in the top 98–99 percentile, and a score of a female first-year matriculant from the same school who falls between 126 and 130 would place her in the 83–95 percentile (assuming similarities in descriptive statistics and score distribution of the JSE in medical school "X" with those reported in Table 7.7).

Tentative Cutoff Scores for the S-Version

For determining tentative cutoff scores for entering medical students to identify the high and low scorers on the JSE, we arbitrarily chose two points on the score distributions: One point was one and half standard deviation above the mean score (to identify the high scorers), and another was one and half standard deviation below the mean score (to identify the low scorers). These cutoff points were separately calculated for men and women. Thus, the cutoff scores for identifying low and high scorers for men were ≤ 96 and ≥ 127, respectively; they were ≤ 102 and ≥ 129, for women. These cutoff scores include approximately 7 % of top scorers and 7 % of bottom scorers in both men's and women's score distributions (Hojat & Gonnella, 2015).

We compared performance measures among high, moderate, and low scorers using the above-mentioned cutoff scores. Results showed a consistent pattern of findings that the low scorers, as compared to the moderate and high scorers, received lower average ratings on clinical competence in six third-year medical school core clerkships (family medicine, internal medicine, obstetrics/gynecology, pediatrics, psychiatry, and surgery) and on the residency program directors' ratings for the factors of the "art" and the "science" of medicine (Hojat, Paskin et al., 2007) given at the end of the first postgraduate training year. However, the results of analysis of variance indicated that the differences, while in the expected direction, were marginally significant for the ratings of clinical competence in the six third-year core clerkships ($F_{(2,2284)} = 2.57$, $p < 0.07$) (Hojat & Gonnella, 2015).

The tentative cutoff scores suggested in this study are not definitive. We need not only more representative samples but also data on well-validated criterion measures to examine the predictive validity of the cutoff scores. We also need more data from representative samples of medical schools at the national level to develop national norm tables and determine cutoff scores for male and female medical school matriculants. Using a similar approach, national norm tables can also be developed for students in other health profession schools, as well as for male and female doctors in different specialties. These ideas set an agenda for future research.

Additional Indicators of Validity of the JSE

The "Contrasted Groups" Method

Other indicators that support the validity of the JSE are based on the notion that a measuring instrument is valid when it can demonstrate group differences or relationships in the expected direction. The expectations are based on previous research, theories, and behavioral tendencies described in the literature. This approach, in which different groups are compared to examine whether the differences in their scores are in the expected direction, is known as validation by the method of "contrasted groups" (Anastasi, 1976).

Expectation of Gender Difference on the JSE Scores in Favor of Women

In a majority of studies, women scored higher than men on measures of empathy (see Chap. 10, and Appendix A). Some authors have suggested that women's behavioral style is generally more "empathizing" than men's style (Baron-Cohen, 2003). Thus, we expected to find a gender difference in favor of women on the JSE scores. Empirical confirmation of this expectation could be regarded as an indicator of the JSE's validity. Consistent with our expectation, in most studies in which the JSE was used, female health professions students and practicing health professionals obtained significantly higher JSE mean scores than their male counterparts. This pattern of gender difference in the JSE scores in favor of women has also been reported in most national and international studies (see Appendix A).

Table 7.10 Gender differences on the JSE scores by matriculating classes

Matriculating class	Men		Women			Effect size[a]
	n	M (SD)	n	M (SD)	t	
2002	120	112.3 (10.1)	101	116.3 (9.3)	3.1**	0.41
2003	105	111.5 (10.8)	113	116.1 (8.6)	3.4**	0.46
2004	103	113.7 (9.6)	121	117.7 (9.6)	3.1**	0.43
2005	126	112.1 (10.2)	121	117.0 (8.6)	4.1**	0.52
2006	107	112.8 (9.2)	140	116.3 (9.3)	3.0**	0.37
2007	132	112.8 (11.7)	116	116.6 (8.6)	2.7**	0.40
2008	120	112.2 (11.9)	117	114.8 (12.3)	1.6***	0.21
2009	111	109.8 (11.5)	128	116.1 (10.3)	4.5**	0.57
2010	124	111.7 (10.8)	128	115.8 (10.4)	3.1**	0.38
2011	125	112.6 (11.0)	127	115.6 (9.0)	2.4*	0.30
2012	128	113.4 (10.9)	124	116.4 (10.2)	2.3*	0.28
Total	1301	112.3 (10.8)	1336	116.2 (9.7)	9.9*	0.40

©2015 Kroger. Reproduced with permission (Hojat & Gonnella, 2015)
Note: $**p < 0.01$, $*p < 0.05$, $***p = 0.10$
[a]Cohen's effect size estimate

In our study of 11 entering classes (between 2002 and 2012) of Jefferson (currently Sidney Kimmel) Medical College (described before in this chapter), we reexamined gender differences on the JSE for each entering class (Hojat & Gonnella, 2015). As reported previously there were 1336 women (51 %) and 1301 (49 %) men in this sample (see Table 7.5). With one exception, women obtained substantially higher mean empathy scores than men in all of our comparisons for different matriculating classes and the differences were statistically significant ($p < 0.01$ by t-test). The exception was the matriculating class of 2008 in which women's higher JSE mean score ($M = 114.8$, $SD = 12.3$) was not significantly different from that for men ($M = 112.2$, $SD = 11.9$) at the conventional level of statistical significance ($t_{(235)} = 1.6$, $p < 0.10$). This is consistent with the previous findings in which the JSE was used (Alcorta-Garza et al., 2005; Fjortoft et al., 2011; Hojat, Mangione, Nasca et al., 2001; Hojat et al., 2002b). The effect size estimates of gender differences varied for different matriculating classes, ranging from a low of 0.21 (for the matriculating class of 2008) to a high of 0.57 (for the matriculating class of 2009). For the entire sample, the effect size estimate was 0.40 (Hojat & Gonnella, 2015). Means and standard deviations of the JSE scores by matriculation year and gender are reported in Table 7.10.

Several plausible explanations have been given for gender differences in empathy, including social learning, genetic predisposition, evolutionary underpinnings, and other factors (Hojat, Mangoine, Nasca et al., 2001; Hojat et al., 2002a, 2002b) (see Chap. 10 for more detailed explanations for gender differences on empathy).

Specialty Interest

Although empathy is the backbone of the patient–clinician relationship in all specialties, there are some specialties that require a higher degree of empathic engagement because of the frequency of encounters, broader consultations, and the provision of continuous care. Based on this notion, some medical education researchers have classified specialties into two broad categories of "people-oriented" and "technology- or procedure-oriented" specialties (Lieu, Schroeder, & Altman, 1989). The so-called people-oriented specialties often require long-term patient-physician relationship with continuous care. The physician–patient relationship often begins as office-based first encounter health or illness appraisals, preventive education or interventions, episodic and long-term comprehensive care of a wide variety of medical problems (e.g., family medicine, general internal medicine, pediatrics), plus obstetrics and gynecology, and psychiatry. The so-called "technology- or procedure-oriented" specialties do not often require long-term continuous care. They primarily involve specialized diagnostic or technical computer-based procedures (e.g., primarily hospital-based specialties such as anesthesiology, pathology, and radiology), and may include specialties that require performing highly skilled and specialized therapeutic techniques or procedures (e.g., surgery and surgical subspecialties), or providing episodic or long-term care of a limited number of medical problems that may include instrumentation and technical interventions with a mix of ambulatory and hospital-based practice (e.g., medical subspecialties such as cardiology, gastroenterology, plus other nonprimary care specialties).

Due to the nature of the patient-physician interpersonal relationship, we expected that those physicians-in-training and in-practice interested in "people-oriented" specialties would outscore those interested in "technology- or procedure-oriented" specialties. Out of 2637 entering medical students in our sample, 75 % ($n = 1979$) specified the specialty they planned to pursue after graduation from medical school (965 were interested in people-oriented, 590 in "technology- or procedure-oriented," and 424 in other specialties). We compared the JSE scores of the three groups by using analysis of covariance to partial out the effect of gender (men = 0, women = 1). Summary results of statistical analysis are reported in Table 7.11.

Consistent with our expectation, those who were interested in pursuing people-oriented specialties obtained a significantly higher JSE mean score ($M = 115.35$) than their classmates who were interested in technology- or procedure-oriented ($M = 112.34$) and other specialties ($M = 114.51$) (adjusted $F_{(2,1973)} = 16.25, p < 0.001$). It is important to notice that the differences observed in this sample of entering medical students who completed the JSE prior to their formal medical education cannot be attributed to their exposure to medical education experiences and training. Instead, the baseline differences can be attributed to a personality attribute developed prior to medical school that prompted some to express interest in different specialties, even though some of these students might change their specialty choice during medical school (Forouzan & Hojat, 1993). The findings regarding higher JSE in those interested in "people-oriented" compared to those interested in

Table 7.11 Means and standard deviations of the JSE by specialty and summary results of analysis of covariance

Specialty	n	M (SD)	F-ratio[a]	p
People oriented[b]	965	115.35 (9.9)	Adjusted $F_{(2,1975)} = 5.79$	<0.001
Technology oriented[c]	590	112.34 (11.02)	Unadjusted $F_{(2,1973)} = 16.25$	<0.01
Other[d]	424	114.51 (10.20)		

[a]Effect of gender was controlled by entering gender as a covariate in statistical analysis. Post hoc mean comparisons showed that technology-oriented<people-oriented; and technology-oriented<other specialties
[b]People-oriented specialties included family medicine, general internal medicine, general pediatrics, obstetrics and gynecology, and psychiatry
[c]Technology-oriented specialties included anesthesiology, pathology, radiology, surgery, and surgical specialties
[d]Other specialties included medical subspecialties, dermatology, emergency medicine, etc.

"technology/procedure-oriented" specialties are in agreement with our previous research findings (Hojat et al., 2002b, Hojat, Zuckerman et al., 2005) and findings reported by others in the USA and abroad (Chen, Lew, Hershman, & Orlander, 2007; Chen, Kirshenbaum, Yan, Kirshenbaum, & Aseltine, 2012; Cheng et al., 2007; Kataoka et al., 2012; Voinescu, Szentagotai, & Coogan, 2009). These findings confirmed our expectation on specialty differences which provide support for the validity of the JSE.

It might be argued that differences in JSE scores at the beginning of medical school could be due to prior undergraduate education. However, in his master's thesis, Smolarz (2005) did not find a significant difference in the JSE scores among first-year medical students who majored in science and non-science disciplines as undergraduates. In other studies with nursing students (Fields et al., 2011; Ward et al., 2009) academic major prior to nursing school did not predict JSE scores in nursing school. Thus, it seems that undergraduate education has no significant link to empathy in health professions students.

Relationships with Relevant Measures (Criterion-Related Validity)

Additional data in support of the validity of the JSE are the positive and significant correlations between scores of the JSE and measures of variables conceptually relevant to empathy, no correlation with measures irrelevant to empathy, and negative correlations with measures of attributes that are conceptually detrimental to empathic engagement. For example, in a study with medical students (Hojat, Zuckerman et al., 2005) we found that the scores on the JSE were significantly and positively correlated with "sociability" scores measured by the short form of the Zuckerman–Kuhlman Personality Questionnaire (ZKPQ) (Zuckerman, 2002).

Empirical evidence showed that a number of personality attributes that are conducive to relationship building, thus relevant to empathy, have been positively correlated with JSE scores including emotional intelligence (Arora et al., 2010; Austin, Evans, Goldwater, & Potter, 2005; Kliszcz, Nowicka-Sauer, Trzeciak, Nowak, & Sadowska, 2006); attitudes toward teamwork and collaboration (Calabrese, Bianco, Mann, Massello, & Hojat, 2013; Van Winkle, Fjortoft, & Hojat, 2012; Ward et al., 2009); desirable professional behavior (Brazeau, Schroeder, Rovi, & Boyd, 2010); therapists' psychological growth (Brockhouse, Msetfi, Cohen, & Joseph, 2011); agreeableness, conscientiousness, extraversion, and openness to experience (Costa et al., 2014); orientation toward integrative patient care (Hojat, Bianco et al., 2015); positive social influence (Hojat, Michalec et al., 2015); peer nomination in clinical and humanistic excellence in medical school (Pohl, Hojat, & Arnold, 2011); patient-centered care (Beattie, Durham, Harvey, Steele, & McHanwell, 2012); friendly and relaxed style of communication (Brown et al., 2011); and cooperativeness and self-directness (Hong, Bahn, Lee, & Moon, 2011).

In a sample of dental students at the University of Washington School of Dentistry, Sherman and Cramer (2005) found positive and significant correlations between scores on the JSE and 18 of 26 measures of attitudes toward clinical competencies. The highest correlation was found between JSE scores and ratings of the following clinical competency: "application of the principles of behavioral sciences that pertain to patient-centered oral health care" ($r = 0.52$).

Furthermore, consistent with views on the effects of early interpersonal relationship experiences on the development of empathy (see Chap. 4) we observed that higher levels of self-reported satisfaction with the early maternal relationship (an indication of a secure mother-child attachment) and satisfactory peer relationships in school (an indication of social skills) were significantly associated with higher scores on the JSE (Hojat, Zuckerman et al., 2005).

Conversely, scores of the JSE yielded negative correlations with personality attributes that are detrimental to positive interpersonal relationship such as measure of aggression-hostility (Hasan, Babar, Chen, Ahmed, & Mitha, 2013); indicators of burnout such as depersonalization and emotional exhaustion (Hojat, Vergare, Isenberg, Cohen, & Spandorfer, 2015; Lamothe, Boujut, Zenasni, & Sultan, 2014); and harm and avoidance (Hong et al., 2011). In our own study (Hojat, Zuckerman et al., 2005), we obtained a significantly negative correlation between the scores on the JSE and the Aggression-Hostility scale of the ZKPQ (Zuckerman, 2002).

In his doctoral dissertation, Reisetter (2003) reported significant correlations between JSE factor scores and subscale scores of the Physician Belief Scale (PBS) (Ashworth, Williamson, & Montano, 1984; McLellan, Jansen-McWilliams, Comer, Gardner, & Kelleher, 1999). For example, a negative correlation ($r = -0.30$) was found between the JSE "Standing in the Patient's Shoes" factor scores of the JSE and the PBS "Burden" subscale (defined as the difficulties perceived by the clinician in addressing the client's psychosocial problems). However, in this study, the correlation between the "Compassionate Care" factor scores of the JSE and the "Belief and Feeling" subscale of the PBS (defined as the clinician's concern about his or her ability to address the client's psychosocial problems) was significant and positive ($r = 0.50$).

Correlations Between Scores on the JSE and the IRI

In a study involving 93 residents in internal medicine at Thomas Jefferson University Hospital (Hojat, Mangione, Kane, & Gonnella, 2005), we examined the relationships between total scores and factor scores (Perspective Taking, Compassionate Care, and Standing in the Patient's Shoes) on the HP-Version and the IRI (see Chap. 5) total and four scale scores (Perspective Taking, Empathic Concern, Fantasy, and Personal Distress). In a study by Yarnold, Bryant, Nightingale, and Martin (1996), it was found that the Perspective Taking and Empathic Concern scales of the IRI were likely to measure empathy, whereas the Personal Distress and Fantasy subscales were likely to measure sympathy. We assumed that the IRI's Perspective Taking and Empathic Concern scales were more relevant to the clinician–patient relationship than were the Personal Distress and Fantasy scales. Therefore, we expected significant but moderate correlations between the JSE total and factor scores and scores on the IRI total and its Perspective Taking and Empathic Concern subscales. Conversely, we expected to obtain trivial correlations between scores on the JSE (and its factors) and scores on the IRI's Personal Distress and Fantasy subscales. A summary of the results is reported in Table 7.12.

As expected, the correlations between scores on the IRI Personal Distress scale on the one hand, and total and factor scores on the JSE on the other hand, were all nonsignificant. Scores on the IRI Fantasy scale yielded modest correlations with scores on the JSE's Perspective Taking and Compassionate Care subscales ($r = 0.24$, $p < 0.05$, and $r = 0.37$, $p < 0.01$, respectively). The highest correlations were found between the scores on the IRI Empathic Concern scale and the JSE Compassionate Care and Perspective Taking factors ($r = 0.41$, $p < 0.01$, and $r = 0.40$, $p < 0.01$, respectively). The correlation between the scores on the perspective taking dimensions of both instruments was $r = 0.35$ ($p < 0.01$), and the correlation between the total scores on the two instruments was $r = 0.45$ ($p < 0.01$).

Table 7.12 Correlations between scores on the JSE and the IRI ($N = 93$ first-year internal medicine residents)

IRI subscales	JSPE factors			
	Perspective taking	Compassionate care	Standing in patient's shoes	Total score
Perspective taking	0.35**	0.31**	0.17	0.40**
Empathic concern	0.40**	0.41**	0.16	0.48**
Fantasy	0.24*	0.37**	0.12	0.35**
Personal distress	0.01	0.02	0.13	0.02
Total score	0.34**	0.40**	0.22*	0.45**

©2005 *Medical Teacher.* Reproduced with permission (Hojat et al., 2005)
*$p < 0.05$; **$p < 0.01$

Therefore, our expectation was confirmed regarding significant correlations of moderate magnitude between total and factor scores on the JSE and scores on the Perspective Taking and Empathic Concern scales of the IRI. Furthermore, our prediction about the lack of relationship between the scores on the JSE and the scores on the IRI Personal Distress subscale was correct (Hojat, Mangione et al., 2005).

Scores on the JSE, Academic Performance, and Clinical Competence

We expected to find a positive and significant relationship between medical students' scores on the S-Version of the JSE and global ratings of their clinical competence in core clinical clerkships. The reason for this expectation was that an ability to communicate with patients and understand their concerns is often considered when assessing global clinical competence. Our expectation was confirmed in a study with third-year medical students in which we found that students with higher scores on the JSE S-Version obtained better ratings of clinical competence than did classmates with lower JSE scores (Hojat, Gonnella, Mangione, Nasca, Veloski et al., 2002).

The lack of convincing evidence precluded a hypothesis that performance on objective (multiple-choice) tests of acquisition of knowledge should be associated with empathy scores. Therefore, we did not expect such an association and, indeed, did not find one (Hojat, Gonnella, Mangione, Nasca, Veloski et al., 2002). Our findings were consistent with those of other researchers (Diseker & Michielutte, 1981; Hornblow, Kidson, & Jones, 1977; Kupfer, Drew, Curtis, & Rubinstein, 1978).

Scores on the JSE and Patient Outcomes

Because the ultimate purpose of medical and all other health professions education is optimal patient outcome, the ultimate criterion measure for the validity of any measure of empathy in patient care should include tangible patient outcome, independent of patients' subjective judgment. In two studies that I will describe in more detail in Chap. 11, we found significant associations between physicians scores on the JSE, and clinical outcomes in diabetic patients. In the first study in the USA (Hojat, Louis, Markham et al., 2011) we showed that physicians with higher JSE scores compared to their counterparts with lower JSE scores had a higher proportion of patients whose disease was under control (evident by the results of medical test such as A1c < 7.0 %, and LDL-C < 100, extracted from patients' electronic records). In another study in Italy (Del Canale et al., 2012), statistically significant associations were found between physicians' scores on the JSE and rates of hospitalization due to metabolic complications (e.g., diabetic ketoacidosis, coma, and hyperosmolar). Findings of these two studies provide undeniable evidence in support of validity of the JSE in predicting clinical outcomes.

Administration and Scoring

All three versions of the JSE can be administered either individually or in groups. Half the items are directly scored according to their Likert weights (1 = Strongly disagree, 7 = Strongly agree) and the other half are reverse scored (1 = Strongly agree, 7 = Strongly disagree). We recommend handling missing data by using the following guidelines: if a respondent fails to answer more than 20 % of the items (four items), the scale should be regarded as incomplete and be excluded from the data analysis. In the case of a respondent with four or fewer unanswered items, we recommend replacing each missing value with the mean score calculated from items completed by the respondent. The scale is "untimed" and takes approximately 5–10 min to complete. We do not recommend a strict time limit for completing the scale.

To assure integrity in scoring and statistical analyses, we have developed scoring instructions that we share with users and strongly encourage them to follow the instructions, and use the text of the items and the order of appearance of the items intact, as well as the 7-point Likert scale for meaningful comparisons of the findings. Also, scannable forms of the three versions of the JSE have been developed and have been used by researchers and processed at our center for scoring and other statistical analyses (information is posted at http://www.jefferson.edu/university/skmc/research/research-medical-education/jefferson-scale-of-empathy.html). Web-based administration of the scale is also available.

A Brief Scale to Measure Patient Perceptions of Physician Empathy

To investigate the relationship between physicians' self-reported scores on the JSE and their patients' perceptions, we developed a brief scale to measure patients' perceptions of physicians' empathic orientation and behavior. Patients complete the Jefferson Scale of Patient Perceptions of Physician Empathy (JSPPPE) (Appendix E) to assess their physician's empathy.

The JSPPPE is a brief scale, containing five Likert-type items that patients can answer in a few minutes after an encounter with a physician or a health care professional. For example, a physician's concern regarding a patient and the patient's family is reflected in the following item: "This physician seems concerned about me and my family." The physician's perspective taking is reflected by the following item: "This physician can view things from my perspective (see things as I see them)." In a study conducted by Kane, Gotto, Mangione, West, and Hojat (2007a, 2007b) with residents in an internal medicine program and in another study by Glaser and colleagues with residents in a family medicine program (Glaser et al., 2007), scores on this scale correlated significantly with selected items from the Physicians' Humanistic Behaviors Questionnaire developed by Weaver, Ow, Walker, and Degenhardt (1993) and also with selected items from a questionnaire measuring patients' appraisal of physicians' performance developed by Matthews and Feinstein (1989).

In the two aforementioned studies of the JSPPPE conducted at Thomas Jefferson University Hospital, data for 225 encounters between patients and resident physicians in the internal medicine residency program (Kane et al., 2007) and 90 encounters between patients and residents in the family medicine residency program (Glaser, Markham, Adler, McManus, & Hojat, 2007) were used. Item–total score correlations of the JSPPPE were statistically significant in both departments (median correlations were 0.78 for family medicine and 0.81 for internal medicine). The item and total scores on the JSPPPE in the Department of Internal Medicine study also yielded significant correlations with scores obtained from a rating form for patients developed by the American Board of Internal Medicine to assess physicians' communicative skills, humanistic qualities, and professionalism (Lipner, Blank, Leas, & Fortna, 2002). The median correlation between the two instruments was 0.64. The internal consistency reliabilities (coefficient alphas) of the patient perceptions scale were in the lower range (0.50s).

In a more recent study with 535 outpatients treated by family physicians (Hojat, Louis et al., 2010), we found that the JSPPPE is a unidimensional scale based on the results of EFA, a finding that was previously reported in another study (Kane et al., 2007). Corrected item-total score correlations of the JSPPPE ranged from 0.88 to 0.94. Cronbach's alpha coefficient ranged from 0.97 to 0.99 for the total sample, and for patients in different gender and age groups (Hojat, Louis et al., 2010) (see Table 7.13). Scores on the JSPPPE were highly correlated with measures of physician–patient trusting relationships ($r > 0.73$). Also, correlation between scores of the JSPPPE and a measure of patient overall satisfaction with the primary care physician (Hojat, Louis et al., 2010) was 0.93 (see Table 7.14).

In addition, we found that higher scores on the JSPPPE were predictive of patients' compliance with their physicians' recommendations (compliance rates >80 %) for preventive care (e.g., colonoscopy for male and female patients, mammogram for female patients, and PSA for male patients) (Hojat, Louis et al., 2010).

The correlation coefficient between patients' ratings of their physicians on the patient perceptions scale and the residents' self-reported empathy (JSE scores) was 0.48 ($p < 0.05$) in the family medicine study (Glaser et al., 2007), but it was only 0.24 (nonsignificant) in the internal medicine study (Kane et al., 2007). Further inspection of data for the Department of Internal Medicine showed that the majority of patients (78 %) gave the highest possible scores to the residents, leading to a highly skewed JSPPPE score distribution with a restricted range of scores. This serious "ceiling effect" would not allow the correlation between residents' self-reported empathy and patients' perceptions of residents' empathy to be fully captured.

In a study of psychiatry residents in Iran who completed the JSE and their standardized patients who completed the JSPPPE (Esfahani, Behzadipour, Nadoushan, & Shariat, 2014), a moderate correlation between the JSE and JSPPPE was observed ($r = 0.39$) which was not statistically significant, probably due to a small sample size according to the study's authors. Consistent with these findings, it was also discovered that although the relationship between physicians' self-report measures of

Table 7.13 Factor coefficients of the Jefferson Scale of Patient Perceptions of Physician Empathy, item-total score correlations, and correlations of each item with scores of patient satisfaction and recommendation ($n = 535$)

Items	Factor coefficients[a]	Item-total score[b]	Patient satisfaction[c]	Recommendation[d]
1. My doctor understands my emotions, feelings, and concerns	0.93	0.94	0.87	0.80
2. My doctor is an understanding doctor	0.92	0.93	0.95	0.89
3. My doctor seems concerned about me and my family	0.92	0.93	0.87	0.82
4. My doctor asks about what is happening in my daily life	0.88	0.91	0.80	0.73
5. My doctor can view things from my perspective (see things as I see them)	0.84	0.88	0.79	0.74

©2010 *International Journal of Medical Education*. Reproduced with permission (Hojat, Louis, Maxwell et al., 2010)
[a]Items are reported by descending order of factor coefficients
[b]Correlation between scores of the item and the rest of the scale
[c]Correlation between scores of the item and scores on the Jefferson Scale of Patient Satisfaction (Hojat, Louis et al., 2010)
[d]Correlation between scores of the item and responses to this anchor item: "I would recommend my doctor to my family and friends"

Table 7.14 Concurrent validity coefficients of the Jefferson Scale of Patient Perceptions of Physician Empathy and criterion measures of patient–physician interpersonal trust by patients' gender and age

	Gender		Age		
Criterion measures	Men ($n = 174$)	Women ($n = 355$)	<56 ($n = 266$)	≥56 ($n = 269$)	Total ($n = 535$)
Patient overall satisfaction with physician[a]	0.94	0.93	0.96	0.90	0.93
I would recommend my doctor to my family and friends	0.88	0.86	0.91	0.80	0.87
My doctor listens carefully to me	0.88	0.91	0.96	0.84	0.91
My doctor spends sufficient time with me	0.79	0.80	0.85	0.75	0.80
My doctor really cares about me as a person	0.93	0.85	0.89	0.87	0.88
I would like my doctor to be present in any medical emergency situation	0.73	0.78	0.80	0.73	0.77
I am satisfied that my doctor has been taking care of me	0.86	0.86	0.90	0.83	0.87

©2010 *International Journal of Medical Education*. Reproduced with permission (Hojat, Louis, Maxwell et al., 2010)
[a]Scores on the Jefferson Scale of Patient Overall Satisfaction with Primary Care physician

empathy (measured by the Hogan's Empathy Scale) and patients' evaluations was positive, it was statistically nonsignificant (Linn et al., 1987). It is interesting to note from the aforementioned findings that the associations between physicians' or medical students' self-reported empathy (JSE scores), and real or standardized patients' perceptions of clinicians' empathy (JSPPPE scores), were mostly moderate or negligible. However, correlations between patients' assessment of clinicians' empathy (JSPPPE scores) and patients' global assessments of clinicians' competence and empathy were found to be larger in magnitude (Grosseman, Hojat et al., 2014; Grosseman, Novack et al., 2014). A possibility exists that patients' views regarding their clinicians' empathic behavior may differ from the clinicians' views of their own empathy. Grosseman and her colleagues raised a question about some physicians' ability to gauge or to communicate their empathic engagement with patients. Further research is needed to explore these and other possibilities.

The link between physicians' self-reported empathy and patients' perceptions of their physicians' empathy could also be strengthened by physicians' efforts to communicate their understanding to their patients (Free, Green, Grace, Chernus, & Whitman, 1985). Measuring patients' perceptions is important because research has shown that their perceptions of clinicians' empathy yield the highest correlations with clinical outcomes, followed by observers' ratings of clinicians' empathy and, finally, by clinicians' self-reported empathy (Bohart, Elliot, Greenberg, & Watson, 2002). Because other factors can contribute to patients' perceptions of clinicians' empathy, including the degree to which patients can cope with their illnesses (Mercer, Watt, & Reilly, 2001), more studies are needed to examine the complex reasons for patients' and clinicians' concordant and discordant views on empathic engagement in clinical encounters.

The associations between clinicians' self-reported empathy and patients' perception of clinician empathy may be confounded by gender and ethnicity. For example, in a few recent studies, standardized patients assessed medical students' empathic engagement by completing the JSPPPE in Objective Structured Clinical Examination (OSCE) stations. Findings showed statistically significant associations between scores of the JSPPPE (completed by standardized patients) and scores of medical students' self-reported empathy (measured by the JSE) (Berg et al., 2015; Berg, Majdan, Berg, Veloski, & Hojat, 2011a, 2011b). However, we noticed that students' gender and ethnicity (Berg et al., 2011b) and their interactions could confound the relationships between self-reported empathy in medical students (measured by the JSE) and standardized patients' assessments of medical students' empathy as measured by the JSPPPE (Berg et al., 2015).

Broad National and International Attention

Over the years, we have been receiving increasing requests from researchers in the USA and abroad for copies of the JSE and for permission to use it. The JSE has enjoyed broad international attention and it has been described as "possibly the

Box 7.2: Translations of the Jefferson Scale of Empathy

Arabic	HP[a]	Lithuanian	HP[a], HPS
Bengali	S[a]	Malay	HPS
Bulgarian	HP[a]	Nepali	S
Catalan	S[a]	Norwegian	HP[a], and S
Chinese	(Simplified), HP[a]	Persian (Farsi)	HP[a] and S[a]
Chinese	(Mainland), HP and S[a]	Polish	HP[a] and S[a]
	(Taiwan), HP[a], S[a], and HPS[a]	Portuguese	(Portugal), HP[a] and S[a]
Croatian	S[a]		(Brazil), HP and S[a]
Czech	HP[a] and S[a]	Romanian	HP[a] and S[a]
Danish	HP[a]	Russian	HP[a]
Dutch	(Flemish, Belgium), S[a]		(Uzbekistan) HP
	(Dutch, The Netherlands), HP and S	Serbian	HP[a], S[a], and HPS[a]
Filipino	HP[a]	Sinhalese	(Sri Lanka) S[a]
Finnish	HP[a], S[a], and HPS[a]	Slovenian	S[a]
French	(Belgium), HP[a]	Spanish	S
	(Canada), HP[a]		(Argentina) HP[a]
	(France), HP[a]		(Chile), HP[a] and S[a]
	(Switzerland) S[a]		(Mexico), HP[a] and S[a]
German	HP[a] and S[a]		(Peru), S[a]
Greek	HP[a]		(Spain), S[a]
Hebrew	HP, S[a]	Swedish	HP
Hindi	HP[a]	Tagalog (Philippines)	HP[a]
Hungarian	HP[a] and S[a]	Tamil (Sri Lanka)	S[a]
Indonesian	HP[a] and S[a]	Thai	HP[a] and S[a]
Italian	HP[a], S[a], and HPS[a]	Turkish	HP[a], S[a], and HPS
Japanese	HP[a], S[a], and HPS[a]	Urdu (Pakistan)	HP and S
Korean	HP[a] and S[a]		

HP health professions/physician version, *S* medical student version, *HPS* health professions student version
[a]PDF available

most researched and widely used instrument in medical education" (Colliver, Conlee, Verhulst, & Dorsey, 2010a, 2010b, p. 1813). As of this writing, we have received a large number of requests from the USA and other countries (see Box 7.2) for information about using the scale, and the JSE has already been translated into 53 languages (see Box 7.3). To ensure the accuracy of translations, we have always strongly recommended using the back-translation procedure (Brislin, 1970; Guillemin, Bombardier, & Beaton, 1993; Geisinger, 1994) to all those who asked us to grant permission to translate the JSE.

Findings from National and International Studies. Interestingly, our findings have been replicated by many other researchers. The patterns of findings of most of

Box 7.3: Interest to Use the Jefferson Scale of Empathy Worldwide

Africa	Algeria	Europe	Albania	Middle East	Iran
	Ghana		Austria		Iraq
	Malawi		Belgium		Israel
	Nigeria		Bulgaria		Jordan
	Rwanda		Croatia		Kuwait
	South Africa		Czech Republic		Lebanon
	Tunisia		Cyprus		Pakistan
			Denmark		Qatar
Asia	Bangladesh		England		Saudi Arabia
	Brunei		Finland		Turkey
	China		France		United Arab Emirates
	India		Germany		
	Indonesia		Greece	North/	Canada
	Japan		Hungary	Central	Costa Rica
	Malaysia		Ireland	America	Guatemala
	Nepal		Italy		Mexico
	Philippines		Latvia		St. Maarten
	Russia		Lithuania		Trinidad and Tobago
	Singapore		Norway		United States
	South Korea		Poland		
	Sri Lanka		Portugal	Oceania	Australia
	Taiwan		Romania		New Zealand
	Thailand		Scotland		
	Uzbekistan		Serbia	South	Argentina
			Slovenia	America	Brazil
			Spain		Chile
			Sweden		Columbia
			Switzerland		Ecuador
			The Netherlands		Peru
			United Kingdom		Uruguay
					Venezuela

the studies in the USA and other countries are similar to those we have reported in our own studies (see Appendix A). The increasing national and international attention to the JSE is reflected in the 189 annotated publications listed in Appendix A. An overall review of findings of the annotated studies in Appendix A provides strong evidence in support of psychometric soundness of the three versions of the JSE in different samples of the health profession students and practitioners, in a variety of health professions disciplines, and in different countries with different educational systems and cultural values. Consistencies in most of the major findings in those studies are amazing. For example, findings generally show that reliability coefficients of the JSE, reflected in the Cronbach's alpha coefficients, in almost all of those studies are in the 0.70s and 0.80s (M=0.78), a well-acceptable range for psychological tests. Also, in most exploratory factor analytic studies of the JSE (reported in Appendix A), three factors of "Perspective Taking," "Compassionate Care," and "Standing in the Patient's Shoes" have emerged, sometimes in different order; and the three-factor model has been confirmed in a number of the confirmatory factor analytic studies.

In many of the studies reported in Appendix A, the mean scores of different versions of the JSE (when there is no remedial/education intervention) hover around 112 (standard deviations hover around 12); and in most of those studies, women outscored men in different versions of the JSE. In addition, in most of those studies with health profession students in the USA, a decline of empathy has been observed during the course of medical and health professions education, particularly at a point in training when curriculum shifts toward the clinical phase that involves patient contact when empathy is most needed. Also, in most of the experimental programs which were developed to enhance empathy, an increase in the JSE mean scores has been observed in the health professions students who were exposed to or participated in the targeted educational programs (see Appendix A). However, in none of the studies with follow-up data were the enhanced empathy scores sustained for a longer time without additional reinforcement.

Information reported in Appendix A and further expansion of the scope of the studies in which the JSE has been used provide a unique opportunity for meta-analytic studies for graduate students' masters theses, or doctoral dissertations, and researchers interested in the topic of empathy in health professions education and in patient care. We hope that in the future, a large and valuable central data bank and a number of meta-analytic studies will be undertaken to summarize findings from different samples, professions, and countries on correlates of empathy in the context of health professions education and patient care, on effective approaches to enhance and sustain empathy among health professions students and practitioners, group differences, changes in empathy as students progress through professional training, etc.

Two Caveats

Attitudes, Orientation, Capacity, and Behavior

When we submitted manuscripts describing the results of our empathy studies to peer-reviewed journals, a few reviewers expressed a legitimate concern about the link between physicians' scores on the JSE and their actual empathic behavior in patient care. If one assumes that the physicians' scores on the JSE indeed reflect their own attitude or orientation toward empathy in physician–patient relationships, and not necessarily their empathic behavior, a convincing argument plus empirical data are needed to establish a link between attitudes and behavior.

Although social psychologists have long debated the link between attitude and behavior, the issue has not been completely settled yet (for a meta-analytic review, see Wallace, Paulson, Lord, & Bond, 2005). When people have formed an attitude or an orientation toward a subject, they are no longer neutral about that subject. In other words, they are likely to take a stand or develop a behavioral tendency consistent with their attitude or orientation (Sherif, Sherif, & Nebergall, 1965). Attitude, orientation, and perception share common cognitive and neural elements that can activate relevant behavior (Prinz, 1997; Viviani, 2002). A concordance between an attitude and behavior is necessary to avoid an unpleasant psychological tension that resembles "cognitive dissonance" (Festinger, 1964), which occurs when a person is caught in a cognitive struggle between opposing motivational forces. Cognitive dissonance research has established that when individuals perform a behavior or make a choice that conflicts with a previously established attitude, the attitude tends to change in the direction that resolves the conflict with the behavior. This process appears to involve rationalization, whereby individuals strategically change their attitudes in order to avoid appearing inconsistent (Lieberman & Matthew, 2007).

Attitudes often generate strong emotions (affective components) and form a cognitive orientation (cognitive components) leading to preferences that ultimately elicit actions (behavioral components) (Rosenberg & Hovland, 1960). Therefore, attitudes, orientations, beliefs, and intentions are all motivating forces that can elicit corresponding behaviors (Fishbein & Ajzen, 1975). For example, acculturation studies have reported that attitudinal changes, even in relation to deeply rooted social institutions, such as marriage and the family, can lead to tangible behavioral changes, such as increased rates of marital discord and divorce (Hojat, Shapurian et al., 2000; Hojat, Shapurian et al., 1999). An abundance of empirical studies have been published about hostile or hateful behaviors resulting from prejudicial attitudes toward members of the opposite sex and toward racial, ethnic, and religious groups. For corroborative proof of such behaviors, one only needs to consult a daily newspaper.

In a recent meta-analysis of 797 studies (Wallace et al., 2005), it was found that the mean of attitude–behavior correlations was 0.41, but the magnitude of the relationship varied, depending on social pressure and perceived difficulty. Considering that the average effect of only 0.21 was found in an analysis of more than 25,000 studies of eight million research participants in social psychology (Richard, Bond, & Stokes-Zoota, 2003), the aforementioned attitude–behavior correlation ($r = 0.41$) seems impressive. These findings suggest that forming an empathic attitude, possessing the capacity to understand others, or developing a tendency or an orientation toward empathic relationships do not necessarily ensure empathic behavior. What is certain, however, is that a higher degree of empathic attitude, tendency, orientation, or capacity will increase the likelihood that these qualities will be manifested as empathic behavior under certain conditions. All measures of empathy, including the JSE, are at best a proxy of empathic behavior. Validity evidence would indicate the extent to which these measures are predictive of actual empathic behavior and optimal clinical outcomes.

Transparency and Social Desirability Response Bias

Respondents can always manipulate their answers on self-report personality tests to produce a more socially desirable result. Edwards (1957), who was the first to systematically study the "social desirability phenomenon," believed that respondents were likely to be unaware of the tendency to show themselves in the most socially acceptable light.

Because most items in the JSE are transparent and thus susceptible to social desirability response bias, they can be answered in a way that is recognized as more socially acceptable. Constructing socially neutral items that measure personal attributes, such as empathy, is difficult to develop, and raises questions about not only the face and content validities of such items but the empirical validity of the test as well. For example, the relevance to empathy of nontransparent items, such as those about an interest in literature and the arts or a sense of humor (used in the JSE), is not necessarily apparent. Indeed, some peer reviewers who evaluated the manuscripts we submitted to professional journals questioned the reasons for including those items in the JSE. (The reasons for including those items were discussed earlier in this chapter.)

The degree to which socially desirable responses to items have a confounding effect on test scores could be a function of the test taker's belief in testing outcomes. For example, when testing is used to screen applicants for employment or college admission, test takers may be more inclined to provide socially acceptable answers to test items that will increase their advantage.

In response to concerns about the possible effect of socially desirable responses in our empathy studies, we offer three explanations. First, the JSE has been administered in "nonpenalizing" situations where the purpose was described as research, not college admission or employment. Respondents were assured that their responses would be confidential and would be used only for research purposes approved by the Institutional Review Board's Research Ethics Committee. This assurance, in itself, could reduce respondents' tendency to give socially desirable responses.

Second, the pattern of relationships in our validity studies, particularly the convergent and discriminant validities (described previously in this chapter), suggests that social desirability response bias, even if operative, did not substantially distort the expected relationships. For example, we observed that the magnitude of the correlation between the JSE scores and a more relevant concept, such as compassion, was twice the magnitude of the correlation between JSE scores and a less relevant concept, such as personal growth (see Table 7.2). Such a correlational pattern would be unlikely to emerge in the presence of the significant confounding effects of social desirability response bias.

Third, we conducted an empirical study to investigate the influence of faking "good impression" responses on the JSE scores (Hojat, Zuckerman et al., 2005). In that study, we administered the JSE and other personality tests, including the ZKPQ, to 422 first-year medical students who matriculated at Jefferson Medical

College. The ZKPQ includes an "Infrequency" scale that was developed to detect intentionally false responses by identifying respondents with an invalid pattern of responses (Zuckerman, 2002). A sample item is "I never saw a person I didn't like." Scores on this scale can be regarded as indicators of social desirability response bias. Attempts to give socially desirable responses were determined by a cutoff score of three, which the test's authors suggested would identify respondents whose patterns of responses were of questionable validity. An examination of the distribution of scores on this scale indicated that less than 5 % of the respondents attempted to give false "good impression" responses or to respond carelessly without regard for the truth (Zuckerman, 2002). The hypothesis that social desirability would not distort the validity of the JSE scores in nonpenalizing testing situations was tested and confirmed.

We recently replicated that study by using a large sample ($n = 2637$) of first-year students who matriculated at Jefferson (currently Sidney Kimmel) Medical College between 2002 and 2013 and completed the JSE and the ZKPQ. In this recent study (unpublished), we found that approximately 6 % of respondents ($n = 169$) attempted to give "good impression" responses determined by their score of 3 or higher on the Infrequency scale of the ZKPQ, which is close to the 5 % figure found in our previous study (Hojat, Zuckerman et al., 2005). We used two approaches to examine the possible effects of social desirability response bias on the outcomes of our research on the JSE. First, we conducted two different sets of statistical analyses. In one set, we included all students in the sample, and in another set we excluded those who according to their scores (≥ 3) on the Infrequency scale attempted to give socially desirable or "good impression" responses. Analyses of data regarding the relationship between scores on the JSE and on scores of the five scales of the ZKPQ clearly demonstrated that research outcomes remained virtually unchanged whether or not respondents who responded carelessly to the instrument were included or excluded in statistical analyses. This finding was expected because of the small proportion of respondents in the sample who scored above the cutoff score of the Infrequency scale. These results also suggest that the magnitude of such descriptive statistics as the mean and median is unlikely to be inflated as a result of respondents' possible faking in nonthreatening testing conditions because of the small proportion of those who scored above the cutoff score.

Second, we used the analysis of covariance (ANCOVA) method to control the effect of giving false responses on the research outcomes by using the "Infrequency" score as a covariate (JSE scores as the dependent variable, gender and scores on the scale of the ZKPQ as the independent variables). Again, we noted no substantial change in the general pattern of results with or without control for social desirability. These findings generally suggest that social desirability response bias does not distort the validity of the JSE scores at least under nonthreatening testing conditions.

These findings were consistent with the results of an earlier study on the heritability of empathy by Matthews, Batson, Horn, and Rosenman (1981), who reported that their derived index of empathy was not affected by social desirability response bias or by scores on a "good impression" scale. Two other studies reported no significant correlations between empathy scores obtained on the Emotional Empathy

Scale and social desirability response bias (Mehrabian & Epstein, 1972; Mehrabian & O'Reilly, 1980). Despite these findings, the confounding effects of giving false "good impression" responses and attempting to present a socially acceptable image in penalizing testing situations (e.g., by applicants for college admission or employment) need to be addressed in further studies.

Recapitulation

The JSE was developed in response to a need for a psychometrically sound instrument specifically designed to measure empathy in the context of health professions education and patient care. Evidence reported in this chapter in support of the validity and reliability of the three versions of the JSE for administration to medical students (S-Version), practicing health professionals (HP-Version), and health professions students other than medical students (HPS-Versions) in a variety of settings in different countries can add to our confidence in using the JSE in studies on empathy among students and practitioners in the health professions.

Chapter 8
The Interpersonal Dynamics in Clinician–Patient Relationships

It is difficult to hate the people with whom you empathize.

—(Walter Stephan & Krystina Finlay, 1999, p. 736)

By far, the most frequently used drug in general practice was the doctor. It was not only the bottle of medicine or the box of pills that mattered, but the way doctor gave them.

—(Michael Balint, 1957, p. 1)

Abstract

- Factors that contribute to interpersonal dynamics in patient care are described, and it is proposed that patients as well as clinicians can benefit from empathic engagement.
- The curing versus caring paradigm and the concept of disease versus illness contribute to the development of attitudes that influence empathic behavior in clinical encounters.
- Certain interpersonal dynamics operate in clinician–patient encounters, including a tendency to bind with others for survival, to comply with the orders of authority figures, and to uncritically accept authority figures, and role expectations as well as clinical environment.
- Important facets of interpersonal psychodynamics and their impact on empathic understanding in clinical encounters are described, and the placebo effect of empathic relationships, cultural factors, personal space, and boundaries in clinician–patient encounters is also discussed.
- Emphasis is placed on how listening with the "third ear" and seeing with the "mind's eye" can enhance empathic understanding in the context of patient care.

Introduction

In Chap. 4, in the general context of human relationships, I described factors that contribute to the development of empathic understanding. This chapter describes the interpersonal dynamics specifically involved in clinical encounters. The way a clinician encounters patients can make a significant difference in patient outcomes.

© Springer International Publishing Switzerland 2016
M. Hojat, *Empathy in Health Professions Education and Patient Care*,
DOI 10.1007/978-3-319-27625-0_8

In support of this notion, Houston (1938) indicated that physicians are themselves therapeutic agents through which cures are affected. The "goodness of the physician" was viewed as a therapeutic agent by Hippocrates, who suggested in the fourth century B.C. that "the patient, though conscious that his condition is perilous, may recover his health simply through his contentment with the goodness of the physician" (cited in DiMatteo, 1979, p. 14).

The moments of understanding and connectedness in clinical encounters, according to Matthews, Suchman, and Branch (1993, p. 973), "[are] often marked by physiological reactions such as gooseflesh or a chill; by an immediacy of awareness of the patient's situation (as if experiencing it from inside the patient's world), by a sense of being part of a larger whole; and by a lingering feeling of joy, peacefulness, or awe. Such moments seem to be therapeutic for the patient and the clinician alike."

Matthews et al. (1993) referred to this powerful interpersonal dynamic, which is beneficial for both clinician and patient, as a "connexion" ("co" for "being together" and "nexus" for "to form a whole") to indicate that the interpersonal dynamics in clinician–patient encounters generate a totality that is greater than the sum of its parts. The importance of empathic relationships in clinician–patient encounters has been discussed in the medical literature (Bylund & Makoul, 2002; Platt & Keller, 1994; Spiro, McCrea Curnen, Peschel, & St. James, 1993; Squier, 1990; Winefield & Chur-Hansen, 2000), and the positive effect of empathy in patient outcomes has been confirmed (see Chap. 10).

In antiquity, medicine was primarily a "craft" (Lewis, 1998), and it was an art when practiced by Greek healers (many of whom were unable to read and write). Medicine was not based on the sciences (mathematics and philosophy in those days); it was based on observation, insight, tradition, and, most importantly, interpersonal relationships (Lewis, 1998).

As Rachel Lewinsohn (1998, p. 1268) rightly stated: "We cannot understand the disease without understanding the patient." The clinician cannot fully understand the patient without entering into the patient's world on the bridge of empathy. Empathy in patient care is bidirectional, affecting both the clinician and the patient. Because of the intrinsic reward associated with establishing a meaningful relationship with others, both clinician and patient can benefit from forming an empathic engagement. However, research attention on the beneficial effects of empathy has focused almost exclusively on the patient's side of the equation; the clinician's side has been the victim of benign neglect.

Benefits of Empathic Relationships for Clinicians

From the perspective of personal life, medicine and other health care professions, although intrinsically self-rewarding, are stressful and often demand a lifestyle that restricts participation in social and family events. Such restrictions can contribute to the discontent of healers who themselves need to be healed. Despite these problems, the good news is that clinicians' satisfaction with their relationships with patients can serve as a buffer against the professional stress, burnout, substance abuse, and even suicide attempts that are reported to be unusually high among health professionals (Sullivan, 1990).

Physicians are not invincible, and research indicates that they are vulnerable to a number of psychosocial problems. For example, physicians are more than twice as likely as the general population to commit suicide (Miller & McGowen, 2000), and divorce rates also are higher among physicians than they are in the general population (Sotile & Sotile, 1996). Research indicates that physicians often do not practice what they preach to their own patients and sometimes are reluctant to seek medical help (Forsythe, Calnan, & Wall, 1999). It is important to note that Miller and McGowen (2000) discovered that physicians who enjoyed the support of social networks (e.g., spouse, family, friends, and acquaintances) were less likely to abuse drugs or to suffer from burnout.

Because physicians often perceive empathic relationships with patients as meaningful interpersonal connections, those relationships can serve as a buffer against dissatisfaction with the health care system and professional burnout. Human life is lived in relationships (Lewis, 1998); thus, physician–patient relationships provide an intrinsically joyful reward that serves as a remedy for the stress of a demanding profession (Zuger, 2004). Empathy has been identified as a protective factor against the stress experienced by clinicians (Shamasundar, 1999) and as a potential factor for their well-being (Hyyppa, Kronholm, & Mattlar, 1991).

Executive physicians who treated patients expressed more satisfaction and happiness with their careers than did executive physicians who did not have an opportunity to treat patients (O'Conner, Nash, Buehler, & Bard, 2002). However, it should be mentioned that the relationship between physicians' satisfaction and number of encounters with patients is not linear after a certain saturation point; too large a patient load was likely to result in distress (Dunstone & Reames, 2001). Nonetheless, satisfactory clinician–patient relationships, reinforced by empathy, can reduce professional stress and contribute positively to physicians' well-being.

Benefits of Empathic Relationships for Patients

Now let us shift our attention to the benefits that patients derive from empathic relationships with their clinicians. In clinical encounters, interpersonal communication is the primary tool for the exchange of information. A large volume of literature is devoted to the beneficial effects of clinician–patient relationships on patients' adherence to treatment regimens, satisfaction with the health care provider and the health care system, the recall and understanding of medical information, the ability to cope with the disease, improvement in quality of life, and physical, mental, and social well-being. Empirical research has shown that physicians' emotional demeanor when communicating with patients resulted in the patients' recalling less information that physician attempted to convey and patients' perceptions of their serious health condition (Shapiro, Boggs, Melamed, & Graham-Pole, 1992).

In the practice of medicine, an empathic physician–patient relationship is regarded as the royal road to optimal care. Illness cannot be understood without understanding the patient, and healing begins not *when* medicine is administered, but *how* it is administered. In addition to a physician's knowledge and clinical skills, effective delivery of health care depends on other factors, such as the quality of clinician–patient interactions (Beisecker & Beisecker, 1990; Di Blasi, Harkness, Ernst, Georgiou, & Kleijnen, 2001). It is obvious that the nature of the physician–patient relationship varies in different clinical encounters. For example, unlike chronic illnesses, which require continuous care, emergency surgical encounters are brief and thus preclude firm establishment of an empathic engagement. As indicated by Mayerson (1976), it might be difficult for a physician in an emergency room to feel empathy for an injured drunken driver who has killed a number of people in a car accident. However, by focusing on the patient's immediate needs and asking what it would be like to be in that situation, the physician may find it easier to make an empathic connection (Mayerson, 1976). Empathic understanding, however, is an important interpersonal capacity of physicians (Squier, 1990) regardless of the duration or nature of clinical encounters. Empathic engagement, according to Spiro (1998), helps healing and improves the medical practice.

Curing Versus Caring, Disease Versus Illness

In rendering treatment, two models of patient care—curing and caring—have been identified (Baumann, Deber, Silverman, & Mallette, 1998; DeValck, Bensing, Bruynooghe, & Batenburg, 2001; Spiro, 1986). In the "curing" model, the emphasis is placed on the biomedical paradigm of disease (see Chap. 6) in identifying the pathophysiology of the disease with the aim of treating the symptoms. In the "caring" model, the emphasis is placed on the biopsychosocial paradigm: The patient is viewed as a whole by focusing on the treatment of illness, not just on removal of the symptoms of disease. A disease can be detected by objective laboratory tests and microscopic examinations (as in the curing model), but detection of illness requires more than that. It is suggested that "cure is directed at disease, and care at patients" (Spiro, 1998, p. 2). The treatment of disease, according to Dr. Francis Peabody (1984), can be entirely impersonal, but the curing the illness requires interpersonal attention and empathy.

Some investigators have argued that medical education and practice traditionally lean toward the curing model, whereas nursing education and practice emphasize the caring model (Baumann et al., 1998; Linn, 1974, 1975; Webb, 1996). Support for this argument is provided in a study in which nursing students were found to be twice as likely as medical students (67 % versus 33 %) to agree that patients' recovery alone should not be the focal point of patient care. Significant differences in rates of agreement also were found between nursing and medical school faculty (89 % and 51 %, respectively) (Linn, 1975). Despite the heavy training of nurse practitioners in diagnostic and treatment procedures, their orientation toward care model was close to the nurses (Linn, 1974). It seems that in medical education more learning opportunities are provided for curing than the caring aspect of patient care. According to Spiro (1998, p. 2) "physicians learn how to *cure* but little about how to *care*."

The notion of professionalism in medical education and practice that places emphasis on the enhancement of empathy and compassionate care in the delivery of health care suggests that the curing and caring models must be integrated in the education of health professionals. Incorporating some of the educational concepts of the caring model from the nursing discipline into the curing model in medical education curricula could help to improve empathy in patient care.

For a better understanding of the nature of the curing and caring models, it is useful to distinguish between "disease" and "illness." A disease is a result of a malfunction or maladaptation of biological and pathophysiological processes that cause organ pathology, whereas an illness represents a personal reaction to the disease (Kleinman, Eisenberg, & Good, 1978; Spiro, 1986). Illness can be experienced in the absence of disease, as indicated by findings that approximately half of all visits to physicians are based on complaints that lack an ascertainable biological reason. These complaints are known as somatization disorders (Hojat, Samuel, & Thompson, 1995; Kleinman et al., 1978), and patients with these disorders turn repeatedly to one physician after another, a phenomenon called "doctor shopping" (Ketterer & Buckholtz, 1989) or "doctor hopping" (Smith, 1991), because they do not experience empathic understanding from their physicians. In a survey of patients in California, 85 % reported that they had changed their physicians in the past 5 years or were thinking of changing their physicians for reasons such as poor communication skills, the physician's inability to inspire confidence in the patient, and so forth (Moser, 1984).

It is argued that empathy in clinical encounters is cost effective because it leads to more accurate and early diagnosis, better compliance, and more efficient treatment planning, thereby avoiding doctor shopping and spiraling costs of unnecessary medical tests and hospitalizations (Bellet & Maloney, 1991; Book, 1991). In addition, a study of patients in primary care and surgical settings showed that the physician–patient visits tended to be more time consuming when physicians did not demonstrate understanding and empathy (Levinson, Gorawara-Bhat, & Lamb, 2000). Thus, an empathic physician–patient engagement can lead to the development of trust, which in turn will lead to better management of illness and containment of costs by preventing doctor shopping or hopping.

Uniqueness of Clinician–Patient Empathic Relationships

The encounter between clinician and patient is a purposeful interpersonal event, and its effectiveness in yielding positive clinical outcomes depends heavily on the clinician's skills in forming an empathic relationship, thus earning the patient's trust. A more positive patient outcome is achieved in a caring model in which clinician and patient establish a mutual understanding about the patient's health problem (Starfield et al., 1981), which has been identified as an important element of patient satisfaction with medical care (Kenny, 1995).

Being empathic is among the ingredients of the ethics of caring (Branch, 2000). The American Medical Association's first Code of Ethics, published in 1847, included the following: "The life of a sick person can be shortened not only by the acts, but also by the words or the manner of a physician. It is, therefore, a sacred duty to guard himself carefully in this respect, and to avoid all things which can have a tendency to discourage the patient and to depress his spirit" (cited in Katz, 1984, p. 20).

An empathic relationship develops when the clinician avoids being arrogant and curbs the sense of superiority and instead becomes friendly, confident, relaxed, unhurried, and capable of communicating his or her empathic understanding and genuine concerns to the patient as well as to the patient's family. Rosenow (1999) argued that physicians who are arrogant in interpersonal contacts are committing a sin that is worse than the sin of greed because arrogance interferes with the development of empathy.

The patient's need to survive, the unequal positions of the clinician and patient in clinical encounters, the atmosphere of patient care, the psychodynamics of interpersonal exchanges in seeking and giving help, and cultural factors and boundaries in patient care suggest that the clinician–patient relationship is unique compared to any other kind of human connection. The following studies provide support for the uniqueness of the clinician–patient relationship.

Bonding for Survival (the Stockholm Syndrome)

In 1973, during a bank robbery in Stockholm, Sweden, two robbers held four people hostage for 6 days. During the ordeal, the hostages developed an attachment to their captors, coming to believe that their captors were protecting them from harm by the police! After the hostages were released and the ordeal was over, one of the hostages began raising funds for the robbers' legal defense! The phenomenon of bonding with captors to reduce the fear of death is known as the "Stockholm syndrome." Although this syndrome may seem to have no relevance to clinician–patient encounters, some psychological factors are common to both situations.

First, bonding occurs in situations where a person's survival depends on the mercy of another person. Second, bonding occurs when a person perceives that the other person is not ignorant and therefore pays some attention to the person. Third, bonding occurs when a person feels isolated from other people. Fourth, bonding occurs when a person perceives that he or she is unable to escape without the help of another person.

Assuming that some or all of the psychological factors underlying the Stockholm syndrome are present when a fearful patient consults a physician for treatment, possible hospitalization, and possible surgery, the similarity between psychological factors characterizing the syndrome and the physician–patient encounter becomes apparent.

The Clinician as an Authority Figure

In rendering help, the clinician is often perceived by the patient as an authority figure. This inequality in relation to power makes the patient more vulnerable to the clinician's influence (Koenig, 2002), which can be strengthened in the presence of empathic understanding.

Obedience to Authority (the Milgram Study)

In a well-known study of obedience conducted at Yale University, Stanley Milgram (1968) used an experimental paradigm to determine if people would be willing to comply with an authority figure's order even when compliance could have painful consequences. The study participants (who played the role of "teachers") were told that they were participating in an experiment to improve learning and memory. Their task was to teach another group of participants (who played the role of "learners"), a list of paired associations. The learners were supposed to recall the associated words. The teachers were instructed to administer an electric shock every time a learner made a mistake and were told that the voltage would increase with each subsequent shock. The experimenter ordered the teachers to increase the intensity of the shock until a learner demanded to terminate the experiment or to continue delivering shocks as long as they liked regardless of the learner's protests. Therefore, the teachers could either comply with the experimenter's orders or refuse to comply and heed the learner's pleas. The experiment was carried out under three different conditions: (1) the teacher and learner were in adjacent rooms, and the teacher could not hear the learner's reactions to the shocks unless the learner expressed distress by pounding on the wall; (2) the teacher and learner were in adjacent rooms, but the teacher could hear the learner's reactions; and (3) the teacher and learner were in the same room. In reality, there were no actual electric shocks, and the experimenter had instructed the learners to pretend that they were experiencing increased pain with each subsequent shock.

Milgram's results showed that approximately two-thirds of the teachers complied with the experimenter's orders and continued to deliver shocks up to the maximum levels although complying was stressful for them and seemingly painful for the learners! The results also indicated that teachers who could hear the learners' screams or see the learners' reactions stopped delivering shocks earlier than did the teachers who were unaware of the learners' reactions. Milgram concluded that visual and auditory cues provided a more complete picture of another person's pain and suffering and thus could increase empathic responses.

Forty-five years after the original Milgram experiment, Burger (2009) conducted a partial replication of the study by limiting the maximum shock level to 150 V (rather than 450 V in the original experiment). It was found that obedience rates were only slightly lower than the original study. Burger (2009) indicated that there was some evidence that scores on the Empathic Concern scale of the IRI affected participants' responses. Although Milgram's research on obedience has been criticized on a number of ethical grounds, it continues to be viewed as a powerful demonstration of compliance with authority. Mehrabian and Epstein (1972) used Milgram's experimental paradigm to examine the construct validity of their Emotional Empathy Scale (see Chap. 5).

Assuming that the physician performs the role of the experimenter in Milgram's study and the patient performs the role of the research participant, the patient is psychologically set to comply with the physician's orders. As an authority figure, the physician has a profound influence on the patient's compliance with the treatment regimen even if the treatment is painful. More important, Milgram's finding that a suffering person's visual and auditory cues can enhance the empathic response in another person suggests that face-to-face clinician–patient encounters have an important advantage that cannot be replaced by any approach to patient care that precludes direct observation of the patient (e.g., computerized medical care, long-distance consultations).

The Milgram's well-known social psychology study has important implications for understanding factors that contribute to turning good people to evil. Could the inconceivable events such as atrocities committed in the Holocaust and brutality of beheading and burning humans by those so-called Islamic State militants be linked to the notion of obedience to authority?

Uncritical Acceptance of Authority (the Doctor Fox Lecture)

An experiment conducted by medical education researchers confirmed the influence that authority figures exerted, even on experts. Naftulin, Ware, and Donnelly (1973) hired a professional actor to deliver a lecture to an audience of 55 physicians, psychologists, social workers, educators, and medical school administrators attending a professional meeting. Introduced as "Dr. Myron L. Fox, a distinguished speaker and an authority on the application of mathematics to human performance," the actor delivered a lecture titled "Mathematical Game Theory as Applied to Physical Education."

The actor knew nothing about the subject. However, the researchers coached him on how to deliver the lecture and conduct the question-and-answer session with excessive use of double-talk, neologisms, and contradictory statements interspersed with humor and meaningless references to unrelated materials. When the researchers subsequently asked members of the audience to assess "Dr. Fox's" presentation, a large number of them highly praised the presentation!

This experiment has relevance to patients' adherence to physicians' orders and supports the notion that a physician's statements are likely to be accepted uncritically by patients, even by medically knowledgeable patients. Some have suggested that the experts' positive assessment of Dr. Fox's presentation was the result, in part, of the professional actor's nonverbal expressions when communicating information (Friedman, Prince, Riggio, & DiMatteo, 1980). This interpretation provides support for the importance of nonverbal communication in enhancing patients' trust in clinical encounters (see Chap. 3).

Role Expectations (the Stanford Prison Experiment)

The expectations of both clinician and patient can influence the process and outcome of their relationship to a significant degree. Role expectations, defined as "patterns of behavior viewed as appropriate or expected of a person who occupies a particular position" (Arnkoff, Glass, & Shapiro, 2002, p. 336), are a result of social learning and cultural factors. The interpersonal dynamics involved in role expectations were examined in a well-known social psychology experiment conducted by Philip Zimbardo and his colleagues at Stanford University in 1971 (Haney, Banks, & Zimbardo, 1973). Although the primary purpose of the experiment was to assess the power of social forces on individuals' behavior, the findings are relevant to clinician–patient encounters.

Twenty-one young healthy male college students were recruited to participate in the Stanford experiment in exchange for receiving money for each day they participated. Ten students were randomly assigned to play the role of prisoners and 11 were assigned the role of prison guards. The participants were told that the purpose was to study a simulated prison.

The mock prison was set up in a basement corridor in the university's psychology building. The prisoners and guards were dressed in different-colored uniforms to distinguish between the two groups. The researchers noticed immediately that the "prisoners" had adopted a generally passive role, and the "guards" had assumed an active role in their interactions with the prisoners.

Although it was made clear to the participants before the experiment began that no verbal abuse or physical violence would be allowed, the situation became so tense because of the guards' increasingly aggressive behavior and the prisoners' suffering that the experiment designed to last for 2 weeks had to be terminated prematurely after only 6 days. Five prisoners suffered from extreme depression, crying, rage, or acute anxiety disorder. When the experiment had to be terminated prematurely because of the aforementioned problems, all the prisoners were delighted, but most of the guards seemed reluctant to give up their role of controlling the prisoners. Although the researchers observed individual differences in the prisoners' coping behaviors and the guards' aggressive behavior, the findings generally suggest that role expectations were the determining factor in eliciting typical behaviors. An interesting observation was that the prisoners with higher empathy scores (a combined score on measures of helpfulness, sympathy, and generosity used in the study) were more resilient than other prisoners during the adversity.

The transformation of good people turning bad due to environmental demands and role expectations has been called the "Lucifer effect" by Zimbardo (2007) (Lucifer is a fallen angel who turned to Satan). Because of the notoriety of the Stanford prison experiment, a commercial movie has recently been made about the entire experiment. The movie benefitted from input and consultation by the experimenter Philip Zimbardo (Chamberlin, 2015).

The relevance of the Stanford experiment to clinical encounters is that physicians and patients have different roles that lead to different behavioral expectations.

As an expert, the physician is often expected to play an active role, and the patient, as a person in need of help, usually plays a submissive role by complying with the physician's orders. It is interesting to note that even physicians who consult a colleague as patients are likely to adopt the patients' role by becoming more passive and less assertive. The role expectations in clinician–patient encounters are determining factors in patient outcomes (Shapiro & Shapiro, 1984; Turner, Deyo, Loeser, von Korff, & Fordyce, 1994). Needless to say, an empathic clinician–patient engagement can lead to more productive expectations.

The Effect of Environment (the Rosenhan Study)

The results of an experiment titled "On Being Sane in Insane Places" conducted by Rosenhan (1973) suggest that the environment in which a clinician encounters a patient creates specific expectations in the minds of both that influence their behavior. Rosenhan instructed a group of eight sane people (three psychologists, a psychiatrist, a pediatrician, a graduate student, a housewife, and a painter) to make appointments with physicians in different hospitals in five different states on the East and West coasts complaining that they were hearing unfamiliar voices in their heads.

All these "patients" used false names and were admitted to the hospitals' psychiatric wards. Upon admission, all the patients behaved normally but were diagnosed by hospital experts as schizophrenics "in remission" and were kept in the hospital for an average of 19 days. Interestingly, many of the hospitals' real patients were able to recognize that nothing was wrong with the study participants, telling them: "You are not crazy" or "You are a journalist or professor" (referring to the fact that the research participants were taking notes).

Rosenhan (1973) reported another experiment that was conducted at a research and teaching hospital whose staffs had been aware of Rosenhan's original study and doubted that such an error could occur in their hospital. The hospital staff was informed that during the next 3 months, one or more pseudopatients would attempt to be admitted to the psychiatric ward. Staff members were asked to specify their level of confidence concerning their judgment regarding whether each patient admitted during the study period was one of the pseudopatients. Among 193 patients admitted during the period, 41 were judged to be pseudopatients with a high level of certainty by at least one staff member, and 23 patients were considered to be suspect by at least one psychiatrist. In reality, no pseudopatients were sent to the hospital during the study! Rosenhan's findings suggest that the patient-care environment creates specific expectations that may influence the dynamics of interpersonal relationships, leading to an exaggerated account of illness or an incorrect diagnosis. Needless to say, an empathic understanding is a useful defense against situational misunderstandings and can lead to more accurate diagnoses and to decisions more consistent with reality.

The Kitty Genovese Tragedy

In March 13, 1964, three hours after midnight, a young and physically petite New York City woman (Catherine "Kitty" Genovese) who was coming back from her work (a bar manager) was brutally attacked on the street near her home by a merciless rapist. She was stabbed repeatedly and viciously, screamed in despair: "Oh my God, he stabbed me! Help me!" She cried for help repeatedly to no avail. Thirty-eight neighbors heard or watched from their windows as a killer stabbed the tiny women to death; none called the police during the assault, nor did anything to prevent the crime. The attacker ran away, when hearing one neighbor shouting "Leave that girl alone!" The attacker came back to finish his evil intent when no one showed up to help the victim. Only one witness called the police after the woman was dead. When the killer after apprehension was asked how he dared to attack a woman in a crowded neighborhood, he replied: "I knew they wouldn't do anything, people never do." (Takooshian, 2014).

The tragedy of Kitty Genovese, raped and killed in two subsequent attacks over a half-hour witnessed by 38 neighbors, has attracted the attention of social psychologists, not only because of its haunting image, but also for defying the well-known "bystander's effect" indicating that in the case of emergency, bystanders are likely to show apathy when other people are present to help. However, in the case of Kitty Genovese no bystander offered help to engender apathy in other witnesses. The entire incident reminded me of the statement attributed to Edmund Burke: "The only thing necessary for the triumph of the evil is for good men to do nothing" (cited in Manning, Levine, & Collins, 2007, p. 561). If only one of those neighbors had had an empathic understanding of that terrified and helpless victim, the evil could have been defeated and the Kitty Genovese's saddening saga would not have been told in here on a discussion of empathic understanding. Empathy can prompt prosocial behavior in response to a call for help.

The Psychodynamics of Clinical Encounters

In addition to altruistic and egoistic motivational factors (Chap. 3), other psychological mechanisms can be involved in clinician–patient encounters. Because the psychological mechanisms involved in any interpersonal communication are complex, scrutinizing the psychodynamics involved in clinician–patient encounters is important to gain a better understanding of the underlying mechanisms that can enhance or impede the relationship. A few of the psychological mechanisms that function in clinical encounters are described in the following sections.

Identification

Among psychological defense mechanisms, identification is commonly associated with empathy (Berger, 1987). Freud (1955, p. 110) referred to the link "from identification by way of imitation to empathy" (cited in Szalita, 1976, p. 147).

Identification is an unconscious mental process in which an individual attempts to satisfy some unmet needs by becoming like another person (Moore & Fine, 1968). To form an empathic relationship, the clinician should experience a sense of temporary oneness with the patient through a transient identification followed by a sense of separateness (Jaffe, 1986). In other words, the clinician should first think *with* the patient (identification, oneness) and then think *about* the patient (empathic separation) (Jaffe, 1986). According to Fenichel (1945), empathy consists of two acts: identification and awareness. Clinicians use the mechanism of identification to understand patients' concerns better while simultaneously becoming aware of their own feelings as well as their patients' feelings. Schwaber (1981) believed that identifying with the patient is a way of truly experiencing the patient's inner world and argued that empathy, although not equivalent to identification, occurs as an outcome of identification.

Identification may sometimes blur the boundaries between clinician and patient (Watson, 2002). Beres and Arlow (1974) proposed that empathy may involve a transient identification with another person's mental activities. In addition, they believed that empathy was mediated by communication of unconscious fantasies shared by the patient and the clinician through both verbal and nonverbal cues emanating from words, gestures, and behaviors. The clinician's understanding of the mechanism of identification can facilitate forming empathic engagement with the patient.

The "Wounded Healer" Effect

Similar to the mechanism of identification, feeling similar to and sharing common characteristics with the patient can influence the empathic engagement between clinician and patient. It has been demonstrated that people who were led to believe that their personality and values were more like those of a "performer" empathized more with the performer who appeared to experience pleasure and pain (Krebs, 1975). According to Decety and Jackson (2004, p. 73), the sense of "self–other overlap" between the helper and the person in need of help can contribute to the enhancement of empathic understanding.

The tendency of health professionals to help those with whom they share common characteristics is described as the "wounded healer" effect (Jackson, 2001). For example, studies have shown that the therapists' own illness can constitute a source of cure for their patients (Cristy, 2001; Holmes, 1992). The notion is that a wounded healer can better understand the experiences of another wounded person by sharing common experiences, by reflection, and by validation of feelings (Laskowski & Pellicore, 2002). I came to grasp the notion of resembling the pain in delivering a child with that of passing a kidney stone after I painfully passed one! I could then recognize, with more empathic understanding, the pain I observed suffered by my wife in the delivery room.

Gustafson (1986) suggested that clinicians who have experienced pain are better able to understand the pain of others and to respond more appropriately. The successful resolution of psychological pain, according to Fussel and Bonney (1990), engenders empathy in the psychotherapist and influences the therapeutic process in a positive manner. Common wounds, according to Means (2002), provide a foundation for shared life experience and contribute to better understanding of patient's concerns, thus connecting clinicians with their patients. The philosophy underlying self-help programs, such as Alcoholics Anonymous (AA), is based on the wounded healer concept from common problems and experiences among participants. It is interesting to note that although perceived similarities between clinician and patient promote empathic understanding, patients' familiarity with their physicians does not predict empathic engagement (Makoul & Strauss, 2003). The fact that familiarity is not an important factor in empathic engagement in clinical situations suggests the unique nature of empathy in clinical encounters.

Transference

In his analysis of psychological illness, Sigmund Freud (1958a) noticed that two psychological phenomena could occur during clinician–patient encounters. One occurred in the patient (transference); the other occurred in the clinician (countertransference). These two phenomena are universal and can shape the nature of clinician–patient relationships (Goldberg, 2000). The transference often develops in the patient in relation to the clinician in ways that mimic an important relationship with a significant other (usually a primary caregiver, a parent, or even a lover) in the patient's past. Transference can be viewed as a repetition of an infantile object relationship that causes the patient to resist the treatment unless the resistance is countered appropriately by the clinician (Gabbard, 1994). Empathy plays an important role in the emergence of transference and in the development of the therapeutic alliance (Book, 1988). The importance of transference in the context of medical care, particularly in the primary care setting, has been discussed by Zinn (1990).

Because the patient unconsciously identifies the clinician with the former significant other, the patient is likely to behave *as if* the clinician is the significant other. The patient's need for understanding and reassurance, especially when experiencing illness and pain, triggers the unconscious tendency to view the clinician as an authoritative parental figure (Novack, 1987), thus increasing the likelihood of transference. The clinician is viewed in the patient's mind as the former significant other, which prompts the patient to reexperience the intense emotions associated with the relationship with the significant other in the past. According to Kohut (1959), this complex phenomenon, called transference in the psychoanalytic literature, plays an active role in the development of empathic engagement in the context of patient care. Awareness of the patient's inner world is possible not only through the senses (hearing, seeing, smelling, and touching) but also through understanding and analysis of the transference phenomenon. Empathic understanding can be enhanced if the clinician handles the phenomenon by an appropriate countertransference.

Countertransference

Transference is by no means confined to the patient. The clinician may, in response, develop mixed feelings toward a patient. The way a clinician handles the patient's transference is called countertransference. Lending oneself to becoming a wise figure to resolve the patient's past frustrations and conflicts is an example of an appropriate countertransference, which would lead to a positive patient outcome. In contrast, a clinician who projects his or her irrationalities and past unresolved conflicts onto the patient's transference relationship is an example of an inappropriate countertransference, which would lead to a negative patient outcome (Katz, 1984). According to Book (1988), difficulties in countertransference arise when the clinician uses empathy defensively to gratify his or her own psychological needs. According to Zinn (1990, p. 293), physicians bring their own "biases and emotional needs to the encounter, resulting in a dynamic interaction that ultimately shapes the outcome of the relationship." Clinicians' awareness of the transference phenomenon and their skill in handling it can empower them to make their interventions more effective even in ambulatory practice settings (Schmidt & Baker, 1986).

By handling the patient's transference properly, the clinician paves the way for an empathic engagement and becomes a secure base the patient can use to resolve past frustrations and explore options for a healthy personal and social life. Although the transference and countertransference phenomena are believed to occur in intense psychoanalytic relationships, their presence in medical consultations cannot be ruled out (Zinn, 1990).

Medical students and physicians tend to eschew probing for psychological factors during interviews with patients for fear of being unable to handle such factors properly (Smith, 1984). The presence of this fear was confirmed in a study with medical students in which it was found that a great majority of them expressed feelings of being unable to handle talking with patients about fears associated with cancer and death because they were afraid of harming the patients (Smith, 1984). Medical educators should pay more attention to teaching medical students and residents the psychodynamics of interpersonal encounters, including transference and countertransference, to improve their understanding of the peculiarities of clinical encounters and to enhance their capacity for empathic engagement with their patients.

Empathy-Enhancing Factors in Clinician–Patient Encounters

A number of factors contribute to the quality of relationships between clinician and patient. Some of the factors that are more relevant to the enhancement of empathy are discussed briefly in the following sections.

The Placebo Effect

White (1991) proposed that once an empathic clinician–patient relationship is formed, the clinician becomes a powerful placebo-like agent, an "X" factor in healing, that has a tangible positive influence on patient outcomes. It is further suggested that the placebo effect of the clinician–patient relationship is independent from any other placebo-like intervention (Hróbjartsson & Gøtzsche, 2001).

The placebo effect, defined as an intervention that simulates medical treatment but is not believed to be a specific treatment for the target condition (Brody, 1985), has a long history in medicine. The existence of the placebo effect is, in itself, a testimony to the notion that psychosocial factors have a tangible influence on the pathophysiology of disease (Spiro, 1986). The reported rate of response to placebos ranges from 15 % to 58 % (Turner et al., 1994). However, the notion that a placebo may be an effective treatment in one-third of cases remains the standard in clinical research (Hróbjartsson & Gøtzsche, 2001) (This rate was first suggested about half a century ago by Beecher, 1955.) Although no convincing evidence exists concerning the underlying mechanisms of the placebo effect, some authors have speculated that expectation, reduced anxiety, learning, and an endorphin-mediating effect may explain the placebo response (Turner et al., 1994). Research suggests that the placebo effect is more pronounced when patients comply with clinician's orders (Turner et al., 1994). Better compliance is a function of clinician–patient empathic engagement (Pumilia, 2002). Thus, through leading to better compliance, the empathic relationship can prompt a more positive placebo effect and a better patient outcome.

Recognition of Nonverbal Cues

In clinician–patient encounters, recognition of nonverbal cues and explicit acknowledgment of patients' feelings, concerns, and experiences are important to establish "rapport" (Matthews et al., 1993), which is the essential element of empathic relationships. Rapport can also be strengthened by physicians' ability to decode and encode nonverbal messages and convey their understanding of those messages to their patients (DiMatteo, 1979). Some nonverbal behaviors that are said to promote rapport include clinicians' efforts to match patients' postures, gestures, respiration rates, tempo and pitch of speech, and language patterns (Matthews et al., 1993). Also, tone of voice, gaze and aversion of gaze, posture, silence, laughter, teary eyes, facial expression, hand and body movements, trembling, touch, physical distance, leaning forward or backward, sighs, sweating, and other signs of distress or comfort are among important nonverbal cues in clinical encounters (Fretz, 1966; Wolfgang, 1979) (see Chap. 3 for a detailed discussion about nonverbal communication in a general context).

Physicians' ability to decode nonverbal cues is an important component in forming empathic relationships with their patients (DiMatteo, 1979). Using the Profile of Nonverbal Sensitivity Test (PONS Test) (Rosenthal, Hall, DiMatteo, Rogers, & Archer, 1979), DiMatteo and associates found that a patient's perception that the physician listened was predicted by the physician's ability to decode nonverbal cues, such as smiles, grimaces, finger tapping, and a high-pitched voice (DiMatteo, Taranta, Friedman, & Prince, 1980).

Other authors have pointed out that leaning forward during interpersonal interactions is perceived as an indication of a warm, intimate, attentive, and empathic relationship (Fretz, 1966; Harrigan & Rosenthal, 1983; Hasse & Tepper, 1972; Trout & Rosenfeld, 1980). Authors have also reported that postural congruency (positioning one's head, hands, and legs in a corresponding manner when interacting with another person) is an indication of nonverbal social rapport among friends, colleagues, and those engaged in conversation with a common goal (Buchheimer, 1963; Trout & Rosenfeld, 1980). Postural congruency may be a remnant of synchronized behavior between mother and child (Chap. 4), a reflection of the understanding and sharing that are important in empathic relationships.

Other components of nonverbal behavior can influence patients' perceptions of rapport during encounters with physicians. For example, the physician who nods his head (indicating agreement and approval), leans toward the patient (indicating attentiveness, accessibility, closeness, and empathic concern), and sits with his hands resting on his lap (indicating openness, confidence in his ability, and readiness to respond), rather than folding his arms across his chest, conveys a positive rapport that opens the gate to more empathic exchanges (Harrigan & Rosenthal, 1983). Arms and legs in the open position convey less defensiveness and a more positive attitude than closed arm and leg positions do (Mehrabian, 1969).

In addition, the degree of eye contact can indicate the nature of clinician–patient empathic engagement. For example, Mehrabian (1969) reported that a higher degree of eye contact is maintained when the interacting pair like, rather than dislike, one another. However, cultural and sex factors help to determine the desirable degree of eye contact in clinician–patient encounters. For example, Mehrabian (1969) indicated that in American culture, people tend to maintain more eye contact when they are dealing with high-status individuals. In some non-Western cultures described as collectivistic (as opposed to individualistic) (Triandis, 1995), direct eye contact between people of the opposite sex or of different status is avoided.

The face is recognized as a primary channel for affective communication (Ekman & Friesen, 1974). Changes in facial expression (e.g., expressions conveying pain) are often accompanied by parallel changes in autonomic arousal and subjective feelings (Vaughan & Lanzetta, 1981). Facial expressions and nonverbal cues often "leak" unconscious messages (DiMatteo et al., 1980). However, when assessing nonverbal cues and detecting deception, one may make more accurate judgments by observing the body rather than the face (Ekman & Friesen, 1974). In psychoanalytic interviews, the psychoanalyst sits behind the patient, who is laying on the couch, to prevent the patient from viewing the analyst's facial expressions and emotional reactions (Slipp, 2000). Hearing hidden messages beyond spoken words with "the third ear" and seeing nonverbal cues emitted often beyond conscious behavior with "the mind's eye" pave the road for empathic engagement in encounters between clinician and patient.

The "Third Ear" and the "Mind's Eye"

For a better understanding of interpersonal dynamics in clinical encounters, clinicians must learn to hear their patients not only with their anatomical ears but also with their "third ear" to get beyond the spoken words. In addition, to enhance their empathic understanding, clinicians must view their patients' inner worlds not only with their anatomical eyes but also with their "mind's eye." The rapport between clinician and patient will be stronger and the empathic understanding between them will become deeper if the clinician listens to the patient's narrative account of illness with the third ear and sees the personal, psychological, social, and cultural factors involved in the patient's interpersonal relationships with the mind's eye. The more that is said, the more that is heard, and the more that is understood, the deeper the relationship becomes (Jackson, 1992). The seeds of empathy are sowed by listening with the third ear and seeing with the mind's eye.

During the nineteenth century, seeing was more prominent than hearing in the realms of sickness and healing (Jackson, 1992). As a result, observation of nonverbal cues was given an important place in the diagnosis and treatment of illness. Waisman (1966) suggested that in clinical medicine, physicians needed to look at the hidden aspects of a patient's illness not only by observation (seeing with the mind's eye) but also by listening with their third ear.

In the therapeutic relationship, listening is a crucial method for acquiring information from the help seeker, for understanding the problem, and for bringing about the help seeker's healing (Jackson, 1992). This tradition is attributed to William Osler, who said: "Listen to the patient, he is telling you the diagnosis" (cited in Jackson, 1992, p. 1630). According to Samuel Coleridge (1802), to submerge ourselves in the thoughts of another being, we must have "the eye of a North American Indian" tracking the footsteps of the enemy upon the leaves that strew the forest, "the ear of a wild Arab" listening to the silent desert, and "the touch of a blind man" feeling the face of a darling child. In the context of patient care, these qualities translate into a clinician's ability to listen with the third ear, to see with the mind's eye, and to possess the capacity for empathy to understand the patient beyond spoken words and observable behavior.

Listening from the "outside" only with one's anatomical ears is insufficient in these encounters. According to Greenson (1960), clinicians must shift their attention to listening and feeling from the "inside." As Jackson (1992) pointed out, such listening can be initiated from an empathically attuned position. Research has demonstrated that teachers who attempt to listen to their students with a third ear by using an empathic response were better able to help them with academic and behavioral problems (Cleghorn, 1978).

Empathy, according to Schwaber (1981), is a "mode of analytic" listening. Similarly, Theodore Reik (1948) pointed out that a clinician must hear not only what the patient's words do say but what the words do not say as well. To achieve that goal, Reik emphasized that the clinician "must learn to listen with the third ear" (p. 144). By listening with the third ear, clinicians can catch what other people feel and think but do not say. Therefore, they need to learn how one person's mind "speaks" to another person in silence. To form an empathic relationship with patients to provide them with optimal care, clinicians must tune in and listen with the third ear to understand what the patients intend to say beyond the spoken word (Good, 1972).

Listening with a third ear can be accomplished by becoming more vigilant during verbal communication with patients, and seeing with the mind's eye can be accomplished better by becoming more observant of nonverbal clues in clinician–patient encounters. Spoken language is more than a vehicle for the transfer of information; it can influence thoughts as well (Hunt & Agnoli, 1991). In a broader context, Lee Whorf (1956) said back in the mid-nineteenth century that language can convey more than perspectives and feelings; it can shape the thoughts of a culture as well. Therefore, in the context of patient care, the voice that can be heard by the anatomical ear can have a more powerful meaning when processed with the third ear. Charles Darwin (1965, p. 354) proposed that the "force of language is much aided by the expressive movements of face and body." Thus, important information about a person's cognitive and affective states can be communicated through nonverbal cues (Lanzetta & Kleck, 1970) that show a wider picture through the mind's eye. Empathic understanding can be enhanced by recognizing hidden and unspoken messages by decoding nonverbal cues with the mind's eye.

Cultural Factors

Culture, defined as "the set of attitudes, values, beliefs and behaviors shared by a group of people, communicated from one generation to the next" (Sternberg, 2004, p. 325), determines how people connect with one another. People in different cultures have strikingly different views of self and others (Markus & Kitayama, 1991) that can influence their help-seeking and help-giving behaviors. Cultural norms, racial or ethnic differences, religious beliefs, sex stereotyping, and other embodied sources of identity can influence empathic engagement in the context of patient care. Comas-Diaz and Jacobsen (1991) postulated that ethnocultural factors can not only influence the individual's presentations and interpretations in clinical encounters, but they can also significantly affect the process and outcomes of patient care.

For a better understanding of interpersonal dynamics of care-seeking and care-giving behaviors, these behaviors must be examined in the cultural context, because culture is inextricably interlinked to any kind of behavior. For example, in a cross-cultural study of care-seeking attitudes, it was found that a Belgian sample expressed less care-oriented and more cure-oriented attitudes toward health care (DeValck et al., 2001). A recent study by Nelson and Baumgarte (2004) showed that unfamiliarity with cultural norms of others reduces empathic understanding mediated by a lack of perspective taking on the part of the observer. Thus, the clinician's familiarity with the patient's culture is another factor that must be considered when studying empathic engagement in patient care. However, little empirical research has been conducted on this topic. Although similarities have been noted in Western and non-Western (e.g., Japanese) cultures with regard to physician–patient communication and patient satisfaction (Ishikawa, Takayama, Yamazaki, Skei, & Katsumata, 2002), it is crucial to recognize that clinician–patient encounters are determined by cultural factors that bring cognitive and affective content as well as therapeutic values, expectations, and goals to the relationship (Kleinman et al., 1978).

Despite the importance of cultural awareness in clinical encounters, a study shows that only 8 % of the medical schools in the USA and no medical school in Canada offer formal courses about cultural issues in patient care (Flores, Gee, & Kastner, 2000). In another study on cross-cultural medical education among a national sample of residents in different specialties in the USA, it was found that although 96 % of the residents indicated that it was important to understand cultural issues when providing care, two-thirds reported that no evaluation was made with regard to their skills in the cross-cultural aspects of communication with patients (Weisman et al., 2005).

Cultural differences can influence the clinician–patient empathic engagement as well as the outcomes of patient care to a significant degree (Hall, Roter, & Katz, 1988; Hooper, Comstock, Goodwin, & Goodwin, 1982; Kleinman et al., 1978; Waxler-Morrison, Anderson, & Richardson, 1990). Cultural differences have been observed in physicians' behavior when revealing cancer diagnoses to patients (Holland, Geary, Marchini, & Tross, 1987). For example, in some cultures, the diagnosis of terminal illnesses is withheld from patients based on the assumption that disclosure may generate such fear that progression of the disease will accelerate (Adib & Hamadeh, 1999; Surbone, 1992; Zahedi, 2011). Evidence suggests that this assumption may not be entirely baseless because increased fear has been reported to be a major factor in "voodoo death" (Cannon, 1957). The power of suggestion often observed in research on hypnosis and imagery is a testimony to the belief that disclosing a serious illness to some patients may result in making their situation worse rather than better.

Hopelessness generated by revealing a fatal diagnosis can cause sudden death among some patients (Richter, 1957). Revealing the diagnosis of a terminal disease is viewed as cruel, inhumane, and unempathic in some cultures but as ethical and empathic in other cultures (Holland et al., 1987). An international survey of oncologists from 20 countries revealed that less than 40 % of physicians in Africa, Hungary, Iran, Panama, Portugal, and Spain would disclose a cancer diagnosis to patients, whereas more than 80 % of physicians in Austria, Denmark, Finland, the Netherlands, New Zealand, Norway, Switzerland, and Sweden would reveal the diagnosis (Holland et al., 1987). Clinical realities are culturally constituted, and the nature of physician–patient relationships varies in different cultures and in different ethnic groups within a culture (Kleinman et al., 1978). Clearly, culture can exert an important influence on the nature and contents of clinician–patient communication. However, empathic understanding is always beneficial in clinical encounters regardless of cultural peculiarities.

Furthermore, despite the highly recommended advice that physicians must share their treatment decisions with patients to obtain the patients' input and compliance, such is not the case in the training and practice of physicians in all cultures. In a study by Ali, Khalil, and Yousef (1993) in which American and Egyptian cancer patients were compared, it was found that Egyptian patients preferred not to be involved in decision making; instead, family had an important role in making decisions. Disclosure of a serious diagnosis was socially unacceptable. Emotional support was considered to be the responsibility of the family, not of the health care provider (Ali et al., 1993). Many Moslem patients, for example, believe in the doctrine of predestination, fatalism, and stoicism. With this group of patients, empathic physician–patient relationships can be better formed when physicians convey to them that it is God's will that provided the opportunity for the patient–physician encounter.

In some cultures, physicians are paternalistic figures who have absolute authority to dictate any treatment they deem necessary regardless of the patient's input. In those authoritarian cultures, the patient-centered approach to medical care is likely to convey a physician's lack of determination and competence! Therefore, because empathic concern has a different connotation in different cultures, clinicians' awareness of their patients' cultural peculiarities can enhance empathic understanding. For this reason, cultural issues must receive serious attention in undergraduate, graduate, and continuing medical education programs.

Personal Space

Everyone knows that most animals display territoriality by marking off certain areas as their own space. Human beings exhibit a similar tendency by establishing an invisible bubble around themselves called "personal space" (Hall, 1966; Sommer, 1969). The boundaries of that space determine the distance individuals need to preserve their privacy. Overcrowding that interferes with one's personal space (or territory) can lead to aggressive behavior (Calhoun, 1962). It is interesting to note that the boundaries of personal space are reduced to a minimum in intimate and empathic relationships (Hall, 1966).

Shamasundar (1999) postulated that interpersonal interactions represent an enmeshment of personal spaces in exchange for affective and cognitive information that results in empathic understanding. Sharing of personal spaces is the essence of an empathic relationship—the more overlap in personal spaces, the deeper the empathic understanding.

The nature of the relationship, gender, personality, and cultural factors determine the desirable amount of personal distance. People who are emotionally disturbed or have low self-esteem tend to maintain more personal space (Shamasundar, 1999). Furthermore, the desirable amount of personal space varies in different individuals and in different cultures. For example, in the USA, a maximum of 18 inches of personal space was observed in most intimate encounters (e.g., romantic relations), and a personal space ranging from one to four feet was considered a desirable distance between friends and acquaintances (Hall, 1966). People who like each other and form empathic relationships with one another tend to maintain less personal space between themselves when conversing than strangers do (Mehrabian, 1969).

Encroaching on a person's personal space can elicit negative attitudes if the relationship is not empathic (Mehrabian, 1969). For example, violation of an individual's personal space can lead to anxiety or irritability and, sometimes, to increased aggression and the breakdown of interpersonal communication. One study found that people sit closer when expecting approval and sit farther away when expecting disapproval (Rosenfeld, 1965). In the context of clinician–patient encounters, a desirable degree of personal space should be maintained to facilitate empathic interpersonal exchanges.

Boundaries

On the basis of Carl Rogers's description of empathic relationships in clinical encounters (Rogers, 1959), one can perceive another person's internal frame of reference "as if" one were the other person. If the "as if" condition is lost, a sense of profound emotional involvement (sympathy) in the clinician–patient relationship can develop, leading to potential risks (see Chap. 1), including the clinician's increased susceptibility to the patient's pain and suffering on the one hand and the patient's dependence on the clinician on the other hand (Chaps. 1 and 3).

In clinician–patient relationships, sharing of emotions always necessitates setting limits or boundaries regarding affective involvement. Although boundaries in clinician–patient encounters are often unspoken and unwritten, they are mutually understood (Gabbard & Nadelson, 1995). Boundaries imply the refraining from intense emotional and erotic involvements. Some boundaries are spelled out in codes of professional ethics. Clinicians violate boundaries when they purposefully exploit the patient's trust and dependency and respond unprofessionally to the patient's desires and expectations. Sexual relationships, dual relationships, receiving inappropriate gifts or services, bartering, unusual time and duration of visits, use of seductive and erotic language, excessive self-disclosure, and inappropriate physical contact are among frequently reported violations of boundaries (Gabbard & Nadelson, 1995). All the aforementioned violations can sabotage the development of an empathic clinician–patient relationship.

The extent of intimacy in clinician–patient relationships is defined by boundaries that prevent the exploitation of both parties (Farber, Novack, & O'Brien, 1997). On the one hand, patients who seek help are vulnerable and tend to form a secure attachment to the clinician who is viewed as an omnipotent authority figure resembling a wise parent (e.g., through the transference mechanism). On the other hand, being human beings, too, and thus vulnerable, clinicians must be vigilant about not bonding with a patient as a result of a strong emotional involvement (e.g., an inability to deal with the patient's transference).

Because "to err is human," errors can be made in clinician–patient relationships (Kohn, Corrigan, & Donaldson, 2000). However, education and the guidelines of professional ethics can minimize the violation of boundaries during encounters with patients (Sage, 2002). Several factors contribute to the maintenance or violation of boundaries in clinician–patient relationships: age, sex, ethnicity, culture, attitudes, developmental and family background, personality, education, and the capacity for empathic understanding.

Transgression of boundaries can occur in all specialties, but the likelihood of transgression is greater in psychological and psychiatric consultations because of the transference arising from the intense emotions generated in such consultations (Gabbard, 1994). Transgressions involving sexual issues are often initiated by patients (Gartrell, Herman, Olarte, Feldstein, & Localio, 1986). The oldest skill in medicine, as Thomas (1985) pointed out, is the physician's laying hands on the patient. Therefore, touching during physical examinations has traditionally been regarded as the opening gate to the diagnosis and sometimes to therapeutic benefits. Touching is not only a reminiscent of maternal stroking that generates a feeling of security but also conveys affection and empathic support (Mayerson, 1976). However, the inappropriate use of touch is certainly a transgression of boundaries that diminishes trust and ruins the empathic relationship.

When medical students and physicians are insufficiently trained with regard to potential transgressions of interpersonal boundaries, medical education is often blamed (Gartrell et al., 1986); but the problem is that the "rules of engagement" concerning identification of boundary transgressions are vague and therefore not easy to teach. Needless to say, empathic engagement in clinician–patient relationships can help to avoid the transgression of boundaries.

Recapitulation

Empathic engagement in the context of patient care is a complex phenomenon driven by many factors operating in the dynamics of the clinician–patient relationship. Factors that bind clinicians and their patients together include the need for human connection, particularly at times of crisis; the need for survival; the clinician's position as an authority figure; role expectations in the patient-care environment; psychological dynamics of clinical encounters; and clinicians' ability to understand patients by listening with the third ear and seeing with the mind's eye. Empathic engagement in patient care can also be influenced by cultural factors, personal space, and boundaries. When two people are empathically connected, there are many factors beyond spoken words and observable behavior that provide the glue for binding them together. Because of the importance of understanding psychodynamics of interpersonal relationships in general, and their implications in clinical encounters, it would be highly desirable to include the topic in the educational curriculum of any health professions education.

Chapter 9
Empathy as Related to Personal Qualities, Career Choice, Acquisition of Knowledge, and Clinical Competence

Man is essentially a bulb with many thousands of roots.

—(George Christoph Lichtenberg, 1742–1799; cited in Strauss, 1968, p. 285)

Abstract

- The link between empathy, personality, selected psychosocial variables, career choice, specialty interest, clinical competence, and patient outcomes is described.
- Empirical research suggests that empathy correlates positively with prosocial and altruistic behaviors and with a number of desirable personal qualities that are conducive to relationship building, including sociability, social skills, likeability, flexibility, tolerance, emotional intelligence, moral judgment, sense of humor, conscientiousness, agreeableness, openness to experiences, positive social influence, personal accomplishment, teamwork, and interprofessional collaboration.
- A number of undesirable personal attributes that are detrimental to positive interpersonal relationships correlate negatively with empathy, including aggression, hostility, externalization, antisocial behaviors, depersonalization, depression, anxiety, conduct disorders, neurotic or psychotic disturbances, lying, stealing, physical abuse, and dogmatism. Also, linked to empathy are factors such as satisfaction with early maternal relationships, selection of a career in medicine for humanistic reasons, and attention to psychosocial issues in medicine.
- Empirical findings suggest that scores on empathy are associated with indicators of clinical competence, and career choice. Health professions students and practitioners who choose the so-called people-oriented specialties are more likely to obtain higher average scores on empathy than those interested in the "procedure- or technology-oriented" specialties.

© Springer International Publishing Switzerland 2016

M. Hojat, *Empathy in Health Professions Education and Patient Care*,

DOI 10.1007/978-3-319-27625-0_9

Introduction

Empathy, like any other personality attribute, varies among individuals with different constitutional, developmental, experiential, and educational backgrounds. This chapter reviews findings regarding the link between empathy, personal qualities, academic attainment, clinical competence, career choice, and tangible patient outcomes.

Psychosocial Correlates of Empathy

Prosocial Behaviors

Prosocial behavior has been defined as a person's voluntary act that can benefit another person (Eisenberg & Miller, 1987). The notion that empathy is a determining factor in altruism and prosocial behavior has been widely discussed and accepted (Aronfreed, 1970; Batson & Coke, 1981; Eisenberg & Miller, 1987; Hoffman, 1981; Staub, 1978).

Some argue that prosocial behavior can be initiated by an egoistic motivation (e.g., the expectation of a reward, an attempt to avoid aversive stimuli or punishment, or an attempt to reduce personal distress by helping others). Others suggest that prosocial behavior can be evoked by an altruistic motivation (e.g., the act of helping to reduce other people's distress, without expecting any reward, even if the act is harmful to oneself). One study found that people who were more empathic behaved more altruistically: that is, they were willing to help others, even when their own welfare was jeopardized (Krebs, 1975). In a later study, teachers' ratings indicated that children's empathy was associated with their helpful behavior (Litvack-Miller, McDougall, & Romney, 1997).

Some authors have argued that empathy-induced helping behavior can be the result of merging the self with others. In certain circumstances, feelings of oneness emerge so that human beings experience others as "we," rather than as "they" (Hornstein, 1978). In these circumstances, we may be psychologically indistinguishable from the others and may understand their experiences better. And when this feeling of oneness emerges, the two shall become one, and, as reported by Lerner and Meindl (1981, p. 227): "If the empathic tie is dominant, it would be natural for us to engage in acts which we or others might label as self-sacrifice or martyrdom." In summarizing their research findings, Batson and Sager et al. (1997, p. 508) reported that "empathy evokes concern for the other, distinct from oneself, that is beyond self-interest."

Prosocial behavior initiated by altruism has been studied in relation to empathy (Eisenberg & Miller, 1987). However, in an earlier meta-analytic review of 11 studies, most of which involved children, the investigators found no consistent link between empathy and prosocial behavior (Underwood & Moore, 1982). This unexpected result can be explained by the finding that the evaluation of empathy in children could be confounded by such factors as validity issues regarding measurements of empathy and the evaluators' gender (Chap. 5). In addition, Eisenberg and Miller (1987) proposed that the association between empathy and prosocial behavior is weaker among children than among adults because emotional or cognitive responses and prosocial behavior become more integrated with age. In a later meta-analytic study of a larger number of research articles involving adults in which empirical studies and doctoral dissertations were reviewed, Eisenberg (1983) reported a significant link between empathy and prosocial behavior.

Individuals with high scores on Mehrabian and Epstein's Emotional Empathy Scale (Chap. 5) were more likely to demonstrate helping behavior than were individuals with low scores (Barnett, Howard, King, & Dino, 1980; Rushton, Chrisjohn, & Fekker, 1981). Cohen and Hoffner (2013) found that empathic concern (measured by the IRI, see Chap. 5) predicted organ donation willingness. In a review of studies on empathy and individual differences, scores on the Emotional Empathy Scale (see Chap. 5) were not only significantly correlated with altruistic behavior but also with greater physiological arousability (greater skin conductance and increased heart rate), more emotionality (a greater tendency to weep), spending more time with and displaying more affection to children, higher moral judgment, more volunteerism, and less aggressive behavior (Mehrabian, Young, & Sato, 1988). It is believed that empathy leads to moral behavior, justice, and preference for fairness (Decety & Cowell, 2015).

College students who scored higher on empathy were more eager than low-scoring students to help neurologically handicapped children who could benefit from a volunteer's efforts (Barnett, Feighny, & Esper, 1983). College students who were members of help-oriented groups, such as those helping the underprivileged, scored higher on the Emotional Empathy Scale than did students who were members of self-interest organizations, such as the biology honors fraternity (Van Orum, Foley, Burns, DeWolfe, & Kennedy, 1981). In a study with prison inmates, the investigators observed that the inmates who volunteered to help disadvantaged individuals in the prison scored higher on Hogan's Empathy Scale than nonvolunteers (Gendreau, Burke, & Grant, 1980).

Personal Qualities

A number of empirical studies have addressed the relationships between empathy, personality, and psychosocial measures. In an earlier empirical study (Kerr & Speroff, 1954), significant correlations were reported between students' scores on a measure of empathy (developed by the study authors) and scores of popularity and likeability measured by a sociometric method developed by Moreno (1934). Also, empathy scores in that study were correlated with the smiles observed at a commencement exercise and with feelings for others. Kerr and Speroff (1954) reported a positive link between empathy scores and automobile salesmen's sales records and their merit rankings. However, a later study by Lamont and Lundstrom (1977) found that the performance of successful industrial salesmen was negatively correlated with scores on Hogan's Empathy Scale but was positively related to a measure of endurance.

In the early 1970s, Hogan and colleagues conducted several studies comparing scores on Hogan's Empathy Scale with scores obtained on other measures of personal qualities. Hogan and Mankin (1970) reported a significant correlation between scores on the Empathy Scale and those on a measure of likeability. Two years later, Hogan and Dickstein (1972) found a significant correlation between empathy and mature moral judgment. A year later, Greif and Hogan (1973) reported a significant link between college students' scores on the Empathy Scale and a personality factor called "person-orientation" they derived from the California Psychological Inventory (Gough, 1987). This finding is consistent with the significant link observed between empathy (measured by the JSE) and "people-oriented" versus "technology- or procedure-oriented" specialty interest in physicians-in-training and in-practice that will be described later in this chapter.

Medical students' scores on Hogan's Empathy Scale were positively and significantly correlated with measures of intellectual efficiency, flexibility, tolerance, good impression, and extraversion, and were significantly but negatively correlated with depression, anxiety, and introversion (Hogan, 1969). The following adjectives had the highest positive correlations with scores on Hogan's Empathy Scale: pleasant, charming, friendly, dreamy, cheerful, sociable, sentimental, imaginative, discreet, and tactful. In contrast, the following adjectives correlated most highly but negatively with scores on Hogan's Empathy Scale: cruel, cold, quarrelsome, hostile, bitter, unemotional, unkind, hard-hearted, argumentative, and opinionated (Hogan, 1969). Hogan's findings paint a picture of an empathic person as one who is emotionally stable and socially mature—that is, a person who possesses the major attributes described as emotional intelligence (Goleman, 1995; Salovey & Mayer, 1990). Indeed, the link between empathy and emotional intelligence has been confirmed in some empirical studies. For example, it has been reported that scores on a measure of emotional intelligence were positively correlated with empathic perspective taking (Schutte et al., 2001). The positive relationship between empathy (measured by the JSE) and emotional intelligence has been confirmed in more recent studies with health profession students (Arora et al., 2010; Austin, Evans, Goldwater, & Potter, 2005; Kliszcz, Nowicka-Sauer, Trzeciak, Nowak, & Sadowska, 2006).

Moral judgment and helping behavior were significantly correlated with scores on Mehrabian and Epstein's Emotional Empathy Scale (Eisenberg-Berg & Mussen, 1978). Students who scored higher on a modified version of the Emotional Empathy Scale were more assertive, less narcissistic, more sensitive, less self-focused, and more concerned about a healthy lifestyle (Kalliopuska, 1992a). It was also reported that people living in the countryside obtained a higher average score on the Emotional Empathy Scale than did those living in towns (Kalliopuska, 1994). In a study with female Japanese physicians, it was found that those who reported living with their parents in an extended family or living close to their parents scored higher on the JSE than those who were living alone or were living in a small nuclear family (Kataoka, Koide, Hojat, & Gonnella, 2012).

Significant and positive correlations have been observed between scores on the IRI and measures of hypnotic susceptibility and self-absorption (Wickramasekera & Szylk, 2003). Among nurses, effective leadership has been linked to scores on the IRI (Mansen, 1993). A meta-analytic study conducted in the late 1980s found that empathy was negatively related to aggressive, antisocial, and externalizing behaviors, such as conduct disorders, lying, and stealing as well as to physical abuse (Miller & Eisenberg, 1988). Physically and emotionally abusive parents scored significantly lower than a comparison group of foster parents on the Perspective Taking, Empathic Concern, and Personal Distress scales of Davis's IRI (Wiehe, 2003). When Hogan's Empathy Scale was administered to incarcerated child molesters, their scores showed deficits in empathy (Marshall & Maric, 1996). The findings in these studies reveal that individuals who are deficient in empathy naturally possess less capacity to understand and respond to the needs of others, including their own children.

Negative relationships were reported between scores on Hogan's Empathy Scale and measures of anxiety, phobia, obsession, and depression (Kupfer, Drew, Curtis, & Rubinstein, 1978), and indicators of neurotic and psychotic disturbances (Hekmat, Khajavi, & Mehryar, 1974, 1975). Scores on Mehrabian and Epstein's Emotional Empathy Scale were inversely related to a measure of psychopathic personality (Sandoval, Hancock, Poythress, Edens, & Lilienfeld, 2000). In addition, negative correlations were reported between scores on Hogan's Empathy Scale and measures of state and trait anxiety (Deardroff, Kendall, Finch, & Sitartz, 1977). Also, scores on the Emotional Empathy Scale were negatively correlated with a measure of narcissism among undergraduate students (Watson, Grisham, Trotter, & Biderman, 1984) and among young baseball players in Finland (Kalliopuska, 1992b).

Symptoms of depression and dogmatism among medical students were negatively correlated with scores on Hogan's Empathy Scale (Streit-Forest, 1982). In a study of medical students at the Louisiana State University Medical Center, perceptions of changes in empathy during medical school (measured by a single item) were strongly associated with students' perceptions of changes in their sensitivity, helpfulness, and concern for patients (Wolf, Balson, Faucett, & Randall, 1989).

In an attempt to validate Hogan's Empathy Scale for medical students at Monash University in Australia, researchers found a significant correlation between students' scores on Hogan's scale and the ratings of peers on students' social skills, sense of humor, and awareness of the impression they made on others (Hornblow, Kidson, & Jones, 1977). Furthermore, medical students in that study obtained higher average empathy scores than did psychiatric patients diagnosed with a personality disorder.

Streit-Forest (1982) studied first-year medical students at the University of Montreal and found that students with a more positive attitude toward the physician–patient relationship and students who chose medicine for humanistic reasons scored highest on Hogan's Empathy Scale. The author also noted that the students who were more likely to watch television in their leisure time scored lower on empathy than did classmates who were more likely to spend their leisure time on a hobby.

In a study with medical students in Canada (Streit, 1980), significant and positive correlations were observed between scores on Hogan's Empathy Scale and scores on the following subtests of the Attitudes Toward Psychosocial Issues in Medicine (Parlow & Rothman, 1974): Doctor–Patient Relations (recognition of the importance of interpersonal clinician–patient relationships in effective patient care), Social Factors (recognition of the importance of social factors as determinants of health and illness), General Liberalism (open-mindedness about social issues outside of medicine), Preventive Medicine (recognition of medicine's role in maintaining health), and Government Role (endorsement of government's involvement in regulating health care costs). In a study with dental students, Sherman and Cramer (2005) found that empathy (measured by the JSE) yielded a statistically significant correlation with students' ratings on willingness to apply the principles of behavioral sciences to oral health care.

In a study with medical students, scores on the Empathic Concern and Perspective Taking scales of the IRI were correlated with a measure of femininity that included such qualities as gentleness, warmth, helpfulness, kindness, understanding emotions, devotion to others, and awareness of other people's feelings (Zeldow & Daugherty, 1987). In another study with medical students, empathy was correlated with a measure of androgyny (Yarnold, Martin, & Soltysik, 1993).

In a study with nurses, social workers, and teachers (Williams, 1989), the respondents' scores on the Emotional Empathy Scale were significantly and positively correlated with both emotional exhaustion and personal accomplishment (measured by the Maslach Burnout Inventory, MBI, 1993). The investigator suggested that high emotional empathy — as opposed to cognitive empathy — may predispose helping professionals to emotional exhaustion that must be mediated by personal accomplishment to avoid depersonalization and burnout (Williams, 1989) (see Chaps. 1 and 6 for the distinction between cognitive and emotional empathy). In a study with medical students, Brazeau, Schroeder, Rovi, and Boyd (2010) reported significant and positive correlation between scores of a measure of cognitive empathy (the JSE) and scores on the Personal Accomplishment scale of the MBI ($r=0.41$), but negative correlation with scores of the Emotional Exhaustion ($r=-0.30$) and Depersonalization ($r=-0.41$) scales of the MBI. Similar patterns of findings were reported in medical students (Hojat, Vergare, Isenberg, Cohen, & Spandorfer, 2015; Lamothe, Boujut, Zenasni, & Sultan, 2014), and by Zenasni et al. (2012) in samples of French general practitioners.

By imagining how other people feel when watching someone whose hand was strapped in a machine, Stotland (1969) demonstrated that perspective taking was a major mechanism that generated empathy. In a later study, Stotland (1978) reported that scores on the Fantasy–Empathy Scale (see Chap. 5) were correlated with altruism, and with more palmar sweat, and more vasoconstriction while study participants were observing others in pain. Stotland attributed this finding to the tendency of more empathic individuals to understand and feel another person's experiences.

Hogan (1969) reported that young delinquents and prison inmates scored approximately one standard deviation lower on the Hogan's Empathy Scale than college students. Hogan (1976) also reported that inmates scored lower on the empathy scale than Air Force officers. Furthermore, incarcerated delinquents scored lower on the Empathy Scale than nondelinquent undergraduate students (Kurtines & Hogan, 1972). Individuals with low scores on the scale were more likely to be deficient in morality. A group of repeat offenders scored lower on Hogan's Empathy Scale than did first-time offenders and research participants from the general public (Deardroff, Finch, Kendall, Liran, & Indrisano, 1975). Also, men with high scores on the Emotional Empathy Scale were influenced to a significantly lesser degree by a female potential coworker's physical attractiveness than were men with low scores (Crouse & Mehrabian, 1977).

Mehrabian et al. (1988) found that empathy measured with the Emotional Empathy Scale was associated with emotional arousability. The investigators explained their findings by suggesting that arousability indicates the degree to which a person's emotions are influenced by events. Similarly, emotional empathy can lead to an individual's tendency to be affected by other people's emotional experiences. Therefore, it followed that scores on emotional empathy (which was viewed as analogous to sympathy in Chap. 1) would be positively linked to arousability.

In our study of 422 first-year medical students (Hojat, Zuckerman et al., 2005), we found that higher scores on the JSE were associated with higher scores on Sociability and lower scores on Aggression–Hostility scales of the short version of the Zuckerman–Kuhlman Personality Questionnaire (ZKPQ) (Zuckerman, 2002). Similar findings were reported by Beven, O'Brien-Malone, and Hall (2004), who found a positive correlation between empathy measured by the Perspective Taking scale of the IRI and a measure of socialization, but found a negative correlation with a measure of impulsivity in a sample of violent offenders. However, in a study with medical students in Kuwait (Hasan, Al-Sharqawi et al., 2013), no significant correlation was found between empathy (measured by the JSE) and scores of the five personality scales of the ZKPQ, but authors reported a negative trend toward an inverse association between empathy and Aggression–Hostility scale scores. Empathy, measured by the JSE, has been linked to the "big five" personality factors such as Agreeableness, Openness to Experience, Conscientiousness, and Extraversion in a sample of 472 medical students in Portugal (Costa et al., 2014).

It is also reported that Empathy (measured by the JSE) could positively predict therapist's psychological growth (Brockhouse, Msetfi, Cohen, & Joseph, 2011). Significant associations have been found between empathy in patient care (measured by the JSE) and friendly and relaxed style of communication in 860 undergraduate health science students in Australia (Brown et al., 2011). Also, significantly positive associations have been reported in a sample of Korean residents in psychiatry (Hong, Bahn, Lee, & Moon, 2011) between empathy in the context of patient care (the JSE scores) and measures of Cooperativeness, Persistence, Self-Directedness, and Reward Dependence, measured by the Cloninger's Temperament and Character Inventory (Cloninger, Svrakic, & Przybeck, 1993). In a study with 229 Chinese nursing students (Xia, Hongyu, & Xinwei, 2011), an inverse relationship was found between the empathy (JSE scores) and the Neuroticism scale of the Eysenck Personality Questionnaire (Eysenck & Eysenck, 1975).

Furthermore, our study of medical students (Hojat, Zuckerman et al., 2005) showed that higher scores on the JSE were associated with higher levels of self-reported satisfaction with early maternal relationships, but not with the paternal relationships. Similar findings have also been reported by Hasan and Al-Sharqawi et al. (2013). These results were consistent with our earlier findings (Hojat, 1998) that medical students' perceptions of satisfaction with the early relationship with their mother were predictors of higher self-esteem; better peer relationships; less loneliness, depression, and anxiety; and more resilience when faced with stressful life events. We did not find such associations with students' perceptions of their early relationship with their father (Hojat, 1998).

In a study of physicians in postgraduate training, we found a significant link between the physicians' perceptions of their early relationship with their mother and their clinical competence in their interpersonal skills and attitudes assessed by the directors of the training programs (Hojat, Glaser, & Veloski, 1996). Again, this link was not observed in relation to the physicians' perceptions of their early relationship with their father. These findings provide support for the developmental aspect of empathy (discussed in Chap. 4) that the quality of the relationship with a primary caregiver (usually the mother) early in life can be a precursor of empathy in adulthood.

At the conceptual level, empathy and interprofessional collaboration have been described as important elements of professionalism in the provision of health care (Veloski & Hojat, 2006). At the empirical level, empathy as measured by the JSE has been found to be significantly associated with orientation toward teamwork and interprofessional collaboration. For example, in a study with 373 osteopathic medical students (Calabrese et al., 2013), statistically significant correlation was found between scores of the JSE and those of the Jefferson Scale of Attitudes Toward Physician-Nurse Collaboration (Hojat et al., 1997; Hojat, Gonnella, Nasca et al., 2003; Hojat, Nasca et al., 2001). Also, in nursing students a statistically significant correlation was observed between scores of the JSE and attitudes toward physician-nurse collaboration (Ward et al., 2009). Similarly, a statistically significant correlation was found in pharmacy as well as medical students (Hojat, Spandorfer, Isenberg, Vergare, & Fassihi, 2012; Van Winkle, Bjork et al., 2012) between scores of the JSE and the Scale of Attitudes Toward Physician-Pharmacist Collaboration (Hojat, Gonnella, Nasca et al., 2003; Van Winkel et al., 2011).

Peer nominations on positive social influence have been found to be associated with empathy in the context of patient care. For example, 630 fourth-year medical students were asked to nominate classmates who had significant positive influences in their professional and personal development. Students who were nominated most were compared to the rest on the JSE. Those with the most number of peer nominations (top 10 %) obtained a significantly higher JSE mean score (Michalec, Veloski, Hojat, & Tykocinski, 2015). In another study (Hojat, Michalec, Veloski, & Tykocinski, 2015), it was found that the top positive social influencers (nominated by their peers at the completion of medical school) scored higher than the rest of their peers on the JSE and on measures of Sociability and Activity (measured by the ZKPQ), but scored lower on experiences of loneliness, measured by a brief version of the UCLA Loneliness Scale (Russell, Peplau, & Cutrona, 1980). These positive social influencers were considered as potential leaders in medicine. In a sample of 255 third-year medical students it was found that students who were nominated by their classmates in six areas of clinical and humanistic excellence, compared to other classmates who were not nominated, obtained a significantly higher JSE mean score (Pohl, Hojat, & Arnold, 2011).

Empathy and Age

The link between empathy and age has been studied with some inconsistent results. For example, younger nurses with a moderate amount of professional experiences expressed more empathy toward elderly patients than older nurses (Pennington & Pierce, 1985). Similarly, younger, less experienced physicians showed more empathic concern for their patients than did older, more experienced physicians (Hall & Dornan, 1988); and in another study, younger Iranian medical students obtained higher JSE scores than their older counterparts (Khademalhosseini, Khademalhosseini, & Mahmoodian, 2014).

On the contrary, older health profession students in Australia demonstrated higher empathy (measured by the JSE) than younger students (Williams, Brown, Boyle et al., 2014; Williams, Brown, McKenna et al., 2014). Similarly, in other studies in which the JSE was used, no significant association was found between empathy and age in nursing students (McKenna et al., 2012): Korean medical students (Park, Roh, Suh, & Hojat, 2015), Iranian residents (Shariat & Kaykhavoni, 2010), Italian residents in hygiene and public health (Soncini et al., 2013), Australian occupational therapy students (Brown et al., 2010), and Malaysian pharmacy students (Hasan, Babar et al., 2013). Findings on most of these studies are limited because of the restriction of range of age in samples of young students. More research is needed to capture the true relationship between empathy and age by using samples with wider range of ages to overcome the aforementioned limitation.

Choice of a Career

A student's choice of a career and interest in a particular specialty can be influenced by a number of variables including constitutional factors, aptitudes, personality, developmental and educational experiences, skills, social trends, role models, cultural factors, and market forces (Bland, Meurer, & Maldonado, 1995; Christodoulou, Lykousras, Mountaokalakis, Voulgari, & Stefanis, 1995; Kassebaum & Szenas, 1994; Richard, Nakamoto, & Lockwood, 2001; Sierles, Vergare, Hojat, & Gonnella, 2004; Weissman, Haynes, Killan, & Robinowitz, 1994). Some empirical studies have reported a link between empathy and career interest. For example, Hogan

(1969) reported that college students majoring in psychology, education, and medicine obtained the highest scores on his Empathy Scale, while engineering and architecture students and military officers obtained the lowest scores. Rovezzi-Carroll and Fitz (1984) found that students majoring in physical therapy scored high on Hogan's Empathy Scale and were more people oriented while those majoring in medical technology were more task oriented, and low in empathy.

Studies with Medical Students

Medical students in Israel scored higher on a Hebrew version of Mehrabian and Epstein's Emotional Empathy Scale than did college students majoring in psychology, social work, economics, physics, and chemistry (Elizur & Rosenheim, 1982). However, the investigators found that the medical students unexpectedly scored lower than the other students in their attention to psychosocial areas related to health and illness. They interpreted this unexpected finding as an indication that medical schools overemphasize achievement in the sciences and fail to devote adequate attention to the development of psychosocial skills. In a Canadian study, medical students who had high scores on Hogan's Empathy Scale had chosen medicine for humanistic reasons, whereas the students who had low scores had chosen medicine for scientific reasons (Streit-Forest, 1982).

A study at Baylor College of Medicine found that medical students interested in family medicine, general internal medicine, and pediatrics obtained the highest mean scores on humanistic attributes (measured by ratings given by standardized patients during the clerkship's Objective Structured Clinical Examinations), whereas students interested in anesthesiology, pathology, radiology, emergency medicine, and physical medicine and rehabilitation obtained the lowest mean score (Coutts-van Dijk, Bray, Moore, & Rogers, 1997). Using the Physician Belief Scale (Ashworth, Williamson, & Montano, 1984), which is a measure of psychosocial orientation in patient care, the researchers found a significant association with empathy scores. A study with medical students at the University of Washington, School of Medicine, found that interaction with patients (a reflection of empathic engagement) was among the major factors that prompted students to choose primary care as their specialty (Burack et al., 1997).

Although Harsch (1989) observed no relationship between medical students' scores on Hogan's Empathy Scale and the specialties they were interested in, a later study with medical students contradicted that report. The researchers who conducted the later study reported that after the effect of gender was controlled in the statistical analyses, the students who expressed interest in pursuing "core" specialties, such as family medicine or pediatrics, scored significantly higher on the Emotional Empathy Scale than did students who were interested in pursuing "non-core" specialties, such as radiology or pathology (Newton et al., 2000). In her doctoral dissertation, Bailey (2001) reported that medical students who planned to pursue a career in specialties requiring extensive and prolonged encounters with patients received significantly higher average scores on the IRI than did their counterparts who planned to pursue procedure-oriented specialties.

None of the aforementioned studies used a validated measure of empathy in the context of patient care. However, there are a number of studies in which the JSE was used to examine associations between medical students' empathic orientation and their specialty interests. For example, in a study with first-year medical students at Jefferson Medical College at Thomas Jefferson University, the JSE was administered on orientation day at the beginning of medical school before students were exposed to formal medical education (Hojat, Zuckerman et al., 2005). Significant association was found between JSE scores and specialty interest in favor of those planning to pursue "people-oriented" specialties. This study was described in more detail in Chap. 7.

The finding of significantly higher JSE mean score being obtained by students who planned to pursue "people-oriented" specialties (compared to those planned to pursue "technology-oriented" specialties) was confirmed in another study of 685 medical students at Boston University School of Medicine (Chen, Lew, Hershman, & Orlander, 2007). However, such association was not observed in a study with 476 health sciences students in Portugal (Magalhäes, Salgueira, Costa, & Costa, 2011). In another study with osteopathic medical students in the USA (Calabrese, Bianco, Mann, Massello, & Hojat, 2013), no statistically significant association was found between empathy (JSE scores) and students' interest in specialty. In his doctoral dissertation research, McTighe (2014) did not find a significant link between scores of the JSE and specialty interest in 717 osteopathic medical students. In another study with 255 third-year medical students at Jefferson Medical College at Thomas Jefferson University (Pohl et al., 2011), students who were nominated by their peers as being excellent in clinical skills and humanistic attributes expressed more interest in pursuing "people-oriented" rather than "technology- or procedure-oriented" specialties.

To address the issue of whether the differences in empathy among students interested in different specialties can be detected when students enter medical school (empathy attributed to personal qualities before being exposed to formal medical education) or after they have been exposed to medical training (empathy attributed to medical education), we administered the JSE to 422 students on orientation day, before they were exposed to the medical school curriculum (Hojat, Zuckerman et al., 2005). We also asked the new students about the medical specialty they planned to pursue after graduating from school. Because some students may have lacked a clear plan regarding a choice of specialty, we presented them with the following four scenarios and asked them to choose the one they were most interested in at that moment:

1. Performing specialized diagnostic procedures or basic or applied laboratory research and major contact with colleagues, not patients: primarily hospital based (e.g., radiology, pathology)
2. Performing highly skilled and specialized therapeutic techniques or procedures; serving as an expert consultant: primarily hospital based, with some office activities (e.g., orthopedic surgery, neurosurgery)

3. Providing episodic or long-term care of a limited number of medical problems, and a mix of ambulatory and hospital-based practice (e.g., cardiology, gastroenterology, dermatology, emergency medicine, psychiatry, obstetrics, and gynecology)
4. Providing first-encounter health or illness appraisal, preventive education and intervention, and episodic and long-term comprehensive care of a wide variety of medical conditions: primarily office based (e.g., family medicine, general internal medicine, general pediatrics)

Our results indicated that students who were interested in Scenario 4 as a career choice obtained the highest mean score on the JSE, followed by students who were interested in Scenario 3, Scenario 2, and finally Scenario 1 (Hojat, Zuckerman et al., 2005). Inferential statistical analyses indicated that students who were interested in Scenario 4 (so-called primary care specialties) obtained a significantly higher JSE mean score than those who were interested in Scenarios 1 and 2 (so-called technology- or procedure-oriented specialties).

These results suggest that some students often come to medical school with a preconceived idea about a career choice that is consistent with their already developed personality. However, the findings cannot eliminate the possibility that educational experiences or the interaction of personal qualities and educational experiences can also influence the choice of medical specialty. In our large-scale study of entering classes between 2002 and 2012 reported in Chap. 7, students' scores on the JSE (administered on the first day of medical school) were significantly associated with students' specialty interest (expressed at the beginning of medical school). As reported in Table 7.11 (Chap. 7), students who expressed an interest in pursuing "people-oriented" specialty after graduation from medical school obtained a significantly higher JSE mean score than others who were interested in pursuing "technology- or procedure-oriented" specialties. The effect of gender was statistically controlled in the aforementioned analyses.

Studies with Physicians and Health Professionals

Truax, Altmann, and Millis (1974) compared the scores of general practitioners, other medical professionals (e.g., nurses), and nonmedical professionals (e.g., clergymen, lawyers) on the Accurate Empathy scale of Truax and Carkhuff's Relationship Questionnaire (see Chap. 5) and on measures of warmth and genuineness. They reported that the general practitioners received the highest scores. These results are consistent with the findings of another study that ongoing interpersonal relationships with patients and their families and interprofessional collaboration with colleagues in other specialties were among the features ascribed to primary care physicians (Hennen, 1975). In a 1983 study comparing physicians in family medicine, internal medicine, and surgery, the family physicians obtained the highest mean score on a humanism scale, the surgeons obtained the lowest mean score, and the mean score of the internists fell in between (Abbott, 1983).

In a survey of 327 physicians representing five graduating classes in the School of Medicine at the University of Missouri-Kansas City, views of a group of primary care physicians were compared with those of a group of non-primary care physicians (Arnold, Calkins, & Willoughby, 1997). The results showed that the primary care physicians assigned significantly higher ratings to such professional qualities as a pleasant personality, the ability to relate to people, and the ability to empathize. Among personal values, the primary care physicians also gave a higher rating to empathy and a lower rating to competition than did the other group.

In one of our studies involving 704 physicians, we noticed that psychiatrists obtained the highest mean score on the JSE, followed by physicians in internal medicine, pediatrics, emergency medicine, and family medicine (Hojat, Gonnella, Nasca, Mangione, Vergare et al., 2002a). The lowest mean scores were obtained by anesthesiologists, orthopedic surgeons, neurosurgeons, and radiologists. When gender was controlled for, the differences in empathy scores among physicians specializing in psychiatry, internal medicine, pediatrics, emergency medicine, and family medicine did not reach the conventional level of statistical significance ($p < 0.05$). However, the psychiatrists' mean score differed significantly from the mean scores of anesthesiologists, orthopedic surgeons, neurosurgeons, radiologists, cardiovascular surgeons, and obstetricians and gynecologists. A higher mean score by psychiatrists was expected because of their specific interpersonal training and findings that showed that they scored high on a measure of tolerance for ambiguity (Geller, Tambor, Chase, & Holtzman, 1993), which facilitates empathic engagement with patients.

In two other studies, we compared two groups of physicians (Hojat, Gonnella, Nasca, Mangione, Veloski et al., 2002b; Hojat, Gonnella, Nasca, Mangione, Vergare et al., 2002a). Group 1 included 462 physicians in "people-oriented" specialties, such as family medicine, general internal medicine, pediatrics, emergency medicine, obstetrics and gynecology, and psychiatry. Group 2 included 242 physicians in "technology- or procedure-oriented" practices, such as anesthesiology, radiology, pathology, surgery, and surgical subspecialties. The physicians in Group 1 outscored their counterparts in Group 2 not only on the total JSE scores, but on all 20 items of the JSE as well (Hojat, Gonnella, Nasca, Mangione, Veloski et al., 2002). However, the differences were statistically significant for only 11 of the 20 items. The results of the two studies remained unchanged when the effect of gender was controlled.

In another study, we compared the JSE scores in three groups: female pediatricians, female physicians in hospital-based specialties (anesthesiology, pathology, and radiology), and female nurse practitioners (Hojat, Fields, & Gonnella, 2003). Physicians in the hospital-based specialties obtained a significantly lower JSE mean scorer than pediatricians and nurse practitioners. In a study with 285 female Japanese physicians, those in "people-oriented" specialties scored significantly higher on the JSE than their counterparts who were practicing "technology- or procedure-oriented" specialties (Kataoka et al., 2012). A study of 352 Italian resident physicians showed that physicians who had health care administrative experiences scored significantly higher on the JSE than those who were only involved in research with no administrative experience (Soncini et al., 2013).

Interestingly, the pattern of malpractice claims against physicians in different specialties has proven to be consistent with research findings on empathy among physicians practicing in different specialties. For example, in a large-scale study involving 12,829 physicians, the following specialists experienced the highest rates of malpractice claims: neurosurgeons, orthopedic surgeons, obstetricians and gynecologists, general surgeons, and anesthesiologists. The lowest rates occurred among specialists in psychiatry, pediatrics, and internal medicine (Taragin et al., 1994). The specialists who experienced low rates of malpractice claims in that study scored highest on the JSE in the aforementioned studies.

Empathy and Acquisition of Factual Knowledge

Few attempts have been made to examine relationships between measures of empathy and indicators of academic attainment. A consistent link between measures of knowledge acquisition and empathy has not been established. For example, a study by Hogan and Weiss (1974) showed a lack of correlation between empathy and academic performance. In another study, scores on a test of empathy developed by the investigators proved to be independent of intelligence, reading level, mechanical comprehension, spatial relations, or aptitude in chemistry and mathematics (Kerr & Speroff, 1954).

In the late 1970s, a study of five classes of medical students at the University of Pittsburgh School of Medicine found that scores on a brief version of Hogan's Empathy Scale and scores on the Medical College Admission Test (MCAT) were positively correlated in one class, negatively correlated in another class, and not correlated at all in the three remaining classes (Kupfer et al., 1978).

At Wake Forest University's Bowman Gray School of Medicine, medical students' scores on Hogan's Empathy Scale were not correlated with either their scores on Parts 1 or 2 of the National Board of Medical Examiners (part of medical licensing examinations) nor with their grades on preclinical and clinical examinations (Diseker & Michielutte, 1981). Furthermore, all correlations between the students' scores on Hogan's Empathy Scale and the Verbal, Quantitative, Science Problems, and General Information subtests of the MCAT were negative and negligible. In our own study of 371 third-year medical students (Hojat, Gonnella, Mangione et al., 2002), we found that the students' scores on the JSE were not significantly correlated with their performance on objective (e.g., multiple choice) tests, such as examinations on sciences basic to medicine in the first two years of medical school; the MCAT's Biological Sciences, Physical Sciences, and Verbal Reasoning subtests; or Steps 1 and 2 of the United States Medical Licensing Examination.

Empathy and Clinical Competence

Significant relationships between empathy and indicators of clinical competence have been reported in some studies. For example, some of these studies involved assessments of medical students by standardized patients. In one study, Colliver, Willis, Robbs, Cohen, and Swartz (1998) reported that the patients' assessments of empathy among fourth-year medical students were associated with indicators of better clinical performance. In another study, Coutts and Rogers (2000) found low correlations between medical students' scores on a measure of humanism in medicine and assessments of their academic performance in medical school. Among these low correlations, the highest one ($r=0.31$) was obtained between the standardized patients' assessment of the students' history-taking skills and the students' "humanism" scores.

In a study with 284 medical students (Berg, Majdan, Berg, Veloski, & Hojat, 2011a), significant associations were observed between students' self-reported JSE scores and ratings of clinical competence given by standardized patients in ten Objective Structured Clinical Examination (OSCE) stations. The associations between measure of empathy and the patients' assessments of students' clinical competence were stronger when standardized patients assessed students' empathic engagement (measured by the Jefferson Scale of Patient's Perception of Physician Empathy, JSPPPE completed by the standardized patients, see Chap. 7), compared to students' self-reported empathy (measured by the JSE). This pattern of findings was observed in a few other studies, as well (Berg, Majdan, Berg, Veloski, & Hojat, 2011b; Berg et al., 2015; Grosseman, Novack et al., 2014). The modest association between medical students' self-reported empathy and standardized patients' assessments of students' clinical skills has been partly attributed to confounding effects of gender and ethnicity of students and standardized patients (Berg et al., 2011b, 2015) and partly to students' inability to gauge the effectiveness of their empathic communications with standardized patients in playing the role of a clinician in simulated clinical encounters (Grosseman, Novack et al., 2014).

In a study with 371 third-year medical students (Hojat, Gonnella, Mangione et al., 2002), we observed a statistically significant link between the students' JSE scores and the faculty's global ratings of students' clinical competence in third-year core clerkships (family medicine, internal medicine, obstetrics and gynecology, pediatrics, psychiatry, and surgery). These results are in agreement with those reported by Colliver et al. (1998). This pattern of findings was expected because the students' understanding of patients' concerns and experiences measured by the JSE could be reflected in their interpersonal communication with patients, a factor usually taken into consideration when assessing students' clinical competence. However, because such personal qualities cannot be measured with objective tests of medical or clinical knowledge, one may not expect to find a significant link between students' empathy scores and measures of knowledge acquisition.

Empathy and Patient Outcomes

A very important evidence in support of validity and utility of measures of empathy in the context of patient care is their ability to predict clinical or patient outcomes. Demonstrating that empathy in patient care is significantly associated with patient outcomes is utterly important because the ultimate goal of medical education and all other health professions is optimal clinical outcomes. We have shown in two empirical studies with diabetic patients in the USA and in Italy that physicians' empathy (measured by the JSE) could significantly predict positive patient outcomes which I will describe in more detail in Chap. 11.

Clinical Importance of the Differences

Differences in empathy among physicians in different specialties do not necessarily indicate a deficiency in empathy in the low-scoring groups. It is important to emphasize this point for two reasons.

First, according to the information available so far, almost all the statistically significant differences in empathy among medical students interested in or physicians practicing in different specialties appear to be moderate at best. Second, the duties involved in the technology- or procedure-oriented specialties obviously are primarily procedural and therefore may not demand a high degree of empathic engagement necessary in the people-oriented specialties. For example, empathic understanding of patients' experiences and emotions, although important in any patient-physician encounter, is more crucial for primary care physicians than for pathologists, radiologists, or anesthesiologists.

Contribution of Personality and Medical Education in Specialty Choice

The question of the unique and interaction effects of personality formed prior to medical school and educational experiences in medical school on specialty interest and empathy is important to be addressed. Our study with medical school matriculants who completed the JSE prior to the beginning of their formal medical education and expressed their specialty interest showed a significant association between JSE scores and specialty interest. This finding indicates that there might be baseline differences in career interests of medical students before they start medical school, prompting them to prefer one specialty over another which can be reflected in their empathy scores.

Obviously, medical school curriculum, observations, and experiences in medical school can also influence specialty interest and empathic orientation toward patient care. For example, in some medical school clerkships and residency programs, such as family medicine, internal medicine, pediatrics, and psychiatry, more emphasis is placed on training in interpersonal skills and physician–patient relationships. Therefore, a stronger empathic orientation could be expected to develop among students or residents who are exposed to such training.

An important question is to tease out the relative contribution of personality formed prior to formal medical education, contribution of medical education, and their interaction in specialty interest and differences in empathic orientation among physicians in different specialties.

Recapitulation

Empathy, like many other personal attributes, is associated with a number of psychosocial variables, clinical competence, and career interest. A large number of desirable personal qualities that are conducive to positive relationship building are positively correlated to measures of empathy. Conversely, a number of undesirable personal attributes, that are detrimental to positive relationships, are negatively linked to measures of empathy. Because of their capacity to engage empathically with patients on a relatively continuous base, individuals with high empathy scores demonstrate greater clinical competence and are more interested in people-oriented (mostly primary care) than technology- or procedure-oriented (mostly hospital based and surgical) specialties.

Chapter 10
Empathy and Gender: Are Men and Women Complementary or Opposite Sexes?

*Then the Lord said: "It is not good for the man to be alone,
I will make him a helper who is just right for him."*

—(Genesis 2:18)

Abstract

- Findings from a large number of gender studies indicate that women in the general population and in health professionals-in-training and in-practice often obtain higher scores than men on self-reported measures of empathy.
- There are some plausible explanations for gender differences in empathy. For example, women are endowed with a greater capacity for social relationship than men, evident by the observations that they often begin showing more sensitivity to social stimuli and emotional signals and demonstrate more care-oriented qualities at an early age.
- Although social learning and cultural values have important role in determining gender differences in social behavior and empathy, other factors such as human evolution history (e.g., sexual selection, parental investment in child rearing, and ancestral division of labor), constitutional dispositions, and hormonal and bio-physiological factors also contribute to the differences.
- Evidence suggests that some of the gender differences could be pre-wired beyond social or observational learning.
- Although in a broader context men and women are more similar than different, accumulated evidence continues to confirm that gender differences in some personal qualities and mental abilities should not be considered as trivial or nonexistent.
- The fact that some of the gender differences are in favor of women (e.g., "communal" inclination, verbal ability) and some in favor of men (e.g., "agentic" inclination, spatial ability) implies that in social skills and mental abilities, men and women should be viewed as "complementary" rather than "opposite" sexes.

© Springer International Publishing Switzerland 2016

M. Hojat, *Empathy in Health Professions Education and Patient Care*,
DOI 10.1007/978-3-319-27625-0_10

Introduction

Differences in personal qualities between men and women have long been discussed, and the implications of those differences have been hotly debated. Although most gender differences have been attributed to social learning, role adaptation, and other sociocultural factors, studies on gender differences in infants and toddlers, before social learning takes place, suggest that some differences may be "prewired"—that is, apart from social learning and sociocultural factors (Cahill, 2005; Campbell, 2008; Carter, 2007; Hall, 1978, 1990; Hittelman & Dickes, 1979; Kimura, 1999; Singer et al., 2006; Van Honk et al., 2011). The role of sexual selection, parental investment, and division of labor during the history of human evolution, and the contribution of hormones and biophysiological function in human behavior must be part of dialogue in any discussion of gender differences.

The issue of gender differences in social behavior and mental abilities is a sensitive topic. One reason for such sensitivity is that in an atmosphere of political correctness, there is a tendency to overlook gender differences for fear of inappropriate social implications and adverse reactions. However, regardless of political correctness, the fact remains that despite many gender similarities, universal variations observed between men and women exist and are part of life.

Research Evidence in the General Population

In addition to the obvious gender differences in physical attributes and reproductive function, empirical evidence consistently indicates that men and women do differ substantially from one another in social behavior and the capacity for empathy. Findings from a large volume of empirical research in the general population indicate that women often outscore men on measures of empathy (Davis, 1983; Eisenberg & Lennon, 1983; Hoffman, 1977; Hogan, 1969; Jose, 1989; Karniol, Gabay, Ochion, & Harari, 1998). Block (1976) reported that the results of most of the studies she examined favored women with regard to empathy. However, Eisenberg and Lennon (1983) reported a significant gender difference in empathy favoring women when the measures of empathy were self-reported inventories. But they noted no gender difference when the measures of empathy were either physiological or unobtrusive observations of behavior. Similarly, Michalska, Kinzler, and Decety (2013) reported gender difference in favor of women when comparisons were made on explicit self-ratings, but not when neurophysiological indicators of empathy were compared.

The controversial findings indicate that women may have an image of themselves as empathic that is reflected in their self-reported measures of empathy. Accordingly, some empathy scholars suggest that women's superiority on self-reported measures of empathy may be due in part to "demand characteristics" that prompt women to respond in a manner that confirms how the researcher expects them to respond (Eisenberg & Lennon, 1983; Ickes, Gesn, & Graham, 2000). However, there are a number of studies in which gender differences were noticed on objective measures, such as physiological reactions and brain activities.

Studies with adults indicate that women are more skillful than men at initiating empathic relationships. They typically exhibit "communal" behaviors (e.g., social sensitivity, caring attitudes, friendliness), whereas men tend to manifest "agentic" behaviors (e.g., controlling, independent, dominant) (Eagly, 1995). Also, Rokeach (1973) found that women place more emphasis on the emotional aspects of their interactions than do men, who instead place more emphasis on the rational aspects. Consistent with Rokeach's findings, a study of undergraduate students found that women differed significantly from men on emotional empathy (akin to sympathy) but not on the perspective taking aspect of cognitive empathy (Riggio, Tucker, & Coffaro, 1989).

Other authors have reported that women tend to adopt care-oriented moral perspective, whereas men tend to have a more justice-oriented moral view (Gilligan, 1982; Gilligan & Attanucci, 1988; Sochting, Skoe, & Marcia, 1994). In a meta-analytic study, Jaffee and Hyde (2000) reported that gender differences in the care-oriented morality favoring women and in justice-oriented mentality favoring men are consistent, but the effect size estimates of differences are not large (see Chap. 7 for a description of the effect size estimates). Gender difference in moral judgment is reflected in their choice in the "runaway trolley" ethical conundrum, which was introduced by Philippa Foot, the British social philosopher. When confronted with a dilemma to divert an out-of-control runaway trolley down to a side track by pulling a signal lever to save five people who are on the train but killing another person who is trapped on the side track (Edmonds, 2015), more men than women choose to pull the signal lever to save five lives, but killing one person. In a brain imaging study (Singer et al., 2006), men and women were engaged in a game in which two confederates who played fairly and unfairly received painful stimuli. Results of the fMRI showed that both men and women exhibit pain-related brain activities. However, empathy-related brain responses significantly reduced in men when observing an unfair person receiving pain, accompanied by increased brain activation in reward-related brain areas, and correlated with an expressed desire for revenge. This pattern of brain activities was not observed in women.

These brain imaging findings suggest that men are more justice oriented than women in perception of others' pain. In a brain activity experiment by Horton (1995), the hypotheses that men and women differ in their empathic responses and that the comforting substrate is located in the right parietal area of the brain were confirmed. Horton (1995) also concluded that the right brain activities of the comforting substrate are more pronounced among women in general and among mothers in particular.

In a brain imaging study, it was noticed that men and women show different brain responses to infant crying and laughing (Seifritz et al., 2003). Correct recognition of infant vocalization is crucial for offspring well-being and survival. Women independent of their parental status, and mothers, in particular, were more sensitive to infant crying than laughing. The gender difference in vocalization recognition is attributed to the variation in biologically based emotional regulation in men and women (Decety & Jackson, 2004). In another study, it was found that at 30 days postpartum, 80 % of mothers, compared to only 45 % of fathers, were able to recognize their own infants' cries (Green & Gustafson, 1983).

In a study of nursing and medical students, the differences in judicial and moral considerations regarding patient care appeared to be explained by gender, rather than by differences in professional roles (Peter & Gallop, 1994). When the students were faced with a hypothetical clinical dilemma, female students, regardless of academic major, were more care oriented than their male counterparts. Gender differences in empathy have been observed among various professionals. In a study of nurses, social workers, and teachers (Williams, 1989), women obtained significantly higher empathy scores than men did on Mehrabian and Epstein's Emotional Empathy Scale (Chap. 5).

Despite their advantage in interpersonal style and empathic capability, women seem to be more vulnerable than men when working under stressful conditions. This differential vulnerability to stress prompts women to appraise stressful events as being more overwhelming than men do (Barnett, Biener, & Baruch, 1987). In our study with medical students, we found that women were more sensitive than men to stressful life events and consequently appraised the same stressful events (e.g., change of health of a family member) as more disturbing than men (Hojat, Gonnella, Erdmann, & Vogel, 2003). These results indicate that although female health professionals have an advantage when it comes to establishing empathic engagement with their patients, vulnerability to professional stress puts them at a disadvantage.

It should also be noted that although empathy enhances patient outcomes (see Chap. 11) and is valued by both clinicians and patients, research shows that empathy is not associated with promotion (Carmel & Glick, 1996), and this may exert more effect on women than men in professional advancement. In one large-scale study involving 5314 medical students, we found that female medical students at the beginning of their medical education expected, on the average, 23 % less financial gain from the practice of medicine than their male counterparts regardless of their planned specialties (Hojat, Gonnella, Erdmann, Rattner et al., 2000). These findings are consistent with the notion that women are more likely than men to choose medicine for altruistic reasons (Gross, 1992) than for financial gain or promotion (Stamps & Boley Cruz, 1994).

Research Evidence in the Health Professions

In a study of 7746 foreign medical school graduate physicians, who were assessed by standardized patients, it was found that female physicians scored significantly higher than their male counterparts on indicators of empathic capacity (e.g., skills in interviewing and counselling, rapport, and personal manner conducive to empathic engagement) (Van Zanten, Boulet, Norcini, & McKinley, 2005). English proficiency of participating physicians was controlled in statistical analyses by their scores on the Test of English as a Foreign Language (TOEFL). In this study, patients also expressed more satisfaction with female than male physicians. In our own studies as well as others with physicians-in-training and in-practice and other health professions students and practitioners in different cultures, gender variations on the JSE scores in favor of women have been frequently observed (Hojat, Mangione, Nasca et al., 2001; Hojat, Gonnella, Mangione et al., 2002; Hojat, Gonnella, Nasca, Mangione, Veloski et al., 2002; Hojat, Gonnella, Nasca, Mangione, Vergare et al., 2002). Chen, Lew, Hershman, and Orlander (2007) and Michalec (2010) reported that female medical students and physicians in the USA, on average, outscored their male counterparts on the JSE. The differences favoring female physicians were particularly pronounced on items that measured the "perspective taking" component of empathy (Hojat, Gonnella, Nasca, Mangione, Veloski et al., 2002). This pattern of gender difference in the JSE has also been observed in osteopathic medical students (Calabrese, Bianco, Mann, Massello, & Hojat, 2013), nursing students (Fields, Mahan, Hojat, Tillman, & Maxwell, 2011; Ward et al., 2009), dental students (Sherman & Cramer, 2005), pharmacy students (Fjortoft, Van Winkle, & Hojat, 2011), and physician assistant students (Mandel & Schweinle, 2012) in the USA and abroad (see Appendix A).

Inconsistent with our findings, however, Kupfer, Drew, Curtis, and Rubinstein (1978) found no gender differences in medical students at the University of Pittsburgh School of Medicine on their scores on an abbreviated version of Hogan's Empathy Scale. In a study of positive role models in medicine, however, female physicians scored higher than their male counterparts on measures of personality facets that were conceptually relevant to empathy, such as openness to new experiences, aesthetics, and feelings (Magee & Hojat, 1998).

Women in other cultures outscored men on the JSE: for example, in Mexican medical students (Alcorta-Garza, Gonzalez-Guerrero, Tavitas-Herrera, Rodrigues-Lara, & Hojat, 2005), Italian medical students (Leombruni et al., 2014), Iranian medical students (Rahimi-Madiseh, Tavakol, Dennick, & Nasiri, 2010; Shariat & Habibi, 2013), Japanese medical students (Kataoka, Koide, Ochi, Hojat, & Gonnella, 2009), Chinese medical students (Wen, Ma, Li, Liu, Xian & Liu, 2013), Korean medical students (Park, Roh, Suh, & Hojat, 2015), medical students in Kuwait (Hasan, Al-Sharqawi et al., 2013; Hasan, Babar, Chen, Ahmed, & Mitha, 2013), Portuguese medical students (Gonçalves-Pereira, Trancas, Loureiro, Papoila, & Caldas-De-Almeida, 2013; Magalhães, Salgueira, Costa, & Costa, 2011), medical students in South Africa (Vallabh, 2011), medical students in Thailand (Jumroonrojana, & Zartrungpak, 2012), medical students in Bangladesh (Mostafa, Hoque, Mosrafa, Rana, & Mostafa, 2014), Caribbean medical students (Youssef, Nunes, Sa, & Williams, 2014), Malaysian pharmacy students (Hasan, Babar, et al., 2013), Taiwanese nursing students (Hsiao, Tsai, & Kao, 2012), nursing students in Greece (Ouzouni & Nakakis, 2012), Australian health professions students (Boyle et al., 2009; Brown et al., 2011; Nunes, Williams, Sa, & Stevenson, 2011), Australian paramedic students (Williams, Boyle et al., 2015), and medical students in England (Austin, Evans, Magnus, & O'Hanlon, 2007).

Also, women obtained higher JSE scores than men in Korean physicians (Suh, Hong, Lee, Gonnella, & Hojat, 2012), Italian physicians (Soncini et al., 2013), and resident physicians in Romania (Voinescu, Szentagotai, & Coogan, 2009). There are a few other studies in which the gender difference on the JSE did not reach the accepted level of statistical significance ($p < 0.05$). For example, no statistically significant gender difference was found in Italian physicians (DiLillo, Cicchetti, Lo Scalzo, Taroni, & Hojat, 2009), dental students in the USA (Hsieh, Herzig, Gansky, & Danley, 2006), Polish medical students (Kliszcz, Nowicka-Sauer, Trzeciak, Nowak, & Sadowska, 2006), Czechoslovakian medical students (Kožen, Tišanská, & Hoschl, 2013), Brazilian medical students (Paro, Daud-Gallotti, Tiberio, Pinto, & Martins, 2012), residents in internal medicine and family medicine in the USA (Grosseman, Hojat et al., 2014), Korean medical students (Hong et al., 2012), medical students in New Zealand (Lim et al., 2013), and nursing students in Australia (McKenna et al., 2012).

In a study with students in the first and final years of a medical school in Poland (Kliszcz, Hebanowski, & Rembowski, 1998), women scored higher than men on both the Emotional Empathy Scale and the IRI (see Chap. 5). A survey of physicians showed that the female physicians rated themselves as more empathic than their male counterparts (Barnsley, Williams, Cockerill, & Tanner, 1999). Similarly, female residents in internal medicine (Day, Norcini, Shea, & Benson, 1989) and family medicine (Abbott, 1983) outscored their male counterparts on a measure of humanism.

In our recent large-scale study of 2637 medical students (1301 men; 1336 women), described in Chap. 7 (also see Hojat & Gonnella, 2015), we examined stability of gender differences on the JSE during a period of 11 years for matriculating students between 2002 and 2012 at Jefferson (currently Sidney Kimmel) Medical College, before students were exposed to formal medical education. Summary results of statistical analysis were presented in Chap. 7 (see Table 7.10). Consistent with the aforementioned findings (also see Appendix A), women consistently obtained higher mean empathy scores than men in all of our comparisons in different matriculating classes. The gender differences in favor of women were all statistically significant, with the exception of only one matriculating class (overall Cohen's effect size = 0.40). These results are in agreement with a great majority of empirical findings on gender difference in empathy in the general population and in health professions students and practitioners. The overwhelming evidence and consistent findings in observational, empirical, and experimental research on differences in empathy between men and women in different samples, settings, and cultures demand plausible explanations.

Plausible Explanations for Gender Differences

Because some of the gender differences are robust regardless of social and cultural differences, the intriguing question is the following: How can those differences be explained? Debate about the reasons for gender differences can be summarized in terms of nature-nurture dichotomy (Eagly & Wood, 1999). Wood and Eagly (2002) suggested that gender differences drive from the interaction between nature and nurture factors, including for example physical differences, reproductive capacity, as well as the social and economic factors in societies. There is a large volume of studies, views, and reviews particularly in social psychology literature in explaining gender differences in terms of social learning, role expectations, and sociocultural factors (more relevant to the nurture aspects of gender differences). Detailed discussion of the contribution of social learning and other social and cultural factors in gender differences is beyond the scope of this book.

Therefore, in this chapter, I will not focus on those findings or theories, related to social learning and social cultural factors that contribute to gender differences; instead, I will briefly present evidence in support of the notion that some aspects of gender differences may be pre-wired (more relevant to the nature aspects of the gender differences), independent from social learning. I will provide brief explanations for gender differences in terms of evolutionary history and hormonal and biophysiological factors. Needless to say that those explanations should not be viewed at all as an argument against the undeniable role of social learning and social-cultural contributions to gender differences.

Evolutionary Underpinnings

In Chap. 3, I indicated that human beings are evolved to make connection for survival purposes. Human beings are endowed with a capacity to understand and a need to be understood. Although manifestations of the aforementioned capacity and need might be different in men and women, evolutionary psychology suggests that men and women in the course of human evolutionary history developed some gender-specific characteristics for better adaptation to survival challenges (Buss, 1995; Tooby & Cosmides, 1990). According to this view, the evolved gender differences are indeed accommodations for survival in the living environment. I will discuss a few aspects of evolutionary theory of gender differences that are more relevant to social behavior and empathic orientation such as mate selection, parental investment, and division of labor.

Mate Selection

The evolutionary explanation of gender differences in sexual selection was initially described by Darwin (1871/1981). There is a large volume of research showing that men and women have different preferences in mate selection for the purpose of survival of the genes (Buss & Schmitt, 1993). For example, studies on mate selection have showed that historically women have higher preference for a mate with higher social status, better access to resources (indicators of better earning potential and more security), and ambitiousness (an indicator of better prospect) (Feingold, 1992). Men, however, place more value on physical attractiveness, and child-bearing capacity in searching for potential mates (Feingold, 1990). In an oft-cited study of 37 cultures, Buss (1989) observed the aforementioned pattern of mate preferences in men and women across all of the studied cultures. These findings confirmed the views in the evolutionary theory that women evolved to prefer mates who are resource providers, and men are evolved to prefer mates who are physically attractive (an indication of the women's health and younger age to bear and rear children).

Aspects of physical appearance such as smooth skin, muscle tone, lively gait, shiny and reddish lips, lustrous hair, curvy hip, and breast shape were proximate cues to a women's age and health that could increase reproduction success (Buss & Barnes, 1986) (at the time in which no birth certificate or medical tests were available to confirm a women's age or health status). Age in men, however, imposes less constraint for reproduction success; thus, preference for signs of younger age in men did not present a great advantage for mate selection However, potential for earning and financial prospect remained a strong selection advantage for women's mate selection. Remnants of the aforementioned mate selection factors are still noticeable in most modern societies. For example, could women's inclination to use make up, beauty parlors, cosmetic surgery, seductive dressing be an evolutionary leftover of retaining physical appeal, an advantage in sexual selection? Or, could the preference for richer male mates with college educations or successful businesses, family fortune, or high ambitious be the remnants of human evolution history to indicate potential for higher social status and better resources, aimed for survival of genes? Eagly and Wood (2013) suggest that changes in romantic mate selection have occurred in some industrial societies as women have entered the labor force and increasingly engaged in paid employment. Gender differences in mate selection contributed to the development of gender specific propensity for social skills and interpersonal behavior.

Maternal Investment

I described in Chap. 4 that during the course of human evolution, mothers have usually been involved more than any other person (including the fathers) in taking care of their own children (Trivers, 1972). Several reasons were described for the unmatched maternal investment (as opposed to paternal investment) including gestation and pregnancy experiences, bearing, weaning, and rearing children (Buss, 2003; Isabella & Belsky, 1991; Smotherman & Robinson, 1994). Also, maternal certainty (as opposed to paternal certainty), scarcity of women's gametes (compared to the abundance of men's sperms), lactation, and breast feeding prompt mothers to invest more than fathers in child care.

Maternal tender loving care and intimate experiences in raising one's own child contributed to women's development of caring attitudes, reflected also in their interpersonal relationships and social behavior. This notion was confirmed in a meta-analytic study by Feingold (1994) in which it was found that women rated themselves as more nurturing than did men. Such unique caring experiences can naturally enhance women's ability in forming empathic engagement. According to Reverby (1987) and Trivers (1972), women's caring attitude toward their offspring, which can be generalized to other humans, has evolutionary roots. Women's caring attitude toward their children often takes precedence over other matters. For example, caring attitudes toward offspring can sometimes interfere with a woman's career advancement in ways that have nothing to do with the barrier known as the "glass ceiling" effect. In support of this notion, Carr, Ash, and Friedman (1998) reported that male and female faculty members of academic medical centers who did not have children showed equivalent career accomplishments, but female faculty members who had children progressed more slowly in their careers because of their involvement with raising children. This phenomenon is an indication of the intrinsic motivation that also prompts professional women to enter into "caring" careers, rather than the prospect of great financial gain. This in turn can contribute to gender differences in empathy.

Division of Labor

Gender roles within the society are not chosen arbitrarily; they are firmly rooted in the human biology that laid the foundation for the genders' historical division of labor. The ancestral division of labor in men and women, determined by the Mother Nature, can provide plausible explanation for the development of gender differences in social skills as well as mental abilities. For example, because of women's advantage to bear and raise children, they naturally developed a propensity for nurturance. Men, because of their greater size, speed, and strength, naturally took the role of hunting, competing for resources, and protection of the family. The division of labor paved the road for gender differences, so that men took on the responsibilities for hunting and scavenging, defending the family against predators and enemies, and making and using weapons, while women took on the responsibilities of gathering, preparing food and clothing, and caring for small children. The division of labor contributed to disparate development of specific areas of the brains of men and women which were more often activated by their gender-specific task during the course of human evolution.

Obviously, those routine and daily activities performed by men and women for a long ancestral history which consistently activated different areas of their brain contributed to pre-wiring their brains differently, providing them with a differing propensity for social behavior and mental abilities. The notion of "neurons that fire together wire together" (Doidge, 2007, p. 63) means that acts or experiences that are repeated enough become embedded in the brain neurons which are activated together simultaneously by performing that act or experience. The set of brain network connections strengthen each time the act or experience is repeated. Hence, propensity for performing that act is "pre-wired" in the brain. On the contrary, lack of experience prevents cells to form a set of network. This notion is reflected in the statements that "neurons that fire apart wire apart" (Doidge, 2007, p. 64). No wonder that men are endowed with better spatial skills (acquired from hunting experiences), and women acquired superior skills in recognizing landmarks (required to locate a gathering spot and returning to the correct place of living). These "pre-wired" gender differences in mental ability have been shown in large volumes of empirical gender studies (Eagly & Wood, 1999; Geary, 1995; Voyer, Voyer, & Bryden, 1995).

Men's "Agentic" and Women's "Communal" Characteristics

No doubt that the human evolutionary history has significantly contributed to the development of distinct psychological qualities in men and women, labeled by Eagly (1987) as the "agentic" personal qualities in men and "communal" personal characteristics in women. Bakan (1966) who coined the terms "agency" and "communion" argues that agency is important for the existence of an individual, and communion is important for the existence of the group in which the individual is a member of. According to Abele and Wojciszke (2007) agency characteristics emerged from striving to expand the self which involves qualities such as dominance and ambition, while communion characteristics emerged from striving for integration in the group and involve qualities such as emotional expressiveness and cooperation. Thus, gender stereotypes are reflected in the two aforementioned agentic and communal characteristics (Abele & Wojciszke, 2007).

Women's historical role as domestic child-rearing individuals requires interpersonal skills that favor development of personality attributes that are linked to tender loving care and social skills, friendliness, concern, compassion, emotional expression, and empathic engagement, described as specific features of the "communal" personality (Eagly & Wood; 1999; Wood & Eagly, 2010). Men's instrumental roles in proving food and security which favor assertiveness and competition are described as specific features of the "agentic" personality (Eagly & Wood, 1999; Wood & Eagly, 2010). Women's communal attributes fosters prosocial behavior such as caring for others, while men's agentic characteristics facilitate some other forms of prosocial behavior such as physical challenges, acts of rescuing, and chivalrous protection (Wood & Eagly, 2010). Women's communal characteristic inspires close relationship, friendliness, perspective taking, and empathy which are indispensable for survival (Abele & Wojciszke, 2007).

The difference between men and women in communal and agentic attributes is reflected in the title of a meta-analytic article on gender differences, "Men and things, women and people." (Su, Rounds, & Armstrong, 2009). Tannen (1990) in her book, "You Just Don't Understand: Women and Men in Conversation," describes the difference in interpersonal style in boys as often doing things together (a feature of agentic attribute), and in girls as often talking together (a feature of communal attribute). In his popular book, "Men Are from Mars, Women Are from Venus" Gray

(1992) suggests that the difference in social behavior and communication between men and women is so wide that they seem to come from different planets!

In the stressful situations women would tend to express their emotions and talk about problem to acquire their mates' support (communal characteristic), but men often prefer not to talk but rather do something about problems (an agentic characteristic). According to Wood and Eagly (2010), women more often use communication to enhance interpersonal relationships due to their communal character. However, men because of their agentic character use communication to achieve tangible outcomes and exert dominance.

Despite the aforementioned gender differences, I must caution that the abovementioned evolutionary determinants of gender behaviors should not lead us to making the fundamental "attribution error." In judging the gender differences, this well-known error can be committed by incorrectly assuming from evolutionary history that gender roles have been fixed for good! In the modern societies, women's domestic role and their maternal investment in nurturing their children on demand and men's role as the sole breadwinners for the family have changed to some extent. The evolutionary advantages in mate selection and division of labor have also been changing in most modern societies. These adjustments, in long run, can insert their effects in the gender role equation formulated by evolution history, and bring about some new gender roles suited to better survival in the modern societies. Consistent with this notion, Zentner and Mitura (2012) studied a large sample of research participants in ten nations and concluded that the historical gender differences in preference for mate selection declined proportionally in nations with a higher gender parity.

However, these findings have been challenged by others (Schmitt, 2012). Changes currently occurring in modern societies include women's out-of-home employment, provision of child care by nonparental sources, and reconstruction of the traditional family structure and function. Over a sufficiently long period of time, this progression may influence the trace of the old history of human evolution by the tracks of modern history, in a way that transforms current gender differences to something more beneficial to survival of the human race. But for now, the impact of the evolutionary history on current social behavior of men and women should not be dismissed.

Hormonal and Biophysiological Differences

Exposure to various sex hormones from the time of conception plays an important role in gender differentiation. The presence of the "Y" chromosome at conception which contributes to the development of testes and male gonads, and its absence which leads to forming ovaries, is the starting point in gender differentiation. Male hormones (e.g., androgens or testosterone, its chief derivative) produces by male testes will have permanent effects on the brain development from inception. Some hormones that are relevant to understanding gender differences include testosterone, oxytocin, and to some extent cortisol. These hormones act as chemical transmitters in the brain that contribute to performance in certain social behaviors.

Higher levels of testosterone for example are associated with dominance, or behaviors that gain or maintain status, which often entail competition, risk taking, thrill seeking, and aggression (Booth, Granger, Mazur, & Kivlighan, 2006), which are consistent with men's agentic characteristic. It is reported that fathers as well as non-father men with lower level of testosterone showed a higher need to respond and more empathic sensitivity to infant cries than fathers with higher testosterone levels (Fleming, Corter, Stallings, & Steiner, 2002). In contrast, higher levels of oxytocin (and low levels of testosterone) are associated with human bonding and attachment, affiliation and friend seeking, nurturance, intimacy, and a propensity for empathic engagement (Campbell, 2008), which are consistent with women's communal attribute.

Some authors have argued that the difference in levels of prenatal testosterone in male and female fetuses supports the notion that the hormone has an important role in forming sex-specific interpersonal styles and verbal ability (Baron-Cohen, 2003; Connellan, Baron-Cohen, Wheelwright, Batki, & Ahluwalia, 2000). For example, a study in which an inverse relationship was found between levels of fetal testosterone and size of the vocabulary in children at 18 and 24 months of age supported the importance of fetal testosterone levels in verbal ability in men and women (Lutchmaya, Baron-Cohen, & Raggatt, 2002).

It is well known that the hormone oxytocin rises in women during childbirth and is released during childbirth and lactation. It has also been shown that women with higher level of oxytocin in early pregnancy and postpartum engage in more intimate behaviors with their babies such as gazing, eye-to-eye contact, affectionate touching, and tender loving care (Feldman, Weller, Zagoor-Sharon, & Levine, 2007). Oxytocin is associated with pair bonding, sexual behavior, maternal care, social attachment, prosocial behavior, and trust in others (Chakrabarti & BaronCohen, 2006; Kosfeld, Heinrichs, Zak, Fischbacher, & Fehr, 2005). It is also reported that oxytocin improves the "mind-reading" ability and adeptness to infer the mental state of others from social cues of the eye region (Domes, Heinrichs, Michel, Berger, & Herpertz, 2007), measured by the Reading the Mind in the Eye Test (Baron-Cohen, Wheelwright, Hill, Raste, & Plumb, 2001), which can facilitate empathic engagement. Hurlemann et al. (2010) reported that oxytocin can enhance social learning and emotional empathy in humans.

Another sex-typed hormone, cortisol, is also implicated in initiation of the parental role, and in gender differences. Hormonal changes have been linked to gender-typed behaviors. Such changes in mothers accompany childbirth and stimulate nursing (Fleming, Ruble, Krieger, & Wong, 1997). It has been observed that anticipation of becoming a father could lead to hormonal changes in men, parallel to the changes that occur in mothers (e.g., in cortisol). Such changes may include a decrease in testosterone (Berg & Wynne-Edwards, 2001). These changes can influence social behavior and empathic orientation.

Inborn Sensitivity to Social Stimuli and Propensity to Social Interaction

Inborn gender differences in responses to social stimuli, prior to any social learning, can be observed in children at an early age. For example, female newborns are more responsive than male newborns to auditory and social stimuli and are able to maintain eye contact for longer periods of time (Hittelman & Dickes, 1979; Osofsky & O'Connell, 1977). Infant's eye contact, recognized as an inducer of maternal caregiving (Hittelman & Dickes, 1979), is a social interaction which is under control of the infant and occurs immediately after birth prior to any social learning. Female neonates also smile more and show less rapid buildup of arousal and excitement (Osofsky & O'Connell, 1977). A study of neonates (mean age 36.7 hours) in which a human face and a mobile were presented simultaneously found that the female infants exhibited a stronger interest in the human face, whereas the male infants showed a greater interest in the mobile (Connellan et al., 2000).

Female newborns have shown less irritability than male newborns (Moss, 1967), and infant girls had less difficulty regulating emotions and displayed less irritation than infant boys when confronted with their mother's expressionless face (the still-face experiment described in Chap. 4) (Weinberg, Tronick, & Cohn, 1999). Obviously, these early differences that are precursor to social development cannot be attributed to socialization and adaptation to gender roles.

It has been reported that girls, compared to boys, show more concern for fairness (Charlesworth & Dzur, 1987), and respond more empathically to the stress of others (Hoffman, 1977). Also, at 1 year of age, girls can show their empathic concern through their sad looks and sympathetic vocalization (Hoffman, 1977).

Perception of Emotions and Decoding of Emotional Signals

Empirical research suggests that from an early age, females seem to be more sensitive to emotional signals than males. For example, female infants exhibit more reactive crying when another crying infant is present than male infants (Sagi & Hoffman, 1976) (in Chap. 5, a reactive crying response was described as an indication of a primitive empathic response).

A significant difference has also been observed in favor of women regarding the transmission and detection of nonverbal emotional cues (Brown & Dunn, 1996; Buck, 1984; Buck, Savin, Miller, & Caul, 1972). In a meta-analytic study, effect sizes of gender differences in sensitivity to nonverbal cues were reported to be in a moderate range of 0.40–0.50 (Hall, 1998). Women's ability to understand emotional cues has been observed in a number of studies in both children and adults (Brown & Dunn, 1996; Davis, 1983, 1994; Eisenberg & Lennon, 1983; Eisenberg & Strayer, 1987a; Feshbach, 1982; Hogan, 1969; Jose, 1989; Litvack-Miller, McDougall, & Romney, 1997).

The ability to perceive the emotions of another person and to "send" and "receive" nonverbal signals through facial expressions and body language (Hall, Carter, & Horgan, 2000; Hall & Gunnery, 2013) contributes significantly to empathic engagement. Yawning for example, as described in Chap. 2 has been linked to empathic ability and social awareness. In a study of naturalistic observations, it was found that the rate of contagious yawning was significantly higher in women than men (Norsica, Demuru, & Palagi, 2016). Also women are more receptive to emotional signals than men (Trivers, 1972), and are more perceptive about their meaning (Baron-Cohen, 2003; Bjorklund & Kipp, 1996; Buss & Schmitt, 1993). Despite the fact that women are generally better at perceiving other people's emotions and are less socially constrained about expressing their emotions, they are not always superior to men in the expression of certain emotions (Brody & Hall, 2008). For example, although women generally are better at expressing fear, sadness, love, and happiness, men are better at expressing anger and hatred (Wagner, Buck, & Winterbotham, 1993), characteristics that are not conducive to empathy. Women have been stereotyped as nurturing and interpersonally oriented (Eisenberg & Lennon, 1983), characteristics that have been identified as central components of female identity (Jack, 1993) and facilitate empathic engagement.

Women not only understand other people's facial expressions better than men, but they are also more facially expressive (Buck, Miller, & Caul, 1974). In one experiment, female pairs were more skillful than male pairs at understanding nonverbal emotional cues (by observing on closed-circuit television the facial expressions of a person who was watching slides with varied emotional content) (Buck et al., 1972). Hall's review (1978) of 75 studies on gender differences in the ability to decode other people's emotional states confirmed women's superiority in decoding visual and auditory cues. Another study (Zuckerman, DePauls, & Rosenthal, 1981) found that women could even detect negative aspects of interpersonal behavior, such as deception, better than men. Obviously, the ability to correctly interpret nonverbal cues and another person's state of mind is relevant to the capacity to form empathic relationships.

Women are more likely than men to exhibit comforting behavior even to strangers in stress (Hoffman, 1977). Women value reciprocity in relationship and endorse cooperation more than men do, whereas men place more value on competition and power (Ahlgren & Johnson, 1979). These characteristics are conducive to empathic engagement in women.

Interpersonal Style, Verbal Ability, Aggressive Behavior, and Caring Attitudes

Men and women have different interpersonal styles. Research has shown that men are more likely to interrupt when women are talking with each other, whereas women are less likely to interrupt when men are talking with each other (McMillan, Clifton, McGrath, & Gale, 1977). In addition, men tend to speak more assertively than women during verbal communication (Kramer, 1974). Taylor et al. (2000) reported that men and women often exhibit different biobehavioral responses to stressful events that reflect differences in their neuroendocrine and physiological systems. The authors suggested that men generally tend to react to stress with the "fight-or-flight" response, whereas women's response tends to be characterized as "tend-and-befriend" (Taylor et al., 2000), a pattern involving nurturing activities developed during human evolution to protect the self and offspring.

Taylor et al. (2000) suggested that the underlying biobehavioral mechanism responsible for this "tend-and-befriend" pattern might be set in motion by the attachment system described in Chap. 4, and by hormones such as oxytocin in conjunction with other female reproductive hormones, and the activities of endogenous opioid peptides. The "tend-and-befriend" approach of social behavior is reflected in typical acts such as taking on the phone for a longer period of time and simple social contacts such as asking for directions without hesitation when lost. Both of these examples are more typical characteristics of women than men. Obviously, these gender differences in interpersonal styles and biobehavioral responses can influence the formation of empathic relationships.

In interpersonal interactions, smiling is the best single predictor of warmth (Bayes, 1972) and an indicator of prosocial behavior and positive affect. Appropriate use of smiling serves as a positive signal in interpersonal communication. A meta-analytic study of gender differences with regard to smiling found that women and adolescent girls were significantly more likely to smile than men and adolescent boys (LaFrance, Hecht, & Paluck, 2003). Based on a meta-analytic study of 20 published articles on gender differences in smiling, Hall (1984) reported a relatively large effect size of 0.63 on gender differences in smiling. Women are generally more expressive and emotional than men (Briton & Hall, 1995; Kring & Gordon, 1998). Women's higher rate of expressing emotion and smiles is an uncomplicated facial signal that can strengthen interpersonal relationships.

Also, women's superiority on tests of verbal ability has been documented in many empirical studies (e.g., see Maccoby & Jacklin, 1974). Girls often begin talking at an earlier age than boys, and they maintain their superior verbal ability thereafter (Rutter et al., 2005). In addition to verbal skills, women surpass men in sociability. For example, Hall (1984) reported that women make more eye contact during interpersonal interactions than age-matched men. Women also tend to understand the social context of certain matters better than men (Willingham & Cole, 1997). For example, female college students identified with story characters to a greater degree than the male students did. The researcher found that such identification correlated positively with scores on the Empathic Concern scale of Davis's Interpersonal Reactivity Index (IRI) (Jose, 1989).

Women's typical characteristic of expressing their emotions (e.g., externalizing) and men's typical characteristic of concealing their emotions (e.g., internalizing) prompt the two sexes to reveal their emotions differently (Buck et al., 1972). An empirical study reported that the men and women who received higher femininity mark on the Gender Role Orientation Inventory (Bem, 1974) also had significantly higher empathy scores on the IRI (Karniol et al., 1998).

Although some gender differences in interpersonal styles and verbal skills can be attributed to socialization and learned sex roles (Eagly, 1995), evidence suggests that these differences may be partially biological in origin (Baron-Cohen, 2003). In a recent study by Singer et al. (2006) using functional magnetic resonance imaging, it was noticed that while both men and women exhibited empathy-related activation in areas that register pain (fronto-insular and anterior cingulated cortices), the empathy-related brain activities were significantly reduced in men when observing a cheater in pain, as described earlier in this chapter.

Although generally no consistent gender difference in anger has been reported, men often show physical aggression more than women, and women often show verbal aggression more than men (Archer, 2004). Verbal aggression and aggressive behavior reflect a negative affect, which interferes with the formation of empathic relationships. Women are generally less likely than men to exhibit aggressive behavior (for a meta-analytic study, see Eagly & Steffen, 1986). Gender differences in the expression of aggression may be attributable not only to hormonal differences but also to social learning and stereotypical sex roles that lead men to become tougher, more assertive, and more behaviorally aggressive than women. However, it is important to note that social learning explains only part of the picture because research indicates that aggression is more pronounced in male than in female children (Hyde, 1984).

Women express aggression in different ways than men and toward different targets. For example, women tend to direct their aggression toward other women, not men (Eagly & Steffen, 1986). Women are more likely than men to show "indirect" aggression often verbally, whereas men are likely to show "direct" physical aggression (e.g., pushing, punching) (Chakrabarti & BaronCohen, 2006). Indirect aggression requires regulation of emotion and better mind reading (Kosfeld et al., 2005) which are conducive to empathic engagement. Daly and Wilson (1988) studied data collected over 700 years on homicide and noticed that male-on-male rate of homicide was 30–40 times more than female-on-female homicide. Women often feel guilty to a greater degree than men about aggressive behavior, so that guilty feeling about aggressive behavior often prohibits women from expressing aggression (Frodi & Macauley, 1977). Control of aggression is a self-regulatory behavior that promotes empathic relationships. By using the "still-face" procedure described in Chap. 4, it was noticed that male infants had greater difficulty than female infants in maintaining emotional regulation (Weinberg et al., 1999), suggesting that women seem to have more control over regulation of their emotions, which leads to better interpersonal interactions.

Social stereotypes often portray men who help others as heroic and chivalrous (e.g., those who risk their own life to save others from harm) and portray women as nurturing and caring (Eagly & Crowley, 1986). A meta-analytic review of the literature revealed that, in general, men were more likely than women to give help and women were more inclined to receive help (Eagly & Crowley, 1986). However, women historically have been more inclined than men to place the needs of others, especially those of their children, above their own (Chodorow, 1978) and are more oriented toward care giving (Gilligan, 1982). Charles Darwin also noticed this quality. In his seminal book, *The Descent of Man*, Darwin (1981) indicated that women exhibit greater tenderness in social relationships than men, and because of their maternal instincts, their tenderness toward their infants is likely to extend toward others.

Gender Differences in the Practice of Medicine

It seems reasonable to speculate that gender differences concerning empathy could influence male and female physicians' styles of practice and provision of patient care, and some empirical studies have confirmed this speculation (Bertakis, Helms, Callahan, Azari, & Robbins, 1995; Bylund & Makoul, 2002; Fruen, Rothman, & Steiner, 1974; Henderson & Weisman, 2001; Maheux, Duford, Beland, Jacques, & Levesque, 1990; Weisman & Teitlebaum, 1985). In examining factors that influence medical students' learning of psychopathology in a psychiatry clerkship, Fabrega, Ulrich, and Keshavan (1994) reported that female medical students showed better achievement due to gender-related factors such as students' ability to assimilate and cope with clinical experiences of the psychiatric clerkship.

Female physicians were more likely than male physicians to engage patients in positive talk, discuss psychological and social issues in health and illness, use more positive statements, engage in more verbal exchanges with patients, and spend a longer time with them (Cooper-Patrick, Gallo, & Gonzales, 1999; Hall, Irish, Roter, Ehrlic, & Miller, 1994; Meeuwesen, Schaap, & Van der Staak, 1991; Roter & Hall, 1997; Roter, Lipkin, & Korsgaard, 1991; Roter, Hall, & Aoki, 2002). On the average, female physicians spent three to four more minutes with their patients than their male counterparts, engaged in more humorous conversations with their patients, and shared more decision-making responsibility with them (Charon, Greene, & Adelman, 1994). Female physicians also are more prevention oriented than their male counterparts (Bertakis et al., 1995; Frank & Harvey, 1996; Maheux et al., 1990). Furthermore, they provide more screening and more preventive counseling about sensitive topics, particularly with female patients (Henderson & Weisman, 2001). These gender differences in practice style, according to Bylund and Makoul (2002), can be the result of the female physicians' tendency to communicate at a higher degree of empathy with their patients than their male counterparts.

Charon et al. (1994, p. 216) observed that female physicians acted as if they were alert to their patients' emotional and daily-life concerns—concerns that otherwise "tend to be muted in medical interactions." Their observation agreed with the idea posed by others that women, more than men, can bring empathy to the healing relationship (Bickel, 1994; Bylund & Makoul, 2002). Charon et al. also found that patients reacted to male and female physicians differently. Patients of both sexes reported that female physicians were more willing to discuss medical topics and probe about personal habits, such as smoking, alcohol, drug use, sex, sleep, psychological issues, family and work problems, finances, and emotional problems.

In a study of patients' satisfaction, both male and female patients gave more favorable ratings to the care they received from female residents than from male residents (Linn, Cope, & Leake, 1984). However, Howell, Gardiner, and Concato (2002) found that although a greater number of patients preferred female over male obstetricians, their satisfaction with medical care was unrelated to a physician's sex. With regard to medical malpractice claims, the fact that female physicians have a better record than male physicians is attributed more to better physician–patient relationships than to taking on less risky patients (Sloan, Mergenhagen, Burfield, Bovjerg, & Hassan, 1989). In the area of clinical competency, our study showed that directors of residency training programs rated female residents higher than their male counterparts on the "socioeconomic aspect of patient care" at the end of the first year of postgraduate medical education (Hojat et al., 1994). These findings suggest that female and male health care providers have different practice styles resulting from their differences in interpersonal style reflected in their empathic engagement with patients.

Complementary or Opposite Sexes?

Despite all gender differences I described in this chapter, a number of meta-analytic studies reported that gender similarities in social behavior are overwhelmingly higher than the overinflated claims of the differences (Eagly & Wood, 2013; Hyde, 2005; Spelke, 2005; Stewart-Williams & Thomas, 2013; Su et al., 2009; Twenge, 1997; Zell, Krizan, & Teener, 2015). Because men and women are similar in many psychosocial qualities, Zell et al. (2015) and Hyde (2005) suggested that in gender research, it would be more desirable to test hypotheses of gender similarities rather than differences. However, despite the fact that the effect size of gender differences is typically small, Zell et al. (2015) suggest that the small differences accumulate when summed across domains. Therefore, differences should not be necessarily considered negligible. Consistent trivial differences can have important consequences that need to be constantly explored.

In her meta-analytic review of 46 studies on psychological and mental ability variables, Hyde (2005) advanced the idea of gender similarities rather than gender differences, and concluded that men and women are alike on most, but not all, psychological and mental ability variables, and declared that gender differences have been substantially overinflated. The modest and sometimes negligible magnitude of gender differences, observed consistently and universally in social skills, mental abilities, emotions, personality, interest, attitudes, and behaviors, does exist. However, such differences should not be considered as an argument for viewing men and women as "opposite" sexes; rather, they should be viewed as the "complementary" genders. For example, women's superiority in communal and men's advantage in agentic characteristics can complement one another to make together a better world. Together, men and women are like a completed jigsaw puzzle.

Recapitulation

A great majority of empirical studies in the general population and in health professions students and practitioners have reported that women outscore men in measures of interpersonal relationships and empathy. The differences in men and women in social behavior and empathy have often been attributed to social learning and sociocultural factors. In this chapter I argued that while the contribution of social learning in gender differences cannot be ignored, there are other evolutionary factors and inborn characteristics that can provide plausible explanations for gender differences in social skills, beyond social learning, gender stereotypical role models, and social and cultural factors. Relying on the human evolutionary history, I proposed that ancestral history in preferred advantages in mate selection, parental investment in child care, division of labor, and hormonal and physiological factors have endowed women with a greater propensity for social skills and empathic engagement. However, some of the current gender differences may cease to exist in the future. Changes currently occurring in modern societies, if continuing over a sufficiently long period of time, require adjustments that can alter the effects of past evolution in gender differences, and transform them into something else for better survival.

Chapter 11
Empathy and Patient Outcomes

The secret of the care of the patient is in caring for the patient.

—(Francis W. Peabody, 1927/1984, p. 818)

The failure to empathize is the basis of most of the unhappy
doctor–patient relationships.

—(Harry A. Wilmer, 1968, p. 248)

Abstract

- The theoretical link between empathy and positive patient outcomes is based on the following assumptions: When an empathic engagement is formed, then a trusting relationship will develop, the constraints of relationship will diminish, and this will lead to a more accurate diagnosis and greater compliance.
- In an empathic engagement, the patient perceives the clinician as a helping member of a social support system with all the beneficial health effects of human connection. All of these should theoretically contribute to optimal patient outcomes, including patients' greater satisfaction with their health care providers, a reduced likelihood of malpractice litigation, and more optimal clinical results.
- Research findings, showing significant associations between scores of a validated measure of physician's empathy and tangible patient outcomes in diabetic patients, present strong evidence in support of the link between the health care provider's empathy and clinical outcomes, independent of patients' subjective assessments.
- The psychosocial and biophysioneurological factors involved in interactions between a clinician and the patient are described as the plausible underlying mechanisms that can explain the link between clinician's empathy and patient outcomes.

Introduction

In this chapter, I briefly discuss the link between empathy and patient outcomes and present some theoretical framework and empirical evidence in support of that link. Presumably, any factor that contributes to enhancement of the clinician–patient

© Springer International Publishing Switzerland 2016   189
M. Hojat, *Empathy in Health Professions Education and Patient Care*,
DOI 10.1007/978-3-319-27625-0_11

relationship, including empathy, should in theory have a beneficial effect on patient outcomes (Mercer & Reynolds, 2002). Although the assumption that an empathic clinician–patient relationship will result in positive patient outcomes is theoretically sound, empirical evidence is needed to verify this assumption, and plausible explanations are required to clarify the underlying mechanisms that establish the link between empathic engagement in patient care and positive clinical outcomes.

A Theoretical Framework

The theoretical link between empathic clinician–patient engagement and positive patient outcomes is based on the assumptions that when an empathic relationship is formed between a clinician and a patient, trust will develop, the truth will emerge, and the result will be reflected in a more precise medical history and thus more accurate diagnostic information and greater compliance. Abundant evidence is available in support of this proposition, some of which was reported in Chap. 8. In addition, in an empathic relationship, the patient perceives a clinician as a trustworthy attachment figure, an omnipotent person of authority similar to a protective wise parent. Therefore, the clinician becomes a secure base from which the patient can explore the unknowns of the illness and disclose real concerns without any constraints. Evidence in support of such beneficial effects of genuine human connection is plentiful, some of which was presented in Chap. 4. Also, when an empathic engagement is formed, the patient views the clinician as a helpful member of a social support system with all of its beneficial effects on his or her physical, mental, and social well-being. Ample evidence is available to support this claim as well, some of which was reported in Chap. 2.

On the basis of the assumptions just described, an empathic clinician–patient relationship paves the road to positive patient outcomes. However, despite the abundance of reports in the medical, psychological, and sociological literature about these assumptions, empirical evidence supporting the direct link between empathy and measurable patient outcomes in medical and surgical care is limited. As I indicated in Chaps. 1 and 6, the dearth of empirical evidence in support of a direct link between empathy and patient outcomes can be attributed to two factors. First, the historical conceptual ambiguity regarding empathy in clinician–patient relationships has been an obstacle to the development of an operational definition of empathy in patient care. A concept that is not well defined does not lend itself to empirical scrutiny. Second, until the development of the Jefferson Scale of Empathy, the lack of a psychometrically sound measure of empathy designed specifically for use in the context of patient care had been an impediment to the empirical investigation of empathy and its outcomes in the context of the health professions education and patient care. However, because empathy is the backbone of clinician–patient relationships, we can safely assume that the majority of research findings about the effects of the quality of physician–patient "relationships" on patient outcomes could be generalizable or applicable to "empathic engagement" in patient care as well.

The Clinician–Patient Relationship and Patient Outcomes

A large volume of research has accumulated in support of the notion that the quality of the clinician–patient relationship can facilitate the process of patient care and thus have a positive influence on patient outcomes (Butow, Maclean, Dunn, Tattersall, & Boyer, 1997; Di Blasi, Harkness, Ernst, Georgiou, & Kleijnen, 2001; Neuwirth, 1997; Roghmann, Hengst, & Zastowny, 1979; Roter et al., 1998; Sanson-Fisher & Maguire, 1980; Staudenmayer & Lefkowitz, 1981; Stewart, 1996; Watts, 2012). The relevance of such research findings to the theme of empathy in patient care is evident if one assumes that empathic engagement is a core ingredient of positive clinician–patient relationships.

The medical literature contains abundant evidence in support of the notion that the quality of clinician–patient relationships has a tangible effect on clinical outcomes. For example, a review of 21 published studies revealed that 16 (76 %) of the articles reported a positive, statistically significant relationship between effective physician–patient communication and health outcomes (Stewart, 1996). Among the elements of effective communication were physicians' empathic engagement, supportive role, and concern about patients' feelings and experiences (Stewart, 1996).

The following sections present some empirical evidence from the medical literature in support of the notion that high-quality clinician–patient relationships positively influence patients' satisfaction and compliance and reduce the likelihood of malpractice litigation.

Patient Satisfaction

Patient satisfaction is a widely recognized outcome measure in health care research (Hall, Roter, & Katz, 1988). The relationship between patients' satisfaction with their health care providers and their recall of and compliance with the providers' medical advice suggests that satisfaction is an important determinant of the outcome of health care (Hall & Dornan, 1988).

Patients' overall satisfaction with their health care providers is often moderately high (in the 70s or 80s on a 100-point scale) (Hall & Dornan, 1988). Interpersonal exchanges between physician and patient have often proved to be significant predictors of patients' satisfaction (Butow et al., 1997). For example, a meta-analytic study found that such factors as nonverbal cues (e.g., touch, forward lean, closer distance, eye contact, nods, gestures), social–emotional conversation (about nonmedical issues), positive talk, and length of encounter contribute to the patients' satisfaction with their health care providers (Hall, Roter, Katz, 1988). Other determinants of patients' satisfaction were patients' participation in the therapeutic process (Speedling & Rose, 1985), commitment to the therapeutic relationship (i.e., willingness to return to the physician for care), the length of time the physicians spent with their patients, and the physicians' willingness to listen and to be accessible when needed (DiMatteo, Prince, & Taranta, 1979).

Moreover, physicians' ability to communicate their concern, warmth, and interest to their patients also leads to patients' satisfaction (Speedling & Rose, 1985). Physicians' general sensitivity to patients' emotions and their ability to express feelings were associated with patients' satisfaction (DiMatteo, Taranta, Friedman, & Prince, 1980). All the qualities of physicians just described are among the ingredients of empathic engagement in patient care.

One can assume that the positive link between physicians' empathy and patient outcomes is the result of empathic engagement that can help patients formulate their health problems more clearly, thus leading to more accurate diagnoses, more acceptable solutions to their health problems, and also to firmer commitment to the treatment regimen (Stiles, Putman, Wolfe, & James, 1979). For example, patients infected with the human immunodeficiency virus (HIV) indicated that the quality of interpersonal relationships with medical staff was an important factor in their satisfaction with the care they received (Stein, Fleisman, Mor, & Dresser, 1993). In another study, patients' perceptions of their physicians' interpersonal and communication skills, rather than physicians' knowledge, contributed more to patients' satisfaction with clinical outcomes (Clearly & McNeil, 1988).

Investigators who conducted a study with residents in internal medicine and their patients noticed that patients' satisfaction was related more to interpersonal relationships reflected in physicians' courtesy and giving of information than to physicians' nonverbal behavior, such as eye contact and body posture (Comstock, Hooper, Goodwin, & Goodwin, 1982).

Reports that patients are generally more satisfied with an empathic health provider (Beckman & Frankel, 1984; Bertakis, Roter, & Putman, 1991; Francis & Morris, 1969; Korsch, Gozzi, & Francis, 1968b; Zachariae et al., 2003) and comply more with physicians who understand them better (Blackwell, 1973; Davis, 1968; Hall et al., 1988; Squier, 1990; Stewart, 1996) provide one explanation for positive clinical outcomes of empathy in patient care. Patients generally view physicians' conduct as a key determinant of their satisfaction with medical care (Moss, 1967). The finding that the physicians' understanding of their patients' perspective is related to the patients' perceptions of being helped (Eisenthal, Emery, Lazare, & Udin, 1979) provides additional support for the link between empathic understanding and improves patient empowerment (Street, Makoul, Arora, & Epstein, 2009). In a factor analytic study, 52 % of the variance in patent's ratings of their satisfaction with medical care was accounted for by the physician's level of interpersonal warmth and respect (Kenny, 1995). In a study with diabetic patients, dieticians' empathic understanding was predictive of the patients' satisfaction and the success of consultations (Goodchild, Skinner, & Parkin, 2005). To summarize, the practice style reflected in a clinician's communication skills and empathic concern leads to more patient's satisfaction.

Adherence and Compliance

Adherence to and compliance with treatment regimens are additional widely used indicators of clinical outcomes (Hall et al., 1988; Kim, Kaplowitz, & Johnston, 2004; Ong, DeHaes, Hoos, & Lammies, 1995; Roter et al., 1998; Sackett & Haynes, 1976; Stewart, 1996). Although the terms "adherence" and "compliance" are often used interchangeably in the literature, their meaning is not identical. For example, compliance reflects a biomedical paradigm of disease that reinforces passivity in patients (Roter et al., 1998) and refers to the patient's acceptance of the clinician's orders or advice without participating in the decision-making process (Kelman, 1958). When the patient follows the clinician's instructions as a participant in the process, however, adherence is the more appropriate term. Adherence implies a more active patient–clinician collaboration involving the patient's choice in planning the treatment (Eisenthal et al., 1979; Roter et al., 1998; Squier, 1990).

Abundant evidence suggests that positive patient–clinician relationships not only contribute to patients' satisfaction with their health care providers and adherence to the providers' advice but also lead to adequate disclosure of problems, all of which can have a significant impact on patient outcomes (Beckman & Frankel, 1984; Butow et al., 1997; Falvo & Tippy, 1988; Sanson-Fisher & Maguire, 1980). Physicians' understanding of their patients was found to be significantly correlated with patients' adhering to treatment and feeling better (Eisenthal et al., 1979). In a pediatric health care setting, investigators reported that mothers of sick children adhered more closely to the care provider's advice when they perceived that the provider attempted to understand their concerns (Francis & Morris, 1969; Korsch, Gozzi, & Francis, 1968a). In a similar study, physicians' empathic understanding, reflected in their expression of positive affect, increased adherence to the physicians' advice among mothers after emergency visits to a children's hospital (Freemon, Negrete, Davis, & Korsch, 1971).

Patients' adherence to treatment reportedly varied from 25 to 94 % depending on several factors, including interactions between physician and patient (Eisenthal et al., 1979). Despite the important benefits patients derived from following their physician's advice, two studies reported that a significant number of patients (30–60 %) failed to follow that advice (Kaplan & Simon, 1990; Luscher & Vetter, 1990). This can be attributed to a lack of empathic engagement. Physicians' empathic skills and interpersonal style have been cited as crucial factors determining whether patients adhere to treatment regimens (DiMatteo et al., 1993). Indicators of a physician's empathy, such as sensitivity, decoding skills, tone of voice, and nonverbal communication, were related to patients' compliance with scheduled appointments (DiMatteo, Hays, & Prince, 1986). Furthermore, in situations where the physician failed to demonstrate empathic engagement, the patient easily forgot their advice and was likely to miss follow-up appointments (Falvo & Tippy, 1988). In addition, physicians who expressed willingness to answer patients' questions without being concerned about the time had a positive influence on patients' adherence to treatment (DiMatteo et al., 1993). These studies suggest that an interpersonal style that reflects a physician's empathic understanding of patients can enhance patients' adherence to treatment.

Malpractice Claims

Research indicates that a problematic physician–patient relationship can increase the likelihood that a patient will initiate a legal action against the physician. A physician's style of communication, in particular, is an important factor in a plaintiff's decision to take such an action (Beckman, Markakis, Suchman, & Frankel, 1994; Hickson, Clayton, Githens, & Sloan, 1992; Levinson, Roter, Mullooly, Dull, & Frankel, 1997; Meyers, 1987; Shapiro, Simpson, & Lawrence, 1989). Empirical evidence suggests that a positive physician–patient relationship reduces not only the actual malpractice claims but also patients' intention to take such action, regardless of the severity of the adverse medical outcomes (Moore, Adler, & Robertson, 2000). In a survey of malpractice attorneys, it was found that more than 80 % of malpractice suits were based on unsatisfactory physician–patient relationships (Avery, 1985).

One study found that physicians who exhibited empathic concern for their patients were better diagnosticians and provided better treatments (Barsky, 1981). Conversely, poor communication skills on the physicians' part, which led to inadequate empathic engagement with patients, proved to be the most important factor prompting patients to file a lawsuit against a physician (Beckman et al., 1994).

In a study examining rates of malpractice claims for different medical specialties, Taragin et al. (1994) controlled for confounding factors (e.g., physicians' age, training, and certification status and the severity of the diseases they treated) and concluded that the variation in claim rates could not be explained by differences in the physicians' academic achievements. Consistent with these findings, researchers in another study found no relationship between malpractice claims against obstetricians and the technical quality of physician's care (Entman et al., 1994).

Among mothers of infants who had been permanently injured or had died, dissatisfaction with the obstetrician's interpersonal style (e.g., not listening, not talking openly, and not discussing long-term outcomes) was a major factor in determining whether the obstetrician was sued (Hickson et al., 1992). Compared with obstetricians who had been sued, those who had never been sued were viewed as concerned, accessible, and willing to talk (Hickson et al., 1994). Other studies have shown that the physician's communication skills and empathic concern are the factors that reduce the risk of malpractice litigation (Beckman et al., 1994; Levinson et al., 1997). A review of allegation transcripts revealed that physicians' failure to understand the perspectives of their patients or their patients' families—an indication of a lack of empathic engagement—was among the important factors that contributed to patients' decisions to sue (Beckman et al., 1994; Levinson et al., 1997).

Clinicians' Empathy and Clinical Outcomes

Although some studies show a link between empathic engagement and patient outcomes in the context of medical and surgical treatments (Luborsky, Chandler, Auerbach, Cohen, & Bacharach, 1971; Nightingale, Yarnold, & Greenberg, 1991), empirical evidence in support of empathic engagement and patient outcomes has been reported more often in the context of psychotherapy (Free, Green, Grace, Chernus, & Whitman, 1985; Gladstein, 1977; Kurtz & Grummon, 1972; Moyers & Miller, 2013). For example, premature termination of therapy has been reported among clients who gave their therapists low ratings on a measure of empathy (Burns & Nolen-Hoeksema, 1992). It is also reported that the therapist's deficiency in empathy is "toxic" to patient outcomes because of its association with high dropout and relapse rates, weaker therapeutic alliance, and less positive change in patients (Moyers & Miller, 2013). Conversely, some reviews of the literature have linked the therapist's empathy, warmth, and genuineness to positive changes in clients (Patterson, 1984). Other reviews have reported positive patient outcomes resulting from empathic engagement between patients and nurses (Bennett, 1995).

Research on psychotherapeutic outcomes, for example, has reported a high level of empathic clinician–patient engagement as the most important factor in the reduction of symptoms (Rogers, Gendlin, Kiesler, & Truax, 1967). Also, therapists' scores on the Accurate Empathy Scale of Truax and Carkhuff's Relationship Questionnaire (see Chap. 5) were significantly higher in successful than in unsuccessful therapy cases. Bacharach (1976) reported that a therapist's empathy was consistently correlated with other qualities such as regard, genuineness, concreteness, and self-disclosure that are associated with treatment outcomes. Some studies have provided evidence supporting the causal role of empathy in psychotherapeutic outcomes (Burns & Nolen-Hoeksema, 1992; Greenberg, Watson, Elliot, & Bohart, 2001). Nonetheless, there are other studies that have not confirmed a direct link between therapists' empathy and positive patient outcomes (Bohart, Elliot, Greenberg, & Watson, 2002; Luborsky et al., 1971; Meltzoff & Kornreich, 1970). The inconsistencies in conceptualization and variation in the measurement of empathy in patient care (see Chaps. 1, 5, and 6) could be among the reasons for inconsistent findings on empathy and patient outcomes reported in the aforementioned studies.

A meta-analytic review found that the typical effect size in studies on empathy and psychotherapy outcomes is in the 0.20s (Bohart et al., 2002). According to the operational definitions of effect sizes (Cohen, 1987; Hojat & Xu, 2004), an effect size of this magnitude is trivial. However, the magnitude of effect size for the relationship between empathy and patient outcomes varies, depending on the conceptualization of empathy (e.g., cognitive or emotional empathy), the instruments for measuring it, the format of the assessment (e.g., self-rated or observer-, peer-, or client-rated), the type of therapy (e.g., group, cognitive, psychoanalytical, behavioral therapy, or eclectic), the therapist's experience, the patient's receptivity, and so on (Bohart et al., 2002).

The aforementioned studies were mostly on the associations between psychotherapists' empathy and patient outcomes. Research on a direct empirical link between physician empathy and the outcomes of medical and surgical treatments is scarce (Stewart, 1996). However, there are some studies on the link between physician empathy and clinical outcomes. For example, it has been reported that internal medicine residents' self-perceived incidents of medical errors were associated with a lower level of their empathy (West et al., 2006). In a study (Sultan, Attali, Gilberg,

Zenasni, & Hartemann, 2011) it was found that physicians' accurate understanding of their diabetic patients' beliefs about their illness (as an indicator of empathic understanding) was associated with better self-care among patients (e.g., improved diet, increased blood glucose self-testing).

Staudenmayer and Lefkowitz (1981) found that physicians' empathic concern (determined by peers' ratings on their sensitivity) was related to the length of hospitalization and concerns about medications: Highly sensitive physicians were more concerned about the side effects of medications and kept their patients (with asthma and other pulmonary problems) in the hospital for longer periods. MacPherson, Mercer, Scullion, and Thomas (2003) reported that the perceptions of acupuncture patients concerning their care providers' empathy were significantly associated with patients' enablement, which in turn was highly correlated with self-reported patient outcomes.

In a study with 1048 fourth-year medical students, empathic engagement, assessed by standardized patients, was significantly correlated with patients' level of comfort and feelings of being important (Colliver, Willis, Robbs, Cohen, & Swartz, 1998). In that study, the students whose empathic engagement was assessed as insufficient (judged to be empathic by less than three of the seven standardized patients) also received lower ratings concerning their skills in history taking and physical examinations (Colliver et al., 1998).

Levinson (1994) reported that patients' satisfaction and adherence to treatment were directly associated with their physicians' empathic skills, whereas patients' dissatisfaction and malpractice claims were associated with their physicians' lack of those skills. In another study, physicians regarded empathic behavior as the most important quality for being a "good physician" for improving patient outcomes; however, the physicians themselves listed empathic behavior as the least important factor for being promoted in the hospital setting (Carmel & Glick, 1996).

An experiment conducted in the General Medicine Clinic at Cook County Hospital in Chicago showed that physicians' empathic, as opposed to sympathetic, responses to patients can lead to different measurable influences on their practice behavior and on patient outcomes (Nightingale et al., 1991). The sample in that experiment consisted of 96 residents and fellows whose preference for responding empathically or sympathetically to patients was determined by the following scenario:

> Your next patient enters the office, sits down, and says: "Doctor, my husband/wife died and I feel terrible!" The English language gives you two basic ways to respond to the patient: (A) "I understand how you feel" or words to that effect, or (B) "I feel sorry for you" or words to that effect. Which do you use?

The "A" option was considered to be an empathic response, and the "B" option was considered to be a sympathetic response. The physicians who chose the empathic response (60 % of the sample) ordered fewer laboratory tests, performed cardiopulmonary resuscitation for a shorter period of time before declaring their efforts unsuccessful, and showed less preference for intubating a hypothetical patient with end-stage lung disease. The investigators concluded that physicians' empathic or sympathetic responses could lead to significant differences in their style of practice and their use of resources. In another study it was reported that empathy can reduce the cost of medical care (Yarnold, Greenberg, & Nightingale, 1991).

In a study on the effect of physicians' empathy on patients' satisfaction and compliance with treatment (Kim et al., 2004), a set of questionnaires was administered to 550 outpatients at a university hospital in South Korea. The results indicated that patients' perceptions of physicians' empathy, measured by a modified version of the Barrett-Lennard's Relationship Inventory (Chap. 5), could have a significant influence on patients' satisfaction and compliance. The researchers concluded that enhancement of physicians' empathic communication skills is among the best approaches to improving patient satisfaction and compliance with treatment. In another study, expressions of empathy and support contributed to patients' satisfaction with their physicians (Thompson, Hearn, & Collins, 1992).

Dubnicki (1977) reported that psychotherapists' high scores on Hogan's Empathy Scale (Chap. 5) were predictive of more accurate prognoses. Kendall and Wilcox (1980) found that when therapists formed an empathic relationship with hyperactive and uncontrolled children, the children's behavior improved. Physicians' empathy, determined by positive interactions between pediatricians and the mothers of sick children, improved the mothers' satisfaction with the children's care and reduced their concern about the illness (Wasserman, Inui, Barriatua, Carter, & Lippincott, 1984). Another study found that physicians' empathy, responsiveness, and reliability were significant determinants of patients' satisfaction with their health care (Bowers, Swan, & Koehler, 1994).

The majority of studies on the link between clinicians' empathy and patient outcomes relied on the clinicians' self-reported empathy. However, it has been suggested that patients' own perceptions of their health care providers' empathy could be a better predictor of clinical outcomes (Free et al., 1985; Kurtz & Grummon, 1972). This was confirmed in a study of 350 patients with the common cold who were treated by six health care providers (five family physicians and one nurse practitioner). Patients completed the Consultation and Relational Empathy (Mercer, Maxwell, Heaney, & Watt, 2004; Mercer, McConnachie, Maxwell, Heaney, & Watt, 2005, see Chap. 5). Results (after adjustment for patients' gender, race, education, optimism, perceived stress, hours since first symptom) showed significant associations between patients' assessment of their health care providers' empathy, and clinical outcomes indicated by shorter duration and reduced severity of cold symptoms along with a positive change in the patients' immune system (Rakel et al., 2009).

Physician Empathy and Tangible Patient Outcomes

The abovementioned studies on the association between clinicians' empathy and patient outcomes are limited for two reasons: (1) empathy of the physician has not been measured by a psychometrically sound instrument with face and content validities, developed specifically to measure empathy in the context of patient care; (2)

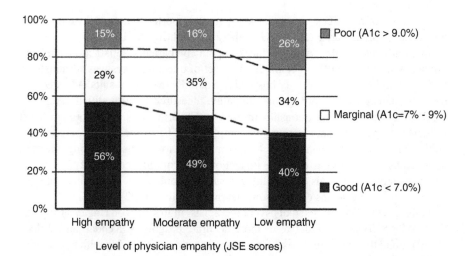

Fig. 11.1 Association between physician (*n*=29) empathy and hemoglobin A1c test results for diabetic patients (*n*=891)

the indicators of patient outcomes have been either subjective or self-reported which could be confounded by judgmental errors.

To the best of our knowledge, there are only two published studies in which a significant association was observed between a validated measure of physician empathy (JSE) and tangible patient outcomes extracted from patients' electronic records, independent from patient's subjective judgment. In the first study (Hojat, Louis, Markham et al., 2011), electronic records of 891 adult patients with diabetes mellitus who were treated by one of 29 family physicians in the USA were examined, and the results of the most recent tests for hemoglobin A1c and low-density lipoprotein cholesterol (LDL-C) were extracted. Positive clinical outcomes were defined as good control of the disease reflected in A1c test results <7.0 % and LDL-C <100. Findings showed that physicians' scores on the JSE could significantly predict clinical outcomes in the diabetic patients. Patients of physicians with high JSE scores were significantly more likely to have good control of their disease (56 % of patients with A1C test results <7.0, and 59 % with LDL-C <100), compared to patients of physicians with low JSE scores (40 % with A1c <7.0, and 44 % with LDL-C <100). The association between physicians' scores on the JSE and patient outcomes (results of A1c and LDL-C) remained statistically significant after controlling for physicians' gender and age, as well as for patients' gender, age, and type of health insurance. Summary results are depicted in Figs. 11.1 and 11.2.

In the second study (Del Canale et al., 2012), electronic records of 20,961 adult patients with type 1 or type 2 diabetes mellitus who were treated by one of 242 primary care physicians (in Parma, Italy) were examined, and information on acute metabolic complications that required hospitalization (e.g., diabetic ketoacidosis,

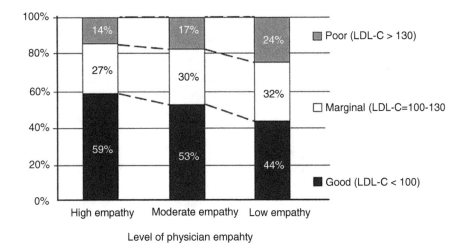

Fig. 11.2 Association between physician ($n=29$) empathy scores and low-density lipoprotein cholesterol (LDL-C) test results for diabetic patients ($n=891$)

coma, and hyperosmolar) and demographic information were extracted. Physicians completed the JSE. Results showed statistically significant associations between physicians' scores on the JSE and rates of hospitalization due to acute metabolic complications in diabetic patients. Rates of disease complication in diabetic patients of physicians who scored high on the JSE (≥ 112), compared to other physicians with moderate scores (111–97) or low JSE scores (<97), were 4.0, 7.1, and 6.5 per 1000, respectively. Summary results are presented in Fig. 11.3.

The association remained statistically significant after controlling for physicians' gender, age, type of practice (solo or group), geographical location of practice (plains, hills, mountains), and also patients' gender, age, and duration of time enrolled with the physician. Similarities in findings of the two aforementioned studies on significant association between physician empathy and patient outcomes are important for the generalization of the findings, given the cultural differences or variation in medical education and the health care systems in the USA and Italy.

Explanations for the Link Between Physician Empathy and Patient Outcomes

Empathic engagement in patient care revolves around reciprocity and mutual understanding which evokes psychosocial and biophysioneurological interactions. Analyses of these interactions can provide plausible explanations for the link between physician empathy and patient outcomes (Hojat, Louis, et al., 2013).

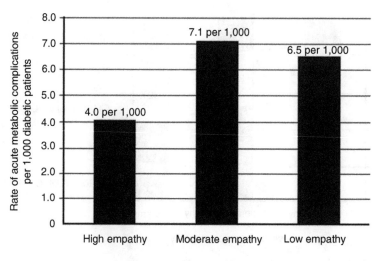

Fig. 11.3 Association between physician empathy ($n = 242$) and acute metabolic complications in their diabetic patients ($n = 20,961$) in Parma, Italy

At the psychosocial level, empathic engagement lays the foundation for a trusting relationship. Constraints in communication will diminish when a trusting relationship is formed. In the security of a trusting relationship, the patient begins to tell the tale of his or her illness without concealment. This in turn leads to a more accurate diagnosis and greater compliance, which ultimately will result in better quality care, and improved patient outcomes (Hojat, Louis et al., 2013).

At the biophysioneurological level, empathic engagement seems analogous to a synchronized dance between the involved parties, orchestrated by biophysioneurological markers. For example, the interpersonal attunement in empathic engagement can activate some prosocial endogenous neuropeptides or hormonal changes such as oxytocin and vasopressin (Heinrichs & Domes, 2008). In addition, it has been shown that a set of neurons, known as the mirror neuron system (MNS), is discharged when observing another person performing a goal-directed act, as if the observer is performing the act (Gallese, 2001; Rizzolatti, Fadiga, Gallese, & Fogassi, 1996). In other words, the same set of neuron cells that are discharged in the acting person will be implicated in the person who observes the act without actually performing it, or feeling the emotions or concerns of the other person. The MNS is believed to play an important role in understanding the experiences of others, which is the key ingredient of empathic engagement in patient care. Thus, subconscious activation of the MNS in empathic engagement in patient care can explain the neurological underpinnings of patient–clinician synchronized connections that can lead to positive patient outcomes.

Over a century ago, Theodore Lipps, who brought the concept of empathy ("ein-fühlung" in the German language) into psychology, proposed that seeing someone else's facial expression triggers the observer to automatically adopt a similar facial expression, known as facial mimicry. These behaviors can be explained by the perception-action model (PAM) formulated by Preston and deWaal (2002). They suggested that perceptions of another person's cognitive, emotional, and somato-sensory states automatically activate representations of those states in the observer, unless inhibited. Thus, the PAM can provide physiological explanations for under-standing of a patient's pain, suffering, experiences, and concerns, which are among components of empathic engagement in patient care (see Chap. 13). The link between the PAM, MNS, and empathy is supported by findings of subconscious mimicry in facial expression, postures, and mannerism; contagious yawning; affect contagion; synchronization in heart rate; mood; and galvanic skin response among interacting individuals, especially among those who are engaged in a goal-directed and meaningful interaction (Hojat, Louis et al., 2013, see also Chap. 13).

In summary, the combined effects of psychosocial and biophysioneurological mechanisms involved in empathic patient–clinician interactions can help in under-standing the mechanisms underlying the beneficial effects of empathic engagement in patient care.

Recapitulation

One can speculate that physicians' positive interpersonal conduct, as an indicator of empathic engagement, is associated with positive patient outcomes, including more accurate diagnoses, greater adherence to treatment regimens, patients' greater satis-faction, and less likelihood of malpractice litigation. Abundant research supports this speculation. Although convincing evidence exists to confirm significant asso-ciations between empathic engagement and patient outcomes, empirical research to verify a direct link between validated measures of empathy in the context of patient care and tangible indicators of patient outcomes is scarce. Two empirical studies of physicians and their diabetic patients in the USA and Italy provided strong evidence in support of positive effects of physician empathy in the control of disease in dia-betic patients. The question of why a health care provider's empathy is associated with patient outcomes was addressed by providing plausible explanations for pos-sible underlying psychosocial and biophysioneurological underpinnings in empathic engagement in patient care.

Chapter 12
Erosion and Enhancement of Empathy

The only thing necessary for the triumph of evil is for good men to do nothing.
—(Edmund Burke, cited in Manning, Levine & Collins, 2007, p. 561).

You couldn't love something you didn't understand.
—(Forrest Carter, 1976, p. 38)

Abstract

- Empathy is viewed as an important element of professionalism in medicine; however, a few obstacles to the development and implementation of empathy exist in medical education and practice.
- Health professions education and the health care system have become very reliant on computer-based diagnostic and therapeutic technology that may limit students' and practitioners' vision about the importance of human connection and empathic engagement in patient care.
- Given the findings that medical students tend to develop a certain cynicism as they progress through their medical education and empathy erodes in medical school and postgraduate medical education, it is timely and important to pay serious attention to enhancing and sustaining empathy in the health professions education and patient care.
- Enhancing and sustaining empathy in health profession education and practice should be considered a mandate that must be acted upon by leaders and educators in the health professions academic centers and heath care institutions.
- Research shows that empathy is an attribute that is amenable to change as a result of targeted educational programs and educational experiences.
- Some approaches used to enhance empathy in the health professionals-in-training and in-practice are described, including improving interpersonal skills, audio- or video-taping of patient encounters, exposure to role models, role playing (e.g., aging game), shadowing a patient (patient navigator), hospitalization experiences, studying literature and the arts, improving narrative skills and reflective writing, theatrical performances, and the Balint method.

© Springer International Publishing Switzerland 2016
M. Hojat, *Empathy in Health Professions Education and Patient Care*,
DOI 10.1007/978-3-319-27625-0_12

- More empirical research is needed to confirm the effectiveness of programs designed to enhance empathy, to examine the long-term effects of such programs, and to develop strategies to sustain enhancement in empathy for a longer period of time.

Introduction

This chapter begins with a discussion of professionalism in medicine and describes some factors that hamper the development of empathy among students and practitioners in the health professions. I also present results of findings of empirical research that suggest that empathy tends to erode during medical and some other health professions education. Then, I describe some of the approaches that psychologists and researchers in health professions education have used to enhance empathy, including ten specific approaches used in undergraduate and graduate medical education to improve and sustain empathy among physicians-in-training.

Professionalism in Medicine

Professionalism in medicine is defined as an array of personal qualities beyond the requisite medical knowledge and procedural skills that health care professionals must possess to deliver high-quality health care to their patients that leads to positive clinical outcomes (Veloski & Hojat, 2006). Medical educators currently are encouraged to make every effort to foster professionalism in medicine by offering programs at the undergraduate, graduate, and continuing education levels.

Although no consensus exists regarding the number and nature of personal qualities required for professionalism in medicine, compassionate care and empathy have frequently been mentioned as its key components (Arnold, 2002; Barondess, 2003; Linn, DiMatteo, Cope, & Robbins, 1987). In his book *Humanism and the Physician*, Edmund Pellegrino (1979) described the empathic way of helping patients as an important aspect of the physician's humanistic attributes. Senior residents at Laval and Calgary Universities in Canada listed empathy, respect, and competence as the three most important elements of professionalism in medicine (Brownell & Cote, 2001).

Cultivating humanistic values, including empathy, is among the important goals of education in the health care professions. The Medical Schools Objectives Project of the Association of American Medical Colleges (2004) includes enrichment of empathy among the educational objectives of medical schools, emphasizing that the schools should strive to produce altruistic physicians who provide compassionate care to patients and demonstrate empathy by conveying their understanding of the patient's perspective. In a position paper, the American Board of Internal Medicine (1983) recommended that humanistic attributes, including empathy, should be instilled in and assessed among residents as an essential part of their medical training.

Despite the consensus regarding the healing potential of empathic encounters in patient care, insufficient attention has been given to enhancement of the capacity for empathy in the design of medical education curriculum. As a result, the concept of empathy in patient care, according to Novack (1987), seems to be fading away in modern medical education. The current system of medical education does not seem to be seriously concerned about physicians' losing their healing touch, treating it instead "as if it were a relic of an unscientific past" (Novack, 1987, p. 346).

The lack of attention to empathy in patient care is partially the result of overreliance on computer-based diagnostic and therapeutic technology and partially the result of changes in the health care system with its ripple effect on medical education and practice. In the biotechnologically advanced atmosphere of patient care, what computers spit out seems to receive more attention from some practitioners who trust the machines more than their skills in detecting clinical signs of disease or their patients' narrative accounts of illness.

Although the pathophysiology of disease may be detected by examining computer output and electronic images, an accurate diagnosis of illness is possible by listening to the patient and conducting physical examinations in clinical encounters (Spiro, 1986). Today, the public pleads desperately for physicians who are more communicative and empathic in their encounters with patients (Fishbein, 1999). Despite the current emphasis on the development of professionalism, enhancement of empathy in the education of health care professionals has not yet received systematic and sufficient attention. According to Girgis and Sanson-Fisher (1995), although most physicians are well equipped to provide high-quality technical services, they are often ill equipped to provide empathic care.

Obstacles to Empathy in Patient Care

Some of the factors that impede the development and implementation of empathy in in-training and in-practice health professionals are described in the following sections.

Cynicism

Most medical students embark on a journey to become physicians with idealism and enthusiasm for curing disease and preventing infirmity. Despite the intention of medical school faculty to nurture these qualities, it is ironic that some have noticed a decline in humanitarianism, enthusiasm, and idealism among students during medical training (Kay, 1990; Maheux & Beland, 1989; Sheehan, Sheehan, White, Leibowitz, & Baldwin, 1990; Silver & Glicken, 1990; Wolf, Balson, Faucett, &

Randall, 1989; Zeldow & Daugherty, 1987). This observation has been supported by empirical research showing that students' empathy tends to erode in medical school (Hojat et al., 2004, 2009) and in postgraduate medical education (Bellini, Baime, & Shea, 2002; Bellini & Shea, 2005).

The effects of medical education on personal qualities were addressed empirically more than five decades ago with some disturbing results (Becker & Geer, 1958; Eron, 1958). One longitudinal study conducted in the 1950s (Eron, 1958) found that medical students became more cynical and less humanitarian as they progressed through medical school, whereas this pattern was not observed among law students! In that study, a typical question used to measure cynicism was "If you don't look out for yourself, nobody else will," and a typical question for measuring humanism was "When I hear about the suffering of a particular individual or group, I want very much to help."

A similar concern about medical students' progression toward cynicism during medical school was raised in the early 1980s (Silver, 1982). Another study found that as many as three-fourths of medical students became more cynical about academic life and the medical profession as they progressed through medical school (Sheehan et al., 1990). This metamorphosis in the character of medical students was likened to the "battered child syndrome" and was attributed to inappropriate treatment of students by the medical schools (Rosenberg & Silver, 1984; Silver & Glicken, 1990). The terms "dehumanization" (Edwards & Zimet, 1976) and "traumatic deidealization" (Kay, 1990) were also used to describe the cynical transformation occurring during medical education.

Several additional studies conducted in the 1980s reported other disturbing findings. A study at the University of Texas Health Science Center in San Antonio found that medical students underwent a significant hedonistic change in personality between the freshman and junior years of medical school: They became less inhibited and more self-indulgent (Burnstein et al., 1980). In a longitudinal study conducted at the same medical center, a decline in students' scores on the "need to understand" scale of a personality inventory also raised concern about the negative influence of medical education on students' personalities (Whittemore, Burstein, Loucks, & Schoenfeld, 1985). Students in the senior year at the Louisiana State University School of Medicine reported that the top two changes in attitude during medical school were more cynicism (76 %) and more concern about making money (60 %) (Wolf et al., 1989).

The alarm bells became even louder in 2002 when a nationwide study found that 61 % of residents in American residency training programs believed that they had become more cynical during their medical education (Collier, MaCue, Markus, & Smith, 2002). Cynicism was more prominent among female residents than it was among male residents (63 % versus 56 %, respectively). Interestingly, however, residents with children reported less cynicism and more humanistic feelings during their medical education (Sanson-Fisher & Maguire, 1980).

In an atmosphere of declining humanism, the emphasis by some modern medical educators placed on "detached concern" and "affective distance" for the purpose of increasing objectivity in clinical decision making is accelerating the dramatic metamorphosis occurring in medical education and patient care (Coulehan & Williams, 2001; Evans, Stanley, & Burrows, 1993; Farber, Novack, & O'Brien, 1997). Although well intended, the advice of those educators can be misinterpreted, thus adding to the factors contributing to the ultimate depletion of empathy's importance in medical education and practice (Ludmerer, 1999; Starr, 1982). Among other factors fueling increased cynicism in medical education are lack of role models (Diseker & Michielutte, 1981; Kramer, Ber, & Moore, 1987) and lack of dedicated educational programs for nourishment of humanistic qualities in patient encounters.

Paradigmatic Shift in the Health Care System

As Gonnella et al. (1993, 1993) suggested, in addition to factors related to physicians and patients, the environment of health care delivery exerts a significant influence on physicians' interpersonal behavior and patient outcomes. Recent developments in the organization, financing, and delivery of health care, notably in the expansion of managed care, cost containment, and the restriction of physicians' autonomy, pose challenges that contribute to physicians' discontent with the practice of medicine and a lack of opportunity for empathic engagement in clinical encounters (Burdi & Baker, 1999; Magee & Hojat, 2001).

Anecdotal reports suggest that financial incentives and insurance regulations in the current environment of health care have forced a number of physicians to trade off their patients' interest against their will. The golden principle that the patient's best interest must be the primary consideration in patient care has lost its priority in such a market-driven health care environment. According to a survey of physicians, the significant decline in the time physicians spent with patients and their inability to control the length of patients' hospital stays and their own work schedules exacerbated their dissatisfaction with the current atmosphere of the health care environment (Burdi & Baker, 1999). When Burdi and Baker (1999) compared a sample of physicians surveyed in 1991 with another cohort-matched sample of physicians surveyed in 1996, they found that the number of physicians who said that they would have chosen medicine if they had been college students declined by 10 % during the 5-year period. This decline reflects the evolving changes in the health care system leading to physician dissatisfaction.

In a survey of 2608 physicians conducted in 2004, 58 % of them said that their enthusiasm for medicine had declined in the past few years, and 87 % said that their morale had declined because of changes in the health care system (Zuger, 2004). The discontent of physicians is an inevitable outcome of the restrictions on their autonomy and use of resources imposed by hospital administrators, the health care system, and the health insurance industry (Hojat, Gonnella, Erdmann, Veloski et al., 2000; Kassirer, 1998; Magee & Hojat, 2001). Physicians' discontent with the practice of medicine, especially among those who have been "wounded" by malpractice allegations, matters because it influences the interpersonal quality of care and empathic engagement in clinical encounters. An analysis of how physicians are depicted in the movies showed that their portrayal as positive figures has declined in recent years. In current films, they are often depicted as greedy, egoistic, uncaring, and unethical (Flores, 2002).

The "time" factor is another impediment caused by the growing emphasis on cost containment that has contributed to shortening the duration spent in clinical encounters, thus hindering the formation of empathic relationships. The medical profession, once the most respected of all professions (Thomas, 1985), is now under siege, and physicians are frequently blamed, often mistakenly, for the problems created by nonphysician managers of health insurance organizations. These structural and functional shifts in the health care delivery system can hamper the potential benefits of forming empathic clinician–patient relationships. The ripple effect of changes in the American health care system has also had a profound effect on medical students (Hojat, Veloski et al., 1999) and nurses (Steinbrook, 2002).

Research shows that physicians' discontent leads to patients' noncompliance with treatment (DiMatteo et al., 1993) and dissatisfaction with their health care providers (Hass et al., 2000; Linn, Yager, Cope, & Leake, 1985). Such discontent among physicians can be reflected in pessimism manifested in their communication with patients. Furthermore, research suggests that pessimism is significantly associated with mortality among physicians as well as their patients (Hollowell & De Ville, 2003).

As a result of the paradigmatic shift described earlier, the health care delivery system has been transformed into a profit-driven enterprise with less emphasis on clinician–patient interactions and more emphasis on financial efficiency (Merlyn, 1998). Diminished prestige, loss of autonomy, and deep personal dissatisfaction are among the outcomes of paradigmatic shifts in health care systems. Research shows a widespread "professional malaise" among physicians who are caught between the desire to provide high-quality care to their patients on the one hand and the need to satisfy the insurers and regulators on the other hand (Zuger, 2004).

According to psychoanalytic theories, this type of approach-avoidance psychic conflict (e.g., a desire to help patients and avoid conflicts with insurers at the same time) can lead to frustration and neurotic-type distress that threatens physicians' physical, mental, and social well-being. Poor clinical management and substandard medical care resulting from a system that restricts physicians' autonomy in dealing with patients inevitably lead to hostile reactions by the public, often directed toward physicians, who themselves are victims of the system's crippling effects.

Added to this paradigmatic shift in the health care delivery system is the dramatic rise in the number of malpractice suits. The inevitable result is greater discontent with medicine among practitioners and even greater dissatisfaction with health care services among patients (Mello et al., 2004). In an atmosphere in which the physician–patient relationship resembles an encounter between consumer and retailer, little room obviously is left for compassion and empathy.

The primary concern of powerful players in the health care system—notably, nonphysicians employed by government agencies, hospital administrators, and the health insurance industry—is cost containment. The new arrangements created by this shift of emphasis have intruded in the clinical autonomy of physicians, led to the inability of physicians to preserve their altruistic image, and eroded the public's trust and support (Schlesinger, 2002). In a hostile atmosphere where physician–patient encounters are based on fear of allegations of malpractice, rather than on trust, the physician–patient relationship is likely to be shaken at best and violated or broken at worst (Thom, Hall, & Pawlson, 2004). As a result of all the changes occurring in the health care system, the adverse effects on the physician–patient relationship are more threatening to the outcomes of care than ever before (Simpson et al., 1991). Needless to say, an empathic relationship is highly unlikely to form in an atmosphere in which physicians view each patient as a potential adversary for malpractice litigation (Mello et al., 2004), while patients view their physicians as uncaring and greedy individuals who cannot be trusted.

In 2002, the American Board of Internal Medicine, the American College of Physicians, the American Society for Internal Medicine, and the European Federation of Internal Medicine jointly published a report titled *Medical Professionalism in the New Millennium: A Physician Charter* (Sox, 2002). The report not only confirmed the existence of the problems described here but also underscored their severity by concluding that the "changes in the health care delivery systems in countries throughout the industrial world threaten the values of professionalism" (p. 234). These trends in medicine, with their ripple effect on medical education, have resulted in brief consultations, the goal of which is to identify one physical problem as the "chief complaint" (Shorter, 1986), thus shifting the attention from the patient as a "whole person" to a disease as a "case." One hopes that the recent attention to professionalism in medical education and practice will bring empathic engagement between physician and patient to the forefront of health care once again.

Overreliance on Biotechnology, Computerized Diagnostic and Therapeutic Procedures

The new millennium offers either the best or the worst clinical care, depending on whether one views the "glass" as half-full or half-empty. The glass is half-full, given the fact the biotechnological developments can certainly help to prevent many diseases worldwide at a rapid pace, to make more accurate diagnoses much earlier than before, and to treat patients more aggressively. The glass is half-empty, however, given the fact that computerized medicine is gradually replacing "the laying on of hands," trivializing the importance of face-to-face encounters between clinician and patient and reducing opportunities to form empathic engagement as a result. Even telephone calls to family physicians (who made home visits in the good old days) are answered by automatic messages instructing desperate patients to call back during office hours, or go to the nearest hospital emergency room for help. Obviously, these trends are not conducive to empathic engagement in patient care.

During visits to a physician's office, patients are often required to undergo a series of laboratory tests, unnecessarily in some cases (Divinagarcia, Harkin, Bonk, & Schluger, 1998; Sandler, 1980), and wait until the physician receives the results and makes a diagnosis, overlooking the clinical signs and symptoms that have been used successfully by physicians for hundreds of years. In this era of overreliance on biotechnology, many physicians tend to view the results of laboratory tests and computerized diagnostic procedures as the holy script—despite the well-known errors associated with the sensitivity and specificity of tests—rather than paying more attention to the patients' clinical signs and illness narrative. Thus, patients are treated as objects for technical services (Coulehan & Williams, 2001) rather than as subjects for human care. This style of dealing with patients defies Peabody's stated purpose of patient care: "The treatment of a disease may be entirely impersonal; the care of a patient must be completely personal" (Peabody, 1984, p. 814). In a survey of patients who either changed their physicians or were thinking of changing their physicians, the following comment made by a patient deserves serious attention in medical education: "Students should be taught to use technology as a backup and not as the primary factor of the examination of the patient" (Cousins, 1985, p. 1423).

The strain in the physician–patient relationship caused by the shift from the patient's trust in the physician's healing touch to the physician's trust in computerized diagnostic and therapeutic procedures has led to the public's perception that physicians have become too "detached" to be concerned about their patients (Mangione et al., 2002). As a result, the medical profession is increasingly faced with the criticism that physicians are losing their human touch (Johnston, 1992). Indeed, a number of studies have supported this view by confirming that medical students, residents, and practicing physicians have become more cynical and less compassionate during medical training and practice (Feudtner, Christakis, & Christakis, 1994; Hojat et al., 2004; Kay, 1990; Lu, 1995; Maheux & Beland, 1989; Self, Schrader, Baldwin, & Wolinsky, 1993; Sheehan et al., 1990; Silver & Glicken, 1990; Wolf et al., 1989; Zeldow & Daugherty, 1987).

The abovementioned issues are only some of the challenges facing medical education and practice today. However, despite all the bad news, the good news is that it is possible to enhance empathy through dedicated educational programs and through demonstrations of its beneficial effects on patient outcomes.

The Amenability of Empathy to Change

A number of studies have shown that during the course of medical education, a students' capacity for empathy can undergo positive, negative, or no change. Although the inconsistent research findings are troublesome and may reflect issues involving conceptualization, measurement, and methodology, the fact that most of the recent studies have noted a change in empathy, either positive as a result of implementing targeted interventions (Hojat, Axelrod, Spandorfer, & Mangione, 2013; Van Winkle, Bjork, et al., 2012; Van Winkle, Fjortoft, & Hojat, 2012) or negative as a result of negative educational experiences and a lack of positive role models (Hojat et al., 2009), indicates that this attribute is amenable to change—welcome news for medical educators.

The State-Versus-Trait Debate

The idea of enhancing empathy during education for the health professions depends heavily on the belief that the capacity for empathy is amenable to change. Thus, it is important to address this issue at the outset because, if empathy proved to be a stable personality trait that cannot be easily changed, discussion of educational programs designed to enhance empathy would be pointless.

Psychologists have long been concerned about the possibility of changing people's motivations, attitudes, values, personality, and behavior. It is generally believed that some human attributes are more resistant to change than others. In the behavioral and social sciences, personal qualities, such as excitability, that are highly stable and difficult to change, are often called *traits*, whereas relatively unstable personality attributes, such as moods, that are easy to change are called *states* (Cole, Martin, & Steiger, 2005). The findings of longitudinal research concerning the stability of the so-called traits are inconsistent. For example, some findings suggest that traits can change over time (Roberts & DelVecchio, 2000), and other findings indicate that traits continue to show stability over a period of 15 years (Caspi & Silva, 1995).

The notion that empathy has an evolutionary root (Chap. 3) suggests that under ordinary circumstances, normal individuals are naturally programmed to demonstrate empathy. The extent to which the potential for empathy can be actualized or enhanced in a particular person depends on the interaction of several factors, including the person's constitutional makeup, early life experiences, motivation, and a facilitating environment as well as exposure to specific educational programs. Therefore, empathy, in my view, is neither a highly stable personality trait nor a state that can be changed without effort. In a sense, empathy resembles the notion of attachment that is rooted in evolutionary, genetic, developmental, experiential, situational, and educational ground, and its deficit can be improved by therapeutic or interventional approaches.

Changes in Empathy During Health Professions Education

Positive Change

Some studies that offered a targeted educational program reported an improvement in empathy. For example, residents who participated in a comprehensive interpersonal skills training course demonstrated greater use of empathy when dealing with patients (e.g., they asked more open-ended questions and provided emotion-related responses) (Kause, Robbins, Heidrich, Abrassi, & Anderson, 1980).

A study of Israeli medical students found that a clerkship in psychiatry improved their scores on Mehrabian and Epstein's Emotional Empathy Scale (Chap. 5) and that the students retained the effect of the program for at least 6 months (Elizur & Rosenheim, 1982). In another study, the investigators noticed that medical students and physicians who participated in an interpersonal skills workshop demonstrated improved empathic engagement, as determined by their increasing use of supportive behaviors, such as listening, responding empathically, and calming patients (Kramer, Ber, & Moore, 1989).

At the University of Missouri School of Medicine in Kansas City, empathy training offered to students in the early years of medical school resulted in increased scores on Carkhuff's Empathic Understanding in Interpersonal Processes Scale (Feighny, Arnold, Monaco, Munro, & Earl, 1998). However, the students' scores on Davis's Interpersonal Reactivity Index (IRI, see Chap. 5) did not increase, probably because of its lower sensitivity in the clinical context. Finally, over the years, training in communication skills provided in various formats (lectures, workshops, and audio- or videotapes) has proven to be useful in improving empathy-related skills (Evans et al., 1993; Fine & Therrien, 1977; Kramer et al., 1989; Sanson-Fisher & Poole, 1978; Winefield & Chur-Hansen, 2000).

Stepien and Baernstien (2006) reviewed articles on empathy education programs in medical schools and found that many of the articles reported an improvement of empathy. However, these authors suggested that research on enhancement of empathy in medical education poses challenges because of the lack of consensus about the conceptualization and definition of empathy, the lack of adequate research designs and control groups, and variation among the instruments used to measure empathy. These limitations may not apply to more recent studies in which a validated measure of empathy (JSE) was used which relies on an operational definition of empathy in the context of patient care which was described in Chaps. 1 and 6 (e.g., Brazeau, Schroeder, Rovi, & Boyd, 2011; Chen, LaLopa, & Dang, 2008; Hojat, Axelrod et al., 2013; Van Winkle, Fjortoft et al., 2012, see also Appendix A).

Negative Change

Another group of studies showed a decline in empathy among medical students and residents during the course of their medical education in the absence of a targeted educational program. For example, after a period of clinical experience, medical students at the Bowman Gray School of Medicine in North Carolina showed a slight decrease in scores on Hogan's Empathy Scale (Diseker & Michielutte, 1981). Another study reported that a sample of medical students developed a hedonistic personality pattern during medical school that contributed to the decline in empathy (Whittemore et al., 1985).

In a study of changes in empathy, humanism, and professionalism during medical education at a major academic center, Marcus (1999) analyzed approximately 400 dreams reported by healthy medical students and house staff and traced the development of empathy and humanistic attitudes in different years of medical education. Marcus reported that identification with cold and uncaring role models; increasing reliance on the technological aspects of treatment, rather than on the humanistic side of patient care; and development of a sense of elitism or of belonging to a privileged group were some of the factors that became noticeable among students in the third year of medical school, as inferred from dream analyses.

At the University of Pennsylvania Hospital, Bellini et al. (2002) administered the IRI (see Chap. 5) to first-year residents in internal medicine and reported a decline in the residents' scores on the Perspective Taking and Empathic Concern scales of the IRI. Conversely, the residents' scores increased on the IRI Personal Distress scale—a result that was not conducive to empathic patient care. A follow-up study 3 years later showed that the decline in scores on the Empathic Concern scale remained throughout the 3 years of the residency program (Bellini & Shea, 2005).

Similar patterns of decline in empathy were found in most of the other studies in which the JSE was used. For example, in a longitudinal study of 456 medical students at Jefferson Medical College, an erosion in empathy was found in the third year of medical school (Hojat et al., 2009). In an earlier longitudinal study of 125 third-year medical students, we also noticed a statistically significant decline in JSE scores from the beginning to the end of the third academic year (Hojat et al., 2004). In a study of residents in internal medicine in three different years of residency at Thomas Jefferson University Hospital, we noticed a progressive decline in JSE scores as the residents progressed from one level of training to the next (Mangione et al., 2002). Although systematic, the observed decline did not reach the conventional level of statistical significance ($p < 0.05$) in this study. Sherman and Cramer (2005) also observed a significant decline in dentistry students' scores on the JSE as the students progressed through dental school.

A number of other researchers have also noticed a statistically significant decline in the JSE scores as medical and other health profession students progress through their education in different cultures (see Appendix A). The unfortunate transformation of health professional students to less empathic beings as they progress through health professions education resembles the notion of the "Lucifer effect" described by Zimbardo (2007) about why good people turn bad as a result of environmental condition he noticed in his well-known Stanford Prison Experiment (see Chap. 8). (Lucifer was a mythological angel who fell from grace to become a Satan.)

In a review article, it is claimed that findings on erosion of empathy among medical and other health profession students have been exaggerated (Colliver, Conlee, Verhulst, & Dorsey, 2010a, 2010b). However, such criticism has not been left unchallenged (Newton, 2010; Hojat, Gonnella, & Veloski, 2010; Sherman & Cramer, 2010). Empirical research findings from a number of studies that have confirmed a decline in empathy during health professions education are deeply troubling and should not be viewed as a trivial matter. To restore respect to the medical profession, the most humanistic profession in existence, the factors that contribute to the decline of empathy and other humanistic values must be investigated seriously. A medical education system that produces physicians who are unable to apply the science of medicine in conjunction with the art of healing represents, in my view, an "unfinished business." The physician who has learned the science of medicine, but has no sense of the art of healing, is, in the words of Saadi (the twelfth-century Persian poet), like "a man who ploughs, but sows no seed."

No Change

There is yet a third group of studies showing no change in empathy during medical education. For example, a course in behavioral science offered to medical students did not change the students' orientation toward viewing the patient as a person (Markham, 1979).

Zeldow and Daugherty (1987) reported that they observed no significant changes in medical students' empathy measured with the Empathic Concern and Perspective Taking subscales of the IRI. A study in which the IRI was administered to nursing students during their third year of nursing education found no change in the students' empathy during the 9-month training period (Becker & Sands, 1988). There are also a number of studies with different health professions students in various cultures who reported no significant changes in the JSE scores as a result of implementation of their educational programs aimed at improving empathy (see Appendix A).

In general, the majority of findings reported in the previous sections indicate that empathy is amenable to either positive or negative changes during professional education. Even the negative findings can be viewed optimistically because if empathy can decline in the absence of appropriate educational programs, it has the potential to increase if appropriate educational remedies are implemented. The possibility of teaching empathy (Spiro, 1992) and other human virtues (Shelton, 1999) during medical and other health professions education has already been discussed. However, do we all agree that educators in the health professions must assume responsibility for improving students' personality, including personal attributes, such as empathy, in addition to imparting knowledge to them and developing their clinical and procedural skills? Although this question may generate some debate concerning the applications of behavioral modification with students and practitioners in the health professions, my own answer is an affirmative one because of my belief that medicine (and all other health professions for that matter) is a public service endeavor and therefore must produce professionals who are fully equipped to better serve the public (Hojat, Erdmann, & Gonnella, 2014). Consequently, in addition to opportunities to acquire up-to-date knowledge and develop fine clinical and procedural skills, medical and all other health professions educational programs should provide students with opportunities to develop personal qualities that lead to optimal patient outcomes (Knight, 1981; Shelton, 1999). That, I believe, must be considered as a mandate not a luxury, not only in health professions education, but also in all other educational programs in any public service disciplines.

As the research findings just described attest, assuming that students in the health professions will automatically develop empathic understanding and other humanistic qualities during their professional education obviously is unrealistic (Hornblow, Kidson, & Ironside, 1988). Therefore, because not everyone develops the capacity for empathy by default, enhancement of empathy among health professions students and practitioners will require targeted educational programs, appropriate experiences, and exposure to humanistic role models.

Approaches to the Enhancement of Empathy

Many approaches have been used to enhance empathy, most of them by social psychologists and some by medical and nursing educators. Among the many approaches to improving empathy are parental training (Gladding, 1978; Therrien, 1979), skill-development workshops (Black & Phillips, 1982; Hatcher et al., 1994; Kremer & Dietzen, 1991; Pecukonis, 1990), perspective-taking exercises (Coke, Batson, & McDavis, 1978), role taking and role playing (Kalisch, 1971; Moser, 1984), communication or interpersonal skill training (Kause et al., 1980; Yedidia et al., 2003), films and videos (Gladstein & Feldstein, 1983; Simmons, Robie, Kendrick, Schumacher, & Roberge, 1992; Werner & Schneider, 1974), role modeling (Dalton, Sunblad, & Hylbert, 1976; Gulanick & Schmeck, 1977; Shapiro, 2002), or a combination of these and other approaches (Beddoe & Murphy, 2004; Benbassat & Baumal, 2004; Erera, 1997; Kipper & Ben-Ely, 1979).

Although didactic teaching methods are effective for improving beginners' empathic communication skills (Gladstein et al., 1987), more advanced techniques, such as role playing, simulation, and audiovisual methods, are useful for advanced training in empathy. In the following sections, I briefly describe some of the approaches used to enhance empathy in the fields of social and counseling psychology and then discuss some of the methods used among students and practitioners in the health care professions.

Social and Counseling Psychology

In early laboratory experiments, social psychologists used the classical conditioning paradigm to demonstrate that empathic responses could be elicited. For example, two studies indicated that watching others who appeared to be receiving electric shocks followed by a warning signal could cause observers to form empathic reactions to the warning signal (Berger, 1962; DiLollo & Berger, 1965). The observers terminated the electric shocks more quickly when they believed that they were able to help (Weiss, Boyer, Lombardo, & Stich, 1973). These studies suggest that the empathic response can be elicited by classical and operant conditioning.

An empathy enhancement program called Parent Effectiveness Training, which included lectures, tape recordings, role playing, and role modeling, was also implemented for parents who wished to improve their parent–child communication (Therrien, 1979). The results showed that parents who participated in the program were able to function at a higher level of empathy, as measured by the Accurate Empathy Scale of Truax and Carkhuff's Relationship Questionnaire. The improvement was maintained over a period of 4 months.

In a series of studies on the use of imagination, Stotland and colleagues demonstrated that when an observer was instructed to "stand in another person's shoes" by simply imagining the pain experienced by a person whose hand was strapped to a machine generating painful heat, the observer exhibited a more intense empathic response than did other observers who passively watched the distressed person's actions and appearance (Stotland, 1969; Stotland, Mathews, Sherman, Hansson, & Richardson, 1978). This finding suggests that a cognitive process of perspective taking or imagining the other person's experience (i.e., standing in the other person's shoes) can elicit empathic responses reflected in the role taker's behavior, heartbeat, and skin conductance.

Imagination has also been used as a method of inducing an empathic response. Two kinds of imagination have been used. One kind was imagining another person in a specific situation (e.g., a person whose parents have been killed in an automobile accident). The question is what the other person might feel and experience (third-person experience). The other kind was imagining oneself experiencing another person's concerns, feelings, and experiences as vividly as possible (first-person experience). Empathic behavior determined by physiological responses or self-reports can be generated by such imaginings.

Since prejudice against specific groups can lead to psychological distance, some psychologists have attempted to reduce prejudice and improve prosocial behavior by enhancing empathy. If an important ingredient of empathy is the ability to understand other people's concern, pain, and suffering, such an understanding can reduce prejudice and bridge the gap between people. Efforts to understand others will diminish hatred toward them, and helping behavior presumably would follow when empathic understanding is formed (Batson, 1991; Batson & Coke, 1981; Davis, 1994).

One approach to understanding others is to read about them—their values, culture, concern, pain, and suffering. Most programs designed to increase cultural sensitivity focus on the simple principle that understanding different cultures reduces prejudice and increases the sense of common identity. When people were asked to read stories about a particular group of sufferers, such as patients with AIDS, homeless people, or prisoners on death row, they developed more positive attitudes toward these groups as their awareness improved (Batson, Polycarpou et al., 1997).

Those who read vignettes about racial discrimination and were instructed to empathize with the victims (by standing in the other person's shoes) improved their attitudes toward the victims (Stephan & Finlay, 1999). When college students participated in a "dialogue group" to discuss diversity, race, and ethnic issues, the researchers observed both short- and long-term improvements in the students' empathic understanding of minority groups (Gruin, Peng, Lopez, & Nagda, 1999; Lopez, Gurin, & Nagda, 1998). Such dialogues concerning people's similarities and differences can create a sense of a common identity that reduces prejudice and increases helping behavior. Research has also demonstrated that people who participate in multicultural educational programs, read relevant materials, watch videos, and engage in conversation with people from other racial, ethnic, and cultural groups increase their insight and their empathic understanding of the views held by those groups (Banks, 1997).

More than three decades ago, Bridgman (1981) suggested that prosocial behavior could be measured by cognitive developmental processes through role taking. In a study based on this suggestion, children from different groups who took the role of a person from another group in specially designed educational programs worked cooperatively together and improved their empathic understanding of each other.

These findings have implications for education in the health professions with regard to not only improving practitioners' understanding of patients and other staff members from diverse sociocultural backgrounds and experiences but also promoting collaboration and teamwork as well. Our studies have shown that when medical students and nurses work together, the students' understanding of the importance of nursing services to patient care increases and their attitudes about collaborative relationships improve significantly (Hojat et al., 1997; Hojat & Herman, 1985).

Krebs (1975) and Stotland and colleagues (Stotland, 1969; Stotland et al., 1978) indicated that taking another person's perspective can lead to increased intensity of the motivation to help and, consequently, to an empathic response. Batson and colleagues reported that empathic behavior could be developed in a two-stage model of training (Batson, Coke, & Pych, 1983; Coke et al., 1978). In Stage 1, adopting the perspective of another person, such as a patient, increased empathic concern. The motivation to help was elicited in Stage 2 as a result of adopting another person's perspective.

Crabb, Moracco, and Bender (1983) developed a training program for lay helpers (church volunteers) based on the micro counseling interviewing technique (Ivey, 1971) and the skilled-helper training method (Egan, 1975) and offered the program to a large group of church volunteers. After administering Carkhuff's Empathic Understanding in Interpersonal Processes Scale to the participants, the authors reported that a large-group format for teaching the skills of empathy can be effective (Crabb et al., 1983).

In another study, undergraduates were taught active listening skills (e.g., identifying expressions of emotion and communicating this understanding verbally) either through training tapes (the self-directed method) or through highly intensive programs presented by teachers (Kremer & Dietzen, 1991). Although both approaches improved the students' empathy skills, the investigators concluded that empathy skills could be taught effectively in a large-group format without intensive programs and with direct contact with a teacher as a necessary component.

Another important finding was that an observer's empathic responses could be demonstrated more vividly when the person observed was involved in a distressing, not pleasant, situation (Stotland et al., 1978). In other words, human beings tend to empathize with people who need help to reduce their pain and suffering, rather than empathize (rejoice) with people who want to share their joy and ecstasy. This finding is relevant to clinician–patient encounters, where there is always a patient in pain and in need of help and a clinician in a position to offer help. Such is the condition in which an empathic relationship is waiting to form.

The Health Professions

Since the 1970s, a number of researchers have argued that empathy is far too important to be taught only to health professionals (Ivey, 1971, 1974). Egan (1975) and Therrien (1979) recommended that everyone should receive empathy training to improve human relationships in general and to face crises of life more effectively. Others have suggested that the capacity for empathy can serve as a foundation for building interpersonal relationships that have a buffering effect against stress and can be an essential step in conflict resolution (Kremer & Dietzen, 1991), regardless of professions.

Researchers in the health professions have attempted to enhance empathy by offering educational programs. Most of the programs address the broader goal of improving students' interpersonal skills and understating which implicitly means enhancement of the capacity for empathy. It is assumed that the capacity for empathy is an essential prerequisite to demonstrate empathic behavior (Book, 1991). The following studies are examples of the training programs designed to enhance empathy among students and practitioners in the health professions.

Helping Professions

In a study at the University of Haifa, social work students participated in an empathy training program developed and implemented for service professionals (Erera, 1997). Designed to enhance participants' sensitivity, the program consisted of four activities: (a) recording students' interviews with clients, (b) reviewing the interviews for the purpose of developing hypotheses or speculating about statements clients made during the interviews, (c) developing hypotheses about the students' statements, and (d) verifying the hypotheses or speculations by analyzing possible reasons for the statements students made during exchanges with clients. For example, "What did the client try to convey by using a specific statement?" or "What did the student infer from the client's statement?" A statistically significant improvement in scores on Mehrabian and Epstein's Emotional Empathy Scale was observed among the students who participated in the program.

Sensitivity to nonverbal cues is an important skill in establishing an empathic clinician–patient relationship. When a group of mental health professionals was exposed to a 90-min program designed to increase their ability to interpret nonverbal cues, the results demonstrated that such skills could be learned (DiMatteo, 1979; Rosenthal, Hall, DiMatteo, Rogers, & Archer, 1979). The brief presentation included information about the importance of nonverbal communication in clinical settings, demonstrations of how one can understand nonverbal expressions of affect by noting changes in tone of voice, and practice in judging emotions by observing facial expressions, bodily movements, and postures. The participants had no difficulty learning the apparent meaning of certain nonverbal cues.

Nursing

In a study designed to improve empathy among nursing students, the students underwent didactic training that involved role playing and exposure to a role model (Kalisch, 1971). Although the investigator noticed an increase in the students' self-reported empathy on Barrett-Lennard's Relationship Inventory, no increase occurred in patients' ratings of the nurses' empathy.

LaMonica, Carew, Winder, Haase, and Blanchard (1976) developed an empathy training program for hospital nursing staff based on Carkhuff's human relationship model (1969). During the brief program, nurses learned to interpret patients' non-verbal behaviors and expressions of anger, engaged in empathic role playing, and practiced responding empathically. Despite a significant increase in the nurses' empathy scores, the authors reported that the majority of participants needed more training.

Layton (1979) attempted to enhance nursing students' empathy by conducting an experiment based on Bandura's observational social learning theory (Bandura, 1977). The students observed interviews with simulated patients that consisted of three components: (a) a modeling component demonstrating the interviewers' empathy (positive modeling) or lack of empathy (negative modeling); (b) a labeling component in which segments of the modeling component were played back, followed by a narrative explaining the presence or absence of empathy depicted on the videotapes; and (c) a rehearsing component, during which the videotapes were stopped briefly after each verbal and emotional expression shown by the patient. During each pause, the students were asked to construct their own responses to the patient's expressions. When the experiment ended, Layton found that the junior-year students' scores on Carkhuff's Empathic Understanding in Interpersonal Processes Scale had improved, whereas the scores of the senior students had not. Layton speculated that one explanation for the disparate results was that the modeling approach may have been more effective for less advanced students.

As a result of extensive work in nursing education and research in the 1960s and 1970s, Orlando (1961, 1972) developed a model of therapeutic encounters proposing that when nurses interacted with patients, they should validate their perceptions to ensure that they had an accurate understanding of the patients' experiences. More than two decades later, Olson and Hanchett (1997) adopted Orlando's model as a suitable method of studying empathy and patient outcomes and hypothesized that if nurses understood their patients' needs accurately and shared that understanding with patients, who in turn confirmed its accuracy, patient outcomes would improve. Accordingly, Olson and Hanchett initiated a study involving 70 staff nurses and 70 patients to test the hypothesis that nurses' empathy would reduce patients' distress and overlap with the patients' perceptions of the nurses' empathy, as measured by the Empathic Understanding subscale of Barrett-Lennard's Relationship Inventory. At the end of the study, the authors reported a moderate but statistically significant relationship between the nurses' self-reported empathy and the patients' perceptions of the nurse's empathy: i.e., the hypothesis was confirmed.

In another study, Beddoe and Murphy (2004) exposed nursing students to an 8-week "mindfulness-based stress reduction" program to explore the program's effects on stress and empathy. At the end of the 8 weeks, the authors reported favorable changes in the students' scores on the Personal Distress and Fantasy subscales of the IRI.

Ten Approaches to Enhance Empathy in Health Professions Education and Practice

In this section, I have selected ten approaches that are more specific to medical (and all other health professions) education and practice (Hojat, 2009). Consistent with our definition of empathy, the common goal of all of these approaches is to improve the understanding of students and practitioners in the health professions in regard to patients' concern, pain, suffering, and experiences.

Improving Interpersonal Skills

Interpersonal skill development is considered as an essential prerequisite to demonstrate empathic behavior (Book, 1991). Researchers in the health professions have attempted to enhance empathy by designing educational programs to improve students' interpersonal skills that implicitly imply enhancement of the capacity for empathy (Evans et al., 1993; Kramer et al., 1989; Poole, & Sanson-Fisher, 1980). Suchman, Markakis, Beckman, and Frankel (1997) developed an interpersonal model of empathic communication in the medical interview. Emphasis in this method is placed on the development of three basic communication skills: "recognition" of patient's negative emotions, concerns, and inner experiences; "exploration" of these emotions, concerns, and experiences; and "acknowledging" them to generate a feeling in the patient of being understood. These three skills correspond, respectively, to the keywords of "cognition," "understanding," and "communicating" in our definition of empathy in the context of patient care. The goal of this training is to form an empathic engagement in the caregiver–care-receiver relationship by the caregiver recognizing an "empathic opportunity" when the care receiver directly or implicitly expresses emotions or concerns. The caregiver responds empathetically by explicitly expressing understanding of the care receiver's concerns, and communicating to the care receiver that his or her concerns are understood.

In responding to the empathic opportunity, many untrained physicians may disregard the patient's concerns, thus missing or terminating an opportunity rather than taking advantage of it. The training focuses on capturing the empathic opportunities that provide the caregiver with "windows of opportunities" (Branch & Malik, 1993) while avoiding pitfalls in missing or terminating them. A caregiver can form and maintain the empathic communication dynamics by continuing the conversation about the patient's concerns (so-called continuer). This can be done by simply nodding the head to reflect understanding and using simple statements such as "I understand your concern; let's work on it together." In addition to verbal cues, sensitivity to nonverbal cues is an important skill in establishing an empathic clinician–patient relationship. Nonverbal communication in clinical settings can be taught by understanding nonverbal expressions of affect. Such nonverbal expressions include changes in tone of voice, eye contact, gaze and aversion of gaze, silence, laughter, teary eyes, facial expressions, hand and body movements, trembling, touch, physical distance, leaning forward or backward, sighs, or other signs of distress or discomfort. These are important nonverbal cues in clinical encounters (Mehrabian, 1972; Wolfgang, 1979). Psychological effects of nonverbal cues such as folded arms (more likely to indicate defensiveness, coldness, rejection, or inaccessibility) or moderately open arms (more likely to convey acceptance and warmth) can also be taught in interpersonal skill training programs (DiMatteo, 1979).

Also, teaching clinicians to try to mirror patients' postures, gestures, respiration rates, tempo and pitch of speech, and language pattern can contribute to forming an empathic engagement (Matthews, Suchman, & Branch, 1993). Winefield and Chur-Hansen (2000) reported that 81 % of medical students who participated in two brief sessions on effective communication with patients felt more prepared to engage in empathic interviews. Yedidia et al. (2003) reported that practicing communication skills and engaging medical students in self-reflection on their performances improved students' overall communication competence as well as their skills in building relationships in patient care. A 5-day communication skill workshop offered to medical students and medical residents in Spain significantly increased scores of participants' empathy (measured by the JSE) compared to a non-participant control group (Fernandez-Olano, Montoya-Fernandez, & Salinas-Sanchez, 2008).

In a randomized clinical trial conducted at the Johns Hopkins University School of Hygiene and Public Health, 69 physicians were assigned to one of the three groups: two experimental groups and one control group (Roter et al., 1995). Physicians in the experimental groups received eight hours of training designed to increase their communication skills and reduce their patients' emotional distress. The patients in one experimental group were actual patients and those in the other group were simulated patients. During the training, the physicians asked patients about their concerns and expectations, reassured them, and acknowledged their psychosocial struggles. The results showed that the empathic skills of the physicians who participated in either training course compared to the control group improved significantly without increasing the time spent with individual patients.

Audio- or Video-Taping of Encounters with Patients

A review and analysis of audio- or video-taping of patient encounters with physicians, nurses, and hospital and office administrators to identify positive and negative interviewing factors is a valuable learning experience for enhancing empathic engagement. Using the interpersonal empathic communication method (Suchman et al., 1997) described above, Pollak et al. (2007) audio-recorded 398 interviews between advanced cancer patients and their oncologists. They found that oncologists responded with empathy to patient concerns only 27 % of the time. Physicians either missed or prematurely terminated the conversation about patients' concerns 73 % of the time. In a similar study, Morse, Edwardsen, and Gordon (2008) reported that only 10 % of physicians responded to empathic opportunities in their communication with lung cancer patients.

Sanson-Fisher and Poole (1978) of the University of Western Australia Medical School exposed 112 medical students to eight audio-taped empathy training sessions and compared them with 23 students without such exposure. After the training, students' scores on the Accurate Empathy scale of Truax and Carkhuff's Relationship Questionnaire increased significantly compared with the scores of a control group of students who did not participate in the program. Audio-taped conversations between patients and physicians can help identify empathic opportunities and physicians' positive responses, as well as demonstrate missed opportunities, or cases in which the concern-related part of the conversation was terminated. This can have valuable educational benefits for enhancing empathy.

By analyzing videotapes of interviews of 87 first-year medical students with simulated patients at Michigan State University School of Medicine, Werner and Schneider (1974) used a variation of a technique called "Interpersonal Process Recall" to enhance medical students' interviewing skills and awareness of patients' affective messages. The students were videotaped as they interacted with simulated patients with various problems. The videotapes were then played back so the students could view interactions with patients and receive critical analyses from instructors and other students about their interactions with the patient. After each tape-recorded interview, the students joined in a group with their faculty instructors to discuss and analyze different sections of the interview. The videotape could be paused, forwarded, and rewound during the analysis. Werner and Schneider (1974) concluded that analysis of the videotape replay made students increasingly aware of their behavior in communicating with patients, and improved students' ability to empathize with patients. They also concluded that the videotape had its greatest impact on students who had the least developed skills for communication.

Exposure to Role Models

Some investigators have suggested that faculty in undergraduate and graduate medical education can serve as role models or mentors to improve students' capacity for empathy (Campus-Outcalt, Senf, Watkins, & Bastacky, 1995; Ficklin, Browne, Powell, & Carter, 1988; Skeff & Mutha, 1998; Wright, 1996). Shapiro (2002) interviewed primary care physicians to discern how empathy can be enhanced in medical students and residents. Role modeling was endorsed by almost all research participants as the most effective approach to teaching empathy. Quill (1987) reported that the practice behavior of the ambulatory preceptors, viewed as role models, exerted a broad influence on the residents. A study of medical students in South Africa (Mclean, 2004) found that as the students progressed through medical school, they selected more faculty members as role models. However, the role models they selected most often were their own parents, and notably their mothers who were described as caring, sympathetic, and self-sacrificing mentors. These findings are consistent with the notion I describe in Chap. 4 that mothers are key figures in the development of a child's capacity for empathy.

Despite the fact that exposure to role models is important in the enhancement of empathy, the results of a mailed survey of medical students at four different medical schools in Canada (Maheux, Beaudoin, Berkson, Des Marchais, & Jean, 2000) raised a question about students' exposure to appropriate role models: 25 % of the second-year students and 40 % of the seniors said that they did not agree that their medical school faculty behaved as humanistic physicians and teachers. In a study of decline in empathy in medical school, students in response to a question about factors that had negatively influenced their views on patient-physician relationships had indicated that inappropriate role models (faculty and attending physicians) was one of the major factors (Hojat et al., 2009).

Role Playing (Aging Games)

About 30 years ago, Hoffman and Reif (1978) described a role-playing game to simulate problems perceived by elderly people. McVey, Davis, and Cohen (1989) adapted the technique and developed the "aging game" to increase medical students' understanding of elderly people's sensory deficits and functional dependency. The game generally consists of three stages. In the first stage, students are instructed to imagine that they are old (e.g., 70–99 years old) and use earplugs to simulate hearing loss.

The second stage begins with a simulation that represents independent living in one area, then proceeds to semi-dependent living in another area, and finally to the third area that simulates dependent living where they are confined to wheelchairs. In each area they are confronted with facilitators who play the role of administrators, physicians, or nurses. As they progress through different game levels, the behaviors of the facilitators become more disrespectful.

Stage 3 is a group discussion of the participants' experiences during the previous stages of the game. Results of the original aging game experiment with 112 medical students at Duke University Medical School showed that the medical students gained an increased understanding and sensitivity to the physical and psychosocial problems of the elderly (McVey et al., 1989). It is suggested that role playing results in the development of awareness and increased understanding of elderly patients (Hoffman, Brand, Beatty, & Hamill, 1985; Menks, 1983). Because understanding is the key ingredient in the definition of empathy, it is expected that improvement in understanding leads to enhancement of empathy. Such a link has been reported by Holtzman, Beck, and Coggin (1978) and Holtzman, Beck, and Ettinger (1981) among medical and dental students, and nurses (Marte, 1988).

Pacala, Boult, Bland, and O'Brien (1995) presented a three hours workshop of a modified version of the aging game to 39 medical students in an ambulatory medicine rotation at the University of Minnesota Medical School. They were then compared with 16 nonparticipating students. Students were asked to assume the identity of elderly persons and used earplugs to simulate hearing loss, heavy athletic stockings to simulate pedal edema, and un-popped popcorn in their shoes to simulate the discomfort of arthritis pain. Scores of a two-item empathy scale (developed by the study authors: "I believe I can truly empathize with older patients" and "I believe I understand what it feels like to have problems associated with aging") increased significantly among participants after completing the workshop.

Varkey, Chutka, and Lesnick (2006) used a variation of the aging game (e.g., students wore heavy rubber gloves to simulate decreased manual dexterity and goggles with films over the lenses to simulate cataracts) with all 84 medical students in two first-year classes. They reported a statistically significant increase in empathy. After 10 years of offering the aging game workshop at the University of Minnesota Medical School, Pacala, Boult, and Hepburn (2006) concluded that despite the burden of required personnel and resources to run the aging game workshops, students benefited greatly from their role-playing experiences by developing a long-lasting awareness and understanding of key issues in elderly patients and geriatric medicine.

In a study with students at Purdue University School of Pharmacy (Chen et al., 2008), students were assigned to simulate the life of an underserved patient with multiple chronic medical conditions who had an economic burden (e.g., homeless), cultural differences (e.g., Hispanic), or a communication barrier (illiterate or hearing-impaired). Participation in this experiment increased students' empathy scores. An examination of remarks by students showed that they grew to become more sensitive to patients whose conditions they simulated, and developed an understanding of the challenges faced by the patients after "walking in a patient's shoes" (Chen et al., 2008). In another study, medical and pharmacy students participated in a workshop which included a theatrical play performed by their classmates who were coached to enact problems and concerns of elderly patients (a variation of the "aging game"). Statistically significant improvement in the JSE scores was observed among students (Van Winkle, Fjortoft, et al., 2012). I will describe this study in more detail in the "Theatrical Performances" section of this chapter.

Shadowing a Patient (Patient Navigator)

The patient navigation program was originally developed at the Harlem Cancer Education and Demonstration Project to help medically underserved cancer patients (Freeman, Muth, & Kerner, 1995). It has been reported that a trained patient navigator, who shadows the patients offering help, contributed to increased satisfaction and decreased anxiety among patients (Ferrante, Chen, & Kim, 2007).

Using the patient navigator paradigm, researchers at the University of Arkansas for Medical Sciences conducted a project in which first-year medical students "shadowed" a patient (with the patient's permission) during visits to a surgical oncologist and observed the patient throughout treatment (Henry-Tillman, Deloney, Savidge, Graham, & Klimberg, 2002). Participants reported that they learned to see patients as people, not as numbers or diseases. Seventy percent of the students said that they experienced feelings of empathy while participating in the program.

In another study, 12 first-year emergency medicine residents at Thomas Jefferson University Hospital were randomly divided into experimental and control groups (Forstater, Chauhan, Allen, Hojat, & Lopez, 2011). Each resident in the experimental group shadowed one patient in the emergency department in the first month of residency training. The control group did not participate in shadowing and followed a routine training schedule. The JSE was completed by all residents 2 and 9 months after the shadowing experiment. No substantial difference was observed on the JSE scores between the two groups 2 months after the experiment (effect size $= 0.02$); however, a larger decline in empathy scores was noticed in the control group compared to the experimental group (effect size $= 0.58$), suggesting that the erosion of empathy may be prevented to some extent by shadowing experiences.

Hospitalization Experiences

Sharing common experiences can influence empathic understanding of the patient. The tendency of health professionals to empathize with those whom they share common experiences has been described as the "wounded healer effect" (Jackson, 2001) (see Chap. 8). Clinicians who have experienced pain have a better understanding of their patients' pain (Gustafson, 1986). Therefore, painful hospitalization experiences can increase one's understanding of the hospitalized patient.

At the University of California-Los Angeles Medical School, healthy second-year medical students who had completed their training in the basic sciences and had no previous history of hospitalization participated in a program designed to examine whether the experience of being hospitalized would increase empathy for hospitalized patients (Wilkes, Milgrom, & Hoffman, 2002). The students were admitted to the hospital under an assumed name. Investigators reported that the pseudo-hospitalization experience was useful because it enhanced students' understanding of patients' problems. Interestingly, the students acting as "new patients" gave the nursing staff more favorable patient encounter ratings than they gave to physicians (Wilkes et al., 2002). Because of the effect of hospitalization on a physician's understanding of patients, Ingelfinger (1980) suggested that actual hospitalization experiences could be used as a criterion for admission to medical schools.

On their first day in the Emergency Medicine Department at the University of Florida Health Sciences Center, 25 residents participated in a study in which they were instructed to register as patients (the admission staff and nurses were not aware of the experiment) (Seaberg, Godwin, & Perry, 1999, 2000). Although the study was brief and ended when the emergency room physician entered the examination room, the results suggested that the experience enhanced residents' empathy, as indicated by their reports that the experiment improved their attitude toward patients in the emergency room.

The Study of Literature and the Arts

In his book, *A History of Medicine*, Castiglioni (1941) quoted Hippocrates as saying, "Where there is a love for man, there is also a love for the arts." The statement indicates that there is a bridge connecting the human heart and the arts together. Numerous authors have proposed that in addition to reading the medical literature, medical students and physicians should read literature unrelated to medicine because it would expose them to a rich source of knowledge and insights about the emotions, pain, and suffering, and perspectives of human beings and would improve their capacity for forming empathic connections (Acuna, 2000; Charon et al., 1995; Herman, 2000; Jones, 1987; Kumagai, 2008; McLellan & Husdon Jones, 1996; Montgomery Hunter, Charon, & Coulehan, 1995; Peschel, 1980; Szalita, 1976) (for an annotated bibliography of works in medical and nonmedical literature, see Montgomery Hunter et al., 1995). In support of the impact of physicians' familiarity with literature and the arts on patient outcomes, Mandell and Spiro (1987, p. 458) suggested that "the humanities will not improve the technical care of our patients, but they may help to civilize that care."

Borrowing from Jungian concepts, Knapp (1984) suggested that by studying classical literature, the reader can develop insight into the "collective unconscious" of the human mind and better understand the archetypal images in myths, legends, literature, and the arts. The simulated worlds presented by famous novels, short stories, poems, plays, paintings, sculptures, music, and films enable us to learn how emotions are expressed in human relationships (Oatley, 2004). Thus, the study of literature and the arts can provide students and practitioners in the health professions with values and experiences in areas of concern in clinical practice, such as aging, death, disability, and dying (Montgomery Hunter et al., 1995). The study of literature and the arts can also aid the development of otherwise hard-to-teach clinical competencies, such as accurate observation, interpretation, imagination, ethical issues, and moral reflection (Montgomery Hunter et al., 1995).

In addition, studying literature and reading poetry not only facilitate clinicians' understanding of other people's feelings and expressions of their inner world but also can be used as an ancillary tool through which both clinician and patient can find different meanings in and ways of expressing emotion, pain, and suffering (Lerner, 1978, 2001). Furthermore, literature and the arts provide clinicians with the ability to use metaphor in encounters with patients that can help them to enhance mutual clinician–patient understanding (Blanton, 1960; Lerner, 2001).

Charon et al. (1995) indicated that in addition to increasing one's understanding of human suffering and ability to use metaphor, studying literature and the arts can help health professionals to "contextualize" and "particularize" the ethical issues in patient care. Other authors have indicated that health professionals can gain new insights into the moral and ethical issues posed by their profession through the lens of literature, poetry, and the arts (Calman, Downie, Duthie, & Sweeney, 1988; Charon et al., 1995; Coles, 1989; Flagler, 1997; Marshall & O'Keefe, 1994; Radley, 1992), and recognize that the discoveries of others can lead to the development of self (Kumagai, 2008). The quandaries and decision-making processes of characters in literary narratives are useful for teaching ethical guidelines to students and practitioners in the health professions (Coles, 1989). The thoughts, feelings, sensations, and intuitions influenced by immersing oneself in literature can serve as a powerful impetus toward understanding the human mind (Schneiderman, 2002).

Reading literature can result in higher mental processes leading to greater imagination and better interpretive skills that reinforce empathic understanding (Calman et al., 1988; Charon et al., 1995; Clouser, 1990; Downie, 1991; Radley, 1992; Starcevic & Piontek, 1997; Younger, 1990). Literature can enrich students' moral education, increase their tolerance for ambiguity, and give them a rich grounding for empathic understanding of their patients. Lancaster, Hart, and Gardner (2002) offered a 1-month course in which medical students read works, such as Tolstoy's *The Death of Ivan Ilych*, which improved their narrative skills. When the course ended, the students assigned their highest rating to the enhancement of empathy as a result of their participation in the course. Shapiro, Morrison, and Boker (2004) noticed a significant improvement in first-year medical students' empathy and attitudes toward humanities after participating in a short course in reading and discussion of poetry, skits, and short stories.

Although it is assumed that engagement with literature can deepen medical students' understanding of illness experiences, increase their capacity for self-reflection, and enhance their capacity for empathy, resistance among medical students to a course on literary inquiry has been observed (Wear & Aultman, 2005). Denying the relevance of studying literature to medicine, discounting the value of literary inquiry to patient care, and distancing the arts from science are among the reasons for medical students' resistance to studying literature and improving their narrative skills (Wear & Aultman, 2005). Students' motivation can be improved by convincing them of the link between literary inquiry and medicine. Despite the importance of humanities in enhancing empathy, only a third of all the medical schools in the USA had incorporated literature into their curriculum as of the mid-1990s (Charon et al., 1995; Jones, 1997; Montgomery Hunter et al., 1995). Other medical schools should be encouraged to follow their lead. The development of professionalism in medicine, according to Wear and Nixon (2002), requires an imaginative immersion into others' stories that can be attained by studying literature and the arts.

Improving Narrative Skills and Reflective Writing

It is said that human beings are storytelling animals (Hurwitz, 2000), that the universe is made of stories (Feldman & Kornfield, 1991), and that physicians are immersed in patients' stories (Steiner, 2005). Humans are described by Dawes

(1999, p. 29) as "the primates whose cognitive capacity shuts down in the absence of a story." It is suggested that the human brain is evolved to process stories better than any other forms of input (Newman, 2003). Narrative, defined by Smith (1981, p. 228) as "someone telling someone else that something happened," is the royal road to a patient's world.

It is physicians' attentive listening to their patients' narratives of illness (narrative skills), rather than "clinical interrogation," (Kleinman, 1995) that opens a window of opportunity to empathic engagement. In clinician–patient encounters, listening to the patient's stories of illness with the third ear while taking the history of the patient's current illness is described as a "narrative communication" that, when skillfully performed, not only has diagnostic value but has therapeutic benefit as well (Adler, 1997). The narrative account of the patient's illness is the beginning of the healing process as well as a pathway to a correct diagnosis (Adler & Hammett, 1973). Patients often carefully monitor the clinician's attentiveness to their illness narrative, detect signs of the clinician's empathic receptiveness, and feel better when the clinician appears to be in tune with the narrative themes (Brody, 1997). In his article "Power of Stories over Statistics," Newman (2003) suggests that narrative skills enable physicians to make empathic connections with their patients.

Clinicians are often witnesses to their patients' pain and suffering: they listen to the patients' stories, and they prepare short narratives of the patients' experiences after taking their history and interviewing them. The clinicians' task, according to Kleinman (1988, p. 50), is "to witness a life story, to validate its interpretation, and to affirm its value." Because the feelings and experiences of others are captured in patients' narratives, their narratives can convey how they view their illness (Bruner, 1990). Evidence suggests that participating in programs on reflective writing and improving narrative skills can improve clinicians' empathic understanding (DasGupta & Charon, 2004; Lancaster et al., 2002; Shapiro & Hunt, 2003). The understanding of patients will improve by adopting their perspectives through their stories, and by narrative skills allowing health care provider to reflect on the nature of patients' concerns and experiences. According to Kumagai (2008), narratives of illness provide an insight into subjective experiences of others, which fosters perspective taking ability, and identification with patients. According to Steiner (2005), clinical stories can be used to inform, share, inspire, educate, and persuade, with implications not only in forming empathic engagement but also in health research (to find a common theme) and in health policy (to formulate compassionate policies).

Clinicians' narrative skills gained by engaging with stories in literature is pivotal when thinking about case histories in ethics (Charon & Montello, 2002). Rita Charon (2001b) has written extensively about narrative medicine and physicians' narrative competence in recognizing and interpreting the predicaments of their patients. She believes that a bridge exists between narrative skills and the capacity for empathy (Charon, 1993) and that the effective practice of medicine requires narrative competence that includes the ability to understand, absorb, interpret, and act based on the stories and plights of patients (Charon, 2000, 2001a).

Narrative competence in medicine can be acquired by reading, writing, studying the arts, and recognizing that all human beings are vulnerable to illness and death

(Charon, 1993). According to DasGupta and Charon (2004), the ability to elicit, interpret, and translate patients' narrative accounts of their illness is the key to empathic communication. Reflective writing and narrative competence offer opportunities for empathic and nourishing medical care (Charon, 2001a). In a study involving 11 second-year medical students, 9 reported that reflective writing (e.g., writing about a personal illness or another person's illness) could enhance their understanding of patients and improve their ability to care for patients (DasGupta & Charon, 2004).

Narrative competence is beneficial not only for the clinicians who write the patients' stories of illness to make accurate diagnoses and select appropriate treatments but for the patients as well. For example, patients with mild or moderately severe asthma or rheumatoid arthritis who wrote about their stressful experiences achieved a significantly better clinical outcome (Smyth, Stone, Hurewitz, & Kaell, 1999). Branch, Pels, and Hafler (1998) suggested that small-group discussions about medical students' narrative reports of critical incidents during encounters with patients could enhance the students' understanding of the clinician–patient relationship.

In another study, 40 staff physicians at the Cleveland Clinic were assigned into the experimental and two control groups (Misra-Hebert et al., 2012). Those in the experimental groups participated in a six-session program on narrative medicine and engaged in guided reflective writing. Physicians in one control group received the assigned course reading materials (which were given to the experimental group) but did not participate in the course sessions (control group 1), and those in the second control group neither received the reading materials nor participated in the course sessions. Quantitative analysis showed improvements in the experimental group compared to the two control groups (using the JSE). Qualitative analysis of physicians' reflective writings in the intervention group showed compassionate solidarity and empathic concern and more exploration of negative rather than positive emotions.

Theatrical Performances

Dramatic performances by real or simulated patients, or by professional actors portraying patients or by health professions students playing a role, have been used to enhance empathy. For example, Shapiro and Hunt (2003) presented medical students at the University of California-Irvine College experiences with AIDS through narrative and song. Another patient, a survivor of ovarian cancer, described her experiences on hearing the diagnosis, undergoing treatment, and coping with the psychological effects of the ordeal and the spiritual journey on which she embarked while dealing with the illness. After the theatrical presentations, the students reported that watching the theatrical performances increased their empathic understanding of patients with AIDS or ovarian cancer.

In another study with 370 medical and pharmacy students at Chicago College of Osteopathic Medicine and at Chicago College of Pharmacy of Midwestern University

(Van Winkle, Fjortoft et al., 2012), students participated in a workshop which included a 10-min theatrical play performed by their classmates who were coached to enact problems and concerns of elderly patients (a variation of the "aging game"). Subsequent to watching the play, students discussed in small groups their perceptions/ feeling about issues of elderly people depicted in the play. Statistically significant increases in the JSE pretest-posttest mean scores were found in both groups of medical and pharmacy students. However, follow-up assessments showed that the improvement in empathy scores did not sustain for a longer time after the workshop.

The performing arts have also been used to increase medical students' understanding of patients' grief (Stokes, 1980) and of death and dying (Holleman, 2000). Dramatic and tragic theatrical performances can generate insights into the observer that arise from climactic intellectual, emotional, or spiritual enlightenment (Golden, 1992). Empathy can arise from the cathartic effects of other peoples' tragedies. In his theory of catharsis, Aristotle explained that observing the hero's tragic experiences can generate a calming effect (a catharsis) that serves to separate the observer from the hero's suffering while understanding the hero's pain. A healthy society needs the performing arts, and students and practitioners in the health care professions need them for the same reason—because they learn about the experiences of others and can experience catharsis by being drawn into their patients' tragic stories while remaining separate from patients (Trautmann Banks, 2002). In other words, empathy can arise from the cathartic effects of these stories.

Another explanation for the beneficial effects of the performing arts on empathy is the involvement of the human mirror neuron system. As I described in Chap. 13, when a person observes another person performing an act, the mirror neuron system is activated in the observer's brain and contributes to empathic understanding of the observed person. It is also well known, particularly from studies involving hypnosis and imagery, that imagination can produce real physiological effects (Wester & Smith, 1984). These neurological and physiological activities may explain how watching theatrical or cinematic performances can induce neurophysiological effects leading to a greater empathic understanding.

There is a new notion of teaching health professions students performing arts to cultivate empathic skills. It is assumed that developing skills to act and think like another human being (e.g., doctors, patients) can improve understanding of those whose acts and thoughts are simulated. The idea seems to be similar to Gestalt-Therapy technique introduced by Frederick Perls (1969/1992). The basic principle in this therapeutic technique is to teach therapists and clients phenomenological awareness (being in the here and now) by placing oneself in another person's shoes, but simultaneously retaining one's own sense of identity. Acting nonjudgmentally as if one is another person, without losing the "as if" condition (Rogers, 1959, 1975), is the guiding acting role to experience another person's feelings and concerns. Based on premises from theater and performing arts education, a technique, called "Facilitated Simulation Education and Evaluation," has recently been introduced to improve interpersonal communication skills and enhance empathic understanding in physicians-in-training (Eisenberg, Rosenthal, & Schlussel, 2015). Currently Dr. Salvatore Mangione and his team at Sidney Kimmel Medical College are undertaking a study to teach different roles to medical students and residents by professional performers and faculty of performing arts to examine if role-performing skills can enhance empathy and tolerance.

Balint Method

The Balint training program was developed by Michael Balint at the Tavistock Institute in London for general practitioners. Balint designed a program to counteract a problem that Houston (1938) had described nearly two decades earlier. It is based on the notion that medical trainees often spend their entire training in the laboratory and the hospital ward where they do not have sufficient opportunity to develop skills in interpersonal aspects of patient care. To compensate for deficits in interpersonal communication and awareness of psychosocial aspects of illness, Balint suggested that they meet in small groups of ten to discuss cases they felt were difficult, particularly in relation to physician-patient relationship (Balint, 1957). The program provides opportunities to enhance understanding of patients' experiences and concerns.

Activities in the original Balint method included one to two hours of unstructured, open, and supportive small group meetings every 1–3 weeks, for 1–3 years. The primary focus in these meetings was on behavioral, cognitive, and emotional issues related to communication between patients, physicians, and other personnel. The discussions (often coordinated by a psychoanalyst or psychologist) focused on the patient as a person rather than his or her disease as a case, and on difficulties experienced in patient-resident encounters. In addition to patient-physician communication, participants were also encouraged to discuss issues related to interprofessional collaboration and hospital administration.

The Balint method, and particularly shorter variations of it, has received attention in some residency programs in the USA, particularly in family medicine (Brock & Salinsky, 1993; Cataldo, Peeden, Geesey, & Dickerson, 2005). In a study of family medicine residents in the USA, no significant difference on the scores of the JSE was observed between those who participated in a Balint training program and those who did not (Cataldo et al., 2005).

Other Approaches to Enhance Empathy in Health Professions Students and Practitioners

There are other innovative approaches used to sustain and enhance empathy among health professions students and practitioners. For example, in an experimental study of 248 second-year medical students at Jefferson (currently Sidney Kimmel) Medical College (Hojat, Axelrod et al., 2013), students were divided into experimental and control groups and participated in a two-phase study. In phase 1, students in the experimental group watched and discussed video clips of patient encounters (selected from commercial movies) meant to enhance empathic understanding; those in the control group watched a documentary film. Ten weeks later in phase 2 of the study, students who were in the experimental group were divided into two groups.

One group attended a lecture on the importance of empathy in patient care, and the other plus those in the control group watched a movie about racism. The JSE was administered pre-post in phase 1 and posttest in phase 2. Results showed a statistically significant increase in the JSE mean scores for the experimental group in phase 1. No significant change in the JSE scores was found in the control group. In phase 2 of the study, the JSE mean score improvement was sustained in the group who attended the lecture on importance of empathy in patient care, but not in the experimental group who watched a movie about racism in this phase of the study. Also, no significant change of empathy was observed in the control group in the second phase of the study. It was concluded that enhancement of empathy in medical students can be sustained by additional educational reinforcements.

In another study 57 residents from 16 family medicine programs (Magee & Hojat, 2010) were offered the opportunity in the second year of their training to choose one of their indigent pregnant patients who was in the second trimester of pregnancy, to receive the free gift of a glider rocking chair. Shortly after the baby was born, ten of the residents agreed to make a prearranged home visit to the mother of the newborn to assist in assembling the chair while talking with the mother in a friendly manner about child care and well-being. Compared to the residents who did not make such a home visit, the simple home visit experience contributed to an impressive increase in posttest JSE scores among those residents who made such a home visit.

In a study conducted at the University of Missouri-Kansas City School of Medicine, medical students participated in a three-stage multidimensional training program on empathy (Feighny et al., 1998). In Stage 1, the students developed a clinical presentation of an illness, such as diabetes, from a patient's perspective (cognitive empathy). In Stage 2, the students tried to experience the situation as if they were patients (emotional empathy). In Stage 3, the students were provided with corrective feedback about their communication skills (behavioral empathy). The investigators noted that the students' scores improved significantly on Carkhuff's Empathic Understanding in Interpersonal Processes Scale but did not change significantly on the IRI. The investigators attributed the discrepancy to the IRI's lack of sensitivity in the context of patient care. In her doctoral dissertation at Iowa University, Stebbins (2005) reported that exposure to interactive interpersonal communication enhanced empathy among second-year osteopathic medical students.

Platt and Keller (1994) developed a program to enhance empathic communication among physicians facing difficult encounters with patients who expressed strong negative emotions (e.g., anger, fear, sadness) and were unwilling to assume responsibility for their own health. During the program, the participants attempted to increase their awareness of a patient's emotional clues by trying to understand the emotion, naming the emotion for the patient to insure that they had identified the emotion correctly, acknowledging and justifying the patient's emotion, and affirming the patient's behavior and offering help. The authors concluded that empathic communication is a teachable and learnable skill.

In summary, the major premise of all of the aforementioned approaches is the improvement of understanding which is the key ingredient in the definition of empathy. Therefore, at a conceptual level, it makes sense to assume that all of these approaches can lead to the cultivation of empathy. However, in their review of the literature on effects of educating for empathy in medicine, Stepien and Baernstien (2006) concluded that most studies that attempted to provide empirical evidence in support of improving empathy suffer from inappropriate design, methodological limitations, uncertainty about conceptualization and measurement of empathy, and small nonrepresentative samples. More convincing empirical evidence is needed to confirm the short- and long-term effects of these programs on health professions education and practice, as well as on the administration of the health care centers, and on health insurance company's policies.

Effectiveness of the Programs

Although some studies cited in this chapter indicate that empathy can be enhanced, some clues suggest that the improvement cannot be sustained without practice or reinforcement (Engler et al., 1981; Hojat, Axelrod et al., 2013). Thus, the popular saying "Use it or lose it" may be applicable to empathy that has been enhanced as a result of an educational program. Furthermore, it is also important to bear in mind that when assessing any educational program designed to enhance empathy, it is desirable to examine not only the short-term but also, more importantly, the long-term effects of the program. Although some studies have indicated that educational training programs designed to enhance empathy may have a relatively long-term effect (Kramer et al., 1989; Poole & Sanson-Fisher, 1980), the long-lasting effect of empathy training programs awaits more empirical scrutiny.

At a conceptual level, it makes sense to believe that targeted educational programs can cultivate empathy. However, Skelton, Macleod, and Thomas (2000) are not satisfied with empirical evidence to verify the truth of this assumption. With regard to this challenge, McManus (1995) suggested that investigators who attempt to conduct empirical assessments of the humanities' contribution to medical outcomes must "bite the bullet" of definition and measurement. However, recent research subsequent to the development of the JSE (Chap. 7) can relieve us, to some extent, of the need to bite that bullet (see Appendix A).

Recapitulation

Although the current emphasis on professionalism in medicine places a high value on enhancement of empathy in patient care, most students in the existing medical education system in the USA do not routinely acquire the skills needed to demonstrate empathy. However, research shows that empathy can be effectively enhanced by targeted educational programs. Counteracting current trends in medical education and practice that are not conducive to empathic engagement in patient care requires a mandate for the development and implementation of educational programs at all levels of training (undergraduate, graduate, and continuing education) in all health professions academic centers and hospitals. Only then will the public be better served and will all health professionals regain the utmost respect they rightly deserve.

Chapter 13
In Search of Neurological Underpinnings of Empathy

Empathy is a biological concept par excellence.

—(Leslie Brothers, 1989, p. 17)

Neurons that fire together wire together.

—(attributed to Carla Shatz, cited in Doidge, 2007, p. 63)

Neurons that fire apart wire apart/neurons out of sync fail to link.

—(cited in Doidge, 2007, p. 64)

Abstract

- During the long evolution history, the human brain has evolved to understand other person's state of mind, feelings, perspectives, and intentions. Such an understanding has survival value and facilitates empathic relationships.
- Evidence suggests that there exists a neurophysiobehavioral substructure in human beings that serves as a precursor and facilitator for understanding others, evident by a newborn's reactive crying, inborn capacity for mimicry and imitation, physiological synchronicity in interpersonal interactions, perception–action coupling, propensity to understand other's state of mind reflected in the theory of mind, and findings of a new line of research on the mirror neuron system.
- Empirical findings from brain imaging studies, brain lesion research, empathy deficiency in neurological disorders (e.g., autism, Asperger's syndrome, alexithymia), and pain research suggest that certain brain areas can be implicated in forming or failing to form empathic connection.
- A search for neurological underpinnings of empathy is highly desirable for better understanding of neurological factors that contribute to the development or otherwise to the arrest of the capacity for empathy. Outcomes of such research will have important educational as well as medical implications.
- From brain imaging research, it can be speculated that certain cortical areas of the brain (e.g., region for cognitive processing in the medial prefrontal cortex, dorsolateral, and mirror neuron region in the premotor areas) could be implicated in cognitive empathic responses.

© Springer International Publishing Switzerland 2016

M. Hojat, *Empathy in Health Professions Education and Patient Care*,

DOI 10.1007/978-3-319-27625-0_13

- Findings also suggest that the regions for emotional processing, the orbitofrontal cortex and older structures of the brain such as the limbic system, and specifically areas known as the pain matrix (e.g., amygdala, insula, anterior cingulate cortex) could be implicated in emotional empathic reactions. However, these speculations await further experimental verification.

Introduction

In recent years, along with the emergence of a new discipline of social cognitive neuroscience, there has been a growing research attention to the neurological underpinnings of empathy. Social cognitive neuroscience is an interdisciplinary branch of science that combines the technology from neuroscience with theories and views from behavioral, social, cognitive, political, and economics sciences to explore the neural bases of perceptions, understanding one's self and others, and social interactions (Coplan & Goldie, 2014; Lieberman, 2007) .

Advancements in brain imaging technology have provided a unique opportunity to examine neural activities associated with cognitive and affective states. Locating the areas of the brain that are implicated in empathic engagement will have important educational and medical implications for enhancing empathy in health professions students and practitioners and for diagnosis and treatment of empathy deficit disorders. Views from the ideomotor principle postulated by William James (1890), neuron cell assembly advanced by Donald Hebb (1946), perception–action coupling proposed by Preston and deWaal (2002), and the discovery of the mirror neuron system (Iacoboni et al., 1999; Rizzolatti, Fadiga, Gallese, & Fogassi, 1996) suggest that neurological activities are involved in empathic engagement. The following factors provide evidence in support of the existence of neurological roots of empathy: universal human capacity for expression and understanding of emotions, mimicry and imitation starting at an early age, synchronization in body postures in interpersonal interactions (see Chap. 3) and in physiological functions (e.g., heartbeat, galvanic skin response), as well as findings on neurological activities in social interactions in general, and in pain research in particular. This chapter examines the theoretical bases and empirical evidence in a search for neurological underpinnings of empathy.

Neuroanatomy

Human brain, according to Keysers (2011), is "wired to be empathic." (p. 216). According to Brothers (1989, p. 11), empathy as a social behavior is a concept that "appears to have a great potential utility in bringing together neural and psychological data." To achieve a better understanding of empathy, we must expand our knowledge about the cellular mechanisms involved in interpersonal relationships.

In an article on a new intellectual framework for psychiatry, Eric Kandel (1998) proposed a basic principle that all mental, cognitive, and emotional processes, without exception, derive from neurological operations of the brain. He further suggested that this principle applies to both individual and social behaviors. Thus, empathy as an attribute that is manifested in interaction with others, falls well within the scope of the brain's neurological operations.

The human brain is a complex command-and-control center for cognition and emotions. Although the three divisions of the brain (brainstem, limbic system, and cerebral cortex) are structurally and evolutionarily distinct, they are closely interconnected through a complex neurological network. The brainstem (reptilian brain), phylogenetically the oldest section of the brain, controls the physiology of survival (e.g., heartbeat, breathing). The next oldest section, the limbic system, wraps around the brainstem and functions as the primary center for emotion and social behavior (MacLean, 1990). The limbic brain has an abundance of opiate receptors that not only can reduce physical pain but also can diminish the excruciating psychological and social pains arising from a broken interpersonal relationship (Lewis, Amini, & Lannon, 2000).

Included in the limbic system are a number of interconnected substructures, such as the amygdala, insula, hippocampus, hypothalamus, and cingulate gyrus. Among the substructures of the limbic system, the role of the amygdala is important in understanding the neurology of social behavior because of its contribution to detect social signals. The amygdala is an almond-shaped structure consisting of a highly interconnected cluster of neurons situated deep in the medial temporal lobes. It is implicated in producing emotional reactions, expressions of emotion and responses to social signals (Milner, Squire, & Kanel, 1998). The amygdala is a gateway to a person's view of the social environment (Nauta & Feirtag, 1986) and plays a crucial role in the fight-or-flight response (Siegel, 1999).

The newest component of the brain, the cerebral cortex, which is largest in humans, has a great deal to do with complex cognitive behavior, abstract thinking, reasoning, language, and other high-level activities of the human brain. One striking change that occurred in the course of the brain's evolution is the tremendous increase in the complexity and size of the cerebral cortex in vertebrates in general and in human beings in particular (Nolte, 1993). The newest layers of the cerebral cortex, the neocortex, stem from complex social living (Keverne, Nevison, & Martel, 1997). These layers allow engagement in voluntary social behavior based on cognitive understanding (akin to empathy as conceptualized in Chaps. 1, 3, and 6).

It appears that cognition is more likely to be linked to cortical activities, whereas emotion is more likely to be associated with subcortical activities and the limbic system (Nathanson, 1996). Most cognition occurs in the thalamic–neocortical axis (the thinking brain), whereas primary emotions are largely registered within the hypothalamic–limbic axis (the feeling brain) (Moore, 1996). Thus, one can speculate that the limbic system is more likely to be implicated in emotional empathy (synonymous to sympathy, see Chaps. 1 and 3), whereas the neocortex is more likely to be implicated in cognitive empathy. (Differences between cognitive and emotional empathy are described in Chaps. 1 and 3, and their implications for patient care are discussed in Chap. 6.) Consistent with this speculation, in a functional fMRI based quantitative meta-analytic study, Fan, Duncan, de Greck, and Northoff (2011) reported that cognitive and emotional empathy can be distinguished by the different regional activation of the brain. They identified the dorsal anterior midcingulate cortex to be recruited more frequently in the cognitive empathy, and the right anterior insula in the emotional empathy. Similar results were reported by Eres, Decety, Louis, and Molenberghs (2015) who found that higher scores on cognitive empathy were associated with greater gray matter density in the midcingulate cortex and adjacent dorsomedial prefrontal cortex, and higher scores on emotional empathy were associated with greater gray matter density in the insula cortex.

A long evolutionary path that resulted in the development of the capacity for bonding and interpersonal relationships must have left durable footprints in the human central nervous system. It is now beyond dispute that our cognition and emotions (empathy and sympathy, respectively) are inextricably woven into the structure and function of the human brain (Damasio, 2003). Behavioral scholars and social cognitive neuroscientists benefiting from the advanced brain imaging technology are positioning themselves to view social and interpersonal behaviors from a neurological perspective (Bennett, 2001).

Using advanced biomedical technology, and brain imaging technology, a new and interesting line of research is shedding light on the uncharted territory of neurology of empathy. New technologies, such as positron emission tomography (PET) and, in particular, functional magnetic resonance imaging (fMRI), allow noninvasive exploration of the human brain at a high level of resolution that helps investigators to understand not only the structural aspects but also the functional activities of the brain that are associated with empathic engagement. However, given the current research findings, we are still far from confidently knowing the neurological roots of empathy. Despite all of the biotechnological advances at the present time, we have only a hint of what the neurological underpinnings of empathy might be.

Theoretical Foundations

The following four theoretical perspectives provide foundations for exploring the neurological underpinnings of empathy.

William James Ideomotor Principle

In his book "Principles of Psychology" William James postulated the ideomotor principle, proposing that mental representation of a movement can lead to the actual movement to some degree. In other words, merely observing or even thinking of an action increases the likelihood of performing the act (James, 1890). The ideomotor principle, according to Iacoboni (2009a) can also account for imitation and mimicry which pave the road to empathic understanding (see Chap. 3). Research findings suggest that those who are good at imitation are better in recognizing emotions in others which is a pillar of empathic understanding (Iacoboni, 2009a). There is a strong tendency in humans for imitation, facial or postural mimicry, to align themselves with others in social interactions (Lieberman, 2007). Thus, a link can be expected between the ideomotor principle, imitation and mimicry, and empathic understanding.

Neuron Cell Assembly Theory

Donald Hebb (1946) postulated that "any two cells or systems of cells that are repeatedly active at the same time will tend to become 'associated', so that activity in one facilitates activity in the other." (p. 70). The Hebb's neuron cell assembly theory indeed can be summarized in the quotation cited in the epigraph of this chapter: "Neurons that fire together wire together" (attributed to Carla Shatz, cited in Doidge, 2007). The notion of firing together-wiring together can also provide neurological explanations for not only the perception–action model (described in the following section), but also for habit formation, observational learning, and the influences of sociocultural and educational experiences on the development of the capacity for empathy.

Perception–Action Model

The perception–action model (PAM), formulated by Preston and deWaal (2002) to describe the ultimate and proximate causes of empathy, specifies that perceptions of another person's cognitive, emotional, and somatosensory states automatically activate representations of those states in the observer, unless inhibited. The integrated PAM is recognized as a function with precursors such as mimicry and imitation (Goubert et al., 2005) which helps to understand mechanisms involved in empathic engagement. Mimicry and imitation (see Chap. 3) are indeed recognized as facilitators of empathic understanding (Iacoboni, 2009a).

Empirical research suggests that perception–action coupling could sometimes function in a peculiar way. For example, in an experiment on perception and activation of motor behavior, research participants performed a scrambled-sentence language task. One group was exposed to words that typically could be associated with elderly people and retirement (e.g., old, gray, bingo, Florida, forgetful, retired). The other group was exposed to neutral words (e.g., thirsty, private, clean). At the end of the experiment, the researchers recorded the time to walk back from the experimental room to the elevator to leave the building. It was noticed that those who were exposed to the words associated with older age walked slower than the other group (Bargh, Chen, & Burrows, 1996). These findings support the PAM, suggesting that words that evoke perceptions that are associated with older age can significantly influence the corresponding motor function of the perceivers, showing that empathic understanding can be reflected in actual behavior.

Consistent with the PAM, Craig and Weiss (1971) suggest that perception of others in pain (e.g., observing a patient in pain) can activate cognitive, emotional, and somatosensory representations of the pain, which in turn has a significant effect on the observer's understanding of the patient's pain and suffering. Over a century ago, Theodore Lipps stated that "when I observe a circus performer walking on a tight rope, I feel I am inside him" (cited in Carr, Iacoboni, Dubeau, Mazziotta, & Lenzi, 2003, p. 5502). This statement is a vivid example of linking the PAM to empathic understanding of others through cognitive, affective, and somatosensory activation. The theory that observation can lead to action is further explained by the mirror neuron system (MNS) which will be discussed in the following section.

The Mirror Neuron System

The ideomotor principle, the neuron cell assembly theory, and the PAM laid the foundation for the discovery of the mirror neuron system (MNS). Indeed, one of my colleagues, Dr. Nuno Sousa, Professor of Neuroscience at Minho University in Portugal, believes that MNS is the underlying substrate of the PAM (personal communication, e-mail dated 8/27/2015). In one of the early studies on the MNS, Di Pellegrino, Fadiga, Fogassi, Gallese, and Rizzolutti (1992) noticed that a set of neurons in primates' brains was activated when primates performed a goal-oriented act (e.g., reaching for an object) and also the same set of neurons were activated when another primate observed the act without performing it.

Subsequent to the observation of Di Pellegrino et al. (1992), neuroscientist Giacomo Rizzolatti and his colleagues at the University of Parma, Italy, were the leading investigators who systematically studied and discovered the mirror neuron system in macaque monkeys (Gallese, Fadiga, Fogassi, & Rizzolatti, 1996; Rizzolatti et al., 1996). They discovered that a specific set of neurons in the ventral premotor cortex of the monkey's brains (known as the F5 area) discharged when the monkey observed another monkey performing hand actions, such as grasping, tearing, and holding or manipulating an object. The same set of neurons (dubbed as "mirror neurons") discharged when the monkey actually performed the hand action (Gallese et al., 1996; Rizzolatti et al., 1996).

Accordingly, Gallese, Keysers, and Rizzolatti (2004, p. 396) concluded that "the observation of an action leads to the activation of parts of the *same* cortical neural network that is implicated during its execution" (emphasis added). This brain mechanism serves as a bridge to the understanding of another's action, and is considered as the neural basis of social cognition (Gallese et al., 2004).

Other studies led by Marco Iacoboni at the University of California at Los Angeles and other neuroscientists demonstrated the existence of a similar system of mirror neurons in humans (Buccino et al., 2001; Gallese, 2003; Hari et al., 1998;

Iacoboni et al., 1999; Iacoboni, 2009b). The results of these studies led to the assumption that a region of the human brain, analogous to the F5 area of a monkey's brain, is activated when we observe actions performed by others *as if* we were performing the actions ourselves. The discovery of the mirror neurons indeed provided the link between social cognition and neuroscience (Gallese et al., 1996; Keysers & Perrett, 2004; Rizzolatti et al., 1996). Research findings on the MNS presented the first convincing neurological evidence to show neurological activities for perception–action coupling (Jackson & Decety, 2004; Rizzolatti & Craighero, 2004).

Brain imaging studies in humans have shown that the mirror neurons matching the hand action, fire in the following sectors of the cortical network: Broca's region, premotor cortex, and posterior parietal cortex (Buccino et al., 2001; Gallese, 2003). Considering the homology between the F5 area of a monkey's brain and Broca's region in the inferior frontal lobe (involved in speech control) of the human brain (Hari et al., 1998; Kohler et al., 2002), one can find similarities in the mirror neuron matching system in monkeys and humans.

Two key studies improved our understanding of the generalized function of the MNS. In the first key study, Umilta et al. (2001) carried out an experiment to examine if mirror neurons are involved in understanding "intention" or the "goal" of an action. This was the first experimental study to explore if the mental representation of an action with intended purpose can trigger the neuron system representing that action and its purpose. In other words, can the intended goal (final part) of the action be inferred when it is hidden from view? In one part of the experiment, the monkey was shown a fully visible action (grasping an object) ("full vision" condition). In the other part of the experiment, the same action was presented to the monkey, but the final grasping of the object was blocked by a screen, thus hidden from being directly observed ("hidden" condition).

The results showed that the majority of the mirror neurons fired in the full vision also responded in the hidden condition, suggesting that mirror neurons were involved in action recognition and could correctly infer the intention of the action (in the hidden condition). Similar results were obtained with human subjects suggesting that the MNS is not only involved in action recognition but also in understanding the intention of others (Iacoboni, 2009b; Iacoboni et al., 2005). These findings generally indicate that the MNS has a mediating role not only in the understanding of others' actions, but also in predicting the goals, intention, and consequences of such actions which are important ingredients of empathic understanding. If monkeys have the capacity to predict the intention of an action, then humans are certainly bestowed with a capacity to understand others' states of mind (mind reading?) (see Chap. 3, for a relevant discussion of the theory of mind).

Another relevant finding with regard to the MNS is that the observed acts must be goal-directed to better recruit mirror neurons, suggesting that random acts or acts performed by robots are less likely to activate the MNS (Tai, Scherfler, Brooks, Sawamoto, & Castiello, 2004). Goal-directed, non-repetitive robot acts, however, can activate the MNS (Gazzola, Rizzolatti, Wicker, & Keysers, 2007). Also, it has been shown that the MNS processes biological (or realistic) and nonbiological (or unrealistic) movements differently. For example, Castiello, Lusher, Mari, Edwards, and Humphreys (2002) reported that the brain reacts differently to a grasping action performed by a human compared to a robotic hand. In addition to humans, monkey's brain encodes the grasping actions performed by a person differently from grasping by a tool or a mechanical device (Castiello, 2003).

The second key study on generalization of the MNS function was conducted by Kohler et al. (2002) in which they found that the MNS in monkeys could recognize actions even from their sound (e.g., ripping a piece of paper, cracking a nut) without seeing the action. The MNS response to the auditory stimulus prompted Rizzolatti and Arbibi (1998) to speculate that the mirror neurons have an evolutionary link to language acquisition. This speculation seems reasonable given that the core area of MNS (F5) in monkey's brains corresponds anatomically to the Broca's area in the human brain which is the language processing center.

Therefore, the mirror neuron system was found to be the key neurophysiological indicator in gestural communication (Kohler et al., 2002) which is another key ingredient of empathic understanding. Further studies showed that not only motor actions and auditory stimulus but also more abstract intentions embedded in the contexts such as drinking a cup of tea in the context of a tea party, or cleaning a cup after the party (Iacoboni et al., 2005) or observation of emotional states (Carr et al., 2003) can also recruit the same areas which contain the MNS. It has also been demonstrated that components of the MNS (including the inferior frontal cortex) are involved in the imitation and expressions of emotions (Carr et al., 2003).

Neurological Roots

Brain studies provide plausible explanations as to why we flinch, wince, cringe, or recoil when observing others in pain and almost "feel" the pain of others (Valeriani et al., 2008). It has been demonstrated that affective brain regions (anterior cingulate cortex and anterior insula) are activated by observing a loved one receiving a painful electric shock (Singer et al., 2004). It is interesting to note that research participants with higher scores on measures of cognitive and emotional empathy (e.g., Interpersonal Reactivity Index, and Balanced Emotional Empathy Scale) showed stronger activations in pain-related areas when observing their partners being subjected to painful stimuli (Singer et al., 2004).

Wicker et al. (2003) discovered that observing another person's expression of emotions such as disgust (produced by unpleasant odors) could activate the neural representation of the emotion, as well. By using fMRI, Wicker and colleagues concluded that anatomical and functional data provided evidence that the insula was the common neural basis of seeing and feeling disgust, which is a pathway to emotional empathy. Heins, Engelmann, Vollberg, and Tobler (2016) found that receiving help from an out-group member elicits a signal in the anterior insular cortex which can contribute to a subsequent increase in empathy for the our-group members.

According to Carr et al. (2003), the insula is a plausible candidate for relaying information about action representation to the area of the limbic system that processes emotional content. Lesions in this circuit can lead to impaired understanding of other people's emotions, thus blocking the pathway to emotional empathy. Therefore, it makes intuitive sense that the observer and the observed person experience similar sensations and emotions that can lead to a common understanding (Goubert et al., 2005) which is the foundation of empathic engagement. Watching a spider crawling on another person's face can make the observer shiver as if the spider were crawling on his or her own face. Keysers et al. (2004) attributed this "tactile empathy" to brain activities in the secondary somatosensory cortex. Gallese (2003, p. 176) proposed that "sensations and emotions by others can also be 'empathized', and therefore *implicitly* understood through a mirror matching mechanism."

The notion that perception of a behavior in another person can activate one's own representation of that behavior is not new (Decety & Jackson, 2004); however, providing objective neurological evidence linking empathy to brain activities is new with broad implications. The mirror neuron system plays an important role in understanding the experiences of others; thus, it opens a gateway to understanding neurological pathways to empathy.

A number of studies suggest that understanding the mental state of others, which is the backbone of empathic engagement, appears to be localized to areas of the frontal cortex (Platek, Keenan, Gallup, & Mohamed, 2004), especially the right frontal lobe (Stuss, 2001). Aspects of cognitive empathy, such as perspective taking and role taking skills, are linked to functions of the frontal lobe, whereas aspects of emotional empathy have been hypothesized to be associated with the orbitofrontal areas (Eslinger, 1998). The prefrontal cortex is particularly vital to empathic engagement, and the dorsolateral region of the frontal cortex are linked to people's ability to understand other people's experiences (more relevant to cognitive empathy), and that the orbitofrontal region of the brain could be related to people's emotional responsiveness and sensitivity to the emotional states of others (more relevant to emotional empathy) (Eslinger, 1998).

The dorsolateral prefrontal cortex is known for its role in decision making and context evaluation (Rahm, 2006). It has been suggested that prefrontal damage may result in impaired perspective taking ability. The medial prefrontal cortex plays a critical role in reading others' intentions (Shallice, 2001). Several authors have demonstrated that theory of mind is associated with a cerebral pattern of activity involving the medial prefrontal cortex. It has been reported that lesions in prefrontal cortex, particularly in orbitoprefrontal area, can lead to "acquired sociopathy" (Shamay-Tsoory, Tomer, Goldsher, Berger, & Aharon-Peretz, 2004).

Both the prefrontal and orbitofrontal cortex are involved in integrating cognitive operations in interpersonal relationships and decision making (de Quervain et al., 2004). Research indicates that dorsolateral lesions are associated with a deficit in empathy as well as impaired cognitive flexibility, whereas patients with orbitofrontal cortex lesions are more impaired in emotional empathy than in cognitive flexibility (Decety & Jackson, 2004). The orbitofrontal cortex has been implicated in the regulation of emotion that contributes to emotional empathic engagement (Cahill, 2005). Singer and Frith (2005) reported that seeing pictures of unknown people getting hurt (e.g., a hand trapped in a car door, or someone's hand being pierced by a needle) elicited brain activities in the affective brain section (anterior cingulate cortex). In their discussion of the "painful side of empathy," these authors suggested that neural activities are elicited even when people think about the pain of others.

In a pain study, using fMRI, Jackson, Meltzoff, and Decety (2005) found that observation of pain in others was associated with significant bilateral changes in activities in the anterior cingulate cortex, the anterior insula, and the cerebellum, which prompted them to conclude that their findings help to understand the neurological mechanisms that are implicated in empathy for pain. Carr et al. (2003) used fMRI to confirm that to form empathic relationships, people need to evoke the representation of actions in the brain associated with the conditions they observe in others. In other words, it is necessary to place oneself in another person's shoes to form empathic understanding. In a review article: "The Functional Architecture of Human Empathy," Decety and Jackson (2004, p. 80) concluded that "part of the neural network mediating pain experiences is shared when empathizing with pain in others." In summing up the findings on neurological underpinnings of empathy, Decety (2015) concluded that circuits connecting the brainstem, amygdala, basal ganglia, anterior cingulate cortex, insula, and orbitofrontal cortex are involved in some forms of empathic responses.

The Role of the Right Hemisphere

A number of studies suggest that the right hemisphere is more involved in empathy than the left hemisphere (Rankin et al., 2006; Ruby & Decety, 2004; Shamay-Tsoory, Tomer, Berger, & Aharon-Peretz, 2003). Interpersonal signals, such as facial expressions of emotion, are recognized best in the right cerebral hemisphere, and, most mechanisms associated with regulating emotions are activated in the right hemisphere as well (Perry et al., 2001). Also, it has been reported that the ability to recognize emotions from facial expressions is impaired in patients whose right hemisphere has been damaged (Kolb & Taylor, 1981). Recognition of facial expressions and empathic understanding were impaired in patients with atrophy of the right temporal lobe (Perry et al., 2001). Greater empathy deficit has been observed in those with anterior temporal lobe atrophy in the right compared to the left hemisphere (Perry et al., 2001). Expression and perception of nonverbal communication appears to be mediated by the right hemisphere, whereas verbal communication is mediated predominantly by the left hemisphere (Siegel, 1999). It is generally believed that the posterior region of the right hemisphere plays a special role in perceptions of emotion and recognition of emotional clues (Buck & Ginsburg 1997a, 1997b).

In an interesting experiment in search of the comforting substrate of the right brain, Horton (1995) hypothesized that the comforting substrate is located in the right hemisphere of the brain. The hypothesis was based on the notion that the calming effectiveness of holding the baby on the left side of the chest against the beating heart is an indication of the baby's specific need to be comforted. In this experiment, Horton (1995) gave the option to 60 research participants to choose between two identical red balls (one on the left and one on the right). Results showed that only 20 % of the right handed subjects chose the left ball. Participants were also given the choice between two identical white teddy bears which were described as grieving because they lost their mothers, were upset and scared, and in need of being soothed. In this experimental condition, the majority of the participants chose the left bear. Also, two-thirds of the participants who were mothers in this study chose the left bear. Results support the view that the comforting attitude has its origin in the right brain (by choosing the left bear) suggesting the possibility that right brain lateralization of the comforting substrate is more pronounced, especially in mothers.

It is also interesting to note that a great majority of mothers regardless of whether they are right- or left-handed (approximately 90 % of people are right handed), carry their infants against the left side of their chest (Salk, 1960). It may be argued that an evolutionary factor prompted mothers to place their infants to the left of their chest closer to their hearts, or to have their dominant right hand free to defend the child against predators. However, from a neurological perspective, placing a child on the left activates the left visual field which can lead to more direct communication to the right hemisphere of the brain (Sieratzki & Woll, 1996). Some believe that this suggests that the right brain may have a more significant role than the left brain in human attachment and interpersonal relationships (Sieratzki & Woll, 1996; Swain, Lorberlaum, Kose, & Strathearn, 2007).

Lesion research showed that while damage to the right hemisphere resulted in greater impairment in cognitive empathy than damage to the left hemisphere, damage to the right prefrontal cortex did not have a significant impairment in emotional empathy (Shamay-Tsoory et al., 2004). Rankin et al. (2006) reported a large scale lesion study of investigating the neural basis of empathy. Their findings suggest that the right anterior temporal and medial frontal regions are neurological roots to empathic behavior. Further support was provided by Tranel, Bechara, and Denburg (2002) who found that the right, compared to the left ventromedial prefrontal cortex, is more directly involved in social behavior and decision-making.

Dementia patients with right-sided brain damage were also more likely than patients with left brain damage to show deficits in empathy and other aspects of interpersonal behavior (Rankin et al., 2006). It has been reported that damage to the right hemisphere is frequently associated with impairment in social interactions (Edwards-Lee & Saul, 1999) and with impaired judgment of facial expressions (Adolphs, Damasio, Tranel, Cooper, & Damasio, 2000). Also, according to Decety and Chaminade (2003), right parietal cortices are involved with the capacity for understanding other's emotions. Rankin et al. (2006) found that empathy scores (measured by the IRI, see Chap. 5) correlated significantly with the volume of the gray matter in the right brain areas. The aforementioned studies generally indicate that the role of the right brain hemisphere seems to be more important in manifesting empathy.

Neurological Impairment and Empathy: Lesion Studies

The inability to recognize one's own emotions and the emotions of others can impair capacity to form empathic relationships. This is often observed in patients with certain developmental, neurological, and psychiatric disorders. If as research suggests, empathy is a function of cellular activities in the brain, it would be reasonable to assume that certain neurological damage in the brain could impair capacity for empathy. This assumption has been supported by studies of patients with brain lesions or certain neurological problems. The well-known case of Phineas Gage is a classic example of impaired social skills associated with lesions of the frontal lobe (Benton, 1991; Damasio, Grabowski, Frank, Galaburda, & Damasio, 1994; Hamilton, 1984). Gage was the foreman of a railroad construction company. In 1848, as a result of an accidental explosion, an iron bar was propelled completely through his skull and landed some 25–30 yards behind him (Macmillan, 2000). Although he recovered physically and survived for $11^1/_2$ years after the injury, he never regained his capacity for forming empathic relationships.

The following neurological conditions have been linked to impairment in the capacity for empathy.

Autism

Of all the developmental disorders, autism is among the best clinical examples for studying the neurological basis of empathy. Poor social skills are among the core features of autistic individuals, and the central pathology of autism is an impaired capacity for empathy (Brothers, 1989). A defect in social interaction is a primary criterion for the diagnosis of autism (Frances, First, & Pincus, 1995). It has been observed that autistic children never respond to their mother's smile, indicating that they do not exhibit a capacity to respond empathically to others (Decety & Jackson, 2004). Autistic infants are born with some deficit in forming attachment and social interactions (Tucker, Luu, & Derryberry, 2005).

Empirical and clinical evidence suggests that compared to the general population, autistic individuals obtain lower scores on tests measuring the ability to understand facial expressions displayed in photographs of people with happy, sad, or fearful faces and display a seriously impaired capacity for empathy (Baron-Cohen, 2003). Autistic children show a profound cognitive impairment to understand the perspectives and intentions of other people, which is a cognitive impairment (Tucker et al., 2005). In a study by Dziobek et al. (2008) using the Multifaceted Empathy Test (MET), it was noticed that adults with Asperger's syndrome (a condition within the autism spectrum disorders, but typically with a milder phenotype), compared to a healthy control group, also displayed impaired empathy, but more pronounced in cognitive empathy rather than emotional empathy. The MET includes a set of pictures depicting individuals in emotionally charged situations (e.g., being threatened). For the assessment of cognitive empathy, participants are asked to infer the mental status on the individual(s) shown in the pictures. For the assessment of emotional empathy, participants are asked to identify and rate their emotional reaction to the event shown in the picture.

Alexithymia

Alexithymia is a condition that impairs patients' perception of other people's affective status. Sufferers usually have difficulty recognizing and labeling emotions and feelings, which are associated with impairment in capacity for empathy (Mann, Wise, Trinidad, & Kohanski, 1994). Guttman and LaPorte (2002) reported that patients with alexithymia score low on empathy measured by the Interpersonal Reactivity Index (Chap. 5). A significant association has been reported between alexithymia and autism (Hill, Berthoz, & Frith, 2004). Most etiological models of alexithymia have proposed a dysfunction of the right hemisphere to account for the characteristic pattern observed in patients with alexithymia (Jessimer & Markham, 1997).

Although no specific brain lesion has been identified as the cause of alexithymia, case studies of patients with alexithymia should be of interest to empathy researchers to examine underlying mechanisms involved in a lack of capacity to recognize emotions which is a main feature of alexithymia.

Other Empathy Deficit Disorders

It has been reported that many pervasive developmental, personality, and neurological disorders such as elective mutism, Tourette's syndrome, anorexia nervosa, schizophrenia, psychopathy, post traumatic brain injury, and stroke are associated with deficits in empathy (Charman et al., 1997; Mullins-Nelson, Salekin, & Leistico, 2006; Rankin et al., 2006). In a study by Grattan and Eslinger (1989), significant empathic change (measured by Hogan's Empathy Scale, see Chap. 5) was associated with brain injury which resulted in acquired disabilities featured by cognitive inflexibility.

Eslinger (1998) reported that more than half of the neurologically damaged patients scored more than two standard deviations below the mean on a measure of empathy. In a study involving patients with neurological damage caused by closed head injuries, ischemic hemispheric strokes, encephalitis, or multiple sclerosis, Eslinger, Satish, and Grattan (1996) found that both cognitive and emotional empathy were impaired by the neurological damage. Brothers (1989) hypothesized that the impairment of empathy observed in certain neurological conditions, such as autism, or in certain lesions of the cortex in the right cerebral hemisphere suggest that empathy has neurophysiological roots.

Evidence presented by Anderson, Bechara, Damasio, Tranel, and Damasio (1999) suggests that individuals with early-onset prefrontal lesions (before 16 months of age) resemble patients with comparable adult-onset lesions in a number of ways. Those individuals failed to acquire complex social knowledge during the regular development period. Unlike adult-onset patients, however, early onset patients could not retrieve complex social knowledge at the factual level, and may never have acquired such knowledge (Anderson et al., 1999).

It has been reported that acquired cerebral damage, such as focal damage to the prefrontal cortex in adulthood and damage to the frontal lobe in early childhood, can disturb social behavior, including the capacity for empathy (Eslinger, 1998). Research showed that empathic understanding was impaired subsequent to focal lesions of the prefrontal cortex (Decety & Jackson, 2004; Eslinger, 1998). Some research findings concerning the neuroanatomical basis of social behavior indicated that after damage to the frontal lobe, patients became profoundly inept in their social behavior in general (Grattan & Eslinger, 1989) and in their capacity for empathy in particular (Eslinger, 1998).

In a study of character changes in patients with multiple sclerosis, a decline in empathy (measured by the Hogan Empathy Scale) was observed that was attributed to a neurogenic frontal lobe syndrome (Benedict, Priore, Miller, Munschauser, & Jacobs, 2001). In another study, it is reported that affective agnosia in patients with lesions in the right temporoparietal area renders patients unable to understand emotions conveyed by vocal quality (Heilman, Scholes, & Watson, 1975). Another condition, aprosodic-agestural syndrome (an inability to express felt emotions through voice intonation), caused by lesions in the right hemisphere, makes patients unable to express themselves through gestures (Ross & Mesulam, 1979). Yet another group of patients includes those with lesions in the left hemisphere that impair the ability for symbolic communication and make patients unable to pantomime.

Empathy deficit is often a feature of psychopathic personality. Although a psychopath may have the skill to understand another person's perspective and have the ability to manipulate others, they often lack concern for the welfare of others and can inflict pain and suffering with no apparent remorse (Tucker et al., 2005); thus, all psychopaths have empathy deficit disorder.

Developmental history of many psychopath patients shows a clear evidence of abuse and neglect in their childhood and a lack of quality attachment with a primary caregiver. However, it is reported that in addition to the aforementioned factors, lesions in prefrontal cortex and particularly in the orbitoprefrontal area can also lead to the "acquired psychopathy" (Shamay-Tsoory et al., 2004; Tucker et al., 2005) with severe empathic deficiency. Rankin, Kramer, and Miller (2005) found that patients with semantic dementia showed low levels of both cognitive and emotional empathy, whereas patients with frontotemporal dementia showed deficits only in cognitive empathy measured by the Interpersonal Reactivity Index. In a study by Shamay-Tsoory et al. (2004), impairment in cognitive empathy (measured by the Interpersonal Reactivity Index) and emotional empathy (measured by Mehrabian and Epstein's Emotional Empathy Scale) was assessed in patients with brain lesions.

It was found that patients with prefrontal lesions (especially those with lesions involving orbitoprefrontal and medial regions) were significantly impaired in both cognitive and affective empathy. In particular, patients with lesions in the prefrontal cortex had significantly low empathy scores. Damage to the right hemisphere resulted in greater impairment in cognitive empathy, whereas damage to the right prefrontal cortex did not exert significant impairment in affective empathy (Shamay-Tsoory et al., 2004).

Gillberg (1992, 1996) grouped conditions that could lead to empathy deficiency in a category labeled "disorders of empathy." Gillberg (1996) assumed that humans have an "empathy quotient" that, like the intelligence quotient (IQ), has a normal distribution in the general population (a bell-shaped curve with a mean of 100 and a standard deviation of 15). Accordingly, Gillberg (1996) suggested that similar to the classification of intellectual abilities (IQ), autism could be arbitrarily classified as an empathic deficiency equivalent to a quotient below 50 (people with an IQ below 50 are classified as either moderately, severely, or profoundly impaired), and Asperger's syndrome (a milder form of autism) would be equivalent to a quotient in the range of 50–70 (people with an IQ between 50 and 70 are classified as mildly impaired).

Empathy for Pain

Neurological underpinnings of empathy have also been explored in a number of pain studies. Understanding the pain and suffering of others is the backbone of empathic relationships in the context of patient care. Neuroimaging studies have generally shown that in mentally healthy people, observing others in pain activates similar brain areas that are implicated in the person in pain (Jackson, Brunet, Meltzoff, & Decety, 2006). Various painful personal experiences, ranging from being pin-pricked to feeling an aching phantom limb or suffering from social loss, are represented in a complex neural network referred to as the 'pain matrix' which is a fluid system jointly activated by pain, composed of several interacting networks including anterior cingulate cortex, anterior insula, as well as frontal and parietal areas (Melzack, 1990).

Pain is an interesting model for incorporating the previously described notions of ideomotor principle, neuron cell assembly, perception–action coupling, and mirror neuron system. A shared representation of others' pain is suggested by the findings that neuron cells in the human cingulate cortex fire when pain is inflicted and when a person observes another person in pain. Empathy for pain can also be a function of the situations, attitudes, and personal relationships. For example, Englis, Vaughan, and Lanzetta (1982) reported that empathy for pain was elicited when the observer had a cooperative (as opposed to competitive) relationship with the person in pain. In a study by Singer et al. (2006), male and female participants engaged in an economic game, with two confederates, who were professional actors in which one confederate played fairly, but the other confederate played unfairly. Brain activities of the participants were recorded when the confederates received painful stimulus to the hand. Both male and female participants showed brain activities in the pain-related brain areas (frontoinsular and anterior cingulate cortices) toward fair players. However, pain-related brain activation was less pronounced for male participants when observing the unfair player receiving pain. These findings suggest that empathic response to pain in men is a function of their attitudes toward social behavior of others in pain. Hein and Singer (2008) reported that the amplitude of perception of other's pain is modulated by the intensity of emotion, characteristics of the suffering person, gender and perceived fairness.

In a pain study, a series of pictures of hands and feet in painful situations and another series of pictures of hands and feet in non-painful situations were shown to research participants (Jackson et al., 2005). The fMRI images showed activation of several brain regions in the observers that are known to play a significant role in pain processing (e.g., anterior cingulate cortex, anterior insula, the cerebellum). Brain regions associated with feeling an emotion can also be influenced by seeing the facial expression of that emotion, a phenomenon described as emotional contagion or sympathy (Singer et al., 2004).

Several neuroimaging studies have demonstrated commonalities in pain matrix activation when subjects experience pain themselves and when they observe others in pain (Morrison, Lloyd, di Pellegrino, & Roberts, 2004). Common areas include thalamus, anterior cingulate cortex, anterior insula, and prefrontal cortex. This is especially true when the person in pain is a significant figure, like a family member, friend, or partner (Holden, 2004). For example, mothers listened to recorded infant cries and white noise control sounds. The fMRI results indicated that the mothers showed significantly greater anterior cingulate cortex activity, hearing the baby cries compared to white noise. This finding demonstrates the plasticity or reactivity of the pain matrix to internal psychological factors.

In another fMRI study, it was observed that the bilateral anterior insula, rostral anterior cingulate cortex, brainstem, and cerebellum were activated when subjects received pain or were signaled that loved ones were experiencing pain. It was also noted that activation intensity in brain areas, when observing others in pain, was correlated with individual empathy scores (Singer et al., 2004).

Evidence also suggests that empathic engagement seems to be more contingent upon the frontocortical brain areas which have been implicated in mentalization and the theory of mind (Nummenmaa et al., 2008; Wellman, 1991). The medial prefrontal cortex has also been implicated in the theory of mind (Gallagher & Frith, 2003) suggesting that this area of the brain may constitute a partial system for empathy (Nummenmaa et al., 2008). The medial prefrontal cortex appears to play a role in the ruminative focus on pain and apprehension about pain's implications.

Sympathetic involvement with a person in pain increased activity in the anterior insula and thalamus, which are involved in processing negative or unpleasant emotions (Nummenmaa et al., 2008). It is also interesting to note that pain-related areas in the anterior cingulate cortex have extensive output connections to premotor areas, a brain region observed to contain much of the MNS in macaque monkeys (Morrison et al., 2004). Some of the same neural activities in the experience of physical pain are also involved in the experience of social pain (e, g., separation, rejection, social exclusion, losing a significant person) (Eisenberger, Leiberman, and Williams 2003). Thus, the expression of being *hurt* by experiencing loneliness, rejection, and separation is not metaphoric only, but real in nature and operates by sharing common neuroanatomical underpinnings with physical pain. Studies have demonstrated that sadness, social exclusion, and physical pain activate similar limbic regions (e.g., anterior cingulate cortex, anterior insula) (Loggia, Mogil, & Bushnell, 2008). It should also be mentioned that in addition to the somatosensory, cognitive and emotional factors, other variables such as genetics, gender, and culture contribute to the perception of pain and to the physicians' approach in the treatment of pain (Grossman & Wood, 1993; Safdar et al., 2009; Weisman & Teitlebaum, 1985).

Avenanti, Bueti, Galati, and Aglioti (2005) showed that empathy for pain increased the BOLD (blood oxygen level-dependent) signal in anterior insula and anterior cingulate cortices, which are part of the affective division of the pain matrix. Neural activity in the affective pain network was also reported in fMRI studies where subjects observed pictures or movies in which potentially painful stimuli were delivered to hands or other human body parts (Jackson et al., 2005; Morrison et al., 2004; Singer et al., 2004).

Approaches to Study the Neurobiophysiology of Pain

Three approaches have often been used in social cognitive neuroscience research in studying perception of pain: (1) studying pain parameters when the person is experiencing pain (self-pain); (2) recording biological, physiological and psychological changes and neurological activities when observing another person in pain and imagining one's own self is actually experiencing the other person's pain (self-perspective, or first-person representation); (3) recording biological, physiological and psychological changes and neurological activities when observing another person in pain, but imagining how that person would experience pain (other-perspective or third-person representation).

Perception of self-pain versus self-perspective of other's pain, versus other-perspective of pain require a distinction between self and others when merging with self, and when separating other's pain from one's own. These different perspectives on pain involve different forms of perceptions, which lead to different consequences (Batson, Early, & Salvarini, 1997). For example, research in social psychology (Batson et al., 2003; Underwood & Moore, 1982) has documented this distinction by showing that self-perspective is likely to induce personal distress (akin to emotional empathy), whereas other-perspective is likely to evoke perspective taking (akin to cognitive empathy).

In the conceptualization of empathy, researchers have often failed to make a distinction between the self- and other-oriented perspective taking (Coplan, 2014). The two types of perspective taking are not only conceptually different, but also recruit different neurological mechanisms. For example, other-oriented perspective taking requires greater mental flexibility and emotional regulation, whereas self-oriented perspective taking is likely to lead to egocentric affective response and emotional exhaustion (Coplan, 2014; Jackson, Brunt, et al., 2006) which is akin to sympathetic reaction. For a true empathic engagement, it is essential to make a clear distinction between self- and other-oriented perspective taking.

One of the earlier experiments on perception of pain in others was conducted by Stotland (1969) in which three groups of participants viewed a subject whose hand was strapped in a heat generating machine. One group was instructed just to watch the event non-judgmentally (neutral observation). The second group was instructed to imagine their own hand strapped in the machine (self-perspective). The third group was told to imagine how the person whose hand was strapped was feeling (other-perspective). It was found that imagining the pain of others could generate cognitive and emotional empathic connections, and produce similar tangible physiological responses which corresponded to perception of pain as predicted by PAM (e.g., palm sweating, galvanic skin response). Data from functional brain imaging studies show that imagining pain in one's self and others, in the absence of any painful stimulus, activates critical brain areas involved in pain perception (Ochsner et al., 2008).

It has been consistently reported that observing someone in pain activates neurons in the observer similar to those that are firing in the person experiencing pain (Botvinick et al., 2005; Jackson et al., 2005). Findings in pain research have generally showed that both the self-perspective and the other-perspective were associated with activation in the neural network involved in pain processing, including the parietal operculum, anterior medial cingulate, and the anterior insula (Derbyshire, 2000; Lamm et al., 2007). However, the self-perspective yielded higher pain ratings and involved the pain matrix more extensively in the secondary somatosensory cortex, the posterior part of the anterior cingulated cortex, and the middle insula (Derbyshire, 2000).

In one study, participants received painful stimuli in some trails, and in other trails participants observed a signal that their partner, who was present in the same room would receive the same stimuli (Singer et al., 2004). The anterior medial cingulated cortex, the anterior insula, and the cerebellum were activated during both conditions. Similar results were reported by Morrison et al. (2004), who applied a moderately painful pinprick stimulus to the fingertips of their participants and in a second condition showed them a video clip showing another person undergoing similar stimulation. Both conditions resulted in common activities in pain-related areas of the cingulated cortex.

In another study, participants were shown photos depicting right hands and feet in painful or neutral situations, and were asked to imagine the level of pain that these situations would generate (Jackson et al., 2005). Significant activation in regions involved in the pain matrix network, notably in the anterior cingulated cortex and the anterior insula was detected. Yet in another study (Lamm et al., 2007), participants were requested to watch the videos adopting two different perspectives, that is, either imagining how they themselves would feel if they were in the place of the other (imagine self), or imagining how the other feels (imagine other). Results supported the view that response to the pain of others can be a function of cognitive and motivational factors. In other words, observing others in pain can either evoke

empathic response and altruistic motivation, or personal distress and egoistic motivation to reduce one's own distress, depending upon the capacity for self–other
differentiation and cognitive appraisal (Lamm et al., 2007). For example, perception of pain via the self-perspective approach is likely to evoke an egoistic motivation to reduce personal distress associated with the activated brain that controls
emotional pain response; whereas the other-perspective approach is likely to insti-
gate an altruistic motivation to help (Batson, 1991; Dovidio, 1991; Goubert et al.,
2005). Altruistic motivation is more aligned with our characterization of cognitively defined empathy, which allows planning; whereas egoistic motivation fits
better with our description of emotionally defined sympathy (or emotional empathy) which is more likely to be spontaneous (see Chap. 1).

Research Challenges

It is important to notice that in neurological research of empathy with the exception of a very few studies (Dziobek et al., 2008; Nummenmaa et al., 2008;
Shamay-Tsoory et al., 2004), no clear distinction has been made between cognitive and emotional empathy (Morelli, Rameson, & Lieberman, 2014) and their
differential motivational factors and specially their different consequences in the
context of patient care (see Chap. 6). No wonder that the results of most of the
studies on neurological underpinnings of empathy are inconsistent because of
conceptual ambiguity (associated with conceptualization and definition) as well
as methodological shortcomings (associated with measurement of the concepts
and research design). Thus, research outcomes cannot be specifically attributed to
only one of the two forms of cognitive or emotional empathy (or empathy and
sympathy, respectively).

It is difficult to dissociate cognitive and emotional empathy within the traditional
pain paradigm because they are somewhat correlated (Jackson et al., 2005), but if
we fail to make such a distinction we can never find the correct answer in our search
for neurological underpinnings of empathy (as opposed to sympathy). The challenge ahead is to propose agreeable conceptualizations and definitions of cognitive
and emotional empathy and their corresponding measurements; and then develop
new research paradigms to evoke cognitive empathic responses in one occasion and
emotional empathic reactions in another (e.g., using event-related brain imaging).
Finally, we can be in a better position to examine similarities and differences in
brain activation in response to scenarios that evoke cognitive or emotional empathy.
Based on the characterization of the two concepts (see Chaps. 1, 3, and 6), and
based on some of the neurological findings reported in this chapter, distinct brain
activations can be expected in cognitive empathic responses (e.g., most likely in the
premotor and prefrontal cortex) and in emotional empathic reactions (e.g., most
likely in amygdala, insular, and cingulate cortex).

Furthermore, brain lesion research may also shed light on the detrimental effects
of damage to cortical or limbic structures on cognitive and emotional empathy,

respectively. Admittedly, this is a very simplistic view of a complex behavioral-social concept (such as empathy), which is certainly more complicated, and convoluted by many biophysioneurological, personal, social, cultural, and educational factors and their interactions. It is a real challenge to tease out the effects of emotion from cognition, and empathy from sympathy in our search for neurological underpinnings of empathy. However, we can hope for the best meaningful outcomes because even the sky is no limit in the realm of scientific inquiry.

Recapitulation

Human beings are evolved to understand and to be understood for survival. Theoretical views on ideomotor principle, neuron cell assembly, perception–action coupling, and mirror neuron system and empirical findings in social cognitive neuroscience support the notion that neurological activities are involved in the process of understanding others and being understood by others. Brain imaging and brain lesion studies, and research findings on brain activities involved in perception of pain provide tangible evidence in support of neurological underpinnings of empathy. Research findings, however, are not consistent, probably due to conceptual ambiguity (e.g., a lack of distinction between cognitive and emotional empathy, or empathy and sympathy, respectively) and methodological shortcomings (e.g., measurement and research design issues). Future explorations on neurological underpinnings of empathy should clarify the conceptual ambiguity, and measurement issues, as well as developing appropriate research paradigms to address neurological underpinnings of empathy. Without such conceptual and methodological rigor, we may never find a satisfactory answer in our search for neurological roots of empathy.

Chapter 14
Parting Thoughts: A Systemic Paradigm of Empathy in Patient Care and Future Directions

Everything in the system is dependent on the previous state of the system.

—(Robert Lilienfeld, 1978, p. 14)

By becoming more and more aware of our roles in patient–doctor relationship—i.e., of our side-effects as drugs—our therapeutic efficiency will grow apace.

—(Michael Balint, 1957, p. 688)

Abstract

- Empathy in health professions education and patient care is viewed from a broader and more comprehensive perspective of systems theory.
- In a systemic paradigm of empathy in patient care, the contributions of major subsets of the system (e.g., clinician-related, nonclinician-related, social learning, and education) and their related elements to clinical encounters that lead to functional or dysfunctional system outcomes are discussed.
- An agenda for future research is outlined which includes: (1) exploration of additional components of empathy in the context of health professions education and patient care; (2) the investigation of additional variables that are beneficial or detrimental to empathy in patient care; (3) consideration of empathy as a criterion for admissions, selection, and employment; (4) the study of empathy as a predictor of career choice, academic and professional success; (5) the development and evaluation of approaches to enhance and sustain empathy in health professions education and patient care; (6) development of approaches to maximize empathy and regulate sympathy; (7) the development of national norm tables and cutoff scores to identify JSE high and low scorers; (8) consideration of patients' and peers' perspectives in outcomes of empathy research; and (9) further explorations of neurological underpinnings of empathy.
- It is suggested that implementation of remedies for enhancing and sustaining empathy is a mandate that must be acted upon, not only by academic medical centers but by all other educational institutions.

© Springer International Publishing Switzerland 2016
M. Hojat, *Empathy in Health Professions Education and Patient Care*,
DOI 10.1007/978-3-319-27625-0_14

Introduction

Empathy is an attribute that is distributed unevenly in the population. Human beings are not created equal with regard to their capacity for empathy. It is a gift bestowed in abundance on some and in only meager amounts on others. It is an endowment that can grow like a tree if the conditions are right. In this book, we embarked on a journey to find out why people differ with respect to their capacity to form empathic connections, how capacity for empathy is developed, how empathy can be quantified in the context of health professions education and patient care, and what are the correlates and clinical outcomes of empathy.

Now that we have come so far, and are approaching the final destination of our journey, I would like to reflect on what I have said so far. We embarked on this journey without even knowing the terrain we hoped to discover. Starting with the confusion reflected in research on the conceptualization and measurement of empathy, we attempted to achieve a better vision by resolving the confusion. We visited empathy's historical roots, developmental trajectories, psychosocial connections, and other related factors along the terrain. In passing along these paths, we learned about the antecedents, development, measurement, and consequences of empathic engagement in the context of health professions education and patient care. Many other terrains remain to be explored, however.

An undefined concept can never be measured, and a well-defined concept is half-measured! On the basis of the premise that research findings are vulnerable to serious challenge when the definition of the phenomenon under study is unclear, I offered a definition of empathy in the context of patient care (Chap. 6) primarily as a cognitive (as opposed to an emotional) attribute. Although I do not expect this conceptual characterization to remain unchallenged, let us hope that it can help, to some extent, to resolve the long-standing and unsettled debate regarding the conceptualization and definition of empathy that has always haunted empathy research.

The concept of empathy as having both cognitive and emotional components, adopted uncritically from social psychology by educators in the health professions, fits poorly with the clinical reality in clinician–patient encounters (Morse et al., 1992). The golden principle of patient care, "Above all, do not harm" (*primum non nocere*), rules out intense emotional engagement between clinician and patient that may jeopardize the outcomes of patient care. In studying empathy in psychology in the context of prosocial behavior, emotions can often facilitate, rather than jeopardize, the positive outcomes. However, as I described in Chaps. 1 and 6, in medical and surgical treatment, emotions must be curbed to maintain objectivity. No wonder that regulation of emotions in patient care was strongly recommended by Sir William Osler (1932) who advised "In the physician or surgeon no quality takes rank with imperturbability [which] means coolness and presence of mind under all circumstances and the physician who has the misfortune to be without it loses rapidly the confidence of his patient." (pp. 3–4). Thus, to achieve optimal patient outcomes, empathy in the context of patient care should be guided primarily by cognition rather than emotion.

Without a distinction between cognition and emotion, we will be wrestling forever with the challenge of how to separate the two in the context of patient care.

With that in mind, we also need to recognize that clinicians cannot remain completely emotionless when dealing with their patients. As part of human nature, emotions always play a role in any kind of human relationship. The challenging issue that remains to be explored is the extent to which emotions would be beneficial and to determine the point from which emotions become detrimental to patient outcomes (see Chaps. 1 and 6).

To avoid more confusion on conceptualization of empathy and sympathy I have used alternative words which are commonly used in empathy literature, namely cognitive empathy (sometimes also recognized as "clinical empathy" in the context of patient care), and emotional (or affective) empathy (synonymous to sympathy). In the definition of empathy in the context of patient care, I placed the emphasis on "understanding" patient's pain, suffering, experiences, and concerns. In the definition of emotional empathy (akin to sympathy), I placed the emphasis on "feeling" of patient's pain and suffering. This distinction, described in details in Chaps. 1, 3, and 6 can help us to clarify, to some extent, the ambiguity associated with the terms, and their respective consequences in patient care, as well as in search for their neurological underpinnings (Chap. 13).

A complex concept, such as empathy, cannot be the subject of scientific inquiries in the absence of an instrument that produces quantifiable results. An instrument intended to measure empathy in patient care cannot pass the litmus test of face and content validity unless its contents are not only consistent with its definition, but also relevant to the context of patient care. In addition, psychometric evidence must provide convincing support for the validity and reliability of the instrument. Let us hope that the Jefferson Scale of Empathy (JSE), the instrument described in Chap. 7, can help us resolve the measurement issues that have caused the uncertainty and have impeded empirical scrutiny of empathy in medical and other health professions education and patient care research.

Complex human attributes are not isolated entities; they always function in relation to other factors. As we learned in previous chapters, empathy is a multifaceted attribute that is deeply rooted in human evolution; it has genetic traces and a long history of development from conception to grave. Furthermore, as was discussed earlier (Chap. 4), environmental, cultural, experiential, and educational factors contribute, independently and interactively, to the makeup of the attribute called empathy. More importantly, empathic engagement, or the lack of it, in the context of patient care can lead to virtually opposite clinical outcomes (Chap. 11).

Despite its deep evolutionary roots and genetic component, the capacity for empathy is amenable to change, positively or negatively, to some extent when the conditions are right or wrong. Therefore, as I discussed in Chap. 12, targeted educational programs, appropriate experiences, and environmental facilitators can enhance the capacity for empathy in health professionals-in-training and in-practice; and detrimental factors can erode it. Frequent reinforcements are also needed to sustain the enhanced orientation toward empathic engagement in patient care (Hojat, Axelrod, Spandorfer, & Mangione, 2013).

Viewed from a broader perspective, a complex concept such as empathy in patient care, requires a comprehensive model to depict its important elements, their interactions, and their outcomes. For that purpose, we can turn to systems theory to present a heuristic paradigm of empathy in the context of patient care.

A Systemic Paradigm of Empathy in Patient Care

The developmental trajectories and outcomes of a complex concept, such as empathy in patient care, can be viewed from the vista of systems theory. According to Pollak (1976), a systemic approach is the professional way of dealing with complexity. A system is defined as a set of interrelated subsets, each with an array of elements, no subset of which is unrelated to any other subset, and each element within a subset is related directly or indirectly to every other element in the system (Ackoff & Emery, 1981). A system will be functional only when all its subsets and all the elements within and between subsets function properly; otherwise, the system will be dysfunctional. A functional system has a purpose. The systemic purpose of empathy in patient care is to enhance mutual understanding between clinician and patient so that the goal of positive and optimal patient outcomes can be achieved.

More than 40 years ago, Gordon Allport (1960) suggested that human personality must be treated as an open system that should be viewed with an open mind. Active systems are often considered to be open systems because they are dynamic and therefore capable of responding and adapting to changes in the environment (Siegel, 1999). The combined functions of the elements within each subset of the system and the interrelationships among subsets prompt the system to generate a totality, a *gestalt*, in which the whole is greater than the sum of its parts. To achieve a better understanding of the antecedents, development, measurement, and outcomes of empathy in patient care, it seems desirable to view the concept of empathy in patient care, its major subsets, and the elements within each subset as an open system.

A complete understanding of any system requires an understanding of the subsets within the system and the nature of their interacting elements. For example, as Bateson (1971) indicated, if the family is viewed as a complex system, then an effective intervention in the context of family therapy requires a complete understanding of all subsets and elements of the system, including the roles, responsibilities, interactions, and functions of all family members within the family structure.

Similarly, in the context of patient care, as described in Chaps. 4 and 8, the act of seeking help brings to the surface a need for connectedness that generates the energy to set the system of empathic engagement in motion. A clinician–patient encounter represents an open system in need of equilibrium brought about by the energy discharged in interpersonal connection. Achieving positive patient outcomes would indicate that the system is functional (i.e., a state of equilibrium), whereas negative patient outcomes would indicate that the system is dysfunctional (i.e., a state of disequilibrium). Empathic engagement in the clinician–patient relationship is the first step in maintaining systemic equilibrium. Figure 14.1 depicts a systemic paradigm of empathy in the context of patient care. It illustrates the major subsets of the system and the major elements within each subset that ultimately determine the functional or dysfunctional outcome of the system.

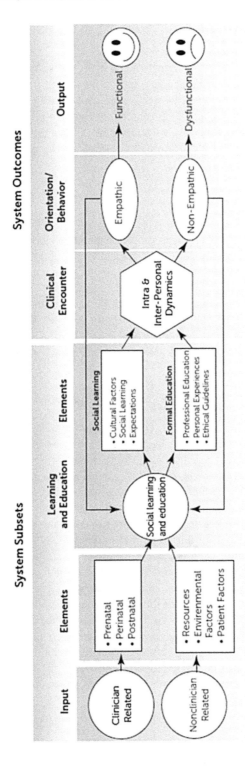

Fig. 14.1 A systemic paradigm of empathy in the context of health professions education and patient care

Major Subsets of the System

Let us elaborate briefly on the paradigm depicted in Fig. 14.1. Assuming that empathy in patient care resembles an open and purposeful system (i.e., a system that is amenable to change for the purpose of positive patient outcomes), the system would be set in motion by two interacting subsets: a clinician-related subset and a nonclinician-related subset (depicted on the left side of the figure as the entry to the model). Social learning and education are other subsets in the system.

The Clinician-Related Subset

This subset consists mainly of elements related to the clinician's personal qualities, which are offshoots of evolutionary, genetic, and constitutional factors (prenatal elements); events during childbirth (perinatal elements) that can contribute to later physical, mental, and social development; and such factors as the early rearing environment, quality of attachment experiences with the primary caregiver, and family environment (postnatal elements) which play significant roles in personality development. These elements, described in Chaps. 3 and 4, are considered to be the bedrock on which a person's capacity for empathy is built.

The Nonclinician-Related Subset

According to Kurt Lewin (1936), manifestations of behavior are a function of personal qualities, environmental demands, and situational factors. In a paradigm of physicians' performance, Gonnella, Hojat, Erdmann, and Veloski (1993b) proposed that in addition to clinician's knowledge, clinical-procedural skills, and personal qualities, other factors that are not related to the clinician and often are not under the clinician's control contribute to patient outcomes. Hence, the term "nonclinician-related subset." The elements of this subset have often been ignored in evaluations of outcomes of health profession education, appraisal of clinicians' performance, and the assessments of patient outcomes. These elements include the availability of (a) human resources, such as technical and professional assistance, and teamwork; (b) technical resources, such as diagnostic and treatment facilities, surgical equipments, and availability of laboratory tests; (c) environmental facilitators, such as physical facilities and facilitating rules and regulations formulated by health care institutions, health insurance agencies, and governmental authorities; and (d) patient factors, such as personality, cultural values, attitudes, and lifestyle; willingness to seek timely help; the severity of the disease, and adherence to preventive guidelines and treatment regimens.

The Social Learning and Educational Subsets

The social learning subset consists mainly of elements related to cultural and social norms and values (e.g., ascribed social roles and modes of social behavior) and expectations (e.g., belief in a supernatural power, in the health care system, in health care providers, and in optimistic or pessimistic expectation of outcomes).

The education subset consists of an array of elements related to formal education and training experiences, such as professional education (e.g., undergraduate, graduate, and continuing education), personal educational experiences (e.g., influence of role models, observations, and clinical experiences, factors in the so called "hidden curriculum," Hafferty, 1998), and professional ethics of conduct (e.g., ethical guidelines of professional organizations, such as the American Medical Association and the American Psychological Association). Targeted educational programs and educational experiences designed to enhance the capacity for empathy (see Chap. 12) also are among the elements of this subset.

The Clinical Encounter

Armed or disarmed with the elements of the aforementioned subsets, a clinician encounters a patient who is in a state of disequilibrium and is reaching out to someone for help. The system of empathic engagement begins to form. The intrapersonal and interpersonal dynamics described in Chap. 8 are triggered into operation during exchanges between the clinician and the patient. To form a functional system, the clinician should be armed with the skills needed to understand the patient's concerns and be motivated (an intrapersonal factor) to communicate this understanding to the patient (an interpersonal factor) with a genuine intention to help. As depicted in Fig. 14.1, all elements of clinician-related, nonclinician-related, social learning, and education subsets come together in clinical encounters that can lead to either empathic or nonempathic clinician–patient engagements that, in turn, ultimately determine patient outcomes that will be positive in a functional system or negative in a dysfunctional system.

Outcomes

The interaction between intrapersonal and interpersonal dynamics described in Chap. 8 brings about cognitive processes that can lead to an orientation or a behavior. When the orientation or behavior is empathic, the likelihood of a positive patient outcome will increase. In this case, the system will achieve its purpose, and we can conclude that the system is functional. However, if the intrapersonal and interpersonal dynamics resting on the clinician-related, nonclinician-related, social learning, and formal educational subsets lead to a nonempathic orientation or behavior, the likelihood of a positive patient outcome will be drastically reduced. In this case, the system will fail to achieve its purpose, and we can conclude that the system is dysfunctional.

However, I must emphasize that because other unpredicted elements may intervene, the pathway to empathic engagement between clinician and patient is more complicated than the model depicted in Fig. 14.1. Nonetheless, I hope that the systemic view of empathy just described can serve as a heuristic paradigm illustrating the major components that set the system in motion and show the complexity of empathy in the context of patient care.

An Agenda for Future Research

Training humane clinicians has long been a concern of education in the health professions. Because of general societal changes that are taking place, particularly in the industrialized world, there is directly or indirectly a weakening occurring of the power of important social support systems (see Chap. 2). Also, due to the changes that are evolving in the health care system and leading toward detached care (see Chap. 12), research on factors that contribute to the understanding and enhancement of empathy in patient care is now more important and timely than ever before.

Research on empathy in patient care deserves serious attention, not only because of its importance in training humane clinicians, but also because of its implications for the selection and education of clinicians. Empirical research on empathy in patient care is still in its infancy; therefore, much more research is needed to enhance our understanding of empathy in patient care. The questions addressed below present only a few of the areas that need to be included in the future research on empathy in patient care.

What Additional Constructs Are Involved in Empathy?

According to the findings determined by our factor analytic studies (Hojat, Gonnella, Nasca, Mangione et al., 2002; Hojat & LaNoue, 2014) and others (see Appendix A), empathy in patient care is a multidimensional concept involving at least three factors: "perspective taking," "compassionate care," and "standing in the patient's shoes." Similar factors that emerged in a factor-analytic study in which the JSE was administered to dental students (Sherman & Cramer, 2005), and in another study with a large sample of medical students in Mexico (Alcorta-Garza, Gonzalez-Guerrero, Tavitas-Herrera, Rodrigues-Lara, & Hojat, 2005) as well as studies by others in the USA and abroad (see Appendix A) have added to our confidence concerning the stability of the factors underlying empathy in different groups of health professionals and in different countries. However, we need more evidence to support the factor structure of empathy in groups of students and practitioners in the various health professions (e.g., nursing, dietetics, psychology, and social work).

It is important to bear in mind that the factors extracted in factor analytic studies obviously are a function of the contents and number of the items that are included in the measuring instruments. Therefore, the three underlying factors of empathy identified by the JSE reflect the contents and intercorrelations of the 20 items included in the instrument. Adding a sufficient number of items to address other factors, such as for example sociability, trust, and ethics could result in a scale with a different underlying factor structure. More important, whether the current factor structure of the JSE saturates the scale to the point where additional factors cannot account for more than a negligible amount of the variance or whether additional factors would contribute significantly to the scale's incremental validity (i.e., increase its criterion-related and predictive validity) needs to be addressed in future research.

What Additional Variables Are Associated with Empathy?

As described in Chap. 9, research has shown that empathy is linked to a number of demographic and psychosocial variables, indicators of clinical competence, and career interests. Evidence also suggests that empathic engagement in patient care is associated with physicians' diagnostic accuracy and patients' adherence to treatment, increased satisfaction with their health care providers, a reduced tendency to file malpractice claims, and more importantly to patient outcomes (Chap. 11). Also, as was described in Chaps. 4 and 8 and depicted in Fig. 14.1, family environment, early attachment relationships, human and material resources, and environmental, social, and cultural factors contribute to the development and manifestation of empathy in patient care situations.

It is important to study empirically and, ideally in prospective longitudinal research designs, the relative contribution of early experiences, the quality of early and late attachment relationships, and social, cultural, educational, and other factors that can significantly predict empathy scores. This line of research would have important implications for the development of programs to retain and enhance the capacity for empathy.

Empathy also was found to predict ratings of clinical competence among medical students and physicians (Chap. 9). However, further research is needed to address other indicators of academic and professional performance that are significantly associated with empathy scores and patient outcomes. It is desirable to use prospective studies to examine the relationship between empathy scores and different measures of academic and professional success or failure (e.g., academic dropout and dismissal, cheating and unethical behavior, disciplinary action against health care providers) at different levels of health professions education.

Furthermore, the findings on gender differences in empathy scores (Chap. 10) call for more empirical research to discern whether the differences are more likely to be related to "intrinsic" gender characteristics or to "extrinsic" sex-role socialization and their interactions. Such research is needed because determining the proportion of the variance in empathy scores that is accounted for by intrinsic or extrinsic factors in the analyses of gender differences is an important issue. The answer would potentially have different implications in relation to the selection and education of health professionals.

Further investigations also are needed on the unique contribution of empathy to accurate diagnoses, improved compliance, better patient satisfaction, reduced malpractice claims (Chap. 11), and other tangible clinical outcomes regarding control of chronic diseases, such as essential hypertension, diabetes mellitus, and treatment of other chronic and acute illnesses. These outcomes are important to be studied, not only because of their impact on mortality and morbidity, but also because of the economic impact on the patients, their families, and society at large. The extent of the short- and long-term impact of empathy enhancement programs for health professions students and practitioners, and empathic engagement in clinical encounters needs to be empirically investigated.

It is also highly desirable, although complicated, to examine the relative contribution of the following factors to the capacity for empathy, as reflected in empathy scores: genetic factors; quality of early attachment relationships; early life experiences (e.g., parental divorce, death in the family, maternal employment, day care experiences); later personal life experiences (e.g., traumatic events, peer relationships, marital relationships, role models); environmental and social factors (e.g., sociopolitical conditions, cultural norms, ascribed roles); cultural and cross-cultural factors, particularly among immigrants; formal education; and the interactions among these and other factors. It is also interesting to explore if the so called "unethical" behavior during medical school (Papadakis et al., 2005) is significantly associated with a lower level of capacity for empathy.

Gonnella and colleagues (Gonnella & Hojat, 2001; Gonnella, Hojat, Erdmann, & Veloski, 1993a, 1993b; Hojat, Erdmann, & Gonnella, 2014) proposed that to achieve optimal patient outcomes, a physician must perform three roles: clinician, educator, and resource manager. Thus, determining the extent to which each of these roles is associated more with capacity for empathy is also important. Furthermore, it would be desirable to investigate the relative contribution of different factors of empathy (e.g., perspective taking, compassionate care, and standing in the patient's shoes) to each of the three roles of a physician as well as to academic and professional success.

Should Empathy Be Considered for Admissions Purposes?

Almost all North American medical schools place great emphasis on applicants' undergraduate grade-point averages and scores on the Medical College Admission Test (MCAT) for screening purposes. Although grade-point averages and MCAT scores are relatively good predictors of a student's academic performance in the early years of medical school (sometimes described as the pre-clinical or pre-clerkship phase of medical school education), they have poor predictive validity regarding a student's performance in the later years of medical school (sometimes described as the clinical phase of medical school education) (Glaser, Hojat, Veloski, Blacklow, & Goepp, 2004; Hojat et al., 2014; Hojat, Erdmann, et al., 2000; Hojat, Veloski, & Zeleznik, 1985). The poor long-term predictive validity of the MCAT is not surprising because the test was developed to predict success in the preclinical component of medical education when attrition is most likely in the US medical schools. In addition, because of the "restriction of the range" issue as a result of attrition in the first two years, the predictive validity coefficients cannot capture the true relationships with indicators of clinical competence in later years of medical school.

It is obvious that the most qualified candidates who wish to embark on a journey to become physicians are those who in addition to medical knowledge and procedural skills possess personal qualities that can generate trust, which ultimately leads to optimal clinical outcomes. However, there is a lingering doubt among medical education leaders about the role of personal qualities in academic success and clinical outcomes. In an article entitled "Building a better physician" Kaplan, Satterfield, and Kington (2012), suggested that just as understanding of biology and chemistry needs some basic background which is often assessed in admission tests to medical schools, we also need to assess candidates' understanding of social and behavioral sciences in applicants and also improve such understanding as part of professional development of physicians-in-training. It is interesting to notice that the Association of American Medical Colleges (AAMC) which sponsors the MCAT, has only recently recognized the importance of the role of psychosocial factors in health and illness. Thus, the AAMC included a new section to the MCAT (starting in 2015) to assess applicants' understanding of psychosocial factors in health and illness.

In addition to understanding psychosocial factors in health and illness, it is important to assess the possession of psychosocial qualities which are pertinent to patient care (Hojat et al., 2014). Research shows that the contribution of such qualities, including empathy, to performance assessments is greater in the clinical than preclinical phase of medical education (for a review see Hojat et al., 2014, also see Chap. 7). Some may argue that personal qualities can be easily assessed from admission interviews, letters of recommendation, essays, and personal statements. However, there is inadequate evidence in support of the validity of such conventional approaches, Some of their shortcomings are described below.

Admissions Interview

Face-to-face interviews are required as part of the admission process in almost all medical schools and residency programs in the USA and Canada. A great majority of these interviews are unstructured with no uniform questions and no standard assessment procedures. It is believed that interviews provide an opportunity to include the human touch in decision-making and that they help in assessing personal qualities (Albanese, Snow, Skochelak, Huggett, & Farrell, 2003). It is claimed that the admissions interviews provide important information in selecting potential students (Eddins-Folensbee, Harris, Miller-Wasik, & Thompson, 2012; Puryear & Lewis, 1981). However, convincing empirical evidence is not yet available to confirm the validity and reliability of admission interviews (Ferguson, James, & Madeley, 2002; Kanter, 2012). Compounding this issue is the fact that medical students themselves, without any training, sometimes perform interviews with new applicants in order to supplement the staff and faculty resources needed for interviewing a large number of applicants. Interestingly, no significant difference has been observed between faculty and students interview ratings (Eddins-Folensbee et al., 2012; Elam & Johnson, 1992; Gelmann & Stewart, 1975).

Although the purpose of interviewing candidates for residency programs is to assess their humanistic qualities, attitudes, motivation, and other personal qualities, guidelines for assessing such qualities are often vague or nonexistent. Interviews are often not structured to assess those human qualities, or the interviewers are not specifically trained to detect them (Hojat et al., 2014). Information on humanistic qualities of candidates is often available from evaluations of students' behavior in clinical clerkships. Letters of evaluation that medical school deans write for graduates not only should summarize the students' academic attainment but also should include assessments of graduates' humanistic qualities when dealing with patients.

Reliance on interviews conducted by untrained staff or students can jeopardize the validity of the selection process by giving advantage to those applicants who play a better role in presenting themselves well in interview settings. The unstructured interviews by untrained interviewers with no standard scoring guidelines may predict nothing other than an applicant's skills in role playing (Musson, 2009). No wonder that the predictive validity of admission interviews has been reported to be disappointingly low (Walton, 1987). It is interesting to note that despite all of the aforementioned limitations, in a national survey with residency program directors in the USA, an applicant's interview was considered as the most important selection criterion (Wagoner, Suriano, & Stoner, 1986). The use of interviews in the undergraduate and graduate selection processes provides a unique opportunity to talk with applicants and may be helpful in observing a candidate's reaction to questions, but uncertainties remain open regarding the validity and practical outcomes of admission interviews (Antonovsky, Anson, & Bernstein, 1979; Green, Peters, & Webster, 1991; Hobfolls & Benor, 1981).

More information about applicants' interpersonal skills and capacity for empathy can be probed during admissions interviews once interviewers are trained todetectassess these qualities. The issue of whether undergraduate elective courses or majors could predict capacity for empathy also needs to be empirically addressed. In addition, the issue of whether training those who interview medical school applicants can lead to the selection of more empathic students needs to be studied.

Letters of Recommendation

Most medical schools in North America require letters of recommendation to be submitted by those who are fairly familiar with the academic performance and personal qualities of the applicants. Letters of evaluation written by medical school deans also play a great role in the selection of candidates for residency. There is no convincing empirical evidence in support of the predictive validity of letters of recommendation in medical schools. In our own empirical study using a multivariate statistical model, we found that the level of recommendation contained in the letters written by undergraduate premedical education advisors did not contribute significantly to the prediction of academic performance in medical school beyond the grades obtained prior to medical school (Zeleznik, Hojat, & Veloski, 1983). Furthermore, it has been reported that letters of recommendation may be biased and flattering with no substantial empirical link to later performance (Walton, 1987). Although one purpose of letters of recommendation is to describe personal qualities of the applicant, our research confirmed that too often these letters fail to add anything about applicant's personality beyond a summary of the student's academic performance (Hojat et al., 2014; Zeleznik et al., 1983). Those who prepare recommendation letters should be advised to include information about applicant's interpersonal skills in the letter.

Personal Statements, Letters of Intent, and Essay

Some medical schools require applicants to write an essay, letter of intent, or some personal statements about, for example, their interest in medicine, career goals, and future plans. There are very few studies on the predictive value of essays or personal statements. In one study, the content of candidates' personal statements was analyzed, and no evidence was found to support its predictive validity (cited in Ferguson et al., 2002). Typically, letters of intent or essays submitted by applicants are evaluated by untrained readers and are assessed on informal criteria (Musson, 2009). Even more questionable is whether candidates themselves, without any help, write the statements, essays, and letters of intent (Musson, 2009). Because of the aforementioned shortcomings, Haque and Waytz (2012) suggest that one appropriate approach for the assessment of personality of physicians-in-training is to administer psychometrically sound instruments for assessing personal qualities pertinent to patient care, including empathy.

Kupfer, Drew, Curtis, and Rubinstein (1978) reported that considering personal qualities, including empathy, when deciding which applicants should be admitted to medical school would lead to excellence in the practice of medicine. Streit-Forest (1982) recommended that once a significant relationship has been established between personal qualities and indicators of academic and professional success, the personal qualities of applicants to medical school should be included among the criteria for admission. In longitudinal studies of medical students, my colleagues and we have shown that measures of personal qualities (e.g., sociability, satisfactory interpersonal relationships, and self-esteem) and measures of academic aptitude (e.g., grade-point averages, and MCAT scores) can equally predict performance measures in the first two years of medical school. However, the measures of personal qualities could predict ratings of clinical performance in the third year of medical school more accurately than grade-point averages or MCAT scores (Hojat et al., 1993; Hojat, Glaser, & Veloski, 1996; Hojat, Vogel, Zeleznik, & Borenstein, 1988). In other words, incremental validity can be improved significantly by including indicators of interpersonal skills and measures of personal qualities in multiple regression models (Hojat et al., 1988, 1993; Zeleznik et al., 1988).

Our research on empathy (using the JSE) has shown that empathy scores are significantly associated with ratings of clinical competence in medical school (Hojat, Gonnella, Mangione, et al., 2002) and with tangible clinical outcomes in the practice of medicine (Del Canale et al., 2012; Hojat, Louis, Markham, et al., 2011). To my knowledge, no empirical study on grade point averages prior to medical school or the MCAT is available to show that science attainment could predict patient outcomes and clinical competence. There is, however, one study in which we showed that the assessments of MCAT's writing samples could significantly predict a student's clinical competence in medical school (Hojat, Erdmann, et al., 2000).

Stern, Frohna, and Gruppen (2005) reported that none of the data on academic performance that are often used for admissions to medical schools could predict medical students' professional behavior. However, in that study, medical students' unprofessional behavior observed by faculty, clerkship directors, and fellow students could be predicted by students' failure to complete required course evaluations and to report immunization compliance. In another study by Papadakis et al. (2005) it was found that disciplinary action taken against physicians by state medical boards was strongly associated with unprofessional behavior recorded in medical school. These findings support the notion that indicators of personal qualities can predict professional behavior beyond measures of academic attainment. Essential humanistic qualities, such as empathy, elude the measures of undergraduate academic achievement that are commonly used when selecting applicants for admission to medical schools.

Undergraduate academic institutions do not routinely provide information about medical school applicants' interpersonal skills or other personal qualities relevant to the capacity for empathy. However, an examination of undergraduate elective courses or baccalaureate majors can provide clues about applicants' interests in humanities and literature which are associated with the capacity for empathy (Chap. 12).

Graduate medical education programs often consider indicators of academic attainment in medical school and scores on medical licensing examinations, such as Step 1 (and Step 2) of the United States Medical Licensing Examinations (formerly the National Board of Medical Examiners), as important determinants in the selection of residents. A residency candidate's personal qualities are often either overlooked or ignored completely.

Jamison and Johnson (1975) suggested that the public would be better served if volunteers for public services were selected on the basis of their capacity for empathy. Because medicine is a public service profession and the professional behavior of physicians includes compassionate care and empathy, should empathy be a criterion for selection of medical students and residents, or even for employment of physicians? This question deserves serious research attention. If further research provides convincing empirical evidence that incorporating empathy into the criteria for selecting applicants to medical schools and residency programs can lead to the advancement of professionalism in medicine, we should set aside our hesitation and include important pertinent personal qualities, such as empathy, when selecting our future health care work force. One positive result could be that health care professionals might regain the respect that has been fading away along with the changes taking place in society in general and in the health care system in particular. Meanwhile, we also need to study the long-term consequences of using empathy as a criterion for selecting applicants to medical schools and residency programs.

Does Empathy Predict Career Choice?

Findings on differences in empathy among physicians in various specialties (Chap. 9) call for further research. The question of whether health professionals choose specific specialties because of differences in their capacity for empathy prior to their professional education or because of effects of their professional education, needs further investigation. The answer to the question will have implications for selection of students and trainees, career counseling, and curriculum development in academic health centers. If empathy predicts career choice and interest in particular specialties, any attempt to select empathic candidates or to enhance empathy could potentially influence the distribution of physicians and other health professionals in the different specialties.

How Can Empathy Be Enhanced and Sustained During Professional Education?

The finding that in the absence of dedicated educational programs, empathy among medical students and residents tends to decline as they progress through medical education (Bellini et al., 2002, 2005; Hojat et al., 2009, 2004, also see Appendix A) raises serious concerns. Consequently, prospective research is needed to investigate whether empathy scores erode *systematically* or *randomly* during the course of medical education. It also is important to determine what factors would contribute to the systematic decline of, or variation in empathy in different individuals at different levels of health profession education. In addition, it is important to determine which factors may be detrimental and which factors may be beneficial to all individuals. If the detrimental and beneficial factors do not affect all individuals equally, determining what individual characteristics or experiences account for the variation would be an important research goal.

Finally, more research is needed to identify the most appropriate methods or the best combinations of approaches for enhancing empathy among students and practitioners (e.g., development of interpersonal skills, exposure to hospitalization experiences, role playing, exposure to role models, specifically targeted video or audio materials, workshops on perspective taking, theatrical approaches, study of literature and the arts, and improvement of narrative skills, etc.; see Chap. 12). Furthermore, both formative and summative evaluations are needed to confirm that programs developed to enhance empathy have achieved their stated goals and that both the short- and long-term effects of such programs have been carefully evaluated.

The unfortunate erosion of empathy reported among the health professionals in-training, and in-practice, raised an alarming red flag that must not be ignored in future research. What are the underlying reasons for this transformation of turning some of the enthusiastic students into cold-hearted practitioners? Is it related to the "Lucifer effect" that Zimbardo (2007) coined (see Chap. 8) in which good-hearted people turn bad as a result of environmental conditions, role expectations, arrogance, sense of belonging to a privileged group, etc.? Added to the seriousness of the erosion of empathy issue is the findings of a meta-analytic study involving 72 samples of American college students including 13,737 participants, reporting that American college students' empathy had declined between 1979 and 2009 on Perspective Taking and Empathic Concern scales of the IRI (Konrath, O'Brien, & Hsing, 2011). The decline was most pronounced after year 2000. Empirical research is needed to explore reasons for these changes. Why is our young generation regressing rather than progressing in their capacity for empathy?

Should We Maximize Empathy and Regulate Sympathy in Patient Care?

Because of their different consequences in patient care, throughout this book, I tried to make a distinction between cognitive empathy (or clinical empathy in the context of patient care) and emotional empathy (or sympathy in the layman's term). Some may argue that the findings on the decline in empathy during health professions education and the practice of patient care could be a result of psychological defense mechanisms to adjust to the emotional drain which is involved in taking care of seriously ill patients. Well, this argument may be true to harden hearts against emotional (not cognitive) empathy. However, I would use a different term: "emotional regulation" (rather than "decline") for such an adjustment in emotional empathy(sympathy). Research indicates that those who are able to regulate their emotions are more likely to form empathic engagement and also act in a heightened moral fashion (Decety & Lamm, 2006; Eisenberg et al., 1994).

In an fMRI study, physicians who practice acupuncture were compared to others while observing animated visual stimuli showing needles being inserted into mouth region, hands and feet of patients (Cheng et al., 2007). Experts in acupuncture knew that such procedure could be painful to their patient, and had learned in their training to regulate their emotions in order not to be distressed and overwhelmed with emotional exhaustion. Thus, as expected, in these acupuncture experts, brain regions involved in emotional aspect of pain processing (e.g., anterior insula and anterior cingulated cortex) did not show increased activation. Instead brain regions associated with emotional regulation and cognitive control (e.g., the medial and dorsolateral prefrontal cortices) showed activation in the expert physicians (Cheng et al., 2007). The control participants, compared to expert physicians showed significantly higher pain intensity, activation of the pain matrix and unpleasant ratings when watching body parts being pricked by needles as opposed to being touched by a Q-tip. Investigators also observed an enhanced self–other distinction in the expert physicians by activation of the right temporoparietal junction, which is known to play a role in self–other differentiation, metacognition, and the theory on mind (Cheng et al., 2007). These findings support the notion that professional training experiences can improve emotional regulation which helps to prevent burnout and emotional exhaustion.

A decline in cognitive empathy (or clinical empathy) is never justifiable and can never be beneficial to either clinician or patient. Thus, the agenda for future research should include studying approaches not only to enhance (or maximize) and sustain cognitive empathy, but also regulate (or optimize) emotions (or emotional empathy) in health professions education and patient care.

Should We Respond to a Need for Norm Data and Cutoff Scores?

As the developers of the JSE, we have been frequently asked by potential national and international users about the availability of norm data and cutoff scores for identifying high and low scorers. For the development of national norm tables and determining cutoff scores, large and representative samples from the target populations are needed. By using a large sample of entering medical students ($n=2637$) who entered Sidney Kimmel (formerly Jefferson) Medical College at Thomas Jefferson University, we developed proxy norm tables and tentative cutoff scores for men and women matriculants separately (Hojat & Gonnella, 2015, also see Chap. 7). Obviously, data from one medical school cannot serve that purpose, instead large scale longitudinal studies are needed with national representative samples of medical and other health professions students, physicians and other practicing health professionals to develop national and international norm tables and cutoff scores by gender, specialties, and country to identify low and high JSE scorers for the purpose of assessments of professional development, admission, and employment.

Do Patients' Perspectives and Peers' Evaluations Contribute to Empathic Outcomes?

Optimal and suboptimal clinician–patient relationships cannot be studied if we fail to understand patients' expectations and perspectives regarding the empathy of their health care providers. In Chap. 11, I pointed out that a large majority of medical malpractice claims filed is the result of patients' negative views of the relationship with their health care providers. Thus, it is important to study clinical outcomes with respect not only to clinicians' self-reported empathy but also to patients' perceptions of their caregivers' empathy and to peers' evaluations of clinicians' empathy.

Furthermore, it is important to examine health care providers' specific behaviors, such as punctuality, sense of humor, nonverbal behavior, and verbal expressions that patients regard as significant determinants of an empathic engagement. The patients' perspectives are particularly important because one key concept in the definition of empathy was clinicians' ability to communicate their understanding to their patients (Chap. 6). Thus, future research should focus on the relationship among three sets of variables: (a) clinicians' self-reported empathy, (b) patients' expectations and perceptions of clinicians' empathy, and (c) peers' evaluations of clinicians' empathy. To enhance our understanding of factors that determine final outcomes of rendering care, the relative contribution of these variables to patient outcomes must be investigated.

What Are the Neurological Underpinnings of Cognitive and Emotional Empathy?

A better understanding of the neurobiological underpinnings of empathy will lead to improving empathy and preventing human abuse and neglect. Brain imaging experiments to find the roots of empathy are just flourishing which will soon shed light on the issues of enhancing and sustaining empathy, and on prevention and treatment of empathy deficit disorders. The discovery of mirror neurons that are activated in the brain when a person sees another person performing a goal-directed act or hears another person who is in distress (Carr, Iacoboni, Dubeau, Mazziotta, & Lenzi, 2003; Kohler et al., 2002) opens a new window for the examination of the neural mechanisms of empathy in human relationships (Chap. 13). With the technical advancements in functional brain imaging, it is now possible to observe and record the neurophysiological indicators of empathy. This exciting new discovery should prove to be extremely valuable in future research designed to identify the structural (neuroanatomical) and functional (neurophysiological) aspects of empathy in the human brain.

In addition, based on the studies cited in Chap. 13, both the limbic system and neocortex areas of the brain have often been implicated in neuroanatomical studies of empathy. However, future research must make a distinction between clinical empathy (described in this book as cognitive empathy) and emotional empathy (or sympathy) and examine whether different areas of the brain are activated by empathic or sympathetic responses. As I suggested in Chap. 13, intuitively one can speculate that the neocortex is more likely to be implicated in cognitive empathy and the limbic system is more likely to be implicated in emotional empathy (sympathy), but this speculation needs further empirical verification.

Recapitulation

We embarked on a journey into the terrain of empathy with the hope of exploring the roads leading to empathy (antecedents) and the paths spreading from empathy (outcomes). Like the wings that evolved to allow birds to fly high in search of food or the long necks that evolved to allow giraffes to feed on leaves high on trees that other species could not reach, empathy, we learned, has evolutionary roots that sprouted for the purpose of survival.

Similarly, we learned that empathy—like hearing, vision, taste, and smell— has neurological and biophysiological underpinnings. Empathy, like human love, connects people more closely, reduces interpersonal space, and fulfills the human need for affiliation, support, and understanding. In the context of patient care, empathy is no longer a vague concept because an operational definition offered in this book has clarified its meaning, and it is no longer an abstract entity because it can be quantified with a valid and reliable instrument described in this book.

Empathy can increase altruistic, prosocial, and helping behaviors; reduce aggressive behavior; encourage avoidance of conflict; improve conflict management; and promote understanding (Larson & Yao, 2005). Medicine, which was considered by the public as one of the most highly respected professions of all, is losing ground (Thomas, 1985) partly because of the failure of medical education to train empathic doctors and partly due to the failure of some doctors to preserve their altruistic image (Schlesinger, 2002). At the turn of twentieth century, George Bernard Shaw equated the image of the medical profession to the faith in God by declaring that "We have not lost faith, but we have transferred if from God to the medical profession." This is no longer the case, given the current image of physicians held by public.

In the past few decades, profound changes in medical education and the health care systems, an imbalance in teaching the science and the art of medicine, unduly financial considerations to contain cost, increasing commercialization of medical care, health insurance policies formulated by nonmedical administrators, the emergence of "defensive" medicine, and loss of the human presence in caring for the patients by its replacement with computerized diagnostic and therapeutic technology have transformed the image of physicians from compassionate healers to technicians and interpreters of medical tests, and eroded the public's trust in medicine (Schlesinger, 2002). Perhaps medicine can regain some of its well-deserved reputation, and physicians can reclaim their altruistic image by greater attention to the role of empathy in the selection, education, practice, and professional development of physicians (Hojat et al., 2014).

In the context of patient care, empathy can eliminate the constraints of the clinician–patient relationship. It can bridge the gap between givers and receivers of help and contribute to the physical, mental, and social well-being of both patient and clinician. Like height, weight, eye color, and type of hair, empathy varies among humans. However, a sense of unity can emerge from variation among human beings once empathic understanding prevails, once one can view the world from the other person's perspective, once one can stand in another person's shoes.

The following saying has been attributed to Albert Einstein: "A person starts to live when he (sic) can live outside himself." Empathic engagement takes a person outside of himself or herself and allows the person to hear others with the third ear and to view the world of others with the mind's eye. Empathic engagement brings unity from diversity, making all of us akin regardless of gender, age, race, culture, religion, or other divisive factors. So, that is why any attempt toward empathic understanding of a fellow human being is a step toward enhancing physical, mental, and social well-being of all in society. Thus, the lesson to be learned is that actual implementation of remedies for enhancement of empathy—not just declaration of their desirability—is a mandate that must be acted upon, not only by teachers and healers of human infirmity, but by all members of the human race for the sake of healing human ills unto eternity.

Appendix A: Annotated Bibliography on the Jefferson Scale of Empathy

> *Science begins in the nothingness of ignorance,*
> *and moves toward truth*
> *by gathering more and more information,*
> *constructing theories as facts accumulate.*
>
> —(Steven Jay Gould, 1981, p. 321)

Since the first publication on psychometrics of the JSE in 2001, there has been an increasing number of empirical, conceptual, and review research published in the USA and abroad in which the JSE was used, reviewed or reported. The following annotated bibliographical list of such studies includes 197 entries, 43 of which are from our own research team at Thomas Jefferson University, the other 154 are from researchers and colleagues from other academic centers either in the USA or abroad. These studies are grouped into the following categories: psychometrics of the JSE (36 entries), correlates of the JSE (40 entries), group comparisons on the JSE scores (22 entries), score changes as students progress through health profession education (24 entries), changes in the JSE scores as a result of an intervention to enhance empathy in health professionals-in-training and in-practice (35 entries), tangible clinical outcomes of physician empathy (2 entries), or a combination of some of the aforementioned categories and other miscellaneous findings (32 entries). There are also a number of doctoral dissertations or theses which were made available to me by their investigators in which the JSE was used as a major instrument (6 entries).

I selected the studies that were written in English (or at least were accompanied by an English abstract) and were accessible to me (either were sent by the study's author or were accessible from journals' websites or publishers without hefty charges!). In each bibliographic entry for empirical studies, I included crucial information such as research participants, major instrument(s) used, intervention if any, and a brief highlight of major findings. These studies of course vary with respect to their quality, some can be ranked as excellent and some may be marginal regarding their quality. However, I tried not to be judgmental with regard to the quality in the selection of the articles. Selection based on quality would be a difficult task, particularly when there are no agreed upon inclusion criteria to judge the merit of the studies. This bibliography not only provides a summary of most of the publications on

© Springer International Publishing Switzerland 2016
M. Hojat, *Empathy in Health Professions Education and Patient Care*,
DOI 10.1007/978-3-319-27625-0

the JSE as of publication date of this book, but also can serve as a source for meta-analytic research on empathy with an important advantage that a uniquely validated instrument was used in all of these studies which is one desirable feature of any meta-analytic research.

Studies on Psychometrics of the JSE

Alcorta-Garza, A., Gonzalez-Guerrero, J. F., Tavitas-Herrera, S. E., Rodrigues-Lara, F. J., & Hojat, M. (2005). Validación de la escala de empatia medica de Jefferson en estudiantes de medicina Mexicanos [Validity of the Jefferson Scale of Physician Empathy among Mexican Medical Students]. *Salud Mental [Mental Health], 28*, 57–63.

> Participants included 1022 first-, third-, and fifth-year medical students (494 women) at the School of Medicine, Autonomous University of Nuevo Leon in Monterrey, Mexico who completed a Spanish translation of the JSE. Results showed that the JSE mean score for the entire simple was 110.4 ($SD = 14.1$). Women obtained a significantly higher JSE mean score ($M = 111.9$, $SD = 13.9$) than men ($M = 109.1$, $SD = 14.1$). Cronbach's alpha coefficient for this sample was 0.74. No significant correlation was observed between scores of the JSE and respondents' ages. Exploratory factor analysis resulted in the same three factors emerged in most studies in the US samples, namely "Perspective Taking," "Compassionate Care," and "Standing in Patient's Shoes."

Di Lillo, M., Cicchetti, A., Lo Scalzo, A., Taroni, F., & Hojat, M. (2009). The Jefferson Scale of Physician Empathy: Preliminary psychometrics and group comparisons in Italian physicians. *Academic Medicine, 84*, 1198–1202.

> Participants included 289 Italian physicians (60 women) from three hospitals in Rome, Italy who completed an Italian translation of the JSE. Results showed that the corrected item-total score correlations of the JSE were all positive and statistically significant, ranging from 0.34 to 0.69. The JSE mean score for the total sample was 115.1 ($SD = 15.5$), and the Cronbach's alpha coefficient was 0.85. Exploratory factor analysis resulted in six factors including Perspective-Taking, Compassionate Care, and Standing in Patient Shoes, plus residual factors. Women obtained a higher JSE mean score ($M = 117.5$, $SD = 14.6$) than did men ($M = 114.5$, $SD = 15.6$), but the difference was not statistically significant. Physicians practicing surgical specialties scored lower ($M = 114.2$, $SD = 15.5$) than their counterparts in medical specialties ($M = 117.5$, $SD = 15.0$). The difference, however, did not reach an accepted level of statistical significance.

Fields, S. K., Mahan, P., Hojat, M., Harris, J., Tillman, P., & Maxwell, K. (2011). Measuring empathy in healthcare profession students using the Jefferson Scale of Physician Empathy: Health Provider-Student Version. *Journal of Interprofessional Care, 25*, 287–293. doi:10.3109/13561820.2011.566648.

> Participants included 265 undergraduate nursing students (233 women) at the College of Health Professions, Armstrong Atlantic State University in Savannah, Georgia, USA who completed the JSE (HPS-Version). Results showed that corrected item-total score correlations were all positive and statistically significant (with the exception of one item), ranging from 0.09 to 0.62, with a median of 0.42. Overall, the JSE mean score for this sample was 111.5 ($SD = 12.2$). Cronbach's alpha coefficient as 0.78, and test–retest reliability with a 3-month interval between testing was 0.58, and it was 0.69 with a 6-month interval. Women scored significantly higher

than men ($M=112.5$, $SD=11.0$ and $M=104.1$, $SD=17.1$, for women and men, respectively). Older students obtained a higher JSE mean score, and no statistically significant associations were found between JSE scores and ethnicity, religiosity, or previous non-nursing degree.

Fjortoft, N., Van Winkle, L. J., & Hojat, M. (2011). Measuring empathy in pharmacy students. *American Journal of Pharmaceutical Education, 75*(6), Article 109. doi:10.5688/ajpe756109.

Participants included 187 first-year pharmacy students at Midwestern University, Chicago College of Pharmacy who completed the JSE-HPS version. Results showed a mean score of 110.7 ($SD=12.1$), and Cronbach's alpha coefficient$=0.84$. Women obtained a significantly higher JSE mean score ($M=112.8$, $SD=11.3$) than did men ($M=106.3$, $SD=13.1$). Corrected item-total score correlations ranged from 0.09 to 0.69, with a median of 0.55. In exploratory factor analysis, based on the scree test, two factors were retained: "perspective-taking" and "compassionate care." It is concluded that psychometric support of the JSE-HPS in pharmacy students can bolster researchers' confidence in using a validated instrument for empathy research in pharmacy education.

Gonnella, J. S., Mangione, S., Magee, M., Nasca, T. J., & Hojat, M. (2005). Empathy scores in medical school and ratings of empathic behavior in residency training 3 years later. *The Journal of Social Psychology, 145*, 663–672.

Participants included 106 physician residents who graduated from Jefferson (currently Sidney Kimmel) Medical College (45 women) who had completed the JSE in the third year of medical school, and their empathy was rated by their program directors 3 years later at the completion of the first-year of residency training. Results showed that the JSE mean score for this sample was 117.8 ($SD=10.9$). A statistically significant association was found between students' self-reported empathy in the third year of medical school (JSE scores) and ratings of their empathy given by the directors of residency training programs approximately 3 years later.

Gonullu, P., & Oztuna, D. (2012). A Turkish adaptation of the student version of the Jefferson Scale of Physician Empathy. *Marmara Medical Journal, 25*, 87–92. doi:10.5472/MMJ.2012.02272.1. Accessible from: http://www.mmj.dergisi.org/pdf/pdf_MMJ_634.pdf.

A Turkish translation of the JSE was administered to 752 (378 women) first- to fifth-year medical students at Ankara University School of Medicine in Turkey. Confirmatory factor analysis confirmed the three-factor model found in most studies with the USA and abroad. Item on "physicians should not allow themselves to be influenced by strong personal bonds between their patients and their family members" did not fit into the model, which was attributed to the possibility of inaccurate translation. Cronbach's alpha coefficients were 0.83, 0.70, and 0.60 for the three factors of Perspective Taking, Compassionate Care, and Standing in Patient's Shoes, respectively. Women scored higher than men on the Perspective Taking factor, but men outscored women on the two other factors.

Hojat, M., Gonnella, J. S., Nasca, T. J., Mangione, S., Veloski, J. J., & Magee, M. (2002). The Jefferson Scale of Physician Empathy: Further psychometric data and differences by gender and specialty at item level. *Academic Medicine* (Suppl.), *77*, s58–s60.

Participants included 704 physicians (26 % women) who completed the JSE. Results of statistical analyses at item level showed that the item mean scores ranged from 4.8 to 6.5 (on a 7-point Likert scale). Although respondents actually used the full range of possible responses (1–7) on all items, respond distributions for each item was skewed toward upper end of the scale.

Corrected item-total score correlations were all positive and statistically significant, ranging from 0.30 to 0.60, with a median of 0.40. Statistically significant differences were observed on six out of the 20 items of the JSE in favor of women; however, effect size estimates of gender differences were modest. Also, statistically significant differences were observed on 11 of the 20 items of the JSE between physicians in "people-oriented" specialties (e.g., family medicine, internal medicine, pediatrics, psychiatry, obstetrics and gynecology, emergency medicine, $n=462$) and "technology-oriented" specialties (e.g., anesthesiology, radiology, pathology, surgery and surgical specialties, $n=242$) in favor of physicians in "people-oriented" specialties (effect size estimates ranged from 0.17 to 0.41).

Hojat, M. Gonnella, J. S., Nasca, T. J., Mangione, S., Vergare, M., & Magee, M. (2002). Physician empathy: Definition, components, measurement, and relationship to gender and specialty. *American Journal of Psychiatry, 159,* 1563–1569.

Participants included 704 physicians (179 women) in the Jefferson Health System affiliated with Thomas Jefferson University Hospital who completed the JSE (HP-Version). Results showed an overall JSE mean score of 120 ($SD=12, M=121$, score range$=50$–140), Cronbach's alpha coefficient of 0.81, and rest-retest reliability of 0.65 (within three to 4 months interval between testing, $n=71$ physicians). Women scored slightly higher than men (for women: $M=120.9, SD=12.2$; for men: $M=119.1, SD=11.8$), but the difference did not reach the level of statistical significance. Psychiatrists obtained the highest JSE mean score ($M=127.0, SD=5.5$), followed by physicians in internal medicine ($M=121.7, SD=10.6$); pediatrics ($M=121.5, SD=12.2$); emergency medicine ($M=121.0, SD=10.7$); and family medicine ($M=120.5, SD=12.6$). The lowest JSE mean scores were obtained by physicians in anesthesiology ($M=116.1, SD=12.0$); orthopedic surgery ($M=116.5, SD=12.9$); neurosurgery ($M=117.3, SD=9.5$); and radiology ($M=117.9, SD=13.1$). Controlling for physicians' gender, psychiatrists obtained a JSE mean score that was significantly higher than those obtained by physicians in anesthesiology, orthopedic surgery, neurosurgery, radiology, cardiovascular surgery, obstetrics and gynecology, and general surgery. Exploratory factor analysis of data resulted in three factors of Perspective Taking, Compassionate Care, and Standing in the Patient's Shoes.

Hojat, M., & LaNoue, M. (2014). Exploration and confirmation of the latent variable structure of the Jefferson Scale of Empathy. *International Journal of Medical Education, 5,* 73–81. doi:10.5116/ijme.533f.0c41.

Participants included 2612 students (1322 women) who entered Jefferson Medical College between 2002 and 2012 and completed the JSE at the entry to medical school. They were divided into two groups: Matriculants between 2002–2007 ($n=1380$) and between 2008 and 2012 ($n=1232$). Data for 2002–2007 matriculants were subjected to exploratory factor analysis (principal component factor extraction with oblique rotation), and data for matriculants of 2008–2012 were used for confirmatory factor analysis (structural equation modeling and root mean square error for approximation). The exploratory factor analysis resulted in three factors of "perspective-taking," "compassionate care," and "walking in patient's shoes" replicating the three-factor model reported in most of the previous studies. The confirmatory factor analysis showed that the three-factor model was an acceptable fit that confirmed the latent variable structure which emerged in the exploratory factor analysis. Corrected item-total scores correlations for the total sample were all positive and statistically significant, ranging from 0.13 to 0.61 with a median of 0.44. Cronbach's alpha coefficient for the total sample was 0.80, ranging from 0.75 to 0.84 for matriculants of different years.

Hojat, M., Mangione, S., Nasca, T. J., Cohen, M J. M., Gonnella, J. S., Erdmann, J. B., Veloski, J. J., & Magee, M. (2001). The Jefferson Scale of Physician Empathy: Development and preliminary psychometric data. *Educational and Psychological Measurement, 61,* 349–365.

This is the first publication on psychometrics of the original version of the Jefferson Scale of Physician Empathy (JSPE). Participants included three groups: 55 physicians, 41 residents, and 193 medical students. Based on an extensive review of the relevant literature, a preliminary version of the JSPE (90 items) was developed, and sent to 100 physicians in 1999 to examine face and content validities (55 responded). Based on feedback received, 45 items were retained after modifications for clarity suggested by the respondents. The modified version plus three scales of the IRI (Perspective Taking, Empathic Concern, and Fantasy), two scales of the NEO PI-R (Warmth and Dutifulness), Faith-in-People (misanthropy) scale, and self-rated personality attributes (sympathy, compassion, etc.) were completed by 41 residents and 183 medical students. Based on the results of factor analysis on item responses from the medical student sample, 20 items with the highest factor coefficients (>0.40) on the grand factor were retained. Mean score of the 20-item JSPE were 118 for both medical student and resident samples ($SD = 11$ and $SD = 12$, respectively). Women scored significantly higher than men. Scores of the 20-item JSPE correlated significantly with scores on perspective taking, empathic concern, and fantasy of the IRI, and with measures of compassion, sympathy, trust, tolerance, personal growth in resident and medical student samples; with scores on the NEO PI-R scales of warmth, and dutifulness, and with scores on the Faith-in-People scale in medical students. These findings provided evidence in support of convergent and discriminant validities of the JSPE. Cronbach's alpha coefficient was 0.87 for residents, and 0.89 for medical students.

Hsiao, C. Y., Tsai, Y. F., & Kao, Y. C. (2012). Psychometric properties of a Chinese version of the Jefferson Scale of Empathy –Health Profession Students. *Journal of Psychiatric and Mental Health Nursing, 20*, 866–873. doi:10.1111/jpm.12024. Accessible from: http://onlinelibrary.wiley.com/doi/10.1111/jpm.12024/pdf.

Participants included 613 Taiwanese undergraduate (second year and fourth year) nursing students (546 women) who completed JSE-HPS version. Content validity was confirmed by 11 experts with an agreement index of 89 %. Corrected item-total score correlations ranged from 0.52 to 0.72 (all positive and statistically significant). The JSE mean score for men was 104.22 ($SD = 16.07$) and 108.57 ($SD = 14.30$) for women which were significantly different. Fourth-year students ($M = 109.22, SD = 13.77$) obtained significantly higher JSE mean score than second-year students ($M = 105.57, SD = 15.91$). Cronbach's alpha coefficient was 0.93 for the entire sample, and test–retest reliability was 0.92. Exploratory factor analysis resulted in three factors: Perspective Taking (Cronbach's alpha coefficient = 0.90), Compassionate Care (Cronbach's alpha coefficient = 0.87), and Standing in Patient's Shoes (Cronbach's alpha coefficient = 0.77).

Jumroonrojana, K., & Zartrungpak, S. (2012). Development of the Jefferson Scale of Physician Empathy-student version (Thai version). *Journal of the Psychiatric Association of Thailand, 57*, 213–224.

Participants included 708 medical students in all 6 years of their medical education at the Faculty of Medicine, Ramathibodi Hospital, and Mahidol University in Thailand who completed a Thai translation of the JSE. Results showed that all item-total score correlations were positive and statistically significant ranging from 0.26 to 0.57. Factor analysis of data resulted in three factors of Compassionate Care, Perspective Taking, and Standing in Patient's Shoes, similar to those emerged in most other factor analytic studies, although in different order. Cronbach's alpha coefficient was 0.79. The JSE mean score for this sample of Thai medical students was 111.31 ($SD = 10.41$). Women outscored men, and the JSE mean score declined significantly as students progressed from pre-clinical to the clinical phase of medical education in this cross-sectional study.

Kataoka, H., Koide, N., Ochi, K., Hojat, M., & Gonnella, J. S. (2009). Measurement of empathy among Japanese medical students: Psychometrics and score differences by gender and level of medical education. *Academic Medicine, 84*, 1192–1197.

Participants included 400 Japanese medical students (103 women) from all 6 years at the Okayama University Medical School in Japan who completed a Japanese translation of the JSE. Results showed that the corrected item-total score correlations were all positive and statistically significant ranging from 0.16 to 0.55 with a median of 0.42. Mean score for the total sample was 104.3 ($SD = 13.1$). Women obtained a significantly higher mean score than men. Cronbach's alpha coefficient was 0.74. The JSE mean score increased from 98.5 in the first year to 107.8 in the last year of medical school in this cross-sections study. Exploratory factor analysis showed five factors: "perspective taking," "compassionate care," "empathic understanding," and two additional factors of "difficulties in taking patient's perspective," and "standing in patient's shoes."

Kliszcz, J., Nowicka-Sauer, K., Trzeciak, B., Nowak, P., & Sadowska, A. (2006). Empathy in health care providers–validation study of the Polish version of the Jefferson Scale of Empathy. *Advances in Medical Sciences, 51*, 219–225. Accessible from: http://www.advms.pl/ms_2006/Kliszcz_J_et%20al_Empathy%20in%20health% 20care%20providers.pdf.

Participants included 405 (324 women) health professional students and practitioners: 118 physicians (95 women), 76 nurses (all women), 149 medical students (91 women), 33 midwifery students (all women), 29 nursing students (all women) who completed the Polish translation of the JSE (S- and HP-versions), the Interpersonal Reactivity Index (IRI), and an Emotional Intelligence Scale. Results showed that the mean scores of the JSE were 112.40 ($SD = 11.40$) and 111.30 ($SD = 16.01$) for students and practicing health professionals, respectively; Cronbach's alpha coefficients were 0.72 and 0.79, respectively. No statistically significant gender difference was observed on the JSE, nor was there a significant difference among the five study samples. In the total sample, statistically significant correlations, although low in magnitude, were found between scores of the JSE and those of the Empathic Concern scale of the IRI ($r = 0.25$); and the Perspective Taking scale of the IRI ($r = 0.26$). However, no statistically significant correlation was found between the JSE scores, and Personal Distress and Fantasy scales of the IRI. Significant correlation was also observed between scores of the JSE and those of the emotional intelligence scale ($r = 0.30$) in the total sample.

Koženým, J., Tišanská, L., & Hoschl, C. (2013). Assessing empathy among Czech medical students: A cross-sectional study. *Československá Psychologie, 57*, 246–254.

Participants included 725 medical students (457 women) at Charles University in Prague, and 871 students (624 women) at Dentistry Palacky University Olomouc in Czechoslovakia who completed a Czechoslovakian translation of the JSE. Results showed that all corrected item-total score correlations were positive and statistically significant, ranging from 0.05 to 0.51. The JSE mean score for the total sample ($n = 1596$) was 99.5 ($SD = 13.08$). No gender difference was observed on the JSE scores. The JSE mean score in this cross-sectional study declined significantly from 106.42 ($SD = 10.42$) in the first year to 98.20 ($SD = 14.22$) in the sixth year of training. Exploratory factor analysis of the JSE resulted in three factors of Perspective-Taking, Compassionate Care, and Empathic Understanding. Cronbach's alpha coefficient for the total sample was 0.76.

Leombruni, P., Di Lillo, M., Miniotti, M., Picardi, A., Alessandri, G., Sica, C., Zizzi, F., Castelli, L., & Torta, R. (2014). Measurement properties and confirmatory factor analysis of the Jefferson Scale of Empathy in Italian medical students. *Perspectives on Medical Education*. Published online: 08 Aug 2014. doi:10.1007/ s40037-014-0137-9.

Participants included 257 medical students (114 men, 143 women) at the University of Turin Medical School who completed an Italian translation of the JSE-S version. Results showed that the JSE mean score for the entire sample was 108.7 ($SD = 10.60$). Women scored significantly higher than men ($M = 110.21$, $SD = 11.47$ for women, $M = 106.83$, $SD = 9.10$ for men) on the total scores of the JSE; however, when compared on the JSE factor scores, women scored significantly higher than men only on the Compassionate Care factor, but not on the Perspective Taking, or Standing in Patient's Shoes factors. Cronbach's alpha coefficient was 0.76 for the entire sample (0.73 for men, and 0.79 for women). Test–retest reliability (2-weeks interval) was 0.72. Confirmatory factor analysis provided support for the three-factor model.

Li, L., Wang, J., Hu, X., & Xu, C. (2015). Empathy in Chinese pharmacy undergraduates: Implication for integrated humanities into professional pharmacy education. *Indian Journal of Pharmaceutical Education and Research, 49*, 31–39. doi: 10.5530/ijper.49.1.5.

Participants included 263 Chinese pharmacy students at Wuhan University of Science and Technology who completed the JSE (HPS-version). Results showed a mean score of 112.58 ($SD = 11.64$), and Cronbach's alpha coefficient of 0.81. No significant gender difference was observed. Exploratory factor analysis resulted in three factors of "perspective taking," "compassionate care," and "standing in patient shoes" which emerged in most of other factor analytic studies of the JSE. The JSE mean score for fourth year students in this cross-sectional study was significant higher ($M = 117.59$) than those for the previous years of pharmacy education. Social activities and humanistic education were the most frequently models suggested by pharmacy students for promoting empathy.

Magalhäes, E., Salgueira A. P., Costa, P., & Costa M. J. (2011). Empathy in senior year and first year medical students: A cross-sectional study. *BMC Medical Education, 11*, 52. doi:10.1186/1472-6920-11-52. Accessible from: http://www.biomedcentral.com/1472-6920/11/52.

Participants included 476 medical students (321 women) at School of Health Sciences, University of Minho in Portugal who completed the Portuguese translation of the JSE-S version. The construct validity of the JSE was cross-validated by using exploratory and confirmatory factor analysis. Exploratory factor analysis resulted in three factors in the Portuguese original model: "compassionate care," "perspective-taking," and "standing in patients' shoes." Empathy scores of students in the final year of medical school were higher than those at the beginning of medical school. Female students scored significantly higher ($M = 112.86$, $SD = 10.81$) than male students ($M = 110.32$, $SD = 10.69$). No significant difference was observed on the JSE scores among those with different specialty preferences. Cronbach's alpha coefficient was 0.77 for this sample.

McMillan, L. R., & Shannon, D. M. (2011). Psychometric analysis of the JSPE nursing student version R: Comparison of senior BSN students and medical students attitudes toward empathy in patient care. *International Scholarly Research Network Nursing*, Article ID 726063. doi:10.5402/2011/726063. Accessible from: http://dx.doi.org/10.5402/2011/726063.

Participants included 598 senior nursing students (88 % women) at University of Auburn School who completed the JSE. Results showed a JSE mean score of 114.57 ($SD = 10.94$) and a Cronbach's alpha coefficient of 0.77 for the entire sample. Exploratory factor analysis initially resulted in five factors; however, two of them marginally met the Kaiser's criterion. Thus three factors were retained which were very similar to those emerged from most other studies with US medical students. Confirmatory factor analysis provided marginal support for the three-factor model.

Mostafa, A., Hoque, R., Mosrafa, M., Rana M., & Mostafa, F. (2014). Empathy in undergraduate medical students of Bangladesh: Psychometric analysis and differences by gender, academic year, and specialty preference. *International Scholarly Research Notices Psychiatry*, Article ID 375439. Accessible from: http://dx.doi.org/10.1155/2014/375439.

Participants included 348 first- through fifth-year medical students (291 women) at Chattagram Maa-O-Shishu Hospital Medical College who completed a Bengali translation of the JSE. Exploratory factor analysis resulted in three factors of "perspective taking," "compassionate care," and "standing in patent's shoes." Corrected item-total score correlations ranged from 0.33 to 0.66, all were statistically significant. Cronbach's alpha coefficient was 0.88. Women obtained higher JSE scores ($M=111.99$, $SD=12.97$) than men ($M=106.72$, $SD=14.33$). No significant association was found between scores of the JSE and specialty interests. In this cross-sectional study, JSE scores increased significantly as students progressed through medical school during the clinical years of medical education.

Paro, H. B. M. S., Daud-Gallotti, R. M., Pinto, I. C., Tiberio, L. F. L. C., & Martins, M. A. (2012). Brazilian version of the Jefferson Scale of Empathy: Psychometric properties and factor analysis. *BMD Medical Education, 12*, 73. doi:10.1186/1472-6920-12-73. Accessible from: http://www.biomedcentral.com/1472-6920/12/73.

Participants included 319 students in their fifth and sixth medical school years at the Sao Paulo University School of Medicine in Brazil who completed a Brazilian translation of the JSE. Results showed that the JSE mean score was 114.95 ($SD=12.41$). Women obtained a higher mean score ($M=116.54$, $SD=12.81$) than did men ($M=113.84$, $SD=12.68$), although the difference was not statistically significant. Cronbach's alpha coefficient was 0.84. Three factors of "compassionate care," "standing in patient's shoes," and "perspective taking" emerged in that order in an exploratory factor analysis (Cronbach's alpha coefficients for these three factors were 0.83, 0.73, and 0.74, respectively).

Preusche, I., & Wagner-Menghin, M. (2013). Rising to the challenge: Cross-cultural adaptation and psychometric evaluation of the adapted German version of the Jefferson Scale of Physician Empathy for students (JSPE-S). *Advances in Health Science Education: Theory and Practice, 18*, 573–587. doi:10.1007/s10459-012-9393-9.

Participants included 516 second-year medical students at the Medical University of Vienna in Austria who completed a German translation of the JSE. Results showed that the JSE mean score was 110.52 ($SD=12.49$). Item-total score correlations were all positive (ranged from 0.13 to 0.68). Cronbach's alpha coefficient was 0.82, and test–retest reliability for 96 students in 6–7 weeks interval was 0.45. An exploratory factor analysis resulted in four factors: "perspective taking," "compassionate care," "standing in patient's shoes," and a residual factor.

Rahimi-Madiseh, M., Tavakol, M., Dennick, R., & Nasiri, J. (2010). Empathy in Iranian medical students: A preliminary psychometric analysis and differences by gender and year of medical school. *Medical Teacher, 32*, e471–e478 (web paper).

Participants included 181 medical students (127 women) at Shahrekord University Medical Science in Iran who completed the JSE (S-Version). Results showed that the JSE mean scores for the sample was 105.1 ($SD=12.9$). Cronbach's alpha coefficient was 0.74. Exploratory factor analysis resulted in three factors: Compassionate Care, Perspective Taking, and Walking in Patient's Shoes, similar to those found in US medical students although in a different order. Women scored higher than men ($M=105.6$ and $M=103.7$, respectively) but the difference was not statistically significant. No significant change in empathy scores was observed in five medical school years in this cross-sectional study.

Roh, M. S., Hahm, B. J., Lee, D. H., & Suh, D. H. (2010). Evaluation of empathy among Korean medical students: A cross-sectional study using Korean version of the Jefferson Scale of Physician Empathy. *Teaching and Learning in Medicine: An International Journal, 22,* 167–171. doi:10.1080/10401334.2010.488191. Accessible from: http://dx.doi.org/10.1080/10401334.2010.488191.

> Participants included 493 medical students (159 women) at Seoul National University College of Medicine in Korea who completed the JSE. Item-total score correlations were all positive and statistically significant, ranging from 0.28 to 0.68 with a median of 0.42. Cronbach's alpha coefficient was 0.84. Cross-sectional comparisons of students in different years of medical school showed that fourth-year students obtained a significantly higher JSE mean score than other students. Exploratory factor analysis of the JSE resulted in the three factors: "perspective taking," "compassionate care," and "standing in patient's shoes" which emerged in the US samples, and in some other international studies. No significant difference was observed between men and women on the JSE mean scores.

Shariat, S. V., Eshtad, E., & Ansari, S. (2010). Empathy and its correlates in Iranian physicians: A preliminary psychometric study of the Jefferson Scale of Physician Empathy. *Medical Teacher, 32,* e417–e421 (web paper). doi:10.3109/01421 59X.2010.498488.

> Participants included 207 general practitioners in Iran who completed the JSE. Results showed that Cronbach's alpha coefficient was 0.78. Exploratory factor analysis resulted in three factors: "perspective taking," "compassionate care," and "standing in patient's shoes." Women scored higher than men, but place of practice and practice setting did not show significant association with scores of the JSE. Regression analysis indicated that practice experiences could significantly predict JSE scores beyond the effect of physicians' ages. Comparisons of mean scores of each item of the JSE in Iran, Japan, the USA showed a similar pattern of findings, with items 2 and 19 showing the highest and items 3 and 18 the lowest mean scores in all three countries. The rank order correlations of the item mean scores were 0.90 (between Iran and the USA), 0.88 (between Japan and the USA), and 0.69 (between Iran and Japan).

Shariat, S. V., & Habibi, M. (2013). Empathy in Iranian medical students: Measurement model of the Jefferson Scale of Empathy. *Medical Teacher, 35,* e913–e918. doi:10.3109/0142159x.2012.714881.

> Participants included 1187 medical students (759 women) from 17 Iranian medical schools who completed the JSE. Results showed that the mean score for the total sample was 101.4 ($SD = 14.5$). Female students scored significantly higher than men ($M = 102.75$, $SD = 13.94$ and $M = 98.94$, $SD = 15.23$, respectively). Cronbach's alpha coefficient was 0.79, and test–retest reliability was 0.95 (2 weeks interval between testing, $n = 31$). A decline in empathy scores was observed as students progressed through medical school in this cross-sectional study. Students in larger medical schools obtained higher JSE mean scores than others in smaller universities. Confirmatory factor analysis provided a satisfactory fitness for the three-factor model (Perspective Taking, Compassionate Care, and Standing in the Patient's Shoes).

Sherman, J. J., & Cramer, A. (2005). Measurement of changes in empathy during dental school. *Journal of Dental Education, 69,* 338–345.

> Participants included 130 dental students (45 women) at the University of Washington School of Dentistry who completed the JSE. Results showed the mean score for total sample was 117.7 ($SD = 14.06$). Women scored ($M = 122.29$, $SD = 12.76$) significantly higher than did men ($M = 115.28$, $SD = 14.17$). No significant association was observed between scores of the JSE and students' race, age, or marital status. Scores of the JSE declined after the first year and remained low throughout fourth year of dental school. Cronbach's alpha coefficient was 0.90,

and the split-half reliability coefficient was 0.87. Scores of the JSE were significantly correlated with 18 out of 26 clinical competency ratings. The largest correlation was obtained between JSE scores and ratings on applying the principles of behavioral sciences that pertain to patient-centered oral health care, and the lowest correlation was obtained with ratings on utilizing business and management skills to conduct an efficient and effective clinical practice. Exploratory factor analysis resulted in four factors of Perspective Taking, Patient's Experiences and Feelings, and Ignoring Emotions in Patient Care.

Stansfield, R.B., Schwartz, A., O'Brien, C.L., Dekhtar, M., Dunham, L., Quirk, M. (2016). Development of a metacognitive effort construct of empathy during clinical training: A longitudinal study of the factor structure of the Jefferson Scale of Empathy. *Advances in Heath Science Education, 21,* 5–17. doi:10.1007/s10459-015-9605-1.

Participants included 4,797 students from 28 medical schools in the United Sates who complete the JSE. They were divided into two groups. One group included students in the preclinical years, and the other included those in clinical years of medical school. Within each group, students were randomly assigned for exploratory factor analysis (EFA), and confirmatory factor analysis (CFA) of the JSE. Despite an unexplained departure from standard scoring of the JSE, results of EFA in preclinical years were almost identical to most factor analytic findings of the JSE reported by others. However, four factors emerged in the clinical years of medical school. The first three factors were similar to those emerged in preclinical years of medical school, but were renamed to avoid confusion with the original model (according to the authors), and the fourth factor called Metacognition. Confirmatory factor analytic results indicated that the 3-factor model was an acceptable fit for the preclinical years, and the 4-factor model was a better fit than the other models for the clinical years of medical school.

Ster, M. P., Ster, B. Petek, D., & Gorup, E. C. (2014). Validation of Slovenian version of Jefferson Scale of Empathy for students. *Slovenian Journal of Public Health, 53,* 89–100. doi:10.2478/sjph-2014-0010.

Participants included 234 first-year medical students (69 % or 162 women) in Slovenia (Ljubljana Medical School) who completed the Slovenian translation of the JSE. Results showed the JSE mean score for this sample was 107.7 (*SD*=12.6), and Cronbach's alpha coefficient was=0.79. Test–retest reliability was 0.70 (*n*=80, 2-week interval between testing). Exploratory factor analysis resulted in factors of Perspective Taking, Compassionate Care, Standing in Patient's Shoes, Interpersonal Relationship, and a residual factor.

Suh, D. H., Hong, J. S., Lee, D. H., Gonnella, J. S., & Hojat. M. (2012). The Jefferson Scale of Physician Empathy: A preliminary psychometric study and group comparisons in Korean physicians. *Medical Teacher, 34,* e464–e468 (web paper). doi:10.3109/0142159x.2012.668632.

Participants included 229 physicians (103 women) in Seoul National University Hospital in Korea who completed a Korean translation on the JSE-HP version. Results showed that the JSE mean score was 98.2 (*SD*=12). Cronbach's alpha coefficient was 0.84. Women scored significantly higher than did men (*M*=100.3, *SD*=11.7 and *M*=96.5, *SD*=12.0, respectively). Exploratory factor analysis resulted in three factors of compassionate care, perspective taking, and a residual factor.

Tavakol, S., Dennick, R., & Tavakol, M. (2011). Psychometric properties and confirmatory factor analysis of the Jefferson Scale of Physician Empathy. *BMC Medical Education, 11,* 54. doi:10.1186/1472-6920-11-54. Accessible from: http://www.biomedcentral.com/1472-6920/11/54.

Participants included 853 medical students (470 women) at the University of Nottingham in England who completed the JSE. Cronbach's alpha coefficient was 0.76. Exploratory factor analysis resulted in three factors entitled "compassionate care," "perspective taking," and "emotional detachment." Confirmatory factor analysis showed that the three-factor model fit well across genders of medical students.

Vallabh, K. (2011). Psychometrics of the student version of the Jefferson Scale of Physician Empathy (JSPE-S) in final-year medical students in Johannesburg in 2008. *South African Journal of Bioethics and Law, 4,* 63–68. Accessible from: http://www.sajbl.org.za/index.php/sajbl/article/view/164/140.

Participants included 158 final year medical students (143 women) who completed the JSE-S at the Faculty of Health Sciences of the University of the Witwatersrand Medical School in South Africa. Results showed that the JSE mean score was 107 ($SD = 10.9$). Women ($M = 109$, $SD = 9.8$) scored higher than men ($M = 104$, $SD = 12$). Item-total score correlations were all positive and statistically significant. Cronbach's alpha coefficient was 0.79. Exploratory factor analysis resulted in three factors of Perspective Talking, Compassionate Care, and Standing in Patient's Shoes.

Veloski, J., & Hojat, M. (2006). Measuring specific elements of professionalism: Empathy, teamwork, and lifelong learning. In D. T. Stern (Ed.). *Measuring medical professionalism* (pp. 117–145). Oxford: Oxford University Press.

In this book chapter, professionalism in medicine is described as personal qualities beyond acquisition of medical knowledge and procedural skills that have relevance to optimal patient outcomes. It is suggested that professionalism is a multi-faceted concept, involving different elements. Three major elements of professionalism are recognized based on a review of relevant literature such as: Empathy in patient care, interprofessional collaboration/teamwork, and lifelong learning. Operational definitions, and measuring instruments for these three elements of professionalism in medicine were provided, and a brief summary of psychometrics support (validity and reliability) of these measuring instruments was reported. The JSE was described as a measure of choice for quantifying empathic orientation/engagement in patient care. The Jefferson Scale of Physician Lifelong Learning was described as the instrument of choice for measuring orientation/attitudes toward lifelong learning, and the Jefferson Scale of Attitudes toward Interprofessional Collaboration (e.g., physician-nurse) was described as a psychometrically sound instrument for measuring teamwork and interprofessional collaboration.

Ward, J., Schaal, M., Sullivan, J., Bowen, M. E., Erdmann, J. B., & Hojat, M. (2009). Reliability and validity of the Jefferson Scale of Empathy in undergraduate nursing students. *Journal of Nursing Measurement, 17,* 73–88. doi:10.1891/1061-3749.17.1.73.

Participants included 333 undergraduate nursing students (284 women) who completed a slightly modified version of the JSE for administration to nursing students. Exploratory factor analysis resulted in three factors "perspective taking," "compassionate care," and "standing in patient's shoes." The JSE mean score for the entire sample was 114.0 ($SD = 11.5$). Cronbach's alpha coefficients were 0.78, 0.83, and 0.72 for the three extracted factors, respectively. The alpha reliability coefficient for the entire sample was 0.77. Corrected item-total score correlations were all positive and statistically significant ranging from 0.20 to 0.64, with a median correlation of 0.44. Female students obtained a significantly higher JSE mean score than did men. No statistically significant associations were observed between JSE scores and ethnicity (white, black, Asian), academic backgrounds (humanities, sciences, business); or marital status. Students with more clinical experiences obtained the highest JSE mean score. A statistically significant correlation ($r = 0.38$, $p < 0.01$) was found between scores of the JSE and a validated measure of attitudes toward teamwork and interprofessional collaboration (Jefferson Scale of Attitudes Toward Physician-Nurse Collaboration).

Wen, D., Ma, X., Li, H., & Xian, B. (2013). Empathy in Chinese physicians: Preliminary psychometrics of the Jefferson Scale of Physician Empathy (JSE) [Letter to the editor]. *Medical Teacher, 35,* 609–610.

> Participants included 1200 Chinese physicians (521 women) who completed a Chinese translation of the JSE. Results showed a JSE mean score of 109.54 ($SD = 11.85$). Exploratory factor analysis resulted in three factors of Perspective Taking, Compassionate Care, and Ability to Stand in Patient's Shoes accounting for 66.2 % of the total variance. Cronbach's alpha coefficient was 0.80.

Williams, B., Brown, T., Boyle, M., & Dousek, S. (2013). Psychometric testing of the Jefferson Scale of Empathy Health Profession Students' version with Australian paramedic students. *Nursing and Health Sciences, 15,* 45–50. doi:10.1111/ j.1442-2018.2012.00719.x.

> Participants included 330 paramedic students (215 women) at Monash University in Australia who completed the JSE-HPS version. Cronbach's alpha coefficient for this sample was 0.75. Exploratory factor analysis resulted in two factors: "compassionate care," and "perspective taking." The two-factor model was appraised in a confirmatory factor analysis for 17 items of the JSE.

Studies on Correlates of the JSE Scores

Austin, E. J., Evans, P., Goldwater, R., & Potter, V. (2005). A preliminary study of emotional intelligence, empathy and exam performance in first year medical students. *Personality and Individual Differences, 39,* 1395–1405. doi:10.1016/j. paid.2005.04.014.

> Participants included 156 first-year medical students (103 women) who completed the JSE, an emotional intelligence (EI) scale, and a "talking with families" scale measuring skills in communicating with patients and their families. Statistically significant correlations that were moderate in magnitudes, were found between scores of the JSE, and EI scale ($r = 0.35$) and talking with families scale ($r = 0.39$). Women scored higher than men on the JSE, and Cronbach's alpha coefficient for the JSE in this sample was 0.85.

Beckman, T. J., Reed, D. A., Shanafelt, T. D., & West, C. P. (2010). Impact of resident well-being and empathy on assessments of faculty physicians. *Journal of General Internal Medicine, 25,* 52–56. doi:10.1007/s11606-009-1152-0.

> Participants included 149 residents at Mayo Clinic enrolled in the Mayo Internal Medicine Well-Being Study who completed the JSE, the Quality of Life (QOL) survey, a measure of depression, Maslach Burnout Inventory (MBI), and a clinical teaching assessment instrument. Results showed a mean score of the JSE of 115.46 ($SD = 12.27$) in this sample. It was found that residents' assessments of faculty teachers are not influenced by scores on well-being including quality of life, burnout, and depression scales. However, scores on the JSE were significantly associated with residents' assessments of faculty.

Berg, K., Blatt, B., Lopreiato, J., Jung, J., Schaeffer, A., Heil, D., Owens, T., Carter-Nolan, P. L., Berg, D., Veloski, J., Darby, E., & Hojat, M. (2015). Standardized patient assessment of medical students empathy: Ethnicity and gender effects in a multi-institutional study. *Academic Medicine, 90,* 105–111. doi:10.1097/ ACM000000000000052.

Participants included 577 students (287 women) from four medical schools in the USA who completed the JSE and two subscales of the IRI. The sample included 373 White students (65 %), 79 (14 %) Black/African American, and 125 (22 %) Asian/Pacific Islander. The students were assessed by 84 standardized patients (SPs) (45 women), 62 (74 %) were White and 22 (26 %) were Black/African American. SPs completed the Jefferson Scale of Patient Perceptions of Physician Empathy (JSPPPE) and Global Ratings of Empathy (GRE). There was a total of 2882 student-standardized patient encounters that were analyzed to examine the effects of ethnicity and gender which could introduce bias in standardized patients assessments of students, and to examine concordance between students' self-reported empathy, and standardized patients assessments of students' empathy. A significant correlation ($r=0.61$, $p<0.001$) was found between scores of the JSE and the IRI. Statistical analyses of patient encounters showed significant interaction effects of gender and ethnicity. Female students, regardless of ethnicity, obtained significantly higher mean score on the self-reported JSE than did men (mean scores for women and men were 114.9 and 109.3, respectively), on SPs' assessments of students' empathy (JSPPPE mean scores were 25.6 and 24.1, respectively), and on the GRE (mean scores 7.4 and 6.9, respectively). Male Black/African American students obtained the lowest SPs' assessments of empathy regardless of the SPs' ethnicity. Black/African American students obtained the highest mean scores on self-reported empathy. It is concluded that the significant interaction effects of ethnicity and gender in clinical encounters and the inconsistencies observed between SPs' assessments of students' empathy and students' self-reported empathy may raise concerns about possible ethnicity and gender biases in the SPs' assessments of students' clinical skills, and thus about the testing fairness in the SPs' assessments of students interpersonal skills.

Berg, K., Majdan, J. F., Berg, D., Veloski, J, & Hojat, M. (2011a). A comparison of medical students' self-reported empathy with simulated patients' assessment of the students' empathy. *Medical Teacher, 33*, 388–391. doi:10.3109/0142159x.2010. 530319.

Participants included 248 third-year students (123 women) at Jefferson (currently Sidney Kimmel) Medical College who completed the JSE-S version, who were assessed by standardized patients (SPs) on empathic engagement using the Jefferson Scale of Patient Perceptions of Physician Empathy (JSPPPE) and a global rating of empathy (GRE) in ten Objective Structured Clinical Examination (OSCE) stations. Correlation between students self-reported empathy (JSE) and SPs' assessments of student empathic engagement (JSPPPE) was statistically significant but low in magnitude ($r=0.19$) indicating that the two measures were not redundant. However, correlations between SPs' assessments of students' empathic engagement (JSPPPE), and their global ratings on students' empathy (GRE) was statistically significant and relatively large in magnitude ($r=0.87$). It was argued that SPs' assessments of well-defined clinical skills such as physical examination, history taking, and laboratory data in the artificial OSCE environment can be more reliable than their assessments of interpersonal and empathic attributes which require a reasonable time to form.

Berg, K., Majdan, J., Berg, D., Veloski, J., & Hojat, M. (2011b). Medical students' self-reported empathy and simulated patients' assessments of student empathy: An analysis by gender and ethnicity. *Academic Medicine, 86*, 984–988. doi:10.1097/ ACM.0b013e3182224f1f.

Participants included 248 third-year medical students (123 women) at Jefferson (currently Sidney Kimmel) Medical College. In Objective Structured Clinical Examinations (OSCE), standardized patients assessed students' empathy by completing the Jefferson Scale of Patient Perceptions of Physician Empathy (JSPPPE), and rated students on a two-item Global Ratings of Empathy (GRE). Results showed that women obtained a significantly higher JSE mean score $(M=110.4,\ SD=11.8)$ than men $(M=106.4,\ SD=13.3,$ effect size$=0.32$). No significant difference on the JSE scores was observed between White and Asian-American students. Consistent with their self-reported empathy (reflected in the JSE scores), women also received higher empathy assessments (reflected in the JSPPPE, effect size$=0.46$) and on global ratings of empathy (reflected in the GRE assessment, effect size$=0.63$) given by standardized patients. However, inconsistent with students' self-reported empathy (JSE scores), standardized patients' assessments on the JSPPPE and GRE were significantly lower for Asian American students, probably indicating an assessment bias against Asian American medical students (effect sizes were 0.56 and 0.43 for the JSPPPE and GRE, respectively).

Brazeau, C. M., Schroeder, R., Rovi, S., & Boyd, L. (2010). Relationship between medical student burnout, empathy, and professionalism climate. *Academic Medicine, 85*, s33–s36. doi:10.1097/ACM.0b013e3181ed4c47.

Participants included 127 fourth-year students at the UMDNJ-New Jersey Medical School who completed the JSE, Maslach Burnout Inventory (MBI), and the Professionalism Climate Instrument (PCI) which measures desirable professional behavior. The JSE mean score for the sample was 113.31 $(SD=13.35)$. Scores on the JSE were significantly $(p<0.01)$ and positively correlated with those from the Personal Accomplishment scale of the MBI $(r=0.44)$, and negatively with scores on Depersonalization scale $(r=-0.41)$ and Emotional Exhaustion scale $(r=-0.30)$ of the MBI. Also, correlation between JSE and PCI scores (desirable professional behavior in medical students) was statistically significant $(r=0.30)$.

Brockhouse, R., Msetfi, R. M., Cohen, K., & Joseph, S. (2011). Vicarious exposure to trauma and growth in therapists: The moderating effects of sense of coherence, organizational support, and empathy. *Journal of Traumatic Stress, 24*, 735–742. doi:10.1002/jts.20704.

Participants included 118 therapists (38 women) in England who completed the JSE, plus a short form of the Sense of Coherence Scale, Perceived Organizational Scale, and the Post Traumatic Growth Inventory. The JSE mean score for the sample was 121.20 $(SD=9.53)$. Results showed that the JSE scores positively predicted the therapists' psychological growth, organizational support did not predict growth, and a strong sense of cohesiveness negatively predicted growth.

Costa, P., Alves, R., Neto, I., Marvão, P., Portela, M., & Costa, M. J. (2014). Associations between medical student empathy and personality: A multi-institutional study. *PLoS One, 9*(3), e89254. doi:10.1371/journal.pone.0089254.

Participants included 472 students (312 women) from three medical schools in Portugal (University of Beira Interior, University of the Algarve, and University of Minho) who completed a Portuguese translation of the JSE (S-version) and the NEO-FFI (a personality inventory for measuring the big five personality factors). A subsample of 334 students was selected with the highest and the lowest JSE mean scores $(M=121.9$ and $M=97.8$, respectively) for statistical analyses. Correlations between the JSE scores and personality factors of Agreeableness $(r=0.31)$, Openness to Experience $(r=0.22)$, Conscientiousness $(r=0.19)$, and Extraversion $(r=0.18)$ were all statistically significant but moderate in magnitude.

Fuertes, J. N., Boylan, L. S., & Fontanella, J. A. (2008). Behavioral indices in medical care outcomes: The working alliance, adherence, and related factors. *Journal of General Internal Medicine, 24*, 80–85. doi:10.1007/s11606-008-0841-4.

Participants included 152 adult outpatients (71 women) from a neurology clinic at Bellevue Hospital in New York who completed a modified version of the JSE, the Physician-Patient Working Alliance Scale, Treatment Adherence Scale, and selected items from the Perceived Utility Scale and the Medical Outcome Study. Results showed significant bivariate correlations between scores of the modified JSE and working alliance ($r=0.73$), perceived utility treatment ($r=0.46$), treatment adherence ($r=0.40$), patient adherence ($r=0.28$), and patient satisfaction scores ($r=0.67$). However, in a multivariate statistical model only working alliance, physician multicultural competence, and treatment adherence could predict patient satisfaction; and physician multicultural competence and treatment adherence could predict patient adherence with treatment.

Glaser, K. M., Markham, F. W., Adler, H. M., McManus R. P., & Hojat, M. (2007). Relationships between scores on the Jefferson scale of physician empathy, patient perceptions of physician empathy, and humanistic approaches to patient care: A validity study. *Medical Science Monitor, 13*, 291–294.

Participants included 36 family medicine residents (23 women) at Thomas Jefferson University Hospital who completed the JSE and their 90 patients who assessed the residents by completing the Jefferson Scale of Patient Perceptions of Physician Empathy (JSPPPE), and a survey about the physicians' humanistic approach to patient care. The mean and standard deviation of the JSE for participating physicians were 118.0 and 9.2, respectively. The mean and standard deviation for the JSPPPE for participating patients were 30.0 and 2.8, respectively. Correlational analyses showed a statistically significant correlation between physician's self-reported JSE scores, and patients' assessments of physician empathy ($r=0.48$). Also, scores on the JSE were significantly and positively correlated with patient assessments of their physician's concern about their feelings ($r=0.55$), taking their wishes into account in making treatment decisions ($r=0.48$), and negatively correlated with patient's perception that their doctor was in hurry ($r=-0.50$).

Grosseman, S., Novack, D. H., Duke, P. Mennin, S., Rosenzweig, S., Davis, T. J., & Hojat, M. (2014). Residents' and standardized patients' perspectives on empathy: Issues of agreement. *Patient Education and Counseling, 96*, 22–28. Accessible from: http://dx.doi.org/10.1016/j.pec.2014.04.007.

Participants included 214 first-year residents in 13 internal medicine or family medicine residency programs who completed the JSE. Each resident was also assessed by five standardized patients who completed the Jefferson Scale of Patient Perceptions of Physician Empathy (JSPPPE). Participating residents also completed the JSPPPE from their own point of view. The JSE mean score was 111.8 ($SD = 11.14$) for the sample. Although women obtained a higher JSE mean score than did men, the difference was not statistically significance. Cronbach's alpha coefficients were 0.80 (for the JSE), 0.91 (for the JSPPPE completed by the standardized patients), and 0.94 (for the JSPPPE completed by residents). A significant correlation was found between scores of the JSE and residents' own view of their empathic engagement with standardized patients ($r=0.43$). However, the obtained correlation between residents' self-reported scores on the JSE, and standardized patients' perceptions of residents' empathy was negligible ($r=0.11$). The authors raised a question about the use of standardized patients in the assessment of residents' empathy and also about residents' ability to gauge the effectiveness of their empathic communications with patients.

Hasan, S., Al-Sharqawi, N., Dashti, F., AbdulAziz, M., Abdullah, A., Shukkur, M., Bouhaimed, M., & Thalib, L. (2013). Level of empathy among medical students in Kuwait University, Kuwait. *Medical Principles and Practice.* Open Access. doi:10.1159/000348300.

Participants were 264 medical students in the Faculty of Medicine at Kuwait University who completed the JSE. Results showed that the JSE mean score was 104.6 ($SD = 16.3$) for this sample. Women obtained a higher JSE mean score than men. Scores on the JSE were positively correlated with students' mother's level of education, higher household income, higher level of satisfaction with early relationship with the mother, and higher levels of perceived stress. Factors such as academic GPAs, specialty interest, marital status of parents, father's education level, and perceived relationships with their father did not significantly correlate with JSE scores. In this cross-sectional study, fourth-year medical students obtained the highest and second-year students the lowest JSE mean scores. However, the difference was not statistically significant. No significant association was found between JSE scores and the five personality factors measured by the ZKPQ; however, a trend toward a significant but negative association was noticed between scores of JSE and those of the Aggression-Hostility factor of the ZKPQ.

Hojat, M., Bianco, J. A., Mann, D., Massello, D., & Calabrese, L. H. (2015). Overlap between empathy, teamwork and integrative approach to patient care. *Medical Teacher, 37*, 755–785. doi:10.3109/0142159x.2014.971722.

Participants included 373 students (197 women) at Ohio University Heritage College of Osteopathic Medicine who completed the JSE-S, the Jefferson Scale of Attitudes Toward Physician-Nurse Collaboration (JSAPNC), and an 11-item survey on orientation toward integrative patient care (IPC) to test the hypothesis that empathy, teamwork and interprofessional collaboration, and an integrative approach to patient care share common denominators. Significant correlations were found among the three measures regardless of participants' gender. Also, a significant multivariate R of 0.60 was obtained in a multivariate regression model in which scores on the JSAPNC, IPC, and gender were predictors of the JSE scores. Although both JSAPNC and IPC contributed significantly to predicting JSE scores, the unique contribution of IPC scores (after partialing out the effect of gender) was substantially higher than that for the JSAPNC. Research hypothesis was confirmed, and it was suggested that implementation of an integrative patient care approach in medical education curriculum may enhance empathy and teamwork among physicians-in-training.

Hojat, M., Gonnella, J. S., Mangione, S., Nasca, T. J., Veloski, J. J., Erdmann, J. B., Callahan, C. A., & Magee, M. (2002). Empathy in medical students as related to academic performance, clinical competence and gender. *Medical Education, 36*, 522–527. doi:10.1046/j.1365-2923.2002.01234.x.

Participants included 371 third-year medical students (173 women) at Jefferson (now Sidney Kimmel) Medical College who completed the JSE. Women obtained a significantly higher JSE mean score ($M = 122$, $SD = 10$) than did men ($M = 119$, $SD = 11$). Statistically significant associations were observed between scores of the JSE and medical school faculty's global ratings of students' clinical competence in six third-year core clerkships (family medicine, internal medicine, obstetrics and gynecology, pediatrics, psychiatry, and surgery). No significant association was found between JSE scores and performance measures on objective examinations of acquisition of factual knowledge.

Hojat, M., Louis, D. Z., Maxwell, K., Markham, F., Wender, R., & Gonnella, J. S. (2010). Patient perceptions of physician empathy, satisfaction with physician, interpersonal trust, and compliance. *International Journal of Medical Education, 1*, 83–87. doi:10.5116/ijme.4d00.b701.

Participants included 535 out-patients (355 women) treated by family physicians in the Department of Family and Community Medicine, Jefferson (currently Sidney Kimmel) Medical College who completed the Jefferson Scale of Patient Perceptions of Physician Empathy (JSPPPE), and a 10-item scale of Patient Overall Satisfaction with Primary Care

Physician. These patients were selected based on the following three criteria: (1) age between 18 and 75 years; (2) had at least two office visits with their primary care physicians during the past 36 months; (3) spent at least two-thirds of the total office visits with the identified primary care physicians. Exploratory factor analysis of the JSPPPE resulted in one prominent component. Corrected item-total score correlations of the JSPPPE ranged from 0.88 to 0.94. Correlation between scores of the JSPPPE and scores on the patient satisfaction scale was 0.93. Scores of the JSPPPE were highly correlated with measures of physician-patient trust ($r = 0.73$). Higher scores of the JSPPPE were significantly associated with patients' compliance with physician's recommendations for preventive tests (colonoscopy, mammogram for female patients, and PSA for male patients) (compliance rates > 80 %). Cronbach's alpha coefficients for the JSPPPE ranged from 0.97 to 0.99 for the total sample, and for patients in different gender and age groups. Findings provide strong evidence in support of the psychometrics of the JSPPPE, and confirmed the link between patient perceptions of physician empathy, satisfaction with care, interpersonal trust, and compliance with physician's recommendations.

Hojat, M., Mangione, S., Kane, G. C., & Gonnella, J. S. (2005). Relationships between scores of the Jefferson Scale of Physician Empathy (JSPE) and the Interpersonal Reactivity Index (IRI). *Medical Teacher, 27*, 625–628. doi:10.1080/0142159050006974.

Participants included 93 first-year internal medicine residents at Thomas Jefferson University Hospital in Philadelphia who completed the JSE and the Interpersonal Reactivity Index (IRI, a measure of cognitive and affective empathy developed for administration to the general population). Results showed a statistically significant correlation between scores of the JSE and total score of the IRI ($r = 0.45$). Higher statistically significant correlations were observed between scores of the JSE and scores of those scales of the IRI that were relevant to patient care such as Empathic Concern ($r = 0.48$) and Perspective Taking ($r = 0.40$). However, correlation between scores of the JSE and those of the IRI's Personal Distress scale (which is a measure of affective or emotional empathy, or sympathy) was negligible ($r = 0.02$). Similarly, no significant correlation was observed between scores of the Personal Distress scale of the IRI and the JSE factor scores of Perspective Taking ($r = 0.01$), Compassionate Care ($r = 0.02$), and Standing in Patient's Shoes ($r = 0.13$). Findings provided support for the validity of the JSE as a measure of cognitive empathy as opposed to sympathy or so-called affective/emotional empathy.

Hojat, M., Michalec, B., Veloski, J., & Tykocinski, M. L. (2015). Can empathy, other personality attributes, and level of positive social influence in medical school identify potential leaders in medicine? *Academic Medicine, 90*, 505–510.

Participants included 666 fourth-year students (338 women) at Sidney Kimmel (formerly Jefferson) Medical College who completed the JSE, the Zuckerman-Kuhlman Personality Questionnaire (ZKPQ), Rosenberg Self-Esteem Scale, and the UCLA Loneliness Scale. They were also asked to identify their classmates (from a class list) who had a positive influence on their professional and personal development by using a peer nomination method. Students with the most number of nominations (top 25 %) were compared to their classmates with the least number of nominations (bottom 25 %) on personality measures. Results showed that top positive influencers obtained statistically significant higher mean scores on engaging personal qualities that were conducive to relationship building (such as JSE scores, Sociability, and Activity scales of the ZKPQ, and Self-Esteem scale). On the contrary, top positive influencers scored significantly lower on disengaging personal qualities that were detrimental to interpersonal relationships such as Neuroticism-Anxiety, Aggression-Hostility, Impulsive Sensation Seeking scales of the ZKPQ, and the UCLA Loneliness Scale.

Hojat, M., Spandorfer, J., Louis, D. Z., & Gonnella, J. S. (2011). Empathic and sympathetic orientations toward patient care: Conceptualization, measurement, and psychometrics. *Academic Medicine, 86,* 989–995. doi:10.1097/ACM. 0b013e31822203d8.

Participants included 201 third-year medical students at Jefferson (currently Sidney Kimmel) Medical College who completed the JSE, the IRI, and responded to four vignettes developed for this study involving a diabetic patient with complications, a rape victim, a patient who had undergone radical prostatectomy and developed complications, and a 16-year-old girl who was pregnant. Students reviewed the vignettes and logged their responses to each scenario on two given Likert scale. One pertained to empathic orientation quantifying the student's inclination toward "understanding" the patient's pain or suffering. The other scale pertained to sympathetic orientation quantifying the student's tendency to "feel" the patient's pain or suffering. A factor analytic study confirmed the construct validity of the empathic and sympathetic orientations. Cronbach's alpha coefficients were 0.79 and 0.84 for measures of empathic and sympathetic orientations, respectively. Scores on empathic orientation were significantly associated with scores of the JSE (a measure of cognitive empathy to understand patient's suffering), but not with scores of the IRI (presumably a measure of sympathy or affective empathy to feel patient's pain and suffering). In contrast, scores on sympathetic orientation were significantly associated with scores of the IRI (feeling a patient's pain and suffering), but not with scores of the JSE. Quantifying empathic and sympathetic orientations in patient care is important for understanding their different consequences in patient care.

Hojat, M., Vergare, M., Isenberg, G., Cohen, M., & Spandorfer, J. (2015). Underlying construct of empathy, optimism, and burnout in medical students. *International Journal of Medical Education, 6,* 12–16. doi:10.5116/ijme.54c3.60cd.

Participants included 265 third-year medical students (130 women) at Sidney Kimmel (formerly Jefferson) Medical College who completed the JSE, the Life Orientation Test-Revised (LOT-R), and the Maslach Burnout Inventory (MBI, which includes three scales of Emotional Exhaustion, Depersonalization, and Personal Accomplishment). Mean and standard deviation of the JSE for this sample were 119.9 and 11.2, respectively. The JSE scores were significantly and positively correlated with scores of the Personal Accomplishment scale of the MBI ($r=0.36$), but inversely correlated with scores of the Depersonalization scale of the MBI ($r=-0.25$). Factor analysis resulted in two factors: "positive personality attributes" that are conducive to relationship building (involving empathy, optimism, and personal accomplishment) and "negative personality attributes" that are detrimental to interpersonal relationships (involving emotional exhaustion, and depersonalization).

Hojat, M., Zuckerman, M., Gonnella, J. S., Mangione, S., Nasca, T., Vergare, M., & Magee, M. (2005). Empathy in medical students as related to specialty interest, personality, and perception of mother and father. *Personality and Individual Differences, 39,* 1205–1215. doi:10.1016/j.paid.2005.04.007.

Participants included 422 first-year medical students (207 women) enrolled at Jefferson Medical College in 2003 and 2004 who completed the JSE, the Zuckerman-Kuhlman Personality Questionnaire (ZKPQ), reported their satisfaction with early relationships with parents, and expressed their interest in a specialty they planned to pursue. Results showed that women obtained a statistically significant higher JSE mean score than men ($M=115.9, SD=8.9$ for women; $M=111.6, SD=10.4$ for men, effect size=0.43). Those who were highly satisfied with their childhood relationships with their mother obtained a significantly higher JSE mean scorer than others. No significant association was observed between reported satisfaction with childhood relationships with the father and JSE scores. The JSE mean score was significantly higher for students interested in pursuing primary care specialties such as general internal medicine, family medicine, general pediatrics ($M=116.6, SD=8.6$) than those who expressed an interest to pursue technology oriented specialties such as orthopedic surgery, neurosurgery, ophthalmology ($M=112.0, SD=10.3$), and hospital-based procedure-oriented specialties such as radiology, pathology, anesthesiology ($M = 108.4$, $SD = 10.1$). Scores on the JSE were significantly but moderately and positively correlated with measures of sociability ($r = 0.15$, $p < 0.01$), and negatively correlated with aggression-hostility scores ($r = -0.13$, $p < 0.01$). No significant correlation was found between JSE scores and personality measures such as neuroticism-anxiety, impulsive sensation seeking, and activity. The effects of gender were controlled in all statistical analyses, and data for 4.9 % of the total study sample with invalid and careless responses to the personality questionnaire (indicated by a high score on a social desirability scale in the ZKPQ) were discarded from final statistical analyses.

Kane, G. C., Gotto, J. L., Mangione, S., West, S., & Hojat, M. (2007). Jefferson Scale of Patient's Perceptions of Physician Empathy: Preliminary psychometric data. *Croatian Medicine Journal, 48*, 81–86.

Participants included 225 patients seen by 166 residents in the internal medicine residency program at Jefferson Hospital Ambulatory Clinic at Thomas Jefferson University Hospital. Patients completed the 5-item Jefferson Scale of Patient Perceptions of Physician Empathy (JSPPPE) to assess their physician's empathic engagement in patient care, and also a patient rating form developed by the American Board of Internal Medicine (ABIM) to measure aspects of physician communication skills, humanistic qualities, and professionalism. A subsample of participating residents ($n = 27$) also completed the JSE. Factor analysis of the JSPPPE resulted in only one reliable factor indicating that the JSPPPE is a unidimensional scale. The mean sore of the JSPPPE was 23.8, $SD = 2.54$, possible range 5–25, actual range in the study sample 10–25. Cronbach's alpha coefficient was 0.58, which is relatively low, probably due to a small number of items. Corrected item-total score correlations were all positive and statistically significant ranging from 0.77 to 0.90, with a median of 0.85. Correlation between JSPPPE scores and assessment on the ABIM patient rating form was 0.75 which was statistically significant, supporting criterion-related validity of the JSPPPE. Correlations between JSPPPE and responses to the following questions were all statistically significant, providing evidence for construct validity of the JSPPPE: "Physicians shows concerns for my feelings and needs" ($r = 0.86$), "Asks me how I feel about my problems" ($r = 0.79$), "Takes my wishes into account" ($r = 0.76$), "Arranges for adequate privacy" ($r = 0.61$), and "is always in a hurry" ($r = -0.50$).

Kiersma, M. E., Chen, A. M. H., Yehle, K. S., & Plake, K. S. (2013). Validation of an Empathy Scale in Pharmacy and Nursing Students. *American Journal of Pharmaceutical Education, 77*. Article 94. doi:10.5688/ajpe77594.

Participants included pharmacy ($n = 158$) and nursing ($n = 58$) students (146 women) who participated in a simulation game (Geriatric Medication Game) in which the challenges of elderly patients were addressed. Participants completed the JSE and another empathy measuring instrument developed by two of the study authors (the Kiersma-Chen Empathy Scale, KCES) before and after participation in the simulation game. Cronbach's alpha coefficients for the JSE before participation in the simulation game were 0.82, 0.79, and 0.82 in pharmacy, nursing, and total samples respectively. These reliability coefficients after the simulation game were 0.80, 0.90, and 0.89, respectively. Correlations between scores of the JSE and the KCES were 0.59 and 0.77 before and after participation in the simulation game.

King, S., & Holosko, M. J. (2012). The development and initial validation of the empathy scale for social workers. *Research on Social Work Practice, 22*, 174–185. doi:10.1177/1049731511417136.

Participants included 271 students (81 % women) in the Master of Social Work program at the University of Georgia who completed the JSE and a newly developed instrument "Empathy Scale for Social Workers." As part of the validity study, the correlation between scores of the JSE and the newly developed instrument for measuring empathy in social workers was examined, and a statistically significant correlation was obtained ($r = 0.34$).

Krasner, M. S., Epstein, R. M., Beckman, H., Suchman, A. L., Chapman, B., Mooney, C. J., & Quill, T. E. (2009). Association of an educational program in mindful communication with burnout, empathy, and attitudes among primary care physicians. *Journal of the American Medical Association, 302*, 1284–1293. doi:10.1001/jama.2009.1384.

> Participants included 70 primary care physicians in Rochester, New York, who participated in a continuing medical education course in mindfulness meditation, self-awareness, reflective writing about clinical experiences, and didactic teaching and discussion. Participants completed a survey which included the JSE, Maslach Burnout Inventory (MBI), Mindfulness Scale, the Profile of Mood State (POMS), a measure of the big five personality factors, and other scales before and after participation in the program. Results showed a significant enhancement in the total scores of the JSE as a result of participation in the program (effect size = 0.45) and in factor scores of the JSE such as Perspective Taking (effect size = 0.38) and Standing in Patient's Shoes (effect size = 0.36). Improvements in mindfulness were significantly correlated with improvements in the Perspective Taking factor scores of the JSE. Also, participation in the program was associated with improvements in personality measures such as Conscientiousness and Emotional Stability.

Lamothe, M., Boujut, E., Zenasni, F., & Sultan, S. (2014). To be or not to be empathic: The combined role of empathic concern and perspective taking in understanding burnout in general practice. *BMC Family Practice, 15*, 15. doi:10.1186/1471-2296-15-15. Accessible from: http://www.biomedcentral.com/1471-2296/15/15.

> Participants included 294 general practitioners in France who completed the JSE to assess cognitive empathy, the Toronto Empathy Questionnaire (TEQ) to assess emotional empathy, and the Maslach Burnout Inventory (MBI). Results showed a JSE mean score of 111.81 ($SD = 10.60$) in this sample of French physicians. Scores on the Standing in Patient's Shoes factor of the JSE were negatively but significantly correlated with scores of the Emotional Exhaustion scale of the MBI ($r = -0.14$). Scores on the Depersonalization scale of the MBI were negatively and significantly correlated with cognitive and emotional empathy. In multiple regression analysis models, lower empathy scores predicted higher burnout scores. Although the correlations were statistically significant, all were low in magnitude. The authors suggested that professionals need to regulate emotional empathy in order to minimize personal distress, compassion fatigue, and burnout.

Lelorain, S., Brédart, A., Dolbeault, S., Cano, A., Bonnaud-Antignac, A., Cousson-Gélie, F., & Sultan, S. (2014). How can we explain physician accuracy in assessing patient distress? A multilevel analysis in patients with advanced cancer. *Patient Education and Counseling, 94*, 322–327. doi:10.1016/j.pec.2013.10.029.

> Participants included 28 physicians (64 % women) mostly medical oncologists (75 %), who completed the JSE, and responded to the following single item to measure their self-efficacy in empathic skills: "In general, I feel competent to detect my patients' emotional distress and needs." In addition, physicians assessed their perceived quality of rapport with their patients. Patients assessed their own emotional distress by using a visual analog scale. Physicians independent from the patient, also subjectively assessed the degree of patient's distress. An index of empathic accuracy was generated by calculating the absolute value of the difference between patients' and physicians' assessments of patient distress. Results showed that neither physicians' self-reported empathy (JSE scores), nor self-reported efficacy in empathic skills could significantly predict an empathic accuracy index. However, physician's self-reported quality of rapport with their patients was associated with better empathic accuracy.

Lelorian, S., Brédart, A., Dolbeault, S., Cano, A., Bonnaud-Antignac, A., Cousson-Gélie, F., & Sultan, S. (2015). How does a physician's accurate understanding of a cancer patient's unmet needs contribute to patient perception of physician empathy? *Patient Education and Counseling, 98*, 734–741. Accessible from: http://dx.doi.org/10.1016/j.pec.2015.03.002.

> Participants included 28 physicians who completed the JSE, and their 201 metastatic cancer patients who completed a survey of physical, psychological, sexual, informational, and support needs. Physicians completed the same survey from the patient perspective. Results showed that physicians self-reported perspective taking, but not compassionate care factor of the JSE was positively related to their understanding of patient's unmet needs.

Lelorain, S., Sultan, S., Zenasni, F., Catu-Pinault, A., Juar, P., Boujut, E., & Rigal, L. (2013). Empathic concern and professional characteristics associated with clinical empathy in French general practitioners. *European Journal of General Practice, 19*, 23–28. doi:10.3109/13814788.2012.709842.

> Participants included 295 French general practitioners who completed a French translation of the JSE and the Toronto Empathy Questionnaire (TEQ). Results showed that empathic concern (measured by the TEQ) was an important component of clinical empathy (measured by the JSE). However, in multiple regression statistical analysis it was found that physician practice characteristics such as consultation length, and attending Balint group could uniquely predict clinical empathy. Clinical experiences did not make a significant contribution to predicting clinical empathy beyond empathic concern.

Lin, C., Li, L., Wan, D., Wu, Z., & Yan, Z. (2012). Empathy and avoidance in treating patients living with HIV/AIDS (PLWHA) among service providers in China. *AIDS Care, 24*, 1341–1348. doi:10.1080/09540121.2011.648602.

> Participants included 1760 health service providers from 40 county hospitals in China who completed a brief (11-item) version of a Chinese translation of the JSE. Results showed that nurses, younger providers, and providers with lower education were more likely to avoid contact with HIV/AIDS patients. Multiple regression analysis showed that higher scores on the JSE were associated significantly and inversely with avoidance attitudes toward HIV/AIDS patients. Findings confirmed that the health providers' empathy (reflected in the JSE scores) plays an important role in providing quality care to HIV-infected and AIDS patients.

Magalhäes, E., Costa P., & Costa, M. (2012). Empathy of medical students and personality: Evidence from the Five-Factor Model. *Medical Teacher, 34*, 807–812.

> Participants included 350 medical students (244 women) from six classes at the School of Health Sciences of the University of Minho in Portugal who completed a Portuguese translation of the JSE and the big-five personality factor survey (NEO-FFI). Correlations between scores of the JSE and those of the big-five personality factors were examined: $r=-0.01$ (with Neuroticism), $r=0.04$ (with Extraversion), $r=0.22, p<0.01$ (with Openness), $r=0.24, p<0.01$ (with Agreeableness), and $r=0.14, p<0.05$ (with Conscientiousness).

Michalec, B., Veloski, J. J., Hojat, M., & Tykocinski, M. (2015). Identifying potential engaging leaders within medical education: The role of positive influence on peers. *Medical Teacher, 37*, 677–683. doi:10.3109/0142159X.2014.947933.

> Participants included 630 fourth-year medical students in three graduating classes at Sidney Kimmel (formerly Jefferson) Medical College at Thomas Jefferson University who were asked to think back to their medical school experiences and respond to the question of "Which of your classmates had significant positive influence on your professional and personal development?"

Students who were selected most (top 10 %) were compared to the rest of the class on scores on the JSE and on selected performance measures. High positive influencers obtained a significantly higher score on the JSE ($M = 117.1$, $SD = 9.0$) than did the other students ($M = 113.5$, $SD = 11.0$). Also, high influencers compared to the rest of their classmates obtained higher clinical competence ratings on six core clerkships in the third year of medical school, and on simulated patients' assessments of their communication and interpersonal skills. No significant difference was found between top influencer and the rest on scores on the MCAT, and medical licensing examinations (Steps 1 and 2 of the USMLE).

Nasr Esfahani, M., Behzadipour, M., Jalili Nadoushan, A., & Shariat, S. V. (2014). A pilot randomized controlled trial on the effectiveness of inclusion of a distant learning component into empathy training. *Medical Journal of the Islamic Republic of Iran, 28*, 1–6.

Participants included 14 first-year residents in psychiatry, divided into two groups. Group 1 attended a 2-day workshop for communication skills. Group 2 viewed the videotape of the workshop and attended a distant learning workshop. Before and after the workshop, the JSE was administered to the residents, the Jefferson Scale of Patient Perceptions of Physician Empathy (JSPPPE) was completed by standardized patients, and an assessment of empathy during residents' interviews with patients was made by board certified psychiatrists' observations of clinical encounters. Although improvement in the JSE scores was observed in Group 1 but not in Group 2, the difference was not statistically significant. Correlations between scores of the JSE and JSPPPE and between JSE and observational assessment of empathy were moderate (0.37 and 0.39, respectively), but they were not statistically significant due to a lack of statistical power and small sample size. A statistically significant correlation was found between scores of the JSPPPE and observational assessments of empathy ($r = 0.85$) which was considered as an evidence in support of the validity of the JSPPPE.

Ogle, J., Bushnell, J., & Caputi, P. (2013). Empathy is related to clinical competence in medical care. *Medical Education, 47*, 824–831. doi:10.1111/medu.12232.

Participants included 57 (20 women) third-year medical students in Australia who completed the JSE. The clinical competence of these students was assessed by Objective Structured Clinical Examinations (OSCE) by medical professionals. Also, students' empathic engagement was rated by an independent observer of the clinical interaction in OSCE stations. Results showed that observers' assessments of clinical competence in OSCE stations were significantly correlated with observers' assessment of students' empathic engagement in OSCE stations. However, no significant association was found between students' self-reported empathy (JSE scores) and observers' assessments of students' empathy in OSCE stations. Significant associations were also observed between observers' assessments of students' empathy and ratings of students' clinical performance. The JSE mean score for this sample was 111.98 ($SD = 11.22$).

O'Sullivan, J., & Whelan, T. A. (2011). Adversarial growth in telephone counsellors: Psychological and environmental influences. *British Journal of Guidance & Counselling, 39*, 307–323. doi:10.1080/03069885.2011.567326.

Participants included 64 telephone counsellors who completed the JSE, Posttraumatic Growth Inventory, and other surveys to examine the level of adversarial growth among these counsellors. Results showed that scores of the JSE were not significant predictors of growth. However, compassion fatigue was significantly associated with posttraumatic growth.

Pohl, C. A., Hojat. M., & Arnold, L. (2011). Peer nominations as related to academic attainment, empathy, personality, and specialty interest. *Academic Medicine, 86*, 747–751. doi:10.1097/ACM.0b013e318217e464.

Participants included 255 third-year medical students (125 women) at Jefferson Medical College (currently Sidney Kimmel Medical College) who completed the JSE, and the Zuckerman-Kuhlman Personality Questionnaire (ZKPQ). Students were asked to nominate classmates whom they considered to be the best in six given areas of clinical and humanistic excellence. Results of comparing those who received at least one peer nomination ($n=155$) with those who received none ($n=100$) showed no significant difference in objective examination grades; however, nominated students obtained a statistically significant higher JSE mean score ($M=115.5$, $SD=9.0$) than their classmates who were not nominated ($M=112.4$, $SD=11.2$, effect size $=0.32$). Also nominated students received higher faculty ratings on clinical competence, and expressed more interest in pursuing "people-oriented" (rather than "technology- or procedure-oriented") specialties. On personality factors, nominated students obtained higher mean score on the Activity factor of the ZKPQ. No statistically significant difference was found between the nominated and not nominated students on other personality factors such as Sociability, Aggression-Hostility, Neuroticism-Anxiety or Impulsive Sensation Seeking.

Reisetter, B. C., Bently, J. P., & Wilkin, N. E. (2005). Relationship between psychosocial physician characteristics and physician price awareness. *Journal of Pharmaceutical Marketing & Management, 17*, 51–76. doi:10.1300/j058v17n01_05.

Participants included 200 primary care and internal medicine physicians (32 women) who completed the JSE, and the Physician Belief Scale (PBS). Physicians were also asked to estimates the cash price for 20 commonly prescribed prescription drugs at the usual quantities dispensed. Results showed that on average, physicians were able to estimates cash price for eight out of 20 sample drugs within ±20 %. Scores on the JSE and PBS did not significantly predict physician price awareness. In a multivariate hierarchical regression analysis, variables such as gender and time spent with patients could significantly explain the variance in accuracy of physicians' awareness of drug costs.

Richards, H. L., Fortune, D. G., Weildmann, A., Sweeney, S. K. T., & Griffiths, C. E. M. (2004). Detection of psychological distress in patients with psoriasis: Low consensus between dermatologist and patient. *British Journal of Dermatology, 151*, 1227–1233. doi:10.1111/j.1365-2133.2004.06221.x.

Participants included five dermatologists (three women) who completed the JSE, and their 43 patients (22 women) with psoriasis who completed the Hospital Anxiety and Depression Scale following their consultations with the dermatologists at the Psoriasis Clinic, Hope Hospital, Salford, Manchester, England. Participating dermatologists also assessed their patient's psychological distress level following the visit by using a 10-point visual analog scale. Results showed that the JSE mean score for participating dermatologists was 114 ($SD=14.2$). The concordance rates between patient's self-reported depression and anxiety and the dermatologists' assessment of the patients' psychological distress was at a lower end of a fair agreement. Dermatologists' JSE scores did not appear to influence their identification of patients' psychological distress.

Weng, H. C., Steed, J. F., Yu, S. W., Liu, Y. T., Hsu, C. C., Yu, T. J., & Chen, W. (2011). The effect of surgeon empathy and emotional intelligence on patient satisfaction. *Advances in Health Sciences Education, 16*, 591–600. doi:10.1007/s10459-011-9278-3.

Participants included 50 surgeons and their 896 outpatients who were scheduled to undergo surgery in Taiwan. A Chinese translation of the JSE and an emotional intelligence test was completed by the surgeons. Patients completed a survey about their satisfaction with their surgeons, and their perception of relationship with the surgeon. In a follow-up telephone interview after surgery, patients were asked to rate their health status on a 7-point scale. Results showed that scores of the JSE were significantly correlated with higher ratings on self-reported health status two weeks after surgery ($r=0.25$, $p<0.05$). Patients satisfaction with their surgeons was also correlated significantly with their self-reported health status after surgery ($r=0.26$, $p<0.05$). No significant association was observed between JSE scores and dimensions of the Chinese test of emotional intelligence. The authors reported that a long-term patient satisfaction with their physicians is influenced more by their physician's empathy rather than physician's emotional intelligence.

Xia, L., Hongyu, S., & Xinwei, F. (2011). Study on correlation between empathy ability and personality characteristics of undergraduate nursing students. *Chinese Nursing Research, 32.*

Participants included 229 undergraduate nursing students from six nursing schools in China who completed a Chinese translation of the JSE, and the Eysenck Personality Questionnaire (EPQ). Correlational analyses showed statistically significant but negative correlations between scores of the Neuroticism scale of the EPQ, with total scores of the JSE, as well as with factor scores on Perspective-Taking, and Compassionate Care of the JSE.

Zenasni, F., Boujut, E., de Vaure, C. B., Catu-Pinault, A., Tavani, J. L., Rigal, L., Juary, P., Magnier, A.M., Falcoff, H., & Sultan, S, (2012). Development of a French-language version of the Jefferson Scale of Physician Empathy and association with practice characteristics and burnout in a sample of general practitioners. *The International Journal of Person Centered Medicine, 2,* 759–766. Accessible from: http://www.ijpcm.org/index.php/IJPCM/article/view/295.

Participants included 308 general practitioners attending a national congress of family medicine in France (150 women) who completed a French translation of the JSE, and the Maslach Burnout Inventory (MBI). Confirmatory factor analysis of the JSE showed an acceptable fit for the three-factor model of the JSE (Perspective Taking, Compassionate Care, Standing in the Patient's Shoes). Scores on the Perspective Taking factor of the JSE were significantly associated with personal experience with psychotherapy, and duration of consultation. Scores on the Compassionate Care factor of the JSE were significantly associated with being female, and living in a coupled relationship. Scores of the Depersonalization scale of the MBI were inversely and significantly correlated with factor scores of the JSE: $r=-0.30$ with the Standing in Patient's Shoes factor scores; $r=-0.26$ with Compassionate Care factor scores, and $r=-0.18$ with Perspective-Taking factor scores. Conversely, scores on the Personal Accomplishment scale of the MBI were positively and significantly correlated with factor scores of the JSE: $r=0.36$ with Perspective Taking, $r=0.18$ with Compassionate Care, and $r=0.21$ with Standing in Patient's Shoes. Also, scores on the Exhaustion scale of the MBI were significantly and inversely correlated with Standing in the Patient's Shoes factor scores of the JSE ($r=-0.15$).

Group Comparisons on the JSE Scores

Aggarwal, R. (2007). Empathy: Do psychiatrists and patients agree? *The American Journal of Psychiatry Resident's Journal, 2,* 2–3.

Participants included ten psychiatrists who completed the JSE and 50 of their patients who completed a modified version of the JSE to reflect their views of their psychiatrist's empathic engagement. Psychiatrists' self-reported JSE mean score was 119.7 ($SD=8.65$), which was significantly higher than that reported by their patients ($M=104.4$, $SD=11.3$). The self-reported JSE mean score was higher for female psychiatrists compared to their male counterparts. Also patients' assessments on empathy of the female psychiatrists were higher than that for male psychiatrists regardless of the patient's gender.

Boyle, M. J., Williams, B., Brown, T., Molloy, A., McKenna, L., Molloy, L., & Lewis, B. (2009). Levels of empathy in undergraduate health science students. *The Internet Journal of Medical Education, 1*. doi:10.5580/1b15.

> Participants included 459 students (81 % women) from six health related disciplines: paramedics, nursing, midwifery, occupational therapy, physiotherapy, and health sciences who completed the JSE. Results showed that women obtained a significantly higher JSE mean score ($M = 109.78$, $SD = 14.73$) than men ($M = 104.76$, $SD = 12.21$). No statistically significant difference on JSE scores was found among students in different disciplines. Cronbach's alpha coefficient for the entire sample was 0.85.

Bucher, J. T., Vu, D. M., & Hojat, M. (2013). Psychostimulant drug abuse and personality factors in medical students. *Medical Teacher, 35*, 53–57.

> Participants included 321 first- to fourth-year students (148 women) at Jefferson (currently Sidney Kimmel) Medical College who anonymously completed the JSE, the Zuckerman-Kuhlman Personality Questionnaire (ZKPQ), and responded to a question about whether they had used psychostimulant medications (e.g., Adderall, Ritalin, dextroamphetamine, and methamphetamine) for medical or non-medical purposes before or during medical school. Those who had used psychostimulant medications for medical reasons ($n=34$) were excluded from statistical analyses. Results for the rest of the sample showed that 14 % had abused psychostimulant drugs for non-medical reasons. Comparisons of psychostimulant drug abusers and the rest showed no statistically significant difference on the JSE scores between the two groups. However, drug abusers obtained a significantly higher mean score on the Aggression-Hostility scale of the ZKPQ. No other statistically significant difference on other scales of the ZKPQ was observed between the two groups.

Dehning, S., Reiß, E., Krause, D., Gasperi, S., Meyer, S., Dargel, S., Müller N., & Siebeck, M. (2014). Empathy in high-tech and high-touch medicine. *Patient Education and Counseling. 95*, 259–264. Accessible from: http://dx.doi.org/10.1016/j.pec.2014.01.013.

> Participants included 56 surgeons (14 women) and 50 psychiatrists (25 women) in the departments of surgery, and psychiatry and psychotherapy at the Ludwig Maximilian University in Munich, Germany who completed the JSE, a short version of the Balanced Emotional Empathy Scale (BEES), and a short version of the Reading the Mind in the Eye Test (RME-R6). Results showed that male psychiatrists scored significantly higher on the JSE ($M=118.0$, $SD=9.86$) than male surgeons ($M=107.5$, $SD=13.84$). The gender difference was not statistically significant between female psychiatrists ($M=115.4$, $SD=14.19$) and female surgeons ($M=114.1$, $SD=7.16$). No statistically significant gender difference was observed on the BEES and RME-R6 results. In addition, analytically trained psychiatrists obtained a significantly higher mean score on the JSE than their behaviorally trained counterparts. Significant correlations were observed between scores of the JSE and the BEES ($r=0.46$) and the RME-R6 ($r=0.31$).

Delgado-Bolton, R., San-Martin, M., Alcorta-Garza, A., & Vivanco, L. (in press). Medical empathy of physicians-intraining who are enrolled in professional training program: A comparative intercultural study in Spain. *Atención Primaria*. Accessible from: http://dx.doi.org/10.1016/j.aprim.2015.10.005.

> Participants included 67 residents from Spain and 32 from Latin America who completed a Spanish translation of the JSE-HP Version. Results showed that the JSE mean score was higher for Spanish ($M=116$, $SD=13$) than the Latin American group ($M=109$, $SD=14$). Cronbach's alpha coefficients were 0.82, and 0.81 for Spanish and the Latin American groups, respectively.

Diaz-Narvaez, V. P., Coronado, A. M.E., Bilbao, J.L., Gonzalez, F., Padilla, M., Howard, M., Silva, G., Alboleda, J., Bullen, M., Utsman, R., Fajardo, E., Alonso, L.M., & Cervantes, M. (2015). Empathy levels of dental students of Central America and the Caribbean. *Health, 7,* 1678–1686. Accessible from: http://dx.doi.org/10.4236/health.2015.712182.

> Participants included 1,834 students from nine dental schools in Colombia, Panama, Costa Rica, and Dominican Republic who complete a Spanish translation of the JSE. The JSE mean scores for students from different dental schools ranged from a high of 111.89 to a low of 100.99. Differences were statistically significant among some of the schools. Cronbach's alpha coefficient for the entire sample was 0.77 (ranged from 0.75 to 0.78 for different dental schools).

Diaz-Narvaez, V. P., Gutierrez-Ventura, F.G., de Villalba, T.V., Salcedo-Rioja, M., Galzadilla-Nunez, A., Hamdan-Rodriguiz, M. (2015). Empathy levels of dentistry students in Peru and Argentina. *Health, 7,* 1268–1274. Accessible from: http://dx.doi.org/10.4236/health.2015.710141.

> Participants included 647 students from three dental schools in Peru and Argentina who completed translated versions of the JSE. Results showed that with a few exceptions, women generally scored a higher mean scores (ranged from 96.5 to 118.6) than men (92.4–120.1) in different universities and in different years of training. Also, empathy scores generally tend to increase as students progress through dental school in this cross-sectional study. However, none of the differences were considered practically important.

Diaz-Narvaez, V.P., Calzadilla-Nunez, A., Carrasco, D., Bustos, A., Zamorano, A., Silva, H., Lopez Tagle, E., Hubermann, J. (2016). Levels of empathy among dental students in five Chilean universities. *Health, 8,* 32–41. Accessible from: http://dx.doi.org/10.4236/health.2016.81005.

> Participants included 1,722 students from five dental schools in Chile who completed the JSE. Results showed that women scores higher (*M*=114.21) than men (*M*=111.42) on the JSE, and mean scores varied from 110.63 to 115.56 in different universities, and empathy scores tend to increase as students progress through dental school in this crosssectional study.

Fields, S. K., Hojat, M., Gonnella, J. S., Mangione, S., Kane, G., & Magee, M. (2004). Comparisons of nurses and physicians on an operational measure of empathy. *Evaluation & The Health Professions, 27,* 80–94. doi:10.1177/0163278703261206.

> Participants included 56 female registered nurses and 42 female physicians at Thomas Jefferson University Hospital who completed the JSE. Comparison of physicians and nurses on the total scores of the JSE showed no statistically significant differences (*M* = 115.7, *SD* = 13.60 in physicians; *M* = 117.2, *SD* = 14.05 in nurses). However, comparisons of the two groups on their responses to the individual items of the JSE showed statistically significant differences between physicians and nurses on five out of 20 items of the JSE (physicians scored higher on two; and nurses scored higher on three items). Cronbach's alpha coefficients were 0.89 and 0.87 for physicians and nurses, respectively.

Grosseman, S., Hojat, M., Duke, P. M., Mennin, S., Rosenzweig, S., & Novack, D. (2014). Empathy, self-reflection, and curriculum choice. *The Interdisciplinary Journal of Problem-Based Learning, 8,* 35–41. Accessible from: http:/dx.doi.org/10.7771/1541-5015.1429.

> Participants included 223 first-year medical students at Drexel University College of Medicine who completed the JSE and the Groningen Reflection Ability Scale. Of this sample, 60 (30 women)

self-selected a problem-based learning curriculum track, and 163 (79 women) self-selected a lecture-based curriculum track. Those who chose the problem-based learning curriculum track scored significantly higher on the JSE ($M = 118.0$, $SD = 8.9$) than their classmates who chose the lecture-based track ($M = 114.0$, $SD = 11.1$). Similar pattern of findings was observed on the Groningen Reflection Ability Scale ($M = 94.6$, $SD = 7.5$; and $M = 92.0$, $SD = 8.2$, respectively). Women scored significantly higher than men on both scales.

Hojat, M., Fields, S. K., & Gonnella, J. S. (2003). Empathy: An NP/MD comparison. *The Nurse Practitioner, 28*, 45–47.

Participants included 32 female nurse practitioners, 37 female pediatricians, and 33 female physicians in hospital-based specialties (anesthesiology, radiology, and pathology) who completed the JSE. Results showed no statistically significant difference on JSE mean scores between nurse practitioners ($M = 124.0$, $SD = 12.3$) and pediatricians ($M = 124.0$, $SD = 9.3$); however, physicians in hospital-based specialties scored significantly lower ($M = 118.0$, $SD = 13.1$) than nurse practitioners and pediatricians. Cronbach's alpha coefficient for nurse practitioners was 0.85.

Hojat, M., Mangione, S., Gonnella, J. S., Nasca, T., Veloski, J. J., & Kane, G. (2001). Empathy in medical education and patient care [Letter to the editor]. *Academic Medicine, 76*, 669.

Participants included 704 physicians affiliated with the Jefferson Health Care System who completed the JSE. Those who were practicing medicine in "people-oriented" specialties (e.g., general internal medicine, family medicine, pediatrics, obstetrics and gynecology, emergency medicine, psychiatry, and medical subspecialties) obtained a significantly higher JSE mean score ($M = 121.0$, $SD = 11.6$) than their counterparts in "technology-oriented" specialties (e.g., anesthesiology, pathology, radiology, surgery and surgical subspecialties) ($M = 117.2$, $SD = 12.1$). Results remained unchanged when the effect of physicians' gender was controlled.

Kataoka, H. U., Koide, N., Hojat, M., & Gonnella, J. S. (2012). Measurement and correlates of empathy among female Japanese physicians. *BMC Medical Education, 12*, 48. doi:10.1186/1472-6920-12-48. Accessible from: http://www.biomedcentral.com/1472-6920/12/48.

Participants included 285 female Japanese physicians who graduated from Okayama University Medical School or were practicing medicine in Okayama University Hospital. They completed a Japanese translation of the JSE (HP Version). Results showed that the JSE mean score for this sample was 110.4 ($SD = 11.9$). Corrected item-total score correlations were all positive and statistically significant, ranging from 0.20 to 0.54 with a median of 0.41. Cronbach's alpha coefficient was 0.80. Physicians who were practicing in "people-oriented" specialties obtained a significantly higher JSE mean score than their counterparts in "procedure or technology-oriented" specialties. Physicians who reported living with their parents in an extended family or living close to their parents, scored higher on the JSE than those who were living alone or were living in a small nuclear family.

McKenna, L., Boyle, M., Brown, T., Williams, B., Molloy, A., Lewis, B., & Molloy, L. (2012). Levels of empathy in undergraduate nursing students. *International Journal of Nursing Practice, 18*, 246–251. doi:10.1111/j.1440-172X.2012.02035.x.

Participants included 106 nursing students (93 % women) at Monash University, Australia who completed in JSE. Results showed a JSE mean score of 107.34 ($SD = 13.74$). No statistically significant association was observed between JSE scores and students' gender, age, and year of training in this cross-sectional study.

Ouzouni, C., & Nakakis, K. (2012). An exploratory study of student nurses' empathy. *Health Science Journal, 6*, 534–552.

> Participants included 279 nursing students (239 women) in the first-, third-, fourth-, and sixth-semester of their nursing education at the Nursing School of the Technological Educational Institute of Lamia in Greece who completed a Greek translation of the JSE. Results showed that women outscored their male classmates. The following groups of students obtained significantly higher JSE mean scores than their other classmates: those who expressed a plan to work as nurses after graduation, those who reported that they were able to understand feelings of others, those who reported receiving emotional support from their nuclear families, those who reported being exposed to training in understanding patient's perspective, those who observed their clinical faculty displaying emotional understanding of the patients, older students, and students who were in higher stages of training.

Park, K. H., Roh, H., Suh, D. H., & Hojat, M. (2015). Empathy in Korean medical students: Findings from a nationwide survey. *Medical Teacher, 37*, 943–948. doi: 10.3109/0142159X.2014.956058.

> Participants included 5343 first- to fourth-year Korean medical students (2056 women) across the country from two types of medical school admission systems: undergraduate admission system ($n = 2624$) and post-baccalaureate admission system ($n = 2719$). Students completed a Korean translation of the JSE. Results showed a JSE mean score of 105.90 ($SD = 12.80$) for the total sample. Women's JSE mean score ($M = 106.95, SD = 11.74$) was significantly higher than men ($M = 105.25, SD = 13.73$). Similar pattern of gender difference was observed in students of both medical school systems. Controlling for gender, significant difference on the JSE was found between students from the two medical school systems in the favor of students in the post-baccalaureate system. No significant association was observed between JSE scores and students' age in both medical school systems. In both systems, students in higher years of medical education scored lower on the JSE.

Shariat, S. V., & Kaykhavoni, A. (2010). Empathy in medical residents at Iran University of Medical Sciences. *Iranian Journal of Psychiatry and Clinical Psychology, 16*, 248–256.

> Participants included 251 residents (41 % women) who were pursuing their residency training in hospitals affiliated with Iran University of Medical Sciences in Tehran, Iran. They completed a Persian (Farsi) translation of the JSE. Results showed no significant gender difference (for men: $M = 100.4, SD = 13.1$; for women: $M = 100.9, SD = 13.3$). Psychiatry residents obtained the highest JSE mean score ($M = 114.2, SD = 14.1$) than other residents. No significant association was found between scores of the JSE and residents' age and level of training.

Soncini, F., Silvestrini, G., Poscia, A., Clorba. V., Conti, A., Murru, C., Rinaldi, A., Zoccali, A., Azzolini, E., & Ziglio, A. (2013). Public health physicians and empathy: Are we really empathic? The Jefferson Scale applied to Italian resident doctors in public health. *European Journal of Public Health, 23*(Suppl. 1), 264–265.

> Participants included 352 Italian resident physicians from residency programs in Italian schools of hygiene and public health who completed an Italian translation of the JSE sent to them by mail (87 % response rate). Results showed an overall mean score of 118.5 ($SD = 13.4, M = 120$, score range 54–120) for this sample. Women obtained a significantly higher JSE mean score ($M = 120.3$) than men ($M = 114.9$), and physicians who had health care administrative experiences scored significantly higher than those who were only involved in research ($M = 120.4$ and $M = 117.1$, respectively). No significant association was found between the JSE scores and physicians' age or level of residency training.

Voinescu, B. I., Szentagotai, A., & Coogan, A. (2009). Residents' clinical empathy: Gender and specialty comparisons—A Romanian study. *Acta Medica Academica, 38*, 11–15. doi:10.5644/ama.v38i1.50.

> Participants included 112 residents (74 % women) in Cluj-Napoca, Romania who completed a Romanian translation of the JSE. Results showed that the JSE mean score for the sample was 113.4 (*SD* = 14.4). Women's JSE mean score (*M* = 114.9, *SD* = 14.75) was significantly higher than men (*M* = 107.2, *SD* = 11.5). Residents in the psychiatry program (*n* = 60) obtained a significantly higher JSE mean score (*M* = 115.8, *SD* = 15.7) than other residents (*M* = 110.4, *SD* = 12.3). Corrected item-total score correlations for the JSE ranged from 0.21 to 0.67 with a median of 0.42. Cronbach's alpha coefficient was 0.84.

Williams, B., Brown, T., Boyle, M., McKenna, L., Palermo, C., & Etherington, J. (2014). Levels of empathy in undergraduate emergency health, nursing, and midwifery students: A longitudinal study. *Advances in Medical Education and Practice, 5*, 299–306. Accessible from: http://dx.doi.org/10.2147/AMEP.S66681.

> Participants included 948 first-, second-, and third-year paramedic, nursing, and midwifery students (798 women) at Monash University in Australia who completed the JSE. Midwifery students scored significantly higher scores on the JSE (*M* = 109.0, *SD* = 17.2), than those in nursing (*M* = 104.0, *SD* = 14.4) and paramedics (*M* = 104.4, *SD* = 14.9). No statistically significant difference was observed on scores of the JSE in students in different years of training. Although women obtained a higher JSE mean score (*M* = 106.6, *SD* = 14.83) than did men (*M* = 100.6, *SD* = 14.41), the difference was not statistically significant. Older students scored higher on the JSE than younger students.

Williams, B., Brown, T., McKenna, L., Boyle, M. J., Palermo, C., Nestel, D., Brightwell, R., McCall, L., & Russo, V. (2014). Empathy levels among health professional students: A cross-sectional study at two universities in Australia. *Advances in Medical Education and Practice, 5*, 107–113. doi:10.2147/AMEP.S57569. Accessible from: http://dx.doi.org/10.2147/AMEP.S57569.

> Participants included 1111 first- to fourth-year health professional students (907 women) studying in health profession disciplines such as medicine, nursing, paramedics, midwifery, occupational therapy, physiotherapy, and nutrition and dietetics from Monash and Edith Cowan universities in Australia who completed the JSE. Exploratory factor analysis of data resulted in three factors of Perspective Taking, Patient Perceptions, and Compassionate Care, somewhat similar to those emerged in most other factor analytic studies of the JSE. No significant difference was observed on scores of the JSE between the two universities: The mean score for students from Monash University was 110.06 (*SD* = 11.76), and that for students from Edith Cowan University was 109.18 (*SD* = 13.31). Cronbach's alpha coefficient for the total sample was 0.78. Women obtained a significantly higher JSE mean score (*M* = 110.86, *SD* = 11.67) than did men (*M* = 105.31, *SD* = 13.47). Paramedic students had significantly lower JSE mean score (*M* = 106.37, *SD* = 12.73) than all other students with the exception of nursing students. A significant increase in the JSE mean score was observed from the first-year (*M* = 108.71, *SD* = 12.52) to second-year (*M* = 111.01, *SD* = 11.94) in this cross-sectional study, but no significant change was found afterward. Students' age was positively associated with JSE scores.

Wilson, S. E., Prescott, J., & Becket, G. (2012). Empathy levels in first- and third-year students in health and non-Health disciplines. *American Journal of Pharmaceutical Education, 76*(2), Article 24. Accessible from: http://www.ncbi.nlm.nih.gov/pmc/articles/PMC3305933/.

Participants included 282 first- and third-year students (190 women) in nursing, pharmacy, and law who completed the JSE at the University of Central Lancashire in England. Results showed that women scored higher than men ($M=103$ and $M=97$, respectively). No significant difference was found between students in nursing and pharmacy programs; however, students in both of these health-related professions obtained significantly higher JSE mean scores than did the law students in both the first- and third-year of their education. In this cross-sectional study, a significant decline was observed in the JSE mean score from the first- to third-year in nursing students ($M=107.9$, $SD=11.9$; $M=101.9$, $SD=14.2$, respectively); however, an increase in the JSE mean score was found in pharmacy students between the first-year ($M=100.3$, $SD=11.8$), and third-year ($M=110.4$, $SD=10.5$); no significant change was noticed on the empathy scores between first- ($M=95.3$, $SD=11.1$) and third-year ($M=94.2$, $SD=13.4$) in law students.

Changes in Empathy During Health Profession Education

Beattie, A., Durham, J., Harvey, J., Steele, J., & McHanwell, S. (2012). Does empathy change in first-year dental students? *European Journal of Dental Education, 16*, e111–e116. doi:10.1111/j.1600-0579.2011.00683.x.

Participants included 66 first-year students (46 women) at the School of Dental Sciences, Newcastle University in England who completed the JSE and the Patient Practitioner Orientation Scale (PPOS, a measure of patient-centered care), before and after a behavioral science course. Results showed a significant increase in the JSE mean score after completion of the behavioral science course. No significant pre–post-course change was observed in PPOS scores. A statistically significant correlation was found between scores on the JSE and the PPOS caring scale ($r=0.36$) in pre-course, but not in post-course testing.

Brown, T., Williams, B., Boyle, M., Molloy, A., McKenna, L., Molloy, L., & Lewis, B. (2010). Levels of empathy in undergraduate occupational therapy students. *Occupational Therapy International, 17*, 135–141. doi:10.1002/oti.297.

Participants included 92 occupational therapy students (91 % women) at Monash University in Australia who completed the JSE. The median JSE score for this sample was 115. No statistically significant association was observed between JSE scores and students' gender, age, or year of training in this cross-sectional study.

Calabrese, L. H., Bianco, J. A., Mann, D., Massello, D., & Hojat, M. (2013). Correlates and changes in empathy and attitudes toward interprofessional collaboration in osteopathic medical students. *The Journal of the American Osteopathic Association, 113*, 898–907. doi:10.7556/jaoa.2013.068.

Participants included 373 first- to fourth-year osteopathic medical students (53 %, $n=197$ women) who completed the JSE and Jefferson Scale of Attitudes Toward Physician-Nurse Collaboration (JSAPNC). A statistically significant correlation of 0.42 was found between scores of the two instruments. Women scored significantly higher than did men on both JSE ($M=117.1$ and $M=111.9$ for women and men, respectively) and the JSAPNC ($M=50.1$ and $M=48.7$, respectively). In contrast to most findings in allopathic medical schools, no statistically significant decline in students' mean scores on the JSE (and JSAPNC) was observed in different medical school years in this cross-sectional study. Inconsistent with the findings in allopathic medical students, no statistically significant difference was found on JSE scores among students who planned to pursue "people-oriented" compared with those interested in "technology/procedure-oriented" specialties. Comparisons of the JSE scores from this study with those in allopathic medical students (reported in other studies) showed no significant difference in the first and second years, but osteopathic medical students had a higher JSE mean score than their allopathic counterparts in the third year and their scores remained relatively high in the fourth year of osteopathic medical school.

Chen, D., Lew, R., Hershman, W., & Orlander, J. (2007). A cross-sectional measurement of medical student empathy. *Journal of General Internal Medicine, 22*, 1434–1438. doi:10.1007/s11606-007-0298-x.

Participants included 658 students at Boston University School of Medicine who completed the JSE-S version. In this cross-sectional study, the JSE mean score was 118.5 in the first year but significantly declined in the third ($M = 112.7$) and remained low in the fourth year of medical school ($M = 106.6$). Women obtained a significantly higher JSE mean score ($M = 116.5$) than men ($M = 112.1$). Students who were interested in pursuing people-oriented specialties scored higher on the JSE than others who were interested in pursuing technology-oriented specialties ($M = 114.6$ and $M = 111.4$, respectively). No substantial association was found between scores of the JSE and students' ages.

Chen, D. C. R., Kirshenbaum, D. S., Yan, J., Kirshenbaum, E., & Aseltine, R. H. (2012). Characterizing changes in student empathy throughout medical school. *Medical Teacher, 34*, 305–311. doi:10.3109/0142159X.2012.644600.

Participants included 1162 students (622 women) at Boston University School of Medicine who completed the JSE at the beginning of medical school and approximately at the end of each academic year. Results showed an upward trend in mean scores of the JSE in preclinical years but a downward trend in clinical years (e.g., JSE mean score in the second year = 116.02, $SD = 12.42$; declined to 113.29, $SD = 12.59$ in the fourth year). Women scored higher than men on the JSE. Those interested in technology-oriented specialties (pathology, radiology, anesthesiology, surgery) obtained a significantly lower JSE mean score than others. Higher level of educational debt was associated with higher empathy scores after adjustment for specialty interest. It was noticed that the decline in empathy was less for students with a higher JSE scores at the beginning of medical school than that for students with lower baseline empathy scores.

Chen, D. C. R., Pahilan, M. E., & Orlander, J. D. (2010). Comparing a self-administered measure of empathy with observed behavior among medical students. *Journal of General Internal Medicine, 25*, 200–202. doi:10.1007/s11606-009-1193-4.

Participants in this cross-sectional study included 167 second-year and 162 third-year students at Boston University School of Medicine who completed the JSE. Their clinical skills, including interactions with patients were assessed by standardized patients in the Objective Structured Clinical Examinations (OSCE). A statistically significant decline in the JSE mean score was noticed when comparing the second-year ($M = 118.68$) and third-year students ($M = 116.08$). However, a statistically significant increase in the average ratings of clinical competence given by standardized patients in OSCE setting was observed ($M = 3.96$ in the second-year, $M = 4.15$ in the third-year). The overall correlation between JSE scores and the OSCE assessment was statistically significant but moderate in magnitude ($r = 0.22$).

Costa, P., Magalhães, E., & Costa, M. J. (2013). A latent growth model suggests that empathy of medical students does not decline over time. *Advances in Health Sciences Education, 18*, 509–522. doi:10.1007/s10459-012-9390-z. Accessible from: http://link.springer.com/article/10.1007/s10459-012-9390-z?null.

Participants included 77 medical students (53 women) at the School of Health Sciences, University of Minho in Portugal who completed a Portuguese translation of the JSE (S-version) three times upon admission, upon completion of the preclinical phase of medical education (third year) and at the start of the clinical phase of medical education (beginning of fourth year). Students also completed the NEO-FFI (a personality inventory for measuring the big five personality factors). Results for the total sample showed no significant decline in empathy scores prior to the clinical phase of medical education. For example, the JSE mean scores taken during preclinical was 111.21 ($SD = 10.80$) and at beginning of the clinical phase of medical education it was 110 ($SD = 10.85$). However, the JSE mean score declined significantly for women from preclinical phase ($M = 113.41$, $SD = 10.57$) to the beginning of clinical phase ($M = 110.77$, $SD = 10.84$). Such significant decline was not observed for men. Although JSE mean score was higher for women as compared to men in all three test administrations, the gender difference was statistically significant only at the end of the preclinical phase of medical education. Scores of the JSE were significantly and positively correlated with those of Openness to Experiences, and Agreeableness personality factors at admission to medical school.

Diaz-Narváez, V. P. D., Palacio, L. M. A., Caro, S. E., Silva, M. G., Castillo, J. A., Bilbao, J. L., & Acosta, J. I. (2014). Empathic orientation among medical students from three universities in Barranquilla, Colombia and one university in the Dominican Republic. *Archivos Argentinos de Pediatria, 112*, 41–49. Accessible from: http://dx.doi.org/10.5546/aap.2014.eng.41.

Participants included 1838 medical students from School of Medicine of Universidad del Norte ($n=345$), Universidad San Martin ($n=283$) and Universidad Libre ($n=695$) in the city of Barranquilla in Colombia and Universidad Central del Este ($n=515$) in the Dominican Republic, who competed the JSE. Mean scores of the JSE for students in different years (years 1–5) within each medical school ranged from a low of 98.2 to a high of 110.7. Differences in JSE scores were observed among medical schools. Empathy scores declined for both men and women as students progressed through medical school in this cross-sectional study, but the decline was not substantial.

Gabard, D. L., Lowe, D. L., Deusinger, S. S., Stelzner, D. M., & Crandall, S. J. (2013). Analysis of empathy in doctor of physical therapy students: A multi-site study. *Journal of Allied Health, 42*, 10–16.

Participants included two cohorts (classes of 2009 and 2010) of students enrolled in the doctor of physical therapy program in five academic institutions (Chapman University, Mount St. Mary's College, University of Colorado, University of Nebraska, and Washington University) who completed a slightly modified version of the JSE (changing "physician" to "physical therapist") in the first, second, and third year of training. The face validity of the modified version was confirmed in a pilot study, and a test–retest reliability coefficient of 0.58 was obtained in a sample of 20 physical therapy students, within 2 weeks interval between testing. Results on institution comparisons showed significant differences on the JSE among entering classes in the five participating institutions ranging from 111.0 ($SD=9.9$) to 120.1 ($SD=8.0$). Within institution comparisons on the JSE scores in the 3 years of training in this cross-sectional study showed mixed results. Comparisons of the JSE scores in the 3 years of study, in the two cohorts, within each institution either did not change significantly, or declined in some students, and increased in others.

Hall, M., Hanna, L.A., Hanna, A., & McDevitt, C. (2015). Empathy in UK pharmacy students: Assessing differences by gender, level in the degree programme, part-time employment and medical status. *Pharmacy Education, 15*, 241–247.

Participants included 318 undergraduate pharmacy students at Queen's University Belfast who completed the JSE-HPS version. Results showed a mean score of 106.19 (SD=11.81), and a Cronbach's alpha coefficient of 0.81. Although women scored higher than men on the JSE, the difference was not statistically significant. Students in the fourth year of training obtained a significantly higher JSE mean score (M=110.26, SD=10.93) than those in the first year (M=104.96, SD=12.39) in this cross-sectional study. No significant difference on the JSE scores was found among those who had a part-time job compared to their counterparts without a job; those who reported chronic health problems compared to others without such problems, and those who were taking medication compared to the rest.

Hojat, M., Mangione, S., Nasca, T. J., Rattner, S., Erdmann, J. B., Gonnella, J. S., & Magee, M. (2004). An empirical study of decline in empathy in medical school. *Medical Education, 38*, 934–941. doi:10.1111/j.1365-2929.2004.01911.x.

Participants included 125 medical students (61 women) who completed the JSE at the beginning and at the end of the third-year of medical school. In this first longitudinal study of change in the JSE scores during medical school, a statistically significant decline in JSE mean score was found when scores at the beginning (M = 123.1, SD = 9.9) and the end of third-year (M = 120.6, SD = 13.9) were compared (effect size of the change = 0.29). Analysis of differences at item level showed significant decline on five of the 20 items of the JSE (effect size estimates ranged from 0.34 to 0.55). Correlation coefficient of scores on the JSE administered at the beginning and end of the academic year was 0.51.

Hojat, M., Vergare, M., Maxwell, K., Brainard, G., Herrine, S. K., Isenberg, G. A., Veloski, J. J., & Gonnella, J. S. (2009). The devil is in the third year: A longitudinal study of erosion of empathy in medical school. *Academic Medicine, 84*, 1182–1191.

Participants in this longitudinal study included 456 students (226 women) in two entering classes at Jefferson (currently Sidney Kimmel) Medical College who completed the JSE five times during their medical school education: at the beginning of medical school and at the end of the fist-, second-, third-, and fourth-year of medical school. Results showed the mean scores of the JSE for both cohorts did not change significantly during the first 2 years of medical school. However, a significant decline in the JSE mean score was observed at the end of the third-year (from M = 115.7 at the end of the second year to M = 108.5 at the end of the third year in the matched cohorts), which persisted until graduation from medical school. Patterns of decline in JSE scores were similar for men and women, and for students interested in pursuing "people-oriented" or "technology- or procedure-oriented" specialties. Possible reasons for erosion of empathy in medical school were described based on students' own reports.

Hong, M., Lee, W. H., Park, J. H., Yoon, T. Y., Moon, D. S., & Lee, S. M. (2012). Changes of empathy in medical college and medical school students: One-year follow up study. *BMC Medical Education, 12*, 122. doi:10.1186/1472-6920-12-122. Accessible from: http://www.biomedcentral.com/1472-6920/12/122.

Participants included 113 students (24 % women) in medical college (6-year curriculum including two years of premedical education) and 113 students (26 % women) in medical school (four year curriculum after completing undergraduate education) at Kyung Hee University. Participants completed a Korean translation of the JSE in 2007 and 2008. They were in the first, second, and third years of medical education. Medical school students' JSE mean score (M = 109.23, SD = 11.06) in the first test administration was significantly higher than those in medical college (M = 106.96, SD = 10.50); however, no significant difference was found between medical school and medical college students in the second test administration one year later. Also, no significant change in empathy scores was observed in the two groups of students from the first to the second test administration, and no significant gender difference was noticed.

Khademalhosseini, M., Khademalhosseini, Z., & Mahmoodian, F. (2014). Comparison of empathy score among medical students in both basic and clinical levels. *Journal of Advances in Medical Education & Professionalism, 2*, 88–91.

> Participants included 260 students (140 women) at Shiraz University of Medical Sciences in Iran who completed a Persian translation of the JSE. Findings of this cross-sectional study showed that students' JSE mean score declined as they progressed from the basic science to clinical science component of medical education. Also, women obtained a significantly higher JSE mean score than men, and younger students scored higher than their older counterparts.

Kimmelman, M., Giacobbe, J., Faden, J., Kumar, G., Pinckney, C. C., & Steer, R. (2012). Empathy in osteopathic medical students: A cross-sectional analysis. *Journal of the American Osteopathic Association, 112*, 347–355.

> Participants included 405 (218 women) osteopathic medical students enrolled in the first-year ($n = 127$), second-year ($n = 105$), third-year ($n = 88$), and fourth-year ($n = 85$) at the University of Medicine and Dentistry of New Jersey, School of Osteopathic Medicine who completed the JSE. Results of comparisons of JSE scores at different years on medical education in this cross-sectional study showed no statistically significant difference. The JSE mean scores were 108.6 ($SD = 15.0$), 111.2 ($SD = 12.6$), 109.4 ($SD = 10.8$), and 107.0 ($SD = 15.2$) for the first, second, third, and fourth years, respectively. No statistically significant association was found between the JSE scores on the one hand, and gender, ethnicity, and specialty interest on the other hand. Comparisons of students' JSE scores from this study sample of osteopathic medical students with published data from allopathic medical students showed that osteopathic students had significantly lower JSE mean scores in the first 2 years, but no significant difference was observed in the last 2 years of medical education.

Lim, B. T., Moriarty, H., Huthwaite, M., Gray, L., Pullon, S., & Gallagher, P. (2013). How well do medical students rate and communicate clinical empathy? *Medical Teacher, 35*, e946–e951. doi:10.3109/0142159X.2012.715783.

> Participants included 72 medical students (39 women) at the University of Otago, Wellington School of Medicine and Health Sciences in New Zealand who completed the JSE at the beginning and end of the fifth-year in which students spend half of their time in clinical setting under supervision. Students also completed the JSE in the sixth-year in which they spend the majority of their time in clinical settings with and without direct supervision. Results of this longitudinal study showed no significant change in JSE scores in the fifth year, but a significant decline in mean JSE scores in the sixth year of medical school education ($M = 114.21$, $SD = 9.46$ at the beginning of the fifth year; $M = 113.55$, $SD = 10.50$ at the end of the fifth year; $M = 82.52$, $SD = 17.87$ in sixth year). No gender difference on the scores of the JSE was observed in this sample.

Mangione, S. Kane, G. C., Caruso, J. W., Gonnella, J. S., Nasca, T. J., & Hojat, M. (2002). Assessment of empathy in different years of internal medicine training. *Medical Teacher, 24*, 370–373.

> Participants included 98 internal medicine residents in the first ($n = 40$), second ($n = 27$), and third ($n = 31$) years of residency training who completed the JSE. Results of this cross-sectional study showed that the JSE mean score declined as residents progressed through training in this cross-sectional study ($M = 117.5$, $SD = 12.4$ in the first year; $M = 114.0$, $SD = 14.3$ in the second year, and $M = 113.5$, $SD = 10.8$ in the third year of training), but the differences did not reached the level of statistical significance. Results remained unchanged when gender was taken into

consideration. A test–retest reliability of 0.72 was obtained for residents who completed the JSE twice within a year of training.

McKenna, L., Boyle, M., Brown, T., Williams, B., Molloy, A., Lewis, B., & Molloy, L. (2011). Levels of empathy in undergraduate midwifery students: An Australian cross-sectional study. *Women and Birth: Journal of the Australian College of Midwives, 24,* 80–84. doi:10.1016/j.wombi.2011.02.003.

Participants included 52 undergraduate female midwifery students in three years of training at Monash University, Australia, who completed the JSE. Results showed a JSE mean score of 109.9 (*SD*=20.9) for the sample. A steady increase in the mean JSE scores was observed in this cross-sectional study as students progressed from the first to the third year of training.

Michalec, B. (2010). As assessment of medical student school stressors on preclinical students' level of clinical empathy. *Current Psychology, 29,* 210–221.

Participants were 329 first-, second-, and third-year US medical students who completed the JSE at the beginning and at the end of the academic year to examine the impact of medical school-specific stressors (e.g., financial worries, lack of time, fear of academic failure, competition, mistreatment by faculty, and interaction with patients) on changes in empathy during the academic year. Results showed that female students outscored their male counterparts, empathy declined in each year, and those who scored high on the JSE were more likely to report that medical school stressors had more negative impact on their lives. Also, changes in scores on the Conscientiousness and Extroversion factors of the NEO-PI-R were found to have unique and significant effects on the JSE scores. It is suggested that while medical school stress may not be the cause of the decline in empathy in medical school, students may be adapting to the stressful medical school environment by "shedding" empathy in order to become less vulnerable to the negative impact of the stressors.

Nunes, P., Williams, S., Sa, B., & Stevenson, K. (2011). A study of empathy decline in students from five health disciplines during their first year of training. *International Journal of Medical Education, 2,* 12–17. doi:10.5116/ijme.4d47.ddb0.

Participants included 355 students (259 women) enrolled in schools of medicine, nursing, dentistry, pharmacy, and veterinary medicine who completed the JSE at the beginning of their professional education and at the end of the academic year. Women scored higher than men, and older students scored higher than their younger counterparts. The highest JSE mean scores were obtained by nursing and dental students. Empathy declined to some extent in all five groups; however, the decline in medical, nursing, and dental students was statistically significant.

Rosenthal, S., Howard, B., Schlussel, Y. R., Herrigel, D., Smolarz, B. G., Gable, B., Vassquez, J., Grigo, H., & Kaufman, M. (2011). Humanism at heart: Preserving empathy in third-year medical students. *Academic Medicine, 86,* 350–358.

Participants included 209 medical students at Robert Wood Johnson Medical School who completed the JSE. In a pre-posttest design, no significant decline in scores of the JSE was observed in students who were exposed in their clerkship to a mandatory "humanism and professionalism" component of the curriculum. The authors concluded that the erosion of empathy in medical school can be prevented by targeted educational programs.

Schwartz, B., & Bohay, R. (2012). Can patient help teach professionalism and empathy to dental students? Adding patient video to lecture course. *Journal of Dental Education, 76,* 174–184.

Participants included 31 second-year and 54 third-year dental students at Schulich School of Medicine and Dentistry, University of Western Ontario in Canada who completed the JSE. Students viewed videos on patient management, and participated in discussion and reflective writing about their experiences. Despite these activities, statistically significant decline in the JSE mean scores were found between the second ($M = 117.13$, $SD = 7.64$) and third-year students ($M = 110.28$, $SD = 16.58$).

Ward, J., Cody, J., Schaal, M., & Hojat, M. (2012). The empathy enigma: An empirical study of decline in empathy among undergraduate nursing students. *Journal of Professional Nursing, 28,* 34–40. doi:10.1016/j.profnurs.2011.10.007.

Participants included 214 undergraduate nursing students (179 women) at the Jefferson School of Nursing, Thomas Jefferson University who completed the JSE twice at the beginning and at the end of the academic year. The JSE mean score for total participants was 114.6 ($SD = 11.8$) at the beginning of the academic year, which declined significantly to 112.7 ($SD = 12.1$) at the end of the academic year. The magnitude of decline during study period was significantly larger among nursing students who were exposed to patient encounters more than for their counterparts with limited clinical experiences. Gender did not significantly contribute to the decline in empathy; however, the magnitude of the decline was significantly larger for Asian students, for those with prior work experiences in clinical settings, and for students with undergraduate major in business.

Williams, B., Boyle, M., & Earl, T. (2013). Measurement of empathy levels in undergraduate parametric students. *Prehospital and Disaster Medicine, 28,* 145–149. doi:10.1017/S1049023X1300006X.

Participants included 94 paramedic students (63 % women) at Monash University, Australia who completed the JSE. Results showed that men obtained a higher JSE mean score ($M = 113.25$) than women ($M = 107.05$) which was inconsistent with most other findings on gender difference. No statistically significant difference was observed in this cross-sectional study among students in the first-, second-, and third-year of training. Students' age was not associated with the JSE scores.

Youssef, F. F., Nunes, P., Sa, B., & Williams S. (2014). An exploration of changes in cognitive and emotional empathy among medical students in the Caribbean. *International Journal of Medical Education, 5,* 185–192. doi:10.5116/ijme.5412. e641.

Participants included 669 first- to seven-year students (438 women) of the Faculty of Medical Sciences at the University of West Indies, St. Augustine, Trinidad and Tobago. The JSE (S-Version), Toronto Empathy Questionnaire, and the Reading the Mind in the Eye Test (this test involves 36 photographs that show the eye region, asking participants to identify the emotion being expressed in the photos) were administered. In this cross-sectional study, a significant decline in the JSE mean scores was found in year 3 compared to years 1 and 2. Women obtained a significantly higher JSE mean score ($M = 106.9$, $SD = 11.59$) than men ($M = 104.3$, $SD = 11.778$). Correlation coefficient between scores of the JSE and Toronto Empathy Questionnaire was statistically significant ($r = 0.48$, $p < 0.001$); however, correlation between scores of the JSE and the Reading the Mind in the Eye Test was statistically significant but negligible in magnitude ($r = 0.08$, $p = 0.04$).

Interventions to Enhance Empathy

Bazarko, D., Cate, R. A., Azocar, F., & Kreitzer, M. J. (2013). The Impact of an innovative mindfulness-based stress reduction program on the health and well-being of nurses employed in a corporate setting. *Journal of Workplace Behavioral Health, 28*, 107–133. doi:10.1080/15555240.2013.779518. Accessible from: http://dx.doi.org/10.1080/15555240.2013.779518.

> Participants included 36 nurses (all women) who participated in an 8-week Mindfulness-Based Stress Reduction (MBSR) program and completed the JSE and five other tests, three times: prior to participation in the MBSR program (Time 1), immediately after completing the program (Time 2), and 4 months after completing the program (Time 3). Results showed a significant improvement in the JSE scores from Time 1 ($M = 116.59$, $SD = 8.98$) to Time 2 ($M = 123.59$, $SD = 9.31$), which was sustained to Time 3 ($M = 123.0$, $SD = 10.48$). A Cronbach's alpha coefficient of 0.78 was obtained for the JSE in this study sample. Participation in the program also contributed to improvement in scores measuring burnout, general health, serenity, mindfulness and self-compassion.

Bombeke, K., Van Roosbroeck, S., De Winter, B., Debaene, L., Schol, S., Van Hal, G., & Van Royen, P. (2011). Medical students trained in communication skills show a decline in patient-centred attitudes: An observational study comparing two cohorts during clinical clerkships. *Patient Education and Counseling, 84*, 310–318. doi:10.1016/j.pec.2011.03.007.

> Participants included 85 medical students; 37 received preclinical communication skills training, and 48 did not. Participants completed the JSE and a set of other measures on attitudes toward patient-centered care and communication skills learning before and after the training. Results showed no statistically significant change in JSE scores in those who participated in the communication skills training and their counterparts who did not.

Bond, A. R., Mason, H. F., Lemaster, C. M., Shaw, S. E., Mullin, C. S., Hollick, E. A., & Saper, R. B. (2013). Embodied health: The effects of mind-body course for medical students. *Medical Education Online, 18*. doi:10.3402/meo.v18i0.20699.

> Participants included 27 first- and second-year medical students at Boston University School of Medicine, who participated in an 11-week elective embodied health course to enhance their well-being and mindfulness. They completed the JSE, and few other tests before and after course. Although an increase in the JSE mean score was observed after completion of the course, the difference did not reach the conventional level of statistical significance. Significant improvements were observed in measures of self-regulation and self-compassion used in the study.

Brazeau, C. M. L. R., Schroeder, R., Rovi, S., & Boyd, L. (2011). Relationship between medical student service and empathy. *Academic Medicine, 86*, s42–s45. doi:10.1097/ACM.0b013e31822a6ae0.

> Participants included 462 medical students (51 % women) from four classes at the UMDNJ-New Jersey Medical School who completed the JSE at graduation. For two classes, the JSE was also administered at the beginning of medical school. Comparison of students who participated in service activities (such as student-run free clinic to render free patient care services) and

those who did not, showed that the former group obtained a significantly higher JSE mean score ($M = 115.18$) than did the latter group ($M = 107.97$) at graduation. It was also found that students who did not participate in any service activities had lower JSE scores both at the beginning and at the end of medical school. Women were more likely than men to participate in service activities (93 % versus 78 %, respectively), and women outscored men on the JSE ($M = 116.12$ and $M = 111.14$, respectively).

Cataldo, K. P., Peeden, K., Geesey, M. E., & Dickerson, L. (2005). Association between Balint training and physician empathy and work satisfaction. *Family Medicine, 37*, 328–331. Accessible from: http://www.stfm.org/fmhub/fm2005/may/kari328.pdf.

> Participants included 182 family physicians who graduated from the Medical University of South Carolina Family Medicine Residency Program. One group of residents voluntarily participated in the Balint training program ($n = 113$), and another group did not ($n = 69$). Mean score of the JSE for residents who participated in the Balint training program was higher ($M = 119.4$, $SD = 8.9$) than that for nonparticipants ($M = 116.7$, $SD = 13.2$), but the difference was not statistically significant. Also, no significant differences were found between the two groups on overall work satisfaction.

Chen, J. T., LaLopa, J., & Dang, D. K. (2008). Impact of patient empathy modeling on pharmacy students caring for the underserved. *American Journal of Pharmaceutical Education, 72*(2), Article 40.

> Participants included 25 students at the School of Pharmacy and Pharmaceutical Sciences, Purdue University, and the University of Connecticut School of Pharmacy who completed the JSE. They completed the patient empathy modeling assignment to enhance their attitudes toward caring for underserved patients. Comparisons of the JSE scores before and after completing the assignment showed statistically significant improvements in 16 out of 20 items of the JSE. The increase in the mean score of the JSE before ($M = 114$, $SD = 9$) and after completing the patient empathy modeling assignment ($M = 119.6$, $SD = 10.5$) was statistically significant. The pretest–posttest increase in the JSE mean score was 6.5 points for students at Purdue University, and it was 5.0 points for those at the University of Connecticut.

Duke, P., Grosseman, S., Novack, D. H., & Rosenzweig, S. (2015). Preserving third-year medical students' empathy and enhancing self-reflection using small group "virtual hangout" technology. *Medical Teacher, 37*, 566–571. doi:10.3109/0142159X.2014.956057.

> Participants included 259 third-year students (123 women) at Drexel University College of Medicine who were invited to participate in a faculty-facilitated, peer small group course of creating virtual classrooms by using social networking and online learning involving narrative self-reflection, group inquiry and discussion, and peer support. Participants completed the JSE and the Groningen Reflection Ability Scale (GRAS) before and after participation in the course. Results showed that empathy can be sustained after the course (reflected in the JSE scores), and self-reflection can be improved (reflected in the GRAS scores), suggesting that the course could prevent erosion of empathy that has been observed in some other studies with third-year medical students, and can foster reflective ability.

Fernandez-Olano, C., Montoya-Fernandez, J., & Salinas-Sanchez, A. S. (2008). Impact of clinical interview training on the empathy level of medical students and medical and residents. *Medical Teacher, 30*, 322–324. doi:10.1080/0142159070180229.

Participants included 203, of which 137 were second-year medical students at the University of Castilla-La Mancha, and 66 were medical residents at the Family and Community Medicine Teaching Unit of Albacete, Spain. Participants were divided into experimental (82 students and 46 residents) and control groups (55 students and 20 residents). The experimental group participated in a 5-day (25 hours) communication skill training workshop. Significant increase in the JSE pre-posttest mean scores was observed in the experimental group (from 119.5 to 125.1, effect size estimate = 0.78) in students and residents regardless of their gender. No significant change in JSE mean scores was observed in residents of the control group; however, a slight increase in scores (from 118.4 to 119.1) was found in students of the control group.

Forstater, A. T., Chauhan, N., Allen, A., Hojat, M., & Lopez, B. L. (2011). An emergency department shadowing experiences for emergency medicine residents: Can it prevent the erosion of empathy? (Abstract). *Academic Emergency Medicine, 18*(10), s2.

Participants included 12 first-year emergency medicine residents at Thomas Jefferson University Hospital who were randomly divided into experimental and control groups. Each resident in the experimental group shadowed one patient in the emergency department in the first month of residency training. The control group did not participate in shadowing and followed a routine training schedule. The JSE was completed by all residents 2 and 9 months after the shadowing experiment. No substantial difference was observed on the JSE scores between the two groups 2 months after the experiment; however, a larger decline in empathy scores was noticed in the control group (−7.2 points, effect size = 1.2) than that in the experimental group (−2.7 points, effect size = 0.22), suggesting that the erosion of empathy may be prevented by shadowing experiences.

Friedrich, B., Evans-Lacko, S., London, J., Rhydderch, D., & Henderson, C. (2013). Anti-stigma training for medical students: The Education not Discrimination project. *British Journal of Psychiatry, 202,* s89–s94. doi:10.1192/bjp.bp.112.114017.

Participants included 1452 medical students (1066 in intervention group, 587 women; 386 in the control group, 216 women) and the rest in the control group in England. Students in the intervention group participated in an anti-stigma training called "Education not Discrimination" (END). Students completed JSE (four items), The Mental Health Knowledge Schedule (measuring stigma-related mental health knowledge), the Community Attitudes toward the Mentally Ill, and a measure of changes in behavior at the beginning of the program, immediate follow up, and 6-month follow up subsequent to the completion of the program. Results showed significant improvements immediately after the END training in the intervention group as compared to the control group, on measures of empathy, mental health knowledge, attitudes toward mentally ill, and the assessment of intended behavior. However, the improvement was not sustained for a longer time 6 months following the intervention.

Ghetti, C., Chang, J., & Gosman, G. (2009). Burnout, psychological skills, and empathy: Balint training in obstetrics and gynecology residents. *Journal of Graduate Medical Education, 1,* 231–235. doi:10.4300/JGME-D-09-00049.1.

Participants included 17 obstetrics and gynecology residents who participated in a Balint training program and completed the JSE, the Maslach Burnout Inventory (MBI), and the Psychological Medicine Inventory before and after completing the program. Results showed no significant change in scorers on the JSE and MBI; however, overall scores on the Psychological Medicine Inventory improved as a result of participation in the Balint program.

Graham, K. L., Green, S., Kurlan, R., & Pelosi, J. S. (2014). A patient-led educational program on Tourette Syndrome: Impact and implications for patient-centered medical education. *Teaching and Learning in Medicine, 26*, 34–39. doi:10.1080/10 401334.2013.857339.

> Participants included 79 medical residents (56 women) in five New Jersey hospitals who completed the JSE (ten items of the Perspective Taking factor) before and after participation in a patient-centered educational program by patient educators involving young patients with Tourette Syndrome who were accompanied by their parent(s). Results of pre-posttest comparison on the JSE scores showed a statistically significant increase in empathic perspective taking.

Gross, N., Nicolas, M., Neigher, S., McPartland, S., Heyes, M., Wrigley, S., & Kurlan, R. (2014). Planning a patient-centered Parkinson's disease support program: Insights from narrative medicine. *Advances in Parkinson's Disease, 3*, 35–39. doi:10.4236/apd.2014.34006. Accessible from: http://dx.doi.org/10.4236/ apd.2014.34006.

> Participants included six health professionals (internist, neurologist, nurses, and speech therapist), six patients with Parkinson disease, and four of their caregivers. Health professionals participated in seven monthly sessions on improving their narrative skills, and completed the JSE before and after completing the narrative skill training sessions. Pretest–posttest scores on the JSE showed an improvement from $M = 120.67$ to $M = 126.00$. No inferential analysis was reported to test the significance of the difference due to a small sample size.

Hojat, M., Axelrod, D., Spandorfer, J., & Mangione, S. (2013). Enhancing and sustaining empathy in medical students. *Medical Teacher, 35*, 996–1001. doi:10.3109/ 0142159X.2013.802300.

> Participants included 248 second-year medical students (126 women) at Jefferson (currently Sidney Kimmel) Medical College who were divided into experimental and control groups, and participated in this two-phase study. In phase 1, students in the experimental group watched and discussed video clips of patient encounters meant to enhance empathic understanding; those in the control group watch a documentary film. Ten weeks later in phase 2 of the study, students who were in the experimental group were divided into two groups. One group attended a lecture on the importance of empathy in patient care, and the other plus those in the control group watched a movie about racism. The JSE was administered pre-post in phase 1 and posttest in phase 2. Results showed a statistically significant increase in the JSE mean scores for the experimental group in phase 1, from $M = 113.0$ ($SD = 11.4$) in pretest to $M = 115.2$ ($SD = 12.3$) in posttest. No significant change in the JSE scores was found in the control group. In phase 2 of the study, the JSE mean score improvement was sustained in the experimental group who attended the lecture on importance of empathy in patient care, but not in the experimental group who watched a movie about racism in this phase of the study. Also, no significant change of empathy was observed in the control group in the second phase of the study. It is concluded that enhancement of empathy in medical students can be sustained by additional educational reinforcements.

Hsieh, N. K., Herzig, K., Gansky, S. A., & Danley, D. (2006). Changing dentists' knowledge, attitudes and behavior regarding domestic violence through an interactive multimedia tutorial. *Journal of American Dental Association, 137*, 596, 603.

> Participants included 174 (40 % women) practicing dentists (86 in the experimental and 88 in the control groups) who completed a slightly modified version of the JSE (adapted for dentists) and a survey of attitudes toward domestic violence in a randomized controlled trial. An educational tutorial was developed to help dentists about their roles in addressing domestic violence experienced by their patients. The experimental group completed the pretest JSE and the

domestic violence survey at the baseline, then was exposed to the tutorial, and subsequently completed the posttests to examine the impact of the tutorial. The control group completed the pretests, then the posttests, and was exposed to the tutorial after completing the posttests. Findings suggest that the tutorial could significantly improve dentists' knowledge of how to help patients affected by domestic violence, but had less effect on questions pertaining to their attitudes toward domestic violence. Scores of the JSE were significantly correlated with those from the domestic violence survey ($r=0.34$ in pretest; $r=0.40$ in posttest). Although women scored ($M=117.28$, $SD=11.02$) higher than men ($M=114.33$, $SD=12.32$), the difference was not statistically significant. The mean JSE score for total participants in pretest was 115.5 ($SD=11.87$). No significant changes in the JSE pretest posttest mean scores were found in the experimental and control groups.

Kazanowski, M., Perrin, K., Potter, M., & Sheehan, C. (2007). The silence of suffering: Breaking the sound barriers. *Journal of Holistic Nursing, 25*, 195–203. doi:10.1177/0898010107305501.

Participants included 30 nursing students who completed the JSE before and after a course on understanding suffering. Results showed a statistically significant increase in the JSE mean scores from $M=118.6$ (pretest) to $M=124.9$ (posttest).

Lim, B. T., Moriarty, H., & Huthwaite, M. (2011). "Being-in-role": A teaching innovation to enhance empathy communication skills in medical students. *Medical Teacher, 33*, e663–e669. doi:10.3109/0142159X2011.611193.

Participants included 149 medical students (84 women) at the University of Otago, Wellington School of Medicine and Health Sciences in New Zealand. They were divided into an intervention ($n=77$), and a control group ($n=72$). All students participated in seminars and workshops in the Psychological Medicine course. The intervention group participated in an additional one-hour actor facilitated teaching innovation on "how to act-in-role" workshop, focusing on enhancing the participants' capacity to connect with the patients. The JSE was completed by students before and after the course. The Behavioral Change Counselling Index (BECCI) to assess students' competence in consultation was completed by students and tutors. Also, assessments were made, using the Objective Structured Clinical Examination (OSCE) by tutors and students. Results showed no significant difference on the JSE pretest scores between the intervention and control groups; however, a statistically significant difference in posttest was observed on the JSE between the two groups in favor of the intervention group. The intervention group obtained significantly higher tutor ratings on the BECCI and in overall OSCE performances. Findings suggest that teaching "how to act-in-role" was effective not only in increasing medical students' self-reported empathy, but also their competence in consultation skills.

Magee, M., & Hojat, M. (2010). Rocking chair and empathy: A pilot study [Letter to the editor]. *Family Medicine, 42*, 466–467.

Participants included 57 residents from 16 family medicine residency programs who completed the pretest JSE; 18 of them completed the JSE posttest. Residents were given the opportunity in the second year of their training to choose one of their indigent pregnant patients who was in the second trimester of pregnancy to receive the fee gift of a glider rocking chair. Shortly after the baby was born in postpartum period, ten of the resident made a prearranged home visit to the mother of the newborn to assist in assembling the chair while talking with the mother in a friendly manner about child care and well-being. Compared to the residents who did not make such a home visit, the simple home visit experience contributed to an impressive increase of about one standard deviation unit in posttest JSE scores among those residents who made such a home visit.

Misra-Hebert, A. D., Isaacson, J. H., Kohn, M., Hull, A. L., Hojat, M., Papp, K. K., & Calabrese, L. (2012). Improving empathy of physicians through guided reflective writing. *International Journal of Medical Education*, *3*, 71–77. doi:10.5116/ijme.4f7e.e332.

> Participants included 40 staff physicians at the Cleveland Clinic who completed the JSE. Twenty physicians were assigned to participate in a six-session program on narrative medicine and engagement in guided reflective writing (intervention group). Ten physicians received the assigned course reading materials but did not participate in the course sessions (control group 1), and ten physicians neither received the reading materials nor participated in the course sessions. Quantitative and qualitative analyses showed improvements in the intervention group compared to the two control groups. Mean scores of the JSE which was administered three times—at the beginning, at session four of the program, and at the completion of the program—showed steady improvement in the intervention group (117.0, 120.7, and 124.6, respectively) compared to those in the control group 1 (114.6, 116.2, and 110.8, respectively) and those in the control group 2 (118.7, 116.2, and 118.9, respectively). Qualitative analyses of physicians' reflective writings in the intervention group showed compassionate solidarity and empathic concern and more exploration of negative rather than positive emotions.

Potash, J. S., Chen, J. Y., Lam, C. L., & Chau, V. T. (2014). Art-making in a family medicine clerkship: How does it affect medical student empathy? *BMC Medical Education*, *14*, 247. doi:10.1186/s12909-014-0247-4. Accessible from: www.biomedcentral.com/1472-6920/14/247.

> Participants included 161 third-year medical students at the University of Hong Kong who were randomly divided into experimental and control groups in their family medicine clerkship. Students in the experimental group participated in a workshop on arts-making involving in writing poems, creating art works, and writing reflective essays. Those in the control group were involved with clinical problem solving. Students in both groups completed the JSE before and after the workshops. Results showed a decrease in the mean scores of the JSE in both groups. For students in the experimental group, the difference between pretest ($M = 106.6$, $SD = 12.4$) and posttest ($M = 102.2$, $SD = 14.3$) was statistically significant. However, in the control group the pretest ($M = 107.2$, $SD = 11.5$) posttest ($M = 106.6$, $SD = 14.7$) difference did not reach the level of statistical significance. No significant association was found between JSE scores and students' gender and age.

Riess, H., Kelley, J., Bailey, R., Dunn, E., & Phillips, M. (2012). Empathy training for resident physicians: A randomized controlled trial of a neuroscience-informed curriculum. *Journal of General Internal Medicine, 27*, 1280–1286. doi:10.1007/s11606-012.2063-z.

> Participants included 99 residents and fellows (52 % women) in surgery, medicine, anesthesiology, psychiatry, ophthalmology, and orthopedics who were randomly assigned to the intervention ($n = 54$) and control groups ($n = 45$). Physicians in the intervention group participated in a postgraduate medical education program grounded in the neurobiology of empathy, and those in the control group followed the standard residency or fellowship training. Participants completed the JSE, the Ekman Facial Decoding Test, and the Balanced Emotional Empathy Scale (BEES). Each participating physician was assessed by multiple patients using the Consultation and Relational Empathy (CARE) scale, measuring empathy in the context of medical consultation. Results showed statistically significant differences in favor of the intervention group on CARE scale and Ekman Facial Decoding Test. Changes observe on the JSE and BEES in the intervention and control groups were not statistically significant.

Riess, H., Kelley, J. M., Bailey, R., Konowitz, P. M., & Gray, S. T. (2011). Improving empathy and relational skills in otolaryngology residents: A pilot study. *Otolaryngology-Head and Neck Surgery, 144*, 120–122. doi:10.1177/0194599810390897.

> Participants included 11 otolaryngology residents (43 % women) who completed the JSE, the Balanced Emotional Empathy Scale (BEES), the Ekman Facial Decoding Test, and the Consultation and Relational Empathy (CARE). They participated in a brief series of empathy training sessions to increase their knowledge of the neurology and physiology of empathy as well as their self-reported empathy. Patients also rated physicians on the CARE at the baseline and completion of training. Pretest–posttest scores on all measures showed an increase in the expected direction. The change of the JSE mean scores before training was 110.1 ($SD = 10.8$), and after training it increased to 114.3 ($SD = 10.7$). However, the difference was not statistically significant. Also increases in mean scores on the BEES and Ekman Facial Decoding Test were not significant. Pretest–posttest difference on physician-reported CARE mean scores reached the level of statistical significance ($p < 0.01$). However, no statistically significant increase was obtained in patient-reported CARE scores.

Schweller, M., Costa, F. O., Antônio, M. Â., Amaral, E. M., & de Carvalho-Filho, M. A. (2014). The impact of simulated medical consultations on the empathy levels of students at one medical school. *Academic Medicine, 89*, 632–637.

> Participants included 124 fourth-year and 123 sixth-year medical students at the State University of Campinas in Brazil who participated in a simulated medical consultation involving simulated patients in four clinical situations followed by debriefing discussions. Participants completed a Brazilian translation of the JSE and the Interpersonal Reactivity Index (IRI) before and after simulated medical consultation experiences. Results of comparing pre-post simulated medical consultations experiences showed statistically significant increases in scores of the JSE in fourth-years students ($M = 115.8$, $SD = 8.8$ pretest, and $M = 121.1$, $SD = 8.6$ posttest, effect size = 0.61) and in sixth-year students ($M = 117.1$, $SD = 10.0$ pretest, and $M = 123.5$, $SD = 9.9$ posttest, effect size = 0.64). Also, statistically significant pretest–posttest improvements were observed in the IRI scores, but with smaller effect sizes (effect size for the fourth-year = 0.19, and it was 0.20 for sixth-year students).

Sheehan, C. A., Perrin, K. O., Potter, M. L., Kazanowski, M. K., & Bennett, L. A. (2013). Engendering empathy in baccalaureate nursing students. *International Journal of Caring Sciences, 6*, 456–464.

> Participants included 99 baccalaureate nursing students who participated in an elective course on understanding suffering, and completed the JSE before and after participating in the course. Results showed a significant increase in the JSE mean score (from $M = 116.96$ in pretest to $M = 123.97$ in posttest) for the total participants.

Van Winkle, L. J., Bjork, B. C., Chandar, N., Cornell, S., Fjortoft, N., Green, J. M., La Salle, S., Lynch, S. M., Viselli, S. M., & Burdick, P. (2012). Interprofessional workshop to improve mutual understanding between pharmacy and medical students. *American Journal of Pharmaceutical Education, 76*(8), Article 150. Accessible from: http://www.ncbi.nlm.nih.gov/pmc/articles/PMC3475779/.

> Participants included 215 first-year pharmacy students and 205 first-year osteopathic medical students at Midwestern University who completed the JSE, and the Scale of Empathy Toward Physician-Pharmacist Collaboration, and participated in an interprofessional development workshop. Results showed that interprofessional collaboration scores of pharmacy students who participated in the workshop increased significantly, and medical students' scores

increased on the factor of shared education of interprofessional collaboration. The collaboration scores of pharmacy students exceeded those of medical students. Statistically significant correlations between scores of the JSE and the Scale of Physician-Pharmacy Collaboration were found in pharmacy students ($r=0.42$) as well as medical students ($r=0.38$).

Van Winkle, L. J., Burdick, P., Bjork, B. C., Chandar, N., Green, J. M., Lynch, S. M., La Salle, S., Viselli, S. M., & Robson, C. (2014). Critical thinking and reflection on community service for a medical biochemistry course raise students' empathy, patient-centered orientation, and examination scores. *Medical Science Educator, 24*, 279–290. doi:10.1007/s40670-014-0049-7.

Participants included 204 first-year osteopathic medical students (45 % women) at Midwestern University who were required to complete a team community project (such as visiting elderly patients with heart failure, diabetes, etc.) and prepare written reports for group discussion. The JSE and Patient-Practitioner Orientation Scale (PPOS) were administered to the students before and after their community service project was completed. Statistical analyses of pretest–posttest data showed a significant increase in the JSE scores, and the PPOS total and Caring subscale scores as a result of participation in the community service program.

Van Winkle, L. J., Fjortoft, N., & Hojat, M. (2012). Impact of a workshop about aging on the empathy scores of pharmacy and medical students. *American Journal of Pharmaceutical Education, 76*(1), Article 9. doi:10.5688/ajpe7619. Accessible from: http://www.ncbi.nlm.nih.gov/pmc/articles/PMC3298407/.

Participants included 370 first-year pharmacy students ($n=187$) at Chicago College of Pharmacy, Midwestern University, and medical students ($n=183$) at Chicago College of Osteopathic Medicine, Midwestern University who completed the JSE and participated in a workshop in which they observed and discussed a 10-min theatrical performance by their classmates who were coached to enact problems and concerns of elderly patients. Comparisons of the JSE scores before and immediately after the workshop showed a significant increase in medical students (from $M=112.9$, $SD=10.9$ to $M=115.0$, $SD=11.9$) and pharmacy students (from $M=110.9$, $SD=12.2$ to $M=113.2$, $SD=13.5$). However, follow up assessments showed that the improvement in empathy scores did not sustain for a longer time after the workshop (26 days after the workshop for medical students: $M=112.7$, $SD=13.9$; and 7 days after the workshop for pharmacy students: $M=110.5$, $SD=17.3$). Pattern of findings was similar for men and women.

Van Winkle, L. J., La Salle, S., Richardson, L., Bjork, B. C., Burdick, P., Chandar, N., Green, J. M., Lynch, S. M., Robson, C., & Viselli, S. M. (2013). Challenging medical students to confront their biases: A case study simulation approach. *Medical Science Educator, 23*, 217–224.

Study participants included 205 first-year osteopathic medical students (47 % women) at Midwestern University who completed the JSE on five occasions. Students watched a play of a simulated patient in prison during a 50-min workshop of a biochemical case of fatigue. Students were expected to relate this patient with a book, "The Immoral Life of Henrietta Lacks," as a required reading at the beginning of medical school to identify biases through critical reflection. No statistically significant differences on the total scores of the JSE were found before or after students' participation in the workshop; however, statistically significant increase in the score of one item of the JSE (on attention to patients' emotions in history taking) was observed after participation in the workshop which was sustained through the study time period.

West, C. P., Dyrbye, L. N., Rabatin, J. T., Call, T. G., Davidson, J. H., Multari, A., Romanski, S. A., Henriksen Hellyer, J. M., Sloan, J. A., & Shanafelt, T. D. (2014).

Intervention to promote physician well-being, job satisfaction, and professionalism: A randomized clinical trial. *JAMA Internal Medicine, 174*, 527–533. doi:10.1001/jamainternmed.2013.14387.

> Participants included 74 physicians in this clinical trial in Department of Medicine at the Mayo Clinic in Rochester, Minnesota. Thirty-seven were assigned to the intervention arm, and 37 to the control arm of the clinical trial. There were also 350 nontrial physicians who responded to annual surveys timed to coincide with the trial surveys. Physicians in the intervention arm of the clinical trial group participated in 19 biweekly facilitated physician discussions incorporating elements of mindfulness, reflection, and shared experiences. The JSE and a set of other instruments were administered to the physicians before starting, during, and after the trial. No statistically significant change was observed in the JSE scores, or measures of stress, symptoms of depression, overall quality of life, job satisfaction, mental and physical well-being, and fatigue. Comparisons on physicians who volunteered to participate in the trail with the nontrial cohort showed that rates of burnout dropped substantially in the trial intervention arm, declined slightly in the trial control arm, but increased in the nontrial cohort. No other significant changes were observed between trial and nontrial physicians.

Williams, B., Brown, T., & McKenna, L. (2013). DVD empathy simulations: An interventional study. *Medical Education, 47*, 1142–1143.

> Participants included 293 (226 women) health professions students from four Australian universities who participated in empathy-oriented DVD simulation workshops. Participants completed the JSE before and after the workshops. Results showed a statistically significant increase in the JSE (from 114.34 before to 120.32 after participation in the workshops).

Williams, B., Brown, T., McKenna, L., Palermo, C., Morgan, P., … Wright, C. (2015). Student empathy levels across 12 medical and health professions: An interventional study. *Journal of Compassionate Health Care, 2*, 4 (open access). doi:10.1186/s40639-015-0013-4.

> Participants included 239 students from 12 different medical and health care professions from four universities in Australia who completed the JSE pre-posttest intervention. Intervention included watching a 20-min DVD simulation showing a teenager with Asperger's syndrome, a young pregnant woman suffering from stroke, an elderly indigenous woman suffering from a suspected neck of femur fracture. Results showed a statistically significant improvement in the JSE scores as a result of participation in the workshop from a mean scores of 114.39 ($SD = 14.56$) in pretest to 120.56 ($SD = 12.48$) in posttest (effect size = 0.22). Women outscored men in pretest and posttest.

Williams, B., Sadasivan, S., Kadirvelu, A., & Olaussen, A. (2014). Empathy level among first year Malaysian medical students: An observational study. *Advances in Medical Education and Practice, 5*, 149–156. doi:10.2147/AMEP.S58094.

> Participants included 122 first-year students (56 % women) at the Jeffrey Cheah School of Medicine and Health Sciences in Malaysia who participated in a workshop to enhance empathic awareness by watching and discussing a video involving a pregnant patient suffering from a stroke. The JSE was completed by participants before and five weeks after the workshop. Results showed a statistically significant improvement in mean score of the JSE from 112.08 ($SD = 10.76$) before to 117.93 ($SD = 13.13$) after the workshop (effect size = 0.48). Women were influenced by the workshop more than men (effect size = 0.54). Cronbach's alpha coefficient for this Malaysian sample was 0.70 before and 0.83 after the workshop.

Worly, B. (2013). Professionalism education of OB/GYN resident physicians: What makes a difference? *Open Journal of Obstetrics and Gynecology*, *3*, 137–141. doi:10.4236/ojog.2013.31A026.

> Participants included 32 obstetrics and gynecology residents at Thomas Jefferson University Hospital who participated in a new professionalism program involving narrative medicine training and a professional development/support group. Twenty residents completed the JSE, the Jefferson Scale of Attitudes Toward Physician-Nurse Collaboration, and the Barry Challenges to Professionalism Questionnaire. Comparisons of scores pre and post program showed no statistically significant changes on the JSE and on the Barry Questionnaire. A significant decline in scores on attitudes toward physician-nurse collaboration was observed.

Yang, K. T., & Yang, J. H. (2013). A study of the effect of a visual arts-based program on the scores of Jefferson Scale of Physician Empathy. *BMC Medical Education*, *13*, 142. Accessible from: http://www.biomedcentral.com/1472-6920/13/142.

> Participants included 110 (92 medical students clerks and 18 first-year residents; 33 women) who completed the JSE. The intervention program in this pretest–posttest study design, included exposing participants to visual arts for appreciation of paintings related to human suffering, and discussion of related arts such as novels, poems, music, and films. The purpose was to help participants to use visual art as a tool for physician competency development and improvement of their interest in the arts. Psychometric findings, using pretest data, supported the three-factor model (exploratory factor analysis). Cronbach's coefficient alpha was 0.81, and the mean score was 110.92 ($SD = 10.3$). The pretest JSE mean score was significantly lower for residents compared to medical students. The JSE mean score increase in the posttest ($M = 111.30$, $SD = 11.57$) was not significantly different from that of pretest scores.

Yaghmaei, M., Monajemi, A., & Soltani-Arabshahi, K. (2014). The effect of storytelling course on medical students' empathy toward patients. *International Journal of Body, Mind & Culture*, *1*, 127–134.

> Study participants included 41 medical students at Zahedan University of Medical Sciences in Iran (16 in the experimental and 25 in the control group). Students in the experimental group participated in ten sessions of storytelling, each lasting two hours in which stories from books and literature about human illness, pain, and suffering, selected by the researchers were described and discussed. Students in both groups completed the JSE before and after the experiment. Those in the experimental groups gained less than one point on the JSE (pretest mean score = 106.7, $SD = 12.78$; posttest mean score = 107.6, $SD = 11.32$); but the JSE mean score declined 5.68 points in the control group (pretest mean score = 105.8, $SD = 15.24$; posttest mean score = 100.12, $SD = 14.04$). However, the pretest–posttest changes in empathy scores were not statistically significant.

Tangible Patient Outcomes of Physician's Empathy

Del Canale, S., Louis, D. Z., Maio, V., Wang, X., Rossi, G., Hojat, M., & Gonnella, J. S. (2012). The relationship between physician empathy and disease complications: An empirical study of primary care physicians and their diabetic patients in Parma, Italy. *Academic Medicine*, *87*, 1243–1249. doi:10.1097/ACM. 0b013e3182628fbf.

Participants included 242 primary care physicians in Parma, Italy who completed an Italian translation of the JSE. Electronic records of 20,961 adult patients with type 1 or type 2 diabetes mellitus who were treated by one of these physicians were examined, and information on acute metabolic complications that required hospitalization (e.g., diabetic ketoacidosis, coma, and hyperosmolar) and demographic information were extracted. Results showed statistically significant associations between physicians' scores on the JSE and rates of hospitalization due to metabolic complications in their diabetic patients. Rates of disease complication in diabetic patients of physicians who scored high on the JSE ($\geq$112), compared to other physicians with moderate scores (111–97) or low JSE scores (<97) were 4.0, 7.1, and 6.5 per 1000, respectively. The association remained statistically significant after controlling for physicians' gender, age, type of practice (solo or group), geographical location of practice (pain, hills, mountain); and also patients' gender, age, and duration of time enrolled with the physician.

Hojat, M., Louis, D. Z., Markham, F. W., Wender, R., Rabinowitz, C., & Gonnella, J. S. (2011). Physicians' empathy and clinical outcomes in diabetic patients. *Academic Medicine*, 86, 359–364. doi: 10.1097/ACM.0b013e3182086fe1.

Participants included 29 family physicians in Department of Family and Community Medicine at Jefferson (currently Sidney Kimmel) Medical College who completed the JSE. Electronic records of 891 adult patients with diabetes mellitus who were treated by one of these physicians were examined, and information on the most recent results of hemoglobin A1c and low-density lipoprotein cholesterol (LDL-C), and selected demographic information were extracted. Positive clinical outcomes were defined as good control of the disease reflected in A1c test results <7.0 % and LDL-C <100. Results showed that physicians' scores on the JSE could significantly predict clinical outcomes in their diabetic patients. Patients of physicians with high JSE scores were significantly more likely to have good control of their disease (56 % had A1c < 7.0, and LDL-C < 100), compared to patients of physicians with low JSE scores (40 % had A1c < 7.0 and LDL-C < 100). The association between physicians' scores on the JSE and patient outcomes remained statistically significant after controlling for physicians' gender and age; and also patients' gender, age, and type of health insurance.

Combined Results and Miscellaneous Findings Using the JSE

Arora, S., Ashrafian, H., Davis, R., Athanasiou, T., Darzi, A., & Sevdalis, N. (2010). Emotional intelligence in medicine: A systematic review through the context of the ACGME competencies. *Medical Education, 44*, 749–764. doi:10.1111/j.1365-2923.2010.03709.x.

In this article, 485 citations were identified from a review of relevant literature in the English language published between January 1980 and March 2009 about measures used to assess emotional intelligence (EI) and its outcomes as related to the six core competencies that constitute the hallmarks of graduate medical education proposed by the Accreditation Council for Graduate Medical Education (ACGME): Patient care, professionalism, system-based practice, interpersonal and communication skills, medical knowledge, and practice-based learning. Sixteen articles were included in the final collection that met the inclusion criteria. Four of these studies examined relationships between EI and empathy (measured by the JSE and the IRI). Results generally suggest that women obtained higher empathy and EI scores than men, and that EI is positively associated with compassionate care, empathic patient care, communication and interpersonal skills, and teamwork and collaboration.

Austin, E. J., Evans, P., Magnus, B., & O'Hanlon, K. N. (2007). A preliminary study of empathy, emotional intelligence and examination performance in MBChB students. *Medical Education, 41*, 684–689. doi:10.1111/j.1365-2923.2007.02795.x.

> Participants included 273 medical students (85 women) in years 1, 2, and 5 of the MBChB program at Edinburg University who completed the JSE and an emotional intelligent (EI) scale. Results showed that women scored significantly higher than did men on the JSE and EI scale. A declining trend in the JSE mean score was observed between years 1 and 2 in women, but an increasing trend in the JSE scores was noticed in men. Cronbach's alpha coefficient for the JSE in this sample was 0.88.

Babar, M. G., Omar, H., Lim, L. P., Khan, S. A., Mitha, S., & Ahmad, S. F. B. (1013). An assessment of dental students' empathy levels in Malaysia. *International Journal of Medical Education, 4*, 223–229. doi:10.5116/ijme.5259.4513.

> Participants included 582 (141 women) first- to fifth-year dental students at two public universities: the University of Malaya, University Technology Mara and one private university: International Medical University. They completed the JSE (HPS) version. Results of exploratory factor analysis (principal component factor analysis) showed three factors of "perspective-taking," "compassionate care," and "standing in patient's shoes" similar to most other findings with US health profession students. The overall Cronbach's alpha coefficient was 0.70. Students enrolled at public universities obtained significantly higher mean JSE scores than their counterparts in the private university. Third-year students obtained the lowest mean empathy scores than those in other years. Students of Indian origin enrolled at public universities and students of Chinese origin enrolled at the private university obtained higher JSE mean scores than other ethnic groups.

Brown, T., Boyle, M., Williams, B., Molloy, A., Palermo, C., McKenna, L., & Molloy, L. (2011). Predictors of empathy in health science students. *Journal of Allied Health, 40*, 143–149.

> Participants included 860 undergraduate health science students (750 women) at Monash University in Australia who completed the JSE, the Listening Style Profile, and the Communication Style Profile. Results showed that the JSE mean score for the sample was 115.5 ($SD = 13.1$). Women scored a significantly higher JSE mean score ($M = 116.4, SD = 12.3$) than did men ($M = 109.5, SD = 15.8$). In multiple regression statistical analyses, gender and factors such as People and Time (of the Listening Style Profile) and Friendly and Relaxed Style of communication (of the Communication Style Profile) predicted the JSE scores.

Colliver, J. A., Conlee, M. J., Verhulst, S. J., & Dorsey, J. K. (2010). Reports of the decline of empathy during medical education are greatly exaggerated: A reexamination of the research. *Academic Medicine, 85*, 588–593.

> This study reviews findings on 11 published studies in which a decline in empathy in medical and dental schools was reported. The JSE was used in five of these studies. Concern was raised about the validity of the empathy measuring instruments used in these studies, and about practical significance of these findings on the ground that response rates in most of these studies were low, and the effect size estimates were not large enough to warrant a strong conclusion that empathy erodes during training. (These critics were not left unchallenged by five researchers including myself, see *Academic Medicine*, 2010, 85, pp. 1812–1813.)

Colliver, J. A., Conlee, M. J., Verhulst, S. J., & Dorsey, J. K. (2010). Rebuttals to critics on studies of the decline of empathy [Letter to the editor]. *Academic Medicine, 85*, 1813–1814.

This is a response to the rebuttals (*Academic Medicine*, 2010, *85*, 1812–1813) by the authors whose studies were reviewed by Colliver et al. (*Academic Medicine*, 2010, *85*, 588–593). Colliver and his colleagues confirmed that the JSE was developed "on an extensive research base and had a solid psychometric foundation—possibly the most researched and widely used instrument in medical education" (p. 1913) [which defies their own criticism about the validity of empathy measuring instruments]. Despite their failure to recognize the empirical evidence presented in other rebuttals (Hojat et al., *Academic Medicine, 85*, 1812–1813) on the link between physicians' scores on the JSE and patient outcomes or physicians' self-reported JSE scores and patients' assessments of physician empathy, Colliver et al. persisted with their unsubstantiated criticisms that the decline in empathy in physicians-in-training reported in several empirical studies has been exaggerated.

Consorti, F., Notarangelo, M. A., Potasso, L. A., & Toscano, E. (2012). Developing professionalism in Italian medical students: An educational framework. *Advances in Medical Education and Practice, 3*, 55–60. doi:10.2147/AMEP.S31228.

The study by researchers at the Faculty of Medicine and Dentistry of the University Sapienza of Rome, Italy summarizes the main issues and experiences in development of professionalism among Italian medical students. The JSE was chosen by investigators as one the three instruments, validated in Italy, for the overall assessment of professionalism in the context of health profession education.

Crandall, S. J., & Marion, G. S. (2009). Commentary: Identifying attitudes towards empathy: An essential feature of professionalism. *Academic Medicine, 84*, 1174–1176.

In this commentary, the authors make some remarks about three empirical studies published in the same issue of the journal with samples of medical students and physicians from the USA, Japan, and Italy in which the JSE was used. It is proposed that decline in empathy in medical education and the practice of medicine can be remedied through the promotion of relationship-centered patient care and interprofessional education and practice.

Dyrbye, L. N., Eacker, A. M., Harper, W., Power, D. V., Massie Jr., F. S., Satele, D., Thomas, M. R., Sloan, J. A., & Shanafelt, T. D. (2012). Distress and empathy do not drive changes in specialty preference among US medical students. *Medical Teacher, 34*, e116–e122. doi:10.3109/0142159x.2012.644830.

Participants included 858 medical students (473 women) at Mayo Clinic College of Medicine, University of Alabama School of Medicine, University of Minnesota Medical School, and University of Washington School of Medicine who completed the JSE and the Maslach Burnout Inventory (MBI) plus a survey to measure symptoms of depression and quality of life. Results showed no significant change of JSE scores in those who did change their specialty interest during medical school ($M = 1186$, $SD = 10.53$) and their counterparts who did not change their interest ($M = 117.6$, $SD = 11.31$). Scores on Depersonalization scale of the MBI declined among those who changed their specialty preference. In a multivariate logistic regression analysis it was found that being male, being a third-year student, and scores on the Depersonalization scale of the MBI independently predicted a change in specialty preference in medical students.

Gonçalves-Pereira, M., Trancas, B., Loureiro, J., Papoila, A., & Caldas-De-Almeida, J. M. (2013). Empathy as related to motivations for medicine in a sample of first-year medical students. *Psychological Reports, 11*, 73–88. doi:10.2466/17.13. PR0.112.1.73-88.

Participants included 202 medical students (136 women) at the Faculty of Medical Sciences, Nova University in Lisbon, Portugal who completed a Portuguese translation of the JSE, plus other instruments for measuring motivation to pursue medicine, and specialty interest. Results showed a mean score of 110 ($SD = 11$) for the total sample. Although women obtained a JSE mean score which was higher than that for men ($M = 110.74$, $SD = 10.50$ for women; $M = 107.79$, $SD = 10.12$ for men), the difference was not statistically significant. Cronbach's alpha coefficient was 0.75. Those who scored high on the people orientation index, as opposed to status/security index of motivation measure, trend to score higher on the JSE. Although the JSE mean score for students who expressed an interest to pursue medical specialties ($M = 110.3$, $SD = 9.3$) and those interested in medico-surgical specialties ($M = 109.72$, $SD = 10.92$) was higher than others who were unsure about their specialty interest ($M = 106.69$, $SD = 9.96$), the difference was not statistically significant.

Hasan, S. H., Babar, M. G., Chen, K. K., Ahmed, S. I., & Mitha, S. (2013). An assessment of pharmacy students' empathy levels in Malaysia. *Journal of Advanced Pharmacy Education & Research*, *3*, 531–540.

Participants included 719 first- to fourth-year pharmacy students (596 women) in a public university (University of Kebangsaan Malaysia, $n = 313$) and a private university (International Medical University, $n = 406$) in Malaysia who completed the JSE (HPS version). Exploratory factor analysis of data resulted in three factors of Perspective Taking, Compassionate Care, and Standing in Patient's Shoes, consistent with most other factor analytic studies of the JSE. Inconsistent with most other studies, men scored higher than women in this Malaysian sample. Students in the private university scored higher on the JSE than did those in the public university. No statistically significant association was observed between the JSE scores and students' ages. A statistically significant decline in empathy mean score was found between second- and fourth-year students in this cross-sectional study. Cronbach's alpha coefficient was 0.70.

Hemmerdinger, H. M., Stoddart, A. D. R., & Lilford, R. J. (2007). A systematic review of tests of empathy in medicine. *BMC Medical Education*, *7*, 24. doi:10.1186/1472-6920-7-24. Accessible from: http://www.biomedcentral.com/1472-6920/7/24.

The authors reported that based on their systematic review of the literature (using Medline, EMBASE, and PsycINFO data bases) on reliability and validity of empathy measuring instruments in medical students and physicians, 50 relevant papers were identified from 1147 citations in the English language. Thirty-six instruments were used in the identified studies. Eight instruments (including the JSE) demonstrated evidence in support of their validity, internal consistency, and reliability. The authors concluded that no empathy measures were found with sufficient evidence of predictive validity for use in medical school admissions.

Gonnella, J. S., Hojat, M., & Veloski, J. J. (2011). AM last page: The Jefferson longitudinal study of medical education. *Academic Medicine, 86*, 404.

In this a one-page snapshot of the Jefferson Longitudinal Study of Medical Education, the history, goals, and scope of the Jefferson Longitudinal Study were briefly described. In this snapshot, the Jefferson Scale of Empathy was described among the major medical education outcomes of the Jefferson Longitudinal Study which contains over 10,600 students and graduates of Jefferson (currently Sidney Kimmel) Medical College at Thomas Jefferson University. The study garnered data from more than 573 postgraduate programs, and inspired over 179 publications in peer-reviewed journals, including a considerable number of publications on empathy in medical education and patient care.

Hojat, M. (2014). Assessments of empathy in medical school admissions: What additional evidence is needed? *International Journal of Medical Education, 5,* 7–10. doi:10.5116/ijme.52b7.5294.

> In this invited editorial it is argued that personality plays an unquestionable role in human behavior and in the care of the patient. The crucial question is which personality attributes are more credible for the assessment of professional development of doctors-in-training and for consideration in the admission of applicants to medical schools. Three requirements are proposed: (1) Conceptual relevancy of personality attributes to clinical competence and patient outcomes, (2) Availability of a psychometrically sound instrument to measure the desirable attribute, and (3) Empirical link of the personality attribute to clinical competence and patient outcomes. Evidence is presented in support of the idea that empathy, as measured by the JSE, seems to be a unique personality attribute than can meet all of the three requirements. It is suggested that for rendering more optimal care, for regaining the lost reputation of the profession of medicine, and for reclaiming a compassionate image of doctors, bold actions must be taken to break free from lingering doubts, persistent skepticism, and a lack of enthusiasm to include assessments of pertinent personality attributes, including empathy measured by the JSE in medical school admission decisions.

Hojat, M. (2009). Ten approaches for enhancing empathy in health and human services cultures. *Journal of Health and Human Services Administration, 31,* 412–450.

> In this article, conceptualization and measurement of empathy in medicine and other health professions are discussed and emphasis is placed on the usefulness of the JSE in quantifying empathy in the context of health profession education and the practice of medicine. The following ten approaches for enhancing empathy in health profession students and practitioners are described: improving interpersonal skills, using audio- or video-taping of encounters with patients, exposure to positive role models, role playing, shadowing a patient, hospitalization experiences, studying literature and the arts, improving narrative skills, theatrical performances, and the Balint method.

Hojat, M., Erdmann, J. B., & Gonnella, J. S. (2014*). Personality assessments and outcomes in medical education and the practice of medicine-AMEE Guide 79.* Dundee, UK: Association for Medical Education in Europe (AMEE). First published in 2013 in *Medical Teacher, 35,* e1267–e1301.

> In a paradigm of physician performance, it is proposed that both "cognitive" (academic performance), and "noncognitive" (personal qualities) components contribute to performance of physicians-in-training and physicians-in-practice. Personality as an important factor of the "noncognitive" component plays a significant role in academic and professional performance outcomes. In this article, 14 personality instruments which were frequently used in medical education research, their strengths and shortcomings, and their major findings relevant to health profession education and practice are described. It is suggested that two conditions must be met for including personality measures for the assessment of applicants to medical school or candidates for postgraduate medical education, as well as in the assessment of professional development of physicians-in-training or in-practice. These include: (1) conceptual relevance to clinical performance and patient outcomes, (2) Strong psychometric support for the instrument's validity (particularly predictive validity) and reliability. It is argued that among the selected personality instruments, the Jefferson Scale of Empathy can successfully meet the two aforementioned conditions. It is suggested that another conceptually relevant personality attribute with reasonable support for its psychometrics is "conscientiousness." It is concluded that the lingering doubts and hesitation to use personality assessments in the selection and professional development of trainees in medicine, can result in a futile and never-ending search for

additional evidence which would be counterproductive. Leaders, admission officers, and faculty in medical and other health profession education are encouraged to take a bold action to incorporate personality assessments as complementary measures in admissions and in professional development of students for the sake of medicine to regain its well-deserved reputation, and to reclaim the altruistic image that physicians used to embody.

Hojat, M., Gonnella, J. S., Mangione, S., Nasca, T. J., & Magee, M. (2003). Physician empathy in medical education and practice: Experience with the Jefferson Scale of Physician Empathy. *Seminars in Integrative Medicine, 1*, 25–41.

This is a report summarizing our experiences in the development and psychometrics of the JSE. Starting with conceptualization and definition of empathy in the context of medical education and patient care, a distinction is made between empathy and sympathy, and their different consequences in patient outcomes. Then we briefly described the step-by-step development of the JSE, and provided evidence in support of its validity and reliability. Our findings at the time of writing this article about gender and specialty differences in the JSE scores were reported. We proposed that empathy is amenable to change and described a few approaches that could help to enhance empathy in physicians-in-training.

Hojat, M., Gonnella, J. S., & Veloski, J. (2010). Rebuttals to critics of studies of the decline of empathy [Letters to the editor]. *Academic Medicine, 85*, 1812.

This is a rebuttal in response to critics by Colliver and his colleagues (2010) about findings of 11 studies in which a decline of empathy during health profession education had been reported. It is argued that Colliver and colleagues failed to recognize the extensive literature on psychometrics of the JSE, used in five of their reviewed studies, and also overlooked the findings that reported a significant association between physicians' empathy to clinical outcomes. Furthermore, it is argued that Colliver and colleagues' suggestion to transform scores on each scale back to the unit of the original Likert scale for addressing the clinical or practical significance of the findings did not make sense due to the fact that the three instruments used in the reviewed studies used three different types of 4-, 7-, and 9-point Likert scales which obviously cannot lead to a "scale free" measure to examine the practical importance of the findings. Instead, it is suggested that a widely used approach for examining the practical or clinical significance of the findings is to calculate the effect size of the differences which yields a "scale free" and an operationally defined index (ranged from 0.29 to 0.64 in the Jefferson studies). It is concluded that the concerns raised by Colliver and colleagues were mostly baseless.

Hojat, M., Louis, D. Z., Maio, V., & Gonnella, J. S. (2013). Empathy and health care quality [Editorial]. *American Journal of Medical Quality, 28*, 6–7. doi:10.1177/1062860612464731.

In this editorial, it is suggested that empathic engagement in patient care evolves around reciprocity and mutual understanding which evokes "psychosocial" and "bioneurological" responses, providing plausible explanations for the significant associations reported in two empirical studies between physician empathy (measured by the JSE) and clinical outcomes in diabetic patients. At the psychosocial level, empathic engagement lays the foundation for a trusting relationship, prompting the patient to tell the tale of his or her illness without concealment. This leads to a more accurate diagnosis and greater compliance. At the bioneurological level, empathic engagement is described as analogous to a synchronized dance between patient and caregiver, orchestrated by bioneurological markers. Also, a set of neurons, known as the mirror neuron system, is discharged by observing actions or emotions of another person which is believed to play a crucial role in understanding the experiences of other human beings, a key ingredient of empathic engagement. Such bioneurological interaction has also been highlighted in the perception-action theory, suggesting that perceptions of another person's cognitive, affective, or somatosensory states automatically activate representations of those states in the observer, unless inhibited. The combined effects of these psychosocial and bioneurological mechanisms provide plausible explanation for the findings that physician's empathic engagement in patient care (reflected in higher JSE scores) paves the road to more optimal clinical outcomes.

Hojat, M., Louis, D. Z., Maxwell, K., & Gonnella, J. S. (2011). The Jefferson Scale of Empathy (JSE): An update. *Health Policy Newsletter, 24*, 5–6. Accessible from: http://jdc.jefferson.edu/cgi/viewcontent.cgi?article = 1727&context = hpn.

This is a brief article highlighting some of the empirical findings on the JSE including associations of JSE scores with gender, clinical competence, long-term predictive validity, specialty choice, peer nomination, objective structured clinical examinations (OSCE), erosion of empathy during medical education, enhancement of empathy by targeted educational programs, patient perceptions of physician empathy, and patient outcomes.

Hong, M., Bahn, G. H., Lee, W. H., & Moon, S. J. (2011). Empathy in Korean psychiatric residents. *Asia-Pacific Psychiatry, 3*, 83–90. doi:10.1111/j.1758-5872.2011.00123x.

Participants included 316 residents (133 women) in 82 psychiatric residency training programs in Korea who completed the JSE and the Cloninger's Temperament and Character Inventory (TCI). Results showed that married residents scored higher on the JSE ($M = 105.2$, $SD = 11.1$) than unmarried residents ($M = 102.0$, $SD = 11.8$). In this cross-sectional study, steady increase in the JSE scores was observed as residents progressed through residency training. It was found that mean scores of the JSE in the third year ($M = 105.2$, $SD = 9.3$) and fourth year ($M = 106.0$, $SD = 13.8$) were higher than those in the first-year ($M = 100.7$, $SD = 11.6$), and second year ($M = 101.2$, $SD = 11.1$) of residency training. Statistically significant positive correlations were found between scores of the JSE and the TCI's personality attributes such as Cooperativeness ($r = 0.39$), Persistence ($r = 0.31$), Self-Directedness ($r = 0.29$), and Reward Dependence ($r = 0.28$). Also, a significantly negative correlation was observed between the JSE and Harm and Avoidance scores of the TCI ($r = -0.26$).

Lee, B. K., Bahn, G. H., Lee, W. H., Park, J. H., Yoon, T. Y., & Baek, S. B. (2009). The relationship between empathy and medical education system, grades, and personality in medical college students and medical school students. *Korean Journal of Medical Education, 21*, 117–124. doi:10.3946/kjme.2009.21.2.117.

Participants included 155 (36 women) medical college (MC) and 137 (83 women) medical school (MS) students who completed a Korean translation of the JSE and the Temperament and Character Inventory (TCI). Results showed no significant gender difference on the JSE scores ($M = 106.8$, $SD = 11.6$ for men and $M = 109.2$, $SD = 11.0$ for women). Also, no significant association was observed between the JSE scores and internal or external motivation to pursue medicine, and interest in the people-oriented and technology-oriented specialties. Students in the medical school system obtained a statistically significant higher JSE mean score ($M = 109.2$, $SD = 11.1$) than their counterparts in the medical college system ($M = 106.6$, $SD = 11.6$). Significant correlations in the 0.30s were found between JSE and Cooperativeness, Self-Directedness, and Reward Dependence scale scores of the TCI.

Mandel, E. D., & Schweinle, W. E. (2012). A study of empathy decline in physician assistant students at completion of first didactic year. *The Journal of Physician Assistant Education, 23*, 16–24.

Participants included 328 (270 women) physician assistant students at the Seton Hall University who completed the JSE within 4 weeks of matriculation, one year later, and approximately one year through their clinical training. Because data were collected anonymously no one-to-one matching in different time points was possible for inferential statistical analyses. The findings showed women obtained a higher JSE mean score than men. Cronbach's alpha coefficient was 0.80. Although a declining trend was observed in empathy scores as students progressed through the physician assistant program, the trend was not substantial. No significant association was found between scores on the JSE and specialty preferences, or with health care experiences prior to matriculating in the physician assistant program.

Neumann, M., Edehäuser, F., Tauschel, D., Fischer M. R., Wirtz, M., Woopen, C., Haramati, A., & Scheffer, C. (2011). Empathy decline and its reasons: A systematic review of studies with medical students and residents. *Academic Medicine, 86,* 996–1009.

In this review study, the authors searched the PubMed, EMBASE, and PsycINFO electronic databases, and identified 669 studies in English, each with a sample size of 30 or greater, published from January 1990 through January 2010 by using keywords "empathy," "medical education," and "change" of which 18 articles were selected which met their selection criteria. None of those articles documented an increase in self-assessed empathy, two reported increase empathy only during early years of medical school but significant declines on entering the clinical phase of medical school. The authors reported that the most valid and reliable measures of self-assessed empathy used most frequently in these studies were the Jefferson Scale of Empathy (JSE) and the Interpersonal Reactivity Index (IRI). The authors concluded that their review of eligible studies, especially those with longitudinal data suggests that empathy declines during medical education, particularly in the clinical phase of medical education, and among those who are interested in patient remote specialties (e.g., procedure-oriented).

Neumann, M., Scheffer, C., Tauschel, D., Lutz, G., Wirtz, M., & Edelhäuser, F. (2012). Physician empathy: Definition, outcome-relevance and its measurement in patient care and medical education. *GMS Zeitschrift Für Medizinische Ausbildung, 29,* 11–21. Accessible from: http://www.ncbi.nlm.nih.gov/pmc/articles/ PMC3296095/.

Participants included 44 medical students (20 women) and 63 from other disciplines (38 women) at the University of Cologne in Germany who completed German translations of the JSE and the Interpersonal Reactivity Index (IRI). Results of psychometric analyses of both the JSE and IRI showed that they are promising tools to evaluate achievement of educational objectives and to assess empathy in German medical students.

Pedersen, R. (2009). Empirical research on empathy in medicine: A critical review. *Patient Education and Counseling, 76,* 307–322. doi:10.1016/j.pec.2009.06.012.

This is a review article on measures of empathy used in health education research. The authors identified 200 publications for their critical review. The JSE and the Jefferson Scale of Patient Perceptions of Physician Empathy (JSPPPE) were among the reviewed instruments. It is concluded that empirical research on empathy in medicine is dominated by relatively narrow quantitative research including physicians' and patients' cognitive understanding and affective experiences to a limited degree.

Spiro, H. (2009). Commentary: The practice of empathy. *Academic Medicine, 84,* 1177–1179.

In this commentary, the author makes some remarks about three empirical studies published in the same issue of the journal, with samples of medical students and physicians from the USA, Japan, and Italy in which the JSE was used. The author maintains that in patient care, the eye is for accuracy to discern diseases, but the ear is for truth to hear patients' complaints. With regard to the findings on decline of the JSE scores in physicians-in-training, the author explained that there is a risk of losing humanities in the crusade for "evidence-based" certainty in medicine than can led to a loss of empathy. It is suggested that in this protocol-based era, selecting medical students as much for their character as their knowledge may be one approach to promote empathy; ensuring that faculty and preceptors serve as reliable role models of empathic understanding for physicians-in-training.

Tavakol, S., Dennick, R., & Tavakol, M. (2011). Empathy in UK medical students: Differences by gender, medical year and specialty interest. *Education for Primary Care*, *22*, 297–303.

Participants included 853 medical students (470 women) at the University of Nottingham Medical School who completed the JSE-S. Three hypotheses were tested: (1) Women would score higher than men on the JSE, (2) Scores of the JSE decline as students progress through medical school in this cross-sectional study, and (3) Students interested in "people-oriented" specialties would score higher on the JSE than students interested in "technology-oriented" specialties. The first and third hypotheses were confirmed, but the second hypothesis was not.

Wen, D., Ma, X., Li, H., Liu, Z., Xian, B., & Liu, Y. (2013). Empathy in Chinese medical students: Psychometric characteristics and differences by gender and year of medical education. *BMC Medical Education, 13*, 130. doi:10.1186/1472-6920-13-130.

Participants included 753 first- to fourth-year Chinese students (476 women) at China Medical University who completed a Chinese translation of the JSE. Exploratory factor analysis resulted in three factors of Perspective Taking, Compassionate Care, and the Ability to Stand in Patient's Shoes, similar to those emerged in a majority of factor analytic studies of the JSE. The JSE mean score for the total sample was 109.60 ($SD = 12.09$), and Cronbach's alpha coefficient was 0.83. Women obtained a significantly higher mean JSE scores ($M = 111.53$, $SD = 10.72$) than men ($M = 106.29$, $SD = 13.53$). No significant association was found between JSE scores and student's age. An upward trend in empathy scores was observed in this cross-sectional study as students progressed through medical school. However, only the difference between the JSE mean score for the fourth-year students was significantly higher ($M = 112.12$, $SD = 13.55$) than that for first-year students ($M = 107.36$, $SD = 13.35$).

Williams, B., Boyle, M., Brightwell, R., Devenish, S., Hartley, P., McCall, M., McMullen, P., Munro, G., O'Meara, P., & Webb, V. (2012). Paramedic empathy levels: Results from seven Australian universities. *International Journal of Emergency Services*, *1*, 111–121. Accessible from: www.emeraldinsight.com/doi/abs/10.1108/20470891211275902.

Participants included 784 paramedic students (449 women) from seven Australian universities who completed the JSE (HPS-Version). Results showed an overall JSE mean score of 106.74 ($SD = 14.8$) for this sample. A statistically significant gender difference was found in favor of women ($M = 108.69$, $SD = 14.65$ for women; $M = 103.81$, $SD = 14.17$ for men). The lowest JSE mean score was obtained by the first-year students ($M = 106.29$, $SD = 15.40$), and the highest by fourth-year students ($M = 110.60$, $SD = 13.71$), but the differences by level of training were not statistically significant. Cronbach's alpha coefficient was 0.83.

Williams, B., Boyle, M., Tozer-Jones, J., Devenish, S., Hartley, P., McCall, M., McMullen, P., Munro, G., & O'Meara, P. (2015). Undergraduate paramedic students' empathy levels: A 2-year longitudinal study. *Journal of Nursing Education and Practice*, 5, 58–64. doi:10.5430/jnep.v5n1p58. Accessible from: http://dx.doi. org/10.5430/jnep.v5n1p58.

> Participants included 1719 undergraduate first-, second-, and third-year paramedic students (979 women) from six Australian universities who completed the JSE (HPS-Version). The overall JSE mean score was 105.92 ($SD = 12.85$). Women obtained a significantly higher JSE mean score than did men ($M = 107.45$ and $M = 103.86$ for women and men, respectively, effect size = 0.28). The JSE scores did not change by level of training in this cross-sectional study. No significant association was found between JSE scores and students' ages.

Yu, J., & Kirk, M. (2009). Evaluation of empathy measurement tools in nursing: Systematic review. *Journal of Advanced Nursing*, 65, 1790–1806. doi:10.1111/ j.1365-2648.2009.05071.x.

> In this review article, based on an extensive literature review of empathy measuring instruments in nursing samples published in 20 years (between 1987 and 2007), 20 tools were identified on which 12 were selected that met the inclusion criteria (e.g., full description of the original development, reported psychometrics properties including validity and reliability, and publication in English language).The JSE was one of the selected tools. However, because only a few early publications (between 2001–2003) about the JSE were reviewed, some specific features of the JSE (e.g., confirmation of the latent variable structure, utility in the assessment of changes, applicability to students as well as practitioners in all health profession disciplines and specialties) could not be captured in this review.

Doctoral Dissertations and Theses

Holub, P. G. (2011). *The influence of narrative in fostering affective development of medical professionalism in an online class* (unpublished doctoral dissertation). Nova Southeastern University, Ft. Lauderdale, FL. ISBN: 978-1-124-43810-8.

> A collection of narratives and learning activities for teaching medical professionalism were presented to health science students in online courses. The JSE was used for quantitative assessment of medical professionalism. Comparisons of the JSE mean score changes showed that the treatment group improved their empathy scores. It is concluded that online exposure to narrative can be beneficial to health science students in enhancing their empathic understanding.

McTighe, A. (2014). *Effects of medical education on empathy in osteopathic medical students* (unpublished doctoral dissertation). Department of Psychology, Philadelphia College of Osteopathic Medicine, Philadelphia, PA, USA.

> Participants included 717 first- to third-year medical students (393 women) at Philadelphia College of Osteopathic Medicine who completed the JSE. Third-year students completed the JSE at the beginning and at the end of the academic year. Results showed that women obtained a significantly higher JSE mean score ($M = 112.3$, $SD = 9.6$) than men ($M = 109.3$, $SD = 10.4$). No statistically significant association was found between the JSE scores, ethnicity, and specialty preference (people-oriented versus technology-oriented specialties). Cross-sectional comparisons of the first-, second-, and third-year students on scores of the JSE showed no statistically significant difference between those in the first ($M = 111.3$, $SD = 9.6$) and in the second-year ($M = 112.4$, $SD = 9.7$); however, a statistically significant decline in the JSE scores was observed in the third-year students ($M = 108.8$, $SD = 10.9$). This decline in the JSE scores was

also observed in a longitudinal study of the third-year students ($M = 111.2$, $SD = 9.6$ at the beginning of the third year; $M = 108.7$, $SD = 10.6$ at the end of the third year).

Montanari, P. (2012). *Psychometric analysis of the Jefferson Scale of Empathy (JSE) health professional students (HPS) version: An Italian validation study with undergraduate nursing students.* Nursing graduation dissertation. Universita degli Studi dell'Aquila, Italy.

> Participants included 797 nursing students (590 women) who completed an Italian translation of the JSE (HPS Version). Exploratory factor analysis of the JSE resulted in three factors of Compassionate Care, Perspective Taking, and Standing in Patient's Shoes. Women obtained a JSE mean score ($M = 113.39$, $SD = 10.37$) which was significantly higher than that for men ($M = 107.25$, $SD = 14.11$). Test–retest reliability within 2 months time interval between testing for 566 nursing students was 0.50.

Moreto, G. (2015). *Evaluating empathy in undergraduate medical students at São Paulo University using two instruments* (unpublished doctoral dissertation). São Paulo University, Brazil.

> Participants included 296 Brazilian medical students who completed translated versions of the JSE and the Interpersonal Reactivity Index (IRI). Results showed that women obtained a significantly higher JSE mean score ($M = 116.3$, $SD = 11.0$) than men ($M = 111.1$, $SD = 13.8$), and those who planned to pursue surgery scored lower ($M = 113.8$, $SD = 12.5$) than others who planned to pursue clinical medicine ($M = 116.2$, $SD = 11.3$). No significant difference was observed in this cross-sectional study on the JSE scores among students in different years of medical school. Students in the clerkship phase of medical school, and those who planned to pursue surgery obtained lower average scores on the affective dimension of the IRI.

Smolarz, B. G. (2005). *Determining the relationship between medical student empathy and undergraduate college major* (master's degree thesis). Albany Medical College, The Graduate College of Union University, Schenectady, NY.

> Participants included 127 first-year medical students at Albany Medical College (74 women) who completed the JSE and the Interpersonal Reactivity Index (IRI). Results showed that women obtained a significantly higher JSE mean score than men ($M = 116.8$ and $M = 110.3$ for women and men, respectively). No statistically significant association was observed between scores on the JSE and medical students' undergraduate major (e.g., science versus nonscience; advanced degrees, combined degree, double major). The pattern of findings was similar for the IRI scores.

Reisetter, B. C. (2003). *Relationship between psychosocial physician characteristics and physician price awareness* (doctoral dissertation). University of Mississippi. Dissertation Dissertation Abstracts International, 63(10-B), 4620.

> Participants included 200 physicians who completed the JSE and the Physician Belief Scale (PBS). Participants were also asked to estimates the cash price for 20 commonly prescribed prescription drugs at the usual quantities dispensed. Results showed that scores on the JSE and PBS did not significantly predict physician price awareness. A statistically significant correlation was found between scores of the JSE's factor of Compassionate Care, and the PBS's Belief and Feeling subtest scores ($r = 0.50$). Also, a statistically significant but negative correlation was observed between scores of the JSE's Standing in Patient's Shoes factor and the PBS's Burden subtest scores.

Appendix B: Jefferson Scale of Empathy, Health Professions Version (JSE HP-Version)

© Springer International Publishing Switzerland 2016   333
M. Hojat, *Empathy in Health Professions Education and Patient Care*,
DOI 10.1007/978-3-319-27625-0

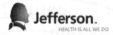

Jefferson Scale of Empathy

Physician/Health Professions (HP - version)

Use a ball-point pen.
Mark one response for each of the items below.

For *ID Code* and *Optional* fields, write numerals completely inside the boxes, one numeral to a box.

Name (optional) _____   ID Code [ ][ ][ ][ ][ ][ ][ ][ ][ ]

Date ____/____/____

Age:
☐ <21   ☐ 21-30   ☐ 31-40   ☐ 41-50   ☐ 51-60   ☐ 61-70   ☐ >70

Gender:
☐ Male   ☐ Female

Physician primary specialty: [Please choose only one]

☐ Anesthesiology ☐ Dermatology ☐ Emergency Medicine
☐ Family Med./General Prac. ☐ Internal Med./Med. specialties ☐ Neurology
☐ Neurosurgery ☐ Obstetrics/Gynecology ☐ Ophthalmology
☐ Otolaryngology ☐ Orthopaedic Surgery ☐ Pathology
☐ Pediatrics ☐ Physical Med./Rehabilitation ☐ Plastic Surgery
☐ Preventive Medicine ☐ Psychiatry ☐ Public Health
☐ Radiology ☐ Surgery/Surgical specialties ☐ Urology
☐ Other _____

Other health professions primary specialty: [Please choose only one]

☐ Community Healthcare Worker ☐ Dentistry ☐ Midwifery
☐ Nursing ☐ Nurse Practitioner ☐ Nutrition/Dietician
☐ Occupational Therapy ☐ Pharmacy ☐ Physician Assistant
☐ Physical Therapy/Physiotherapy ☐ Podiatry ☐ Psychology/Counseling
☐ Public Health Worker ☐ Speech Therapy/Audiology ☐ Social Worker
☐ Other _____

Optional field #1.. [ ][ ][ ][ ]

Optional field #2.. [ ][ ][ ][ ]

Please continue on the back --- Do not write below this line

||||| S E L F - S C O R E |||||

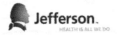

Jefferson Scale of Empathy

Physician/Health Professions (HP - version)

Instructions: Using a ball-point pen, please indicate the extent of your agreement or disagreement with *each* of the following statements by marking the appropriate circle to the right of each statement.

Please use the following 7-point scale (*a higher number on the scale indicates more agreement*):
Mark one and only one response for each statement.

1-------2-------3-------4-------5-------6-------7
Strongly Disagree   **Strongly Agree**

	1	2	3	4	5	6	7

1. My understanding of how my patients and their families feel does not influence medical or surgical treatment........................ ○ ○ ○ ○ ○ ○ ○

2. My patients feel better when I understand their feelings. .... ○ ○ ○ ○ ○ ○ ○

3. It is difficult for me to view things from my patients' perspectives................ ○ ○ ○ ○ ○ ○ ○

4. I consider understanding my patients' body language as important as verbal communication in caregiver-patient relationships................ ○ ○ ○ ○ ○ ○ ○

5. I have a good sense of humor that I think contributes to a better clinical outcome. .... ○ ○ ○ ○ ○ ○ ○

6. Because people are different, it is difficult for me to see things from my patients' perspectives................ ○ ○ ○ ○ ○ ○ ○

7. I try not to pay attention to my patients' emotions in history taking or in asking about their physical health................ ○ ○ ○ ○ ○ ○ ○

8. Attentiveness to my patients' personal experiences does not influence treatment outcomes. .... ○ ○ ○ ○ ○ ○ ○

9. I try to imagine myself in my patients' shoes when providing care to them. .... ○ ○ ○ ○ ○ ○ ○

10. My patients value my understanding of their feelings which is therapeutic in its own right................ ○ ○ ○ ○ ○ ○ ○

11. Patients' illnesses can be cured only by medical or surgical treatment; therefore, emotional ties to my patients do not have a significant influence on medical or surgical outcomes. .... ○ ○ ○ ○ ○ ○ ○

12. Asking patients about what is happening in their personal lives is not helpful in understanding their physical complaints. .... ○ ○ ○ ○ ○ ○ ○

13. I try to understand what is going on in my patients' minds by paying attention to their non-verbal cues and body language................ ○ ○ ○ ○ ○ ○ ○

14. I believe that emotion has no place in the treatment of medical illness. .... ○ ○ ○ ○ ○ ○ ○

15. Empathy is a therapeutic skill without which success in treatment is limited. .... ○ ○ ○ ○ ○ ○ ○

16. An important component of the relationship with my patients is my understanding of their emotional status, as well as that of their families................ ○ ○ ○ ○ ○ ○ ○

17. I try to think like my patients in order to render better care. .... ○ ○ ○ ○ ○ ○ ○

18. I do not allow myself to be influenced by strong personal bonds between my patients and their family members. .... ○ ○ ○ ○ ○ ○ ○

19. I do not enjoy reading non-medical literature or the arts................ ○ ○ ○ ○ ○ ○ ○

20. I believe that empathy is an important therapeutic factor in medical or surgical treatment. .... ○ ○ ○ ○ ○ ○ ○

Appendix C: Jefferson Scale of Empathy, Medical Student Version (JSE S-Version)

© Springer International Publishing Switzerland 2016
M. Hojat, *Empathy in Health Professions Education and Patient Care*,
DOI 10.1007/978-3-319-27625-0

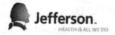

Jefferson Scale of Empathy

Medical Student version (S - version)

Use a <u>ball-point pen</u>. Mark one response for each item below.
For *ID Code*, write numerals completely inside the boxes, one numeral to a box.
Leave *Optional* fields blank unless otherwise instructed.

Name _____   **ID Code** .... ☐☐☐☐☐☐☐☐☐

Date ____/____/_____

Age:

☐ < 22   ☐ 22-24   ☐ 25-27   ☐ 28-30   ☐ 31-33   ☐ 34-36   ☐ > 36

Gender:

☐ Male   ☐ Female

Year of Medical School:

☐ 1st year   ☐ 2nd year   ☐ 3rd year   ☐ 4th year   ☐ > 4th year

Which specialty do you plan to pursue? [Please choose only <u>one</u>]

☐ Anesthesiology	☐ Dermatology	☐ Emergency Medicine
☐ Family Med./General Prac.	☐ Internal Med. (see below)	☐ Neurology
☐ Neurosurgery	☐ Obstetrics/Gynecology	☐ Ophthalmology
☐ Otolaryngology	☐ Orthopaedic Surgery	☐ Pathology
☐ Pediatrics	☐ Physical Med./Rehabilitation	☐ Plastic Surgery
☐ Preventive Medicine	☐ Psychiatry	☐ Public Health
☐ Radiology	☐ Surgery (see below)	☐ Urology
☐ Other _____	☐ Undecided	

Medical Sub-specialty: [Please choose <u>one</u> if your primary specialty interest is Internal Medicine]

☐ Cardiology	☐ Critical Care/Pulmonary	☐ Endocrinology
☐ General Internal Medicine	☐ Gastroenterology	☐ Hematology/Oncology
☐ Infectious Disease	☐ Nephrology	☐ Rheumatology
☐ Other _____	☐ Undecided	

Surgical Sub-specialty: [Please choose <u>one</u> if your primary specialty interest is Surgery]

☐ Cardiothoracic	☐ Colorectal	☐ General Surgery
☐ Transplant	☐ Trauma/Critical Care	☐ Vascular
☐ Other _____	☐ Undecided	

Optional field #1 .... ☐☐☐☐

Optional field #2 .... ☐☐☐☐

Please continue on the back   ---   Do not write below this line

S E L F - S C O R E

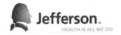 **Jefferson.** HEALTH IS ALL WE DO

Jefferson Scale of Empathy

Medical Student version (S - version)

Instructions: Using a ball-point pen, please indicate the extent of your agreement or disagreement with *each* of the following statements by marking the appropriate circle to the right of each statement.

Please use the following 7-point scale (*a higher number on the scale indicates more agreement*):
Mark <u>one and only one</u> response for each statement.

1-------2-------3-------4-------5-------6-------7
Strongly Disagree   **Strongly Agree**

	1	2	3	4	5	6	7
1. Physicians' understanding of their patients' feelings and the feelings of their patients' families does not influence medical or surgical treatment.	○	○	○	○	○	○	○
2. Patients feel better when their physicians understand their feelings.	○	○	○	○	○	○	○
3. It is difficult for a physician to view things from patients' perspectives.	○	○	○	○	○	○	○
4. Understanding body language is as important as verbal communication in physician-patient relationships.	○	○	○	○	○	○	○
5. A physician's sense of humor contributes to a better clinical outcome.	○	○	○	○	○	○	○
6. Because people are different, it is difficult to see things from patients' perspectives.	○	○	○	○	○	○	○
7. Attention to patients' emotions is not important in history taking.	○	○	○	○	○	○	○
8. Attentiveness to patients' personal experiences does not influence treatment outcomes.	○	○	○	○	○	○	○
9. Physicians should try to stand in their patients' shoes when providing care to them.	○	○	○	○	○	○	○
10. Patients value a physician's understanding of their feelings which is therapeutic in its own right.	○	○	○	○	○	○	○
11. Patients' illnesses can be cured only by medical or surgical treatment; therefore, physicians' emotional ties with their patients do not have a significant influence in medical or surgical treatment.	○	○	○	○	○	○	○
12. Asking patients about what is happening in their personal lives is not helpful in understanding their physical complaints.	○	○	○	○	○	○	○
13. Physicians should try to understand what is going on in their patients' minds by paying attention to their non-verbal cues and body language.	○	○	○	○	○	○	○
14. I believe that emotion has no place in the treatment of medical illness.	○	○	○	○	○	○	○
15. Empathy is a therapeutic skill without which the physician's success is limited.	○	○	○	○	○	○	○
16. Physicians' understanding of the emotional status of their patients, as well as that of their families is one important component of the physician-patient relationship.	○	○	○	○	○	○	○
17. Physicians should try to think like their patients in order to render better care.	○	○	○	○	○	○	○
18. Physicians should not allow themselves to be influenced by strong personal bonds between their patients and their family members.	○	○	○	○	○	○	○
19. I do not enjoy reading non-medical literature or the arts.	○	○	○	○	○	○	○
20. I believe that empathy is an important therapeutic factor in medical treatment.	○	○	○	○	○	○	○

Appendix D: Jefferson Scale of Empathy, Health Professions Student Version (JSE HPS-Version)

© Springer International Publishing Switzerland 2016
M. Hojat, *Empathy in Health Professions Education and Patient Care*,
DOI 10.1007/978-3-319-27625-0

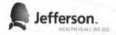 **Jefferson.**
HEALTH IS ALL WE DO

Jefferson Scale of Empathy

Health Professions Student version (HPS- version)

Use a **ball-point pen**. Mark one response for each item below.
For *ID Code*, write numerals completely inside the boxes, one numeral to a box.

Name (optional) _____   **ID Code**............ ☐☐☐☐☐☐☐☐☐

Date ___/___/_____

Age:
☐ < 19   ☐ 19 - 21   ☐ 22- 24   ☐ 25 - 27   ☐ 28 - 30   ☐ 31 - 33   ☐ 34 - 36
☐ 37 - 39   ☐ 40 - 42   ☐ 43 - 45   ☐ 46 - 48   ☐ 49 - 51   ☐ >51

Gender:
☐ Male   ☐ Female

What is your degree program?
☐ Bioscience/Medical technology   ☐ Counseling/Psychology   ☐ Dentistry
☐ Diagnostic Imaging   ☐ Nursing   ☐ Nurse Practitioner
☐ Occupational Therapy   ☐ Ophthalmology/Optometry   ☐ Pharmacy
☐ Physical Therapy   ☐ Physician Assistant   ☐ Public Health
☐ Other _____

Year in this program:
☐ 1st year   ☐ 2nd year   ☐ 3rd year   ☐ 4th year   ☐ > 4th year

Please leave *Optional* fields blank unless otherwise instructed.

Optional field #1 .... ☐☐☐

Optional field #2 .... ☐☐☐

PLEASE CONTINUE ⇨⇨⇨

S E L F · S C O R E

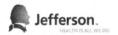 **Jefferson.**
HEALTH IS ALL WE DO

Jefferson Scale of Empathy

Health Professions Student version (HPS-version)

Instructions: Using a ball-point pen, please indicate the extent of your agreement or disagreement with *each* of the following statements by marking the appropriate circle to the right of each statement.

Please use the following 7-point scale (*a higher number on the scale indicates more agreement*):
Mark <u>one and only one</u> response for each statement.

1-------2-------3-------4-------5-------6-------7
Strongly Disagree   **Strongly Agree**

	1	2	3	4	5	6	7
1. Health care providers' understanding of their patients' feelings and the feelings of their patients' families does not influence treatment outcomes.	○	○	○	○	○	○	○
2. Patients feel better when their health care providers understand their feelings.	○	○	○	○	○	○	○
3. It is difficult for a health care provider to view things from patients' perspectives.	○	○	○	○	○	○	○
4. Understanding body language is as important as verbal communication in health care provider - patient relationships.	○	○	○	○	○	○	○
5. A health care provider's sense of humor contributes to a better clinical outcome.	○	○	○	○	○	○	○
6. Because people are different, it is difficult to see things from patients' perspectives.	○	○	○	○	○	○	○
7. Attention to patients' emotions is not important in patient interview.	○	○	○	○	○	○	○
8. Attentiveness to patients' personal experiences does not influence treatment outcomes.	○	○	○	○	○	○	○
9. Health care providers should try to stand in their patients' shoes when providing care to them.	○	○	○	○	○	○	○
10. Patients value a health care provider's understanding of their feelings which is therapeutic in its own right.	○	○	○	○	○	○	○
11. Patients' illnesses can be cured only by targeted treatment; therefore, health care providers' emotional ties with their patients do not have a significant influence in treatment outcomes.	○	○	○	○	○	○	○
12. Asking patients about what is happening in their personal lives is not helpful in understanding their physical complaints.	○	○	○	○	○	○	○
13. Health care providers should try to understand what is going on in their patients' minds by paying attention to their non-verbal cues and body language.	○	○	○	○	○	○	○
14. I believe that emotion has no place in the treatment of medical illness.	○	○	○	○	○	○	○
15. Empathy is a therapeutic skill without which a health care provider's success is limited.	○	○	○	○	○	○	○
16. Health care providers' understanding of the emotional status of their patients, as well as that of their families is one important component of the health care provider - patient relationship.	○	○	○	○	○	○	○
17. Health care providers should try to think like their patients in order to render better care.	○	○	○	○	○	○	○
18. Health care providers should not allow themselves to be influenced by strong personal bonds between their patients and their family members.	○	○	○	○	○	○	○
19. I do not enjoy reading non-medical literature or the arts.	○	○	○	○	○	○	○
20. I believe that empathy is an important factor in patients' treatment.	○	○	○	○	○	○	○

THANK YOU!

Appendix E: Jefferson Scale of Patient Perceptions of Physician Empathy (JSPPPE)

© Springer International Publishing Switzerland 2016
M. Hojat, *Empathy in Health Professions Education and Patient Care*,
DOI 10.1007/978-3-319-27625-0

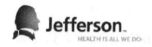

Jefferson Scale of Patient Perceptions of Physician Empathy

Instructions: We would like to know the extent of your agreement or disagreement with *each* of the following statements *about your physician named below.* Please use the following 7-point scale and write your rating number from 1 to 7 on the <u>underlined</u> space before each statement (1 means that you Strongly Disagree, and 7 means you Strongly Agree with the statement, a higher number indicates more agreement).

1-------2-------3-------4-------5-------6-------7
Strongly Disagree   *Strongly Agree*

Dr. (Name of the physician here)_____

---

1. __ Can view things from my perspective (see things as I see them).

2. __ Asks about what is happening in my daily life.

3. __ Seems concerned about me and my family.

4. __ Understands my emotions, feelings and concerns.

5. __ Is an understanding doctor.

References

AAMC (Association of American Medical Colleges). (2004). Medical School Objectives Project. Retrieved from: http://www.aamc.org/meded/msop.

Abbott, L. C. (1983). A study of humanism in family physicians. *The Journal of Family Practice, 16*, 1141–1146.

Abele, A. E., & Wojciszke, B. (2007). Agency and communion from perspective of self versus others. *Journal of Personality and Social Psychology, 93*, 751–763.

ABIM (American Board of Internal Medicine). (1983). Evaluation of humanistic qualities in the internist. *Annals of Internal Medicine, 99*, 720–724.

Ackoff, R. L., & Emery, F. E. (1981). *On purposeful systems*. Seaside, CA: Intersystems.

Acuna, L. E. (2000). Don't cry for us Argentinians: Two decades of teaching medical humanities. *Journal of Medical Ethics: Medical Humanities, 26*, 66–70.

Adams, G. R., Jones, R. M., Schvaneveldt, J. D., & Jenson, G. O. (1982). Antecedents of affective role-taking behaviour: Adolescent perceptions of parental socialization styles. *Journal of Adolescence, 5*, 259–265.

Adib, S. M., & Hamadeh, G. N. (1999). Attitudes of the Lebanese public regarding disclosure of serious illness. *Journal of Medical Ethics, 25*, 399–403.

Adler, H. M. (1997). The history of the present illness as treatment: Who's listening, and why does it matter? *The Journal of the American Board of Family Practice, 10*, 28–35.

Adler, H. M. (2002). The sociophysiology of caring in the doctor-patient relationship. *Journal of General Internal Medicine, 17*, 874–882.

Adler, H. M., & Hammett, V. B. O. (1973). The doctor-patient relationship revisited: An analysis of the placebo effect. *Annals of Internal Medicine, 78*, 595–598.

Adolphs, R., Damasio, H., Tranel, D., Cooper, G., & Damasio, A. R. (2000). A role for somatosensory cortices in the visual recognition of emotion as revealed by three-dimensional lesion mapping. *Journal of Neuroscience, 20*, 2683–2690.

Adolphs, R., Tranel, D., Damasio, H., & Damasio, A. R. (1994). Impaired recognition of emotion in facial expression following bilateral damage to human amygdala. *Nature, 372*, 669–672.

Aggarwal, R. (2007). Empathy: Do psychiatrists and patients agree? *The American Journal of Psychiatry Resident's Journal, 2*, 2–3.

Agosta, C. (1984). Empathy and intersubjectivity. In J. Lichtenberg, M. Borenstein, & D. Silver (Eds.), *Empathy II* (pp. 43–61). Hillsdale, NJ: Analytic Press.

Ahlgren, A., & Johnson, D. W. (1979). Sex differences in cooperative and competitive attitudes from the 2nd to the 12th grades. *Developmental Psychology, 15*, 45–49.

Ainsworth, M. D. S. (1985a). Attachment across the life span. *Bulletin of the New York Academy of Medicine, 61*, 792–812.

Ainsworth, M. D. S. (1985b). Patterns of infant-mother attachment: Antecedents and effects on development. *Bulletin of the New York Academy of Medicine, 61*, 771–791.

Ainsworth, M. D. S., Blehar, M. C., Waters, E., & Wall, S. (1978). *Patterns of attachment: A psychological study of the strange situation.* Hillsdale, NJ: Erlbaum.

Albanese, M. A., Snow, M. H., Skochelak, S. E., Huggett, K. N., & Farrell, P. M. (2003). Assessing personal qualities in medical school admissions. *Academic Medicine, 78*, 313–321.

Alcorta-Garza, A., Gonzalez-Guerrero, J. F., Tavitas-Herrera, S. E., Rodrigues-Lara, F. J., & Hojat, M. (2005). Validación de la escala de empatia medica de Jefferson en estudiantes de medicina Mexicanos [Validity of the Jefferson Scale of Physician Empathy among Mexican medical students]. *Salud Mental [Mental Health], 28*, 57–63.

Ali, N. S., Khalil, H. Z., & Yousef, W. (1993). A comparison of American and Egyptian cancer patients' attitudes and unmet needs. *Cancer Nursing, 16*, 193–203.

Allport, F. H. (1924). *Social psychology.* Boston: Houghton Mifflin.

Allport, G. W. (1960). The open system in personality theory. *Journal of Abnormal and Social Psychology, 61*, 301–310.

Amini, F., Lewis, T., Lannon, R., Louie, A., Baumbacher, G., McGuinness, T., et al. (1996). Affect, attachment, memory: Contributions toward psychobiologic integration. *Psychiatry, 59*, 213–239.

Anastasi, A. (1976). *Psychological testing.* New York: Macmillan.

Anderson, S. W., Bechara, A., Damasio, H., Tranel, D., & Damasio, A. R. (1999). Impairment of social and moral behavior related to early damage in human prefrontal cortex. *Nature Neuroscience, 2*, 1032–1037.

Anthony, A. A., & Wain, H. J. (1971). An investigation of the outcome of empathy training for medical corpsmen. *Psychological Aspects of Disability, 18*, 86–88.

Antonovsky, A., Anson, O., & Bernstein, J. (1979). Interviewing and the selection of medical students: The experience of five years of Beersheba. *Innovation in Education & Training International, 16*, 328–334.

Arbuckle, J. J., & Wothke, W. (1999). *Amos 4.0 user's guide.* Chicago, IL: SPSS.

Archer, J. (1988). *The behavioural biology of aggression.* Cambridge: Cambridge University Press.

Archer, J. (2004). Sex differences in aggression in real-world settings: A meta-analytic review. *Review of General Psychology, 8*, 291–322.

Aring, C. D. (1958). Sympathy and empathy. *Journal of the American Medical Association, 167*, 448–452.

Arnkoff, D. B., Glass, C. R., & Shapiro, S. (2002). Expectations and preferences. In J. C. Norcross (Ed.), *Psychotherapy relationships at work: Therapist contributions and responsiveness to patients* (pp. 335–356). Oxford: Oxford University Press.

Arnold, L. (2002). Assessing professional behavior: Yesterday, today, and tomorrow. *Academic Medicine, 77*, 28–37.

Arnold, L., Calkins, E. V., & Willoughby, T. L. (1997). Antecedent and concurrent correlates of primary care practice. *Teaching and Learning in Medicine, 9*, 192–199.

Aronfreed, J. (1970). The socialization of altruistic and sympathetic behavior: Some theoretical and experimental analyses. In J. Macauley & L. Berkowitz (Eds.), *Altruistic and helping behavior* (pp. 103–126). New York: Academic Press.

Aronson, E., & Patnoe, S. (1997). *Jigsaw classroom.* New York: Longman.

Arora, S., Ashrafian, H., Davis, R., Athanasiou, T., Darzi, A., & Sevdalis, N. (2010). Emotional intelligence in medicine: A systematic review through the context of the ACGME competencies. *Medical Education, 44*, 749–764. doi:10.1111/j.1365-2923.2010.03709.x.

Ashcroft, J., & Straus, A. (1993). *Families first: Report of the National Commission on America's Urban Families.* Washington, DC: National Commission on America's Urban Families.

Ashworth, C. D., Williamson, P., & Montano, D. (1984). A scale to measure physician beliefs about psychosocial aspects of patient care. *Social Science & Medicine, 19*, 1235–1238.

Astin, H. S. (1967). Assessment of empathic ability by means of a situational test. *Journal of Counseling Psychology, 14*, 57–60.

Austin, E. J., Evans, P., Goldwater, R., & Potter, V. (2005). A preliminary study of emotional intelligence, empathy and exam performance in first year medical students. *Personality and Individual Differences, 39*, 1395–1405. doi:10.1016/j.paid.2005.04.014.

Austin, E. J., Evans, P., Magnus, B., & O'Hanlon, K. N. (2007). A preliminary study of empathy, emotional intelligence and examination performance in MBChB students. *Medical Education, 41*, 684–689. doi:10.1111/j.1365-2923.2007.02795.x.

Avenanti, A., Bueti, D., Galati, G., & Aglioti, S. (2005). Transcranial magnetic stimulation highlights the sensorimotor side of empathy for pain. *Nature, Neuroscience, 8*, 955–960.

Avery, J. K. (1985). Lawyers tell what turns some patients litigious. *Medical Malpractice Review, 2*, 35–37.

Ax, A. F. (1964). Goals and methods of psychophysiology. *Psychophysiology, 1*, 8–25.

Ayra, D. K. (1993). To empathize or to dissociate—A physician's dilemma. *Journal of the Royal Society of Medicine, 86*, 3.

Babar, M. G., Omar, H., Lim, L. P., Khan, S. A., Mitha, S., & Ahmad, S. F. B. (2013). An assessment of dental students' empathy levels in Malaysia. *International Journal of Medical Education, 4*, 223–229. doi:10.5116/ijme.5259.4513.

Bacharach, M. H. (1976). Empathy: We know what we mean, but what do we measure? *Archives of General Psychiatry, 33*, 35–38.

Baggaley, A. R. (1983). Deciding on the ratio of number of subjects to number of variables in factor analysis. *Multivariate Experimental Clinical Research, 6*, 81–86.

Bailey, B. A. (2001). Empathy in medical students: Assessment and relationship to specialty choice. *Dissertation Abstracts International, 62*(6-A), 2024.

Bakan, D. (1966). *The duality of human existence*. Reading, PA: Addison-Wesley.

Baldwin, D. A., & Baird, J. A. (2001). Discerning intentions in dynamic human action. *Trends in Cognitive Science, 5*, 171–178.

Balint, M. (1957). *The doctor, his patient and the illness*. New York: International Universities Press.

Ballou, J. W. (1978). *The psychology of pregnancy*. Lexington, MA: Lexington Books.

Bandura, A. (1977). *Social learning theory*. Englewood Cliffs, NJ: Prentice Hall.

Banks, J. A. (1997). *Educating citizens in a multicultural society*. New York: Teachers College Press.

Bargh, J. A., Chen, M., & Burrows, L. (1996). Automaticity of social behavior: Direct effects of trait construct and stereotype-activation on action. *Journal of Personality and Social Psychology, 71*, 230–244.

Barnett, M. A. (1987). Empathy and related responses to children. In N. Eisenberg & J. Strayer (Eds.), *Empathy and its development* (pp. 146–162). New York: Cambridge University Press.

Barnett, R. C., Biener, L., & Baruch, G. K. (1987). *Gender and stress*. New York: Free Press.

Barnett, M. A., Feighny, K. M., & Esper, J. A. (1983). Effect of anticipated victim responsiveness and empathy upon volunteering. *The Journal of Social Psychology, 119*, 211–218.

Barnett, M. A., Howard, J. A., King, L. M., & Dino, G. A. (1980). Antecedents of empathy: Retrospective accounts of early socialization. *Personality & Social Psychology Bulletin, 6*, 361–365.

Barnsley, J., Williams, A. P., Cockerill, R., & Tanner, J. (1999). Physician characteristics and the physician-patient relationship: Impact of sex, year of graduation, and specialty. *Canadian Family Physician, 45*, 935–942.

Baron-Cohen, S. (2003). *The essential difference: The truth about the male and female brain*. New York: Basic Books.

Baron-Cohen, S., & Wheelwright, S. (2004). The empathy quotient: An investigation of adults with Asperger syndrome or high functioning autism, and normal sex differences. *Journal of Autism and Developmental Disorders, 34*, 163–175.

Baron-Cohen, S., Wheelwright, S., Hill, J., Raste, Y., & Plumb, I. (2001). The "Reading the Mind in the Eye" test, revised version: A study with adults, and adults with Asperger syndrome or high functioning autism. *Journal of Child Psychology and Psychiatry, 42*, 241–251.

Barondess, J. A. (2003). Medicine and professionalism. *Archives of Internal Medicine, 163*, 145–149.

Barrett-Lennard, G. T. (1962). Dimensions of therapist response as causal factors in therapeutic change. *Psychological Monographs, 76,* 1–36.

Barrett-Lennard, G. T. (1986). The relationship inventory now: Issues and advances in theory, method and use. In L. S. Greenberg & W. M. Pinsof (Eds.), *The psychotherapeutic process: A research handbook* (pp. 439–476). New York: Guilford.

Barsky, A. J. (1981). Hidden reasons some patients visit doctors. *Annals of Internal Medicine, 94,* 492–498.

Bartholomew, K., & Horowitz, L. (1991). Attachment styles among adults: A test of four-category model. *Journal of Personality and Social Psychology, 61,* 226–244.

Basch, M. F. (1983). Empathic understanding: A review of the concept and some theoretical considerations. *Journal of the American Psychoanalytic Association, 31,* 101–126.

Basch, M. F. (1996). Affect and defense. In D. L. Nathanson (Ed.), *Knowing feeling: Affect, script, and psychotherapy* (pp. 257–269). New York: W.W. Norton.

Bateson, G. (1971). A systems approach. *International Journal of Psychiatry, 9,* 242–244.

Batson, C. D. (1991). *The altruism question: Toward a social psychological answer.* Hillsdale, NJ: Erlbaum.

Batson, C. D., Batson, J. G., Singlsby, J. K., Harrell, K. L., Peeka, H. M., & Todd, R. M. (1991). Empathic joy and the empathy-altruism hypothesis. *Journal of Personality and Social Psychology, 61,* 413–426.

Batson, C. D., & Coke, J. S. (1981). Empathy: A source of altruistic motivation for helping? In J. P. Rushton & R. M. Sorrentino (Eds.), *Altruism and helping behavior: Social personality, and developmental perspectives* (pp. 167–211). Hillsdale, NJ: Erlbaum.

Batson, C. D., Coke, J. S., & Pych, V. (1983). Limits on the two-stage model of empathic mediation of helping: A reply to Archer, Diaz-Loving, Gollwitzer, Davis, and Foushee. *Journal of Personality and Social Psychology, 45,* 895–898.

Batson, C. D., Early, S., & Salvarini, G. (1997). Perspective taking: Imagining how another feels versus imagining how you would feel. *Personality and Social Personality Bulletin, 23,* 751–758.

Batson, C. D., Fultz, J., & Schoenrade, P. A. (1987). Distress and empathy: Two qualitatively distinct vicarious emotions with different motivational consequences. *Journal of Personality, 55,* 19–39.

Batson, C. D., Lishner, D. A., Carpenter, A., Dublin, L., Hajusola-Webb, S., Stocks, E. L., … Sampat, B. (2003). As you would have them do unto you: Does imagining yourself in the other's place stimulate moral action? *Personality and Social Psychology Bulletin, 29,* 1190–1201.

Batson, C. D., Polycarpou, M. P., Harmon-Jones, E., Imhoff, H. J., Mitchener, E. C., Bednar, L. L., … Highberger, L. (1997). Empathy and attitudes: Can feeling for a member of a stigmatized group improve feelings toward the group? *Journal of Personality and Social Psychology, 72,* 105–118.

Batson, C. D., Sager, K., Garst, E., Kang, M., Rubchinsky, K., & Dawson, K. (1997). Is empathy-induced helping due to self-other merging? *Journal of Personality and Social Psychology, 73,* 495–509.

Baumann, A. O., Deber, R. B., Silverman, B. E., & Mallette, C. M. (1998). Who cares? Who cures? The ongoing debate in the provision of health care. *Journal of Advanced Nursing, 28,* 1040–1045.

Bavelas, J. B., Black, A., Lemery, C. R., & Mullett, J. (1986). "I show how you feel": Motor mimicry as a communicative act. *Journal of Personality and Social Psychology, 50,* 322–329.

Bayes, M. A. (1972). Behavioral cues of interpersonal warmth. *Journal of Consulting and Clinical Psychology, 39,* 333–339.

Bazarko, D., Cate, R. A., Azocar, F., & Kreitzer, M. J. (2013). The Impact of an innovative mindfulness-based stress reduction program on the health and well-being of nurses employed in a corporate setting. *Journal of Workplace Behavioral Health, 28,* 107–133. doi:10.1080/155 55240.2013.779518. Retrieved from: http://dx.doi.org/10.1080/15555240.2013.779518.

Beattie, A., Durham, J., Harvey, J., Steele, J., & McHanwell, S. (2012). Does empathy change in first-year dental students? *European Journal of Dental Education, 16*, e111–e116. doi:10.1111/j.1600-0579.2011.00683.x.

Becker, H. S., & Geer, B. (1958). The fate of idealism in medical school. *American Sociological Review, 23*, 50–56.

Becker, H., & Sands, D. (1988). The relationship of empathy to clinical experience among male and female nursing students. *Journal of Nursing Education, 27*, 198–203.

Beckman, H. B., & Frankel, R. M. (1984). The effect of physician behavior on the collection of data. *Annals of Internal Medicine, 101*, 692–696.

Beckman, H. B., Markakis, K. M., Suchman, A. L., & Frankel, R. M. (1994). The doctor-patient relationship and malpractice: Lessons from plaintiff depositions. *Archives of Internal Medicine, 154*, 1365–1370.

Beckman, T. J., Reed, D. A., Shanafelt, T. D., & West, C. P. (2010). Impact of resident well-being and empathy on assessments of faculty physicians. *Journal of General Internal Medicine, 25*, 52–56. doi:10.1007/s11606-009-1152-0.

Beddoe, A. E., & Murphy, S. O. (2004). Does mindfulness decrease stress and foster empathy among nursing students? *Journal of Nursing Education, 43*, 305–312.

Beecher, H. K. (1955). The powerful placebo. *Journal of the American Medical Association, 159*, 1602–1606.

Beisecker, A. E., & Beisecker, T. D. (1990). Patient information-seeking behaviors when communicating with doctors. *Medical Care, 28*, 19–28.

Bellet, P. S., & Maloney, M. J. (1991). The importance of empathy as an interviewing skill in medicine. *Journal of the American Medical Association, 266*, 1831–1832.

Bellini, L. M., Baime, M., & Shea, J. A. (2002). Variation of mood and empathy during internship. *Journal of the American Medical Association, 287*, 3143–3146.

Bellini, L. M., & Shea, J. A. (2005). Mood change and empathy decline persist during three years of internal medicine training. *Academic Medicine, 80*, 164–167.

Belsky, J. (1988). The "effects" of infant day care reconsidered. *Childhood Research Quarterly, 3*, 235–272.

Bem, S. L. (1974). The measurement of psychological androgyny. *Journal of Consulting and Clinical Psychology, 42*, 155–162.

Benbassat, J., & Baumal, R. (2004). What is empathy, and how can it be promoted during clinical clerkships? *Academic Medicine, 79*, 832–839.

Benedict, R. H. B., Priore, R. L., Miller, C., Munschauser, F., & Jacobs, L. (2001). Personality disorder in multiple sclerosis correlates with cognitive impairment. *Journal of Neuropsychiatry & Clinical Neurosciences, 13*, 70–76.

Bennett, J. A. (1995). "Methodological notes on empathy": Further considerations. *Advances in Nursing Science, 18*, 36–50.

Bennett, M. J. (2001). *The empathic healer: An endangered species.* San Diego, CA: Academic Press.

Benton, A. L. (1991). The prefrontal region: Its early history. In H. Levin, H. M. Eisenberg, & A. L. Benton (Eds.), *Frontal lobe function and dysfunction* (pp. 3–32). New York: Oxford University Press.

Beres, D., & Arlow, J. A. (1974). Fantasy and identification in empathy. *Psychoanalytic Quarterly, 43*, 26–40.

Berg, K., Blatt, B., Lopreiato, J., Jung, J., Schaeffer, A., Heil, D., … Hojat, M. (2015). Standardized patient assessment of medical students empathy: Ethnicity and gender effects in a multi-institutional study. *Academic Medicine, 90*, 105–111. doi:10.1097/ACM0000000000000529.

Berg, K., Majdan, J. F., Berg, D., Veloski, J., & Hojat, M. (2011a). A comparison of students' self-reported empathy with simulated patients' assessment of the students' empathy. *Medical Teacher, 33*, 388–391. doi:10.3109/0142159x.2010.530319.

Berg, K., Majdan, J., Berg, D., Veloski, J., & Hojat, M. (2011b). Medical students' self-reported empathy and simulated patients' assessments of student empathy: An analysis by gender and ethnicity. *Academic Medicine, 86*, 984–988. doi:10.1097/ACM.0b013e3182224f1f.

Berg, S. J., & Wynne-Edwards, K. E. (2001). Changes in testosterone, cortisol, and estradiol levels in men becoming fathers. *Mayo Clinic Proceedings, 76*, 582–592.

Berger, S. M. (1962). Conditioning through vicarious instigation. *Psychological Review, 69*, 450–466.

Berger, D. M. (1987). *Clinical empathy*. Northvale, NJ: Jason Aronson.

Berkman, L. F. (1995). The role of social relations in health promotion. *Psychosomatic Medicine, 57*, 245–254.

Berkman, L. F. (2000). Which influences cognitive function: Living alone or being alone? *Lancet, 355*, 1291–1292.

Berkman, L. F., Glass, T., Brissette, I., & Seeman, T. E. (2000). From social integration to health: Durkheim in the new millennium. *Social Science & Medicine, 51*, 843–857.

Berkman, L. F., Leo-Summers, L., & Horwitz, R. I. (1992). Emotional support and survival after myocardial infarction. *Annals of Internal Medicine, 117*, 1003–1009.

Berkman, L., & Syme, S. (1979). Social networks, host resistance, and mortality: A nine-year follow-up of Alameda County residents. *American Journal of Epidemiology, 109*, 186–204.

Berkowitz, L. (1984). Some effects of thoughts on anti and prosocial influences of media events: A cognitive-neoassociation analysis. *Psychological Bulletin, 95*, 410–427.

Bertakis, K. D., Helms, L. J., Callahan, E. J., Azari, R., & Robbins, J. A. (1995). The influence of gender on physician practice style. *Medical Care, 33*, 407–416.

Bertakis, K. D., Roter, D., & Putman, S. M. (1991). The relationship of physician medical interview style to patient satisfaction. *Journal of Family Practice, 32*, 175–181.

Beutler, L. E., Johnson, D. T., Neville, C. W., & Workman, S. N. (1973). Some sources of variance in "Accurate Empathy" ratings. *Journal of Consulting and Clinical Psychology, 40*, 167–169.

Beven, J. P., O'Brien-Malone, A., & Hall, G. (2004). Using the Interpersonal Reactivity Index to assess empathy in violent offenders. *International Journal of Forensic Psychology, 1*, 33–41.

Bickel, J. (1994). Special needs and affinities of women medical students. In E. S. More & M. A. Milligan (Eds.), *The empathic practitioner: Empathy, gender, and medicine* (pp. 237–249). New Brunswick, NJ: Rutgers University Press.

Bjorklund, D. F., & Kipp, K. (1996). Parental investment theory and gender differences in the evolution of inhibition mechanism. *Psychological Bulletin, 100*, 163–188.

Black, D. M. (2004). Sympathy reconfigured: Some reflections on sympathy, empathy and the discovery of values. *International Journal of Psychoanalysis, 85*, 579–595.

Black, H., & Phillips, S. (1982). An intervention program for the development of empathy in student teachers. *Journal of Psychology: Interdisciplinary & Applied, 112*, 159–168.

Blackman, N., Smith, K., Brokman, R., & Stern, J. (1958). The development of empathy in male schizophrenics. *Psychiatric Quarterly, 32*, 546–553.

Blackwell, B. (1973). Drug therapy, patient compliance. *New England Journal of Medicine, 289*, 249–252.

Blakemore, S. J., Bristow, D., Bird, G., Frith, C., & Ward, J. (2005). Somatosensory activations during the observation of touch and a case of vision-touch synaesthesia. *Brain, 128*, 1571–1583.

Bland, C. J., Meurer, L. N., & Maldonado, G. (1995). Determinants of primary care specialty choice: A non-statistical meta-analysis of the literature. *Academic Medicine, 70*, 620–641.

Blanton, S. (1960). *The healing power of poetry*. New York: Crowell.

Blass, C. D., & Hech, E. J. (1975). Accuracy of accurate empathy ratings. *Journal of Counseling Psychology, 22*, 243–246.

Blazer, D. G. (1982). Social support and mortality in an elderly community population. *American Journal of Epidemiology, 115*, 684–694.

Block, J. H. (1976). Assessing sex differences: Issues, problems, and pitfalls. *Merrill-Palmer Quarterly, 22*, 283–308.

Bloom, B. L., Asher, S. J., & White, S. W. (1978). Marital disruption as a stressor: A review analysis. *Psychological Bulletin, 85*, 867–894.

Blumenthal, J. A., Burg, M. M., Barefoot, J., Williams, R. B., Haney, T., & Zimet, G. (1987). Social support, Type A behavior, and coronary artery disease. *Psychosomatic Medicine, 49*, 331–340.

Blumgart, H. L. (1964). Caring for the patient. *New England Journal of Medicine, 270*, 449–456.

Bohart, A. C., Elliot, R., Greenberg, L. S., & Watson, J. C. (2002). Empathy. In J. C. Norcross (Ed.), *Psychotherapy relationships that work: Therapist contributions and responsiveness to patients* (pp. 89–108). Oxford: Oxford University Press.

Bolognini, S. (1997). Empathy and "empathism". *International Journal of Psychoanalysis, 78*, 279–293.

Bombeke, K., Van Roosbroeck, S., De Winter, B., Debaene, L., Schol, S., Van Hal, G., & Van Royen, P. (2011). Medical students trained in communication skills show a decline in patient-centred attitudes: An observational study comparing two cohorts during clinical clerkships. *Patient Education and Counseling, 84*, 310–318. doi:10.1016/j.pec.2011.03.007.

Bond, A. R., Mason, H. F., Lemaster, C. M., Shaw, S. E., Mullin, C. S., Hollick, E. A., & Saper, R. B. (2013). Embodied health: The effects of mind-body course for medical students. *Medical Education Online, 18.* doi:10.3402/meo.v18i0.20699.

Book, H. E. (1988). Empathy: Misconceptions and misuses in psychotherapy. *American Journal of Psychiatry, 145*, 420–424.

Book, H. E. (1991). Is empathy cost efficient? *American Journal of Psychotherapy, 45*, 21–30.

Book, A. S., Starzyk, K. B., & Quinsey, V. L. (2001). The relationship between testosterone and aggression: A meta-analysis. *Aggression and Violent Behavior: A Review Journal, 6*, 579–599.

Booth, A., Granger, D. A., Mazur, A., & Kivlighan, K. T. (2006). Testosterone and social behavior. *Social Forces, 85*, 167–191.

Borgenicht, L. (1984). Richard Selzer and the problem of detached concern. *Annals of Internal Medicine, 100*, 923–934.

Borke, H. (1971). Interpersonal perception of young children: Ego-centrism or empathy. *Developmental Psychology, 5*, 263–269.

Boruch, R. F. (1982). Evidence and inference in research on mass psychogenic illness. In M. J. Colligan, J. W. Pennebaker, & L. R. Murphy (Eds.), *Mass psychogenic illness: A social psychological analysis* (pp. 101–125). Hillsdale, NJ: Erlbaum.

Boscarino, J. A. (1995). Post-traumatic stress and associated disorders among Vietnam veterans. The significance of combat exposure and social support. *Journal of Trauma Stress, 8*, 317–336.

Botvinick, M., Jha, A. P., Bylsma, L. M., Fabian, S. A., Solomon, P. E., & Prkachin, K. M. (2005). Viewing facial expression of pain engages cortical areas involved in the direct experience of pain. *Neuroimage, 25*, 312–319.

Bowers, M. R., Swan, J. E., & Koehler, W. F. (1994). What attributes determine quality and satisfaction with health care delivery? *Health Care Management Review, 19*, 49–55.

Bowlby, J. (1973). *Attachment and loss (Vol. 2): Separation: Anxiety and anger.* New York: Basic Books.

Bowlby, J. (1980). *Attachment and loss (Vol. 3): Loss: Sadness and depression.* New York: Basic Books.

Bowlby, J. (1982). *Attachment and loss (Vol. 1): Attachment.* New York: Basic Books.

Bowlby, J. (1988). *A secure base: Parent-child attachment and healthy human development.* New York: Basic Books.

Boyd, R. W., & DiMascio, A. (1957). Social behavior and automatic physiology: A sociophysiological study. *Journal of Nervous and Mental Disease, 120*, 207–212.

Boyle, M. J., Williams, B., Brown, T., Molloy, A., McKenna, L., Molloy, L., & Lewis, B. (2009). Levels of empathy in undergraduate health science students. *The Internet Journal of Medical Education, 1.* Retrieved from: https://ispub.com/IJME/1/1/9959.

Branch, W. T. (2000). The ethics of caring and medical education. *Academic Medicine, 75*, 127–132.

Branch, W. T., & Malik, T. K. (1993). Using windows of opportunities in brief interviews to understand patients' concerns. *Journal of the American Medical Association, 169*, 1667–1668.

Branch, W. T., Pels, R. J., & Hafler, J. P. (1998). Medical students' empathic understanding of their patients. *Academic Medicine, 73*, 360–362.

Brazeau, C. M. L. R., Schroeder, R., Rovi, S., & Boyd, L. (2010). Relationship between medical student burnout, empathy, and professionalism climate. *Academic Medicine, 85*, s33–s36. doi:10.1097/ACM.0b013e3181ed4c47.

Brazeau, C. M. L. R., Schroeder, R., Rovi, S., & Boyd, L. (2011). Relationship between medical student service and empathy. *Academic Medicine, 86*, s42–s45. doi:10.1097/ACM.0b013e31822a6ae0.

Bretherton, I. (1987). New perspectives on attachment relations: Security, communication, and internal working models. In J. Osofsky (Ed.), *Handbook of infant development* (pp. 1061–1100). New York: John Wiley & Sons.

Bridgman, D. L. (1981). Enhanced role taking through cooperative interdependence: A field study. *Child Development, 52*, 1231–1238.

Brislin, R. W. (1970). Back-translation for cross-cultural research. *Journal of Cross-Cultural Psychology, 1*, 185–216.

Briton, N. J., & Hall, J. A. (1995). Beliefs about female and male nonverbal communication. *Sex Roles, 32*, 79–90.

Brock, C. D., & Salinsky, J. V. (1993). Empathy: An essential skill for understanding the physician-patient relationship in clinical practice. *Family Medicine, 25*, 245–248.

Brockhouse, R., Msetfi, R. M., Cohen, K., & Joseph, S. (2011). Vicarious exposure to trauma and growth in therapists: The moderating effects of sense of coherence, organizational support, and empathy. *Journal of Traumatic Stress, 24*, 735–742. doi:10.1002/jts.20704.

Brody, H. (1985). Placebo effect: An examination of Grunbaum's definition. In L. White, B. Tursky, & G. E. Schwartz (Eds.), *Placebo: Theory, research, and mechanisms* (pp. 37–58). New York: Guilford Press.

Brody, H. (1997). Placebo response, sustained partnership, and emotional resilience in practice. *Journal of the American Board of Family Practice, 10*, 72–74.

Brody, L. R., & Hall, J. A. (2008). Gender and emotion in context. In M. Lewis & J. Haviland (Eds.), *Handbook of emotions* (3rd ed., pp. 395–408). New York: Guilford.

Brothers, L. (1989). A biological perspective on empathy. *American Journal of Psychiatry, 146*, 10–19.

Brown, T., Boyle, M., Williams, B., Molloy, A., Palermo, C., McKenna, L., & Molloy, L. (2011). Predictors of empathy in health science students. *Journal of Allied Health, 40*, 143–149.

Brown, J., & Dunn, J. (1996). Continuities in emotional understanding from 3 to 6 years. *Child Development, 67*, 789–802.

Brown, T., Williams, B., Boyle, M., Molloy, A., McKenna, L., Molloy, L., & Lewis, B. (2010). Levels of empathy in undergraduate occupational therapy students. *Occupational Therapy International, 17*, 135–141. doi:10.1002/oti.297.

Brownell, A. K., & Cote, L. (2001). Senior residents' views on the meaning of professionalism and how they learn about it. *Academic Medicine, 76*, 734–737.

Bruner, J. (1990). *Acts of meaning*. Cambridge, MA: Harvard University Press.

Bryant, B. K. (1982). An index of empathy for children and adolescents. *Child Development, 53*, 413–425.

Buccino, G., Binkofski, F., Fink, G. R., Fadiga, L., Fogassi, L., Gallese, V., ... Freund, H. J. (2001). Action observation activates premotor and parietal areas in a somatotypic manner: An fMRI study. *European Journal of Neuroscience, 13*, 400–404.

Bucher, J. T., Vu, D. M., & Hojat, M. (2013). Psychostimulant drug abuse and personality factors in medical students. *Medical Teacher, 35*, 53–57.

Buchheimer, A. (1963). The development of ideas about empathy. *Journal of Counseling Psychology, 10*, 61–70.

Buck, R. (1984). *The communication of emotion*. New York: Guilford Press.

Buck, R., & Ginsburg, B. (1997a). Communicative genes and the evolution of empathy: Selfish and social emotions as voices of selfish and social genes. *Annals of the New York Academy of Sciences, 807*, 481–483.

Buck, R., & Ginsburg, B. (1997b). Communicative genes and the evolution of empathy. In W. Ickes (Ed.), *Empathic accuracy* (pp. 17–43). New York: Guilford.

Buck, R., Miller, R. E., & Caul, W. F. (1974). Sex, personality, and physiological variables in the communication of affect via facial expression. *Journal of Personality and Social Psychology, 30*, 587–596.

Buck, R. W., Savin, V. J., Miller, R. E., & Caul, W. F. (1972). Communication of affect through facial expressions in humans. *Journal of Personality and Social Psychology, 23*, 362–371.

Burack, J. H., Irby, D. M., Carline, J. D., Ambrozy, D. M., Ellsbury, K. E., & Stritter, F. T. (1997). A study of medical students' specialty-choice pathways: Trying on possible selves. *Academic Medicine, 72*, 534–541.

Burdi, M. D., & Baker, L. C. (1999). Physicians' perceptions of autonomy and satisfaction in California. *Health Affairs, 18*, 134–145.

Burger, J. M. (2009). Replicating Milgram: Would people still obey today? *American Psychologist, 64*, 1–11. doi:10.1037/a0010932.

Burlingham, D. (1967). Empathy between infant and mother. *Journal of the American Psychoanalytic Association, 15*, 764–780.

Burns, D. D., & Nolen-Hoeksema, S. (1992). Therapeutic empathy and recovery from depression in cognitive-behavioral therapy: A structural equation model. *Journal of Consulting and Clinical Psychology, 60*, 441–449.

Burnstein, A. G., Loucks, S., Kobos, J., Johnson, G., Talbert, R. L., & Stanton, B. (1980). A longitudinal study of personality characteristics of medical students. *Journal of Medical Education, 55*, 786–787.

Bush, L. K., Barr, C. L., McHugo, G. J., & Lanzetta, J. T. (1989). The effects of facial control and facial mimicry on subjective reactions to comedy routines. *Motivation and Emotion, 13*, 31–52.

Bushnell, M. C., Duncan, G. H., Hofbauer, R. K., Ha, B., Chen, J. I., & Carrier, B. (1999). Pain perception: Is there a role for primary somatosensory cortex? *National Academy of Sciences, 96*, 7705–7709.

Buss, D. M. (1989). Sex differences in human mate preferences: Evolutionary hypotheses tested in 37 cultures. *Behavioral and Brain Sciences, 12*, 1–49.

Buss, D. M. (1995). Psychological sex differences: Origins through sexual selection. *American Psychologist, 50*, 164–168.

Buss, D. M. (2003). *The evolution of desire: Strategies of human mating.* New York: Basic Books.

Buss, D. M., & Barnes, M. (1986). Preferences in human mate selection. *Journal of Personality and Social Psychology, 50*, 559–570.

Buss, D. M., & Schmitt, D. P. (1993). Sexual strategies theory: An evolutionary perspective on human mating. *Psychological Review, 100*, 204–232.

Butow, P. N., Maclean, M., Dunn, S. M., Tattersall, M. H. N., & Boyer, M. J. (1997). The dynamics of change: Cancer patients' preferences for information, involvement and support. *Annals of Oncology, 8*, 857–863.

Bylund, C. L., & Makoul, G. (2002). Empathic communication and gender in the physician-patient encounter. *Patient Education and Counseling, 48*, 207–216.

Bylund, C. L., & Makoul, G. (2005). Examining empathy in medical encounters: An observational study using the empathic communication coding system. *Health Communication, 18*, 123–140.

Cacioppo, J. T., Hawkley, L. C., Crawford, E., Ernst, J. M., Burleson, M. H., Kowalewski, R. B., … Berntson, G. G. (2002). Loneliness and health: Potential mechanisms. *Psychosomatic Medicine, 64*, 401–417.

Cahill, L. (2005). His brain, her brain. *Scientific American, 292*, 40–47.

Calabrese, L. H., Bianco, J. A., Mann, D., Massello, D., & Hojat, M. (2013). Correlates and changes in empathy and attitudes toward interprofessional collaboration in osteopathic medical students. *The Journal of the American Osteopathic Association, 113*, 898–907. doi:10.7556/jaoa.2013.068.

Calhoun, J. B. (1962). Population density and social pathology. *Scientific American, 206*, 3–10.

Calman, K. C., Downie, R. S., Duthie, M., & Sweeney, B. (1988). Literature and medicine: A short course for medical students. *Medical Education, 22,* 265–269.

Campbell, A. (2008). Attachment, aggression, and affiliation: The role of oxytocin in female social behavior. *Biological Psychology, 77,* 1–10.

Campbell, D. T., & Fiske, D. W. (1959). Convergent and discriminant validation by the multitrait-multimethod matrix. *Psychological Bulletin, 56,* 81–105.

Campos, J., & Sternberg, C. (1981). Perception, appraisal and emotion in the onset of social referencing. In M. E. Lamb & L. R. Sherrod (Eds.), *Infant social cognition* (pp. 273–314). Hillsdale, NJ: Erlbaum.

Campus-Outcalt, D., Senf, J., Watkins, A. J., & Bastacky, S. (1995). The effects of medical school curricula, faculty role models, and biomedical research on choice of generalist physician career: A review and quality assessment of the literature. *Academic Medicine, 70,* 611–619.

Cannon, W. (1957). "Voodoo" death. *Psychosomatic Medicine, 19,* 182–190.

Carkhuff, R. (1969). *Helping and human relations: Selection and training* (Vol. 1). New York: Holt, Rinehart & Winston.

Carmel, S., & Glick, S. M. (1996). Compassionate-empathic physicians: Personality traits and social-organizational factors that enhance or inhibit this behavior pattern. *Social Science and Medicine, 43,* 1253–1261.

Carr, P. L., Ash, A. S., & Friedman, E. H. (1998). Relation of family responsibilities and gender to the productivity and career satisfaction of medical faculty. *Annals of Internal Medicine, 129,* 532–538.

Carr, L., Iacoboni, M., Dubeau, M. C., Mazziotta, J. C., & Lenzi, G. L. (2003). Neural mechanisms of empathy in humans: A relay from neural systems for imitation to limbic areas. *Proceedings of the National Academy of Sciences of the United States of America, 100,* 5497–5502. doi:10.1073/pnas.0935845100.

Carter, F. (1976). *The education of little tree.* Albuquerque: University of New Mexico Press.

Carter, C. S. (2007). Sex differences in oxytocin and vasopressin: Implications for autism spectrum disorders? *Behavior and Brain Research, 176,* 170–186.

Case, R. B., Moss, A. J., Case, N., McDermott, M., & Eberly, S. (1992). Living alone after myocardial infarction: Impact on prognosis. *Journal of the American Medical Association, 267,* 515–519.

Caspi, A., & Silva, P. A. (1995). Temperamental qualities at age three predict personality traits in young adulthood: Longitudinal evidence from a birth cohort. *Child Development, 66,* 486–492.

Castiello, U. (2003). Understanding other people's actions: Intention and attention. *Journal of Experimental Psychology, 29,* 416–430.

Castiello, U., Lusher, D., Mari, M., Edwards, M., & Humphreys, G. (2002). Observing a human or a robotic hand grasping an object: Differential motor priming effects. In W. Prinz & B. Hommel (Eds.), *Common mechanisms in perception and action: Attention and performance XIX* (pp. 315–333). New York: Oxford University Press.

Castiglioni, A. (1941). *A history of medicine.* New York: Knopf.

Cataldo, K. P., Peeden, K., Geesey, M. E., & Dickerson, L. (2005). Association between Balint training and physician empathy and work satisfaction. *Family Medicine, 37,* 328–331. Retrieved from: http://www.stfm.org/fmhub/fm2005/may/kari328.pdf.

Cattle, R. B. (1966). The scree test for the number of factors. *Multivariate Behavioral Research, 1,* 245–276.

Chakrabarti, B., & BaronCohen, S. (2006). Empathizing: Neurocognitive developmental mechanisms and individual differences. *Progress in Brain Research, 156,* 403–417.

Chamberlin, J. (2015). Social psychology on the silver screen. *Monitor on Psychology, 46,* 16–17.

Chaminade, T., Meltzoff, A., & Decety, J. (2002). Does the end justify the means? A PET exploration of the mechanisms involved in human imitation. *Neuroimage, 15,* 318–328.

Charlesworth, W. R., & Dzur, C. (1987). Gender comparisons of preschoolers' behavior and resource utilization in group problem-solving. *Child Development, 58,* 191–200.

Charman, T., Swettenham, J., Baron-Cohen, S., Cox, A., Baird, G., & Drew, A. (1997). Infants with autism: An investigation of empathy, pretend play, joint attention, and imitation. *Developmental Psychology, 33*, 781–789.

Charon, R. (1993). The narrative road to empathy. In H. Spiro, M. G. McCrea Curnen, E. Peschel, & D. St. James (Eds.), *Empathy and the practice of medicine* (pp. 147–159). New Haven: Yale University Press.

Charon, R. (2000). Medicine, the novel, and the passage of time. *Annals of Internal Medicine, 132*, 63–68.

Charon, R. (2001a). Narrative medicine: A model for empathy, reflection, profession, and trust. *Journal of the American Medical Association, 286*, 1897–1902.

Charon, R. (2001b). Narrative medicine: Form, function, and ethics. *Annals of Internal Medicine, 134*, 83–87.

Charon, R., Greene, M. G., & Adelman, R. (1994). Woman readers, woman doctors: A feminist reader-response theory of medicine. In E. S. More & M. A. Milligan (Eds.), *The empathic practitioner: Empathy, gender, and medicine* (pp. 205–221). New Brunswick, NJ: Rutgers University Press.

Charon, R., & Montello, M. (2002). *Stories matter: The role of narrative in medical ethics*. New York: Routledge.

Charon, R., Trautmann Banks, J., Connelly, J. E., Hunsaker Hawkins, A., Montgomery Hunter, K., Hudson Jones, A., … Poirer, S. (1995). Literature in medicine: Contribution to clinical practice. *Annals of Internal Medicine, 122*, 599–606.

Chartrand, T. L., & Bargh, J. A. (1999). The chameleon effect: The perception-behavior link and social interaction. *Journal of Personality and Social Psychology, 76*, 893–910.

Chase-Lansdale, P. L., Wakschlag, L. S., & Brooks-Gunn, J. (1995). A psychological perspective on the development of caring in children and youth: The role of the family. *Journal of Adolescence, 18*, 515–556.

Chen, D. C. R., Kirshenbaum, D. S., Yan, J., Kirshenbaum, E., & Aseltine, R. H. (2012). Characterizing changes in student empathy throughout medical school. *Medical Teacher, 34*, 305–311. doi:10.3109/0142159X.2012.644600.

Chen, J. T., LaLopa, J., & Dang, D. K. (2008). Impact of patient empathy modeling on pharmacy students caring for the underserved. *American Journal of Pharmaceutical Education, 72*(2). Article 40.

Chen, D., Lew, R., Hershman, W., & Orlander, J. (2007). A cross-sectional measurement of medical student empathy. *Journal of General Internal Medicine, 22*, 1434–1438. doi:10.1007/s11606-007-0298-x.

Chen, D. C. R., Pahilan, M. E., & Orlander, J. D. (2010). Comparing a self-administered measure of empathy with observed behavior among medical students. *Journal of General Internal Medicine, 25*, 200–202. doi:10.1007/s11606-009-1193-4.

Cheng, Y., Lin, C. P., Liu, H. L., Hsu, Y. Y., Lim, K. E., Hung, D., & Decety, J. (2007). Expertise modulates the perception of pain in others. *Current Biology, 17*, 1708–1713.

Chessick, R. D. (1992). *What constitutes the patient in psychotherapy: Alternative approaches to understanding humans*. Northvale, NJ: Jason Aronson.

Chinsky, J. M., & Rappaport, J. (1970). Brief critique of the meaning and reliability of "Accurate Empathy" ratings. *Psychological Bulletin, 73*, 379–382.

Chismar, D. (1988). Empathy and sympathy: The important difference. *Journal of Value Inquiry, 22*, 257–266.

Chlopan, B. E., McCain, M. L., Carbonell, J. L., & Hagen, R. L. (1985). Empathy: Review of available measures. *Journal of Personality and Social Psychology, 48*, 635–653.

Chodorow, N. (1978). *The reproduction of mothering: Psychoanalysis and sociology of gender*. Berkeley, CA: University of California Press.

Chow, K. L., Riesen, A. H., & Newell, F. W. (1957). Degeneration of retinal ganglion cells in infant chimpanzees reared in darkness. *Journal of Comparative Neurology, 107*, 27–42.

Christenfeld, N., & Gerin, W. (2000). Social support and cardiovascular reactivity. *Biomedicine and Pharmacotherapy, 54*, 251–257.

Christodoulou, G. N., Lykousras, L. P., Mountaokalakis, T., Voulgari, A., & Stefanis, C. N. (1995). Personalities of psychiatric versus other medical trainers. *Journal of Nervous and Mental Disease, 183*, 330–340.

Ciechanowski, P. S., Russo, J. E., Katon, W. J., & Walker, F. A. (2004). Attachment theory in health care: The influence of relationship style on medical students' specialty choice. *Medical Education, 38*, 262–270.

Clark, K. B. (1980). Empathy—A neglected topic in psychological research. *American Psychologist, 35*, 187–190.

Clearly, P. D., & McNeil, B. J. (1988). Patient satisfaction as an indicator of quality care. *Inquiry, 25*, 25–36.

Cleghorn, S. M. (1978). Empathy: Listening with the third ear. *Tennessee Education, 8*, 7–11.

Cliffordson, C. (2002). The hierarchical structure of empathy: Dimensional organization and elations to social functioning. *Scandinavian Journal of Psychology, 43*, 49–59.

Cloninger, C. R., Svrakic, D. M., & Przybeck, D. M. (1993). A psychobiological model of temperament and character. *Archives of General Psychiatry, 50*, 975–990.

Clouser, K. D. (1990). Humanities in medical education: Some contributions. *Journal of Medical Philosophy, 15*, 289–301.

Cohen, J. (1987). *Statistical power analysis for the behavioral sciences*. Hillsdale, NJ: Erlbaum.

Cohen, S. (1988). Psychological models for the role of social support in the etiology of physical disease. *Health Psychology, 7*, 269–297.

Cohen, S. (2004). Social relationship and health. *American Psychologist, 59*, 676–684.

Cohen, E. L., & Hoffner, C. (2013). Gifts of giving: The role of empathy and perceived benefits to others and self in young adults' decisions to become organ donors. *Journal of Health Psychology, 18*, 128–138.

Cohen, S., & Matthews, K. A. (1987). Social support, type A behavior, and coronary artery disease. *Psychosomatic Medicine, 49*, 325–330.

Coke, J. S., Batson, C. D., & McDavis, K. (1978). Empathic mediation of helping: A two-stage model. *Journal of Personality and Social Psychology, 36*, 752–766.

Cole, D. A., Martin, N. C., & Steiger, J. H. (2005). Empirical and conceptual problems with longitudinal trait-state models: Introducing a trait-state-occasion model. *Psychological Methods, 10*, 3–20.

Coleridge, S. T. (1802). Letter to William Sotheby, July 13th. In E. L. Griggs (Ed.), *Collected letters of Samuel Taylor Coleridge* (Vol. 2). Oxford, UK: Oxford University Press (Reprinted in 1956).

Coles, R. (1989). *Call of stories: Teaching and moral imagination*. Boston: Houghton-Mifflin.

Collier, V. U., MaCue, J. D., Markus, A., & Smith, L. (2002). Stress in medical residency: Status quo after a decade or reform? *Annals of Internal Medicine, 136*, 384–390.

Colligan, M. J., & Murphy, L. R. (1982). A review of mass psychogenic illness in work settings. In M. J. Colligan, J. W. Pennebaker, & L. R. Murphy (Eds.), *Mass psychogenic illness: A social psychological analysis* (pp. 33–52). Hillsdale, NJ: Erlbaum.

Collins, F. S. (1999). Shattuck lecture—Medical and societal consequences of the human genome project. *New England Journal of Medicine, 341*, 28–37.

Colliver, J. A., Conlee, M. J., Verhulst, S. J., & Dorsey, J. K. (2010a). Rebuttals to critics of studies of the decline on empathy [Letter to the editor]. *Academic Medicine, 85*, 1813–1814.

Colliver, J. A., Conlee, M. J., Verhulst, S. J., & Dorsey, J. K. (2010b). Reports of the decline of empathy during medical education are greatly exaggerated: A reexamination of the research. *Academic Medicine, 85*, 588–593.

Colliver, J. A., Willis, M. S., Robbs, R. S., Cohen, D. S., & Swartz, M. H. (1998). Assessment of empathy in a standardized-patient examination. *Teaching and Learning in Medicine, 10*, 8–10.

Colman, A. M. (2001). *A dictionary of psychology*. London, UK: Oxford University Press.

Comas-Diaz, L., & Jacobsen, F. M. (1991). Ethnocultural transference and countertransference in the therapeutic dyad. *American Journal of Orthopsychiatry, 61*, 392–402.

Comstock, L. M., Hooper, E. M., Goodwin, J. M., & Goodwin, J. S. (1982). Physician behaviors that correlate with patient satisfaction. *Journal of Medical Education, 57*, 105–112.

Connellan, J., Baron-Cohen, S., Wheelwright, S., Batki, A., & Ahluwalia, J. (2000). Sex differences in human neonatal social perception. *Infant Behavior & Development, 23*, 113–118.

Consorti, F., Notarangelo, M. A., Potasso, L. A., & Toscano, E. (2012). Developing professionalism in Italian medical students: An educational framework. *Advances in Medical Education and Practice, 3*, 55–60. doi:10.2147/AMEP.S31228.

Cooper-Patrick, L., Gallo, J. J., & Gonzales, J. J. (1999). Race, gender and partnership in the patient-physician relationship. *Journal of the American Medical Association, 282*, 583–589.

Coplan, A. (2014). Understanding empathy: Its features and effects. In A. Coplan & P. Goldie (Eds.), *Empathy: Philosophical and psychological perspectives* (pp. 3–18). New York: Oxford University Press.

Copland, A., & Goldie, P. (Eds.). (2014). *Understanding empathy: Its features and effects.* New York: Oxford University Press.

Costa, P., Alves, R., Neto, I., Marvão, P., Portela, M., & Costa, M. J. (2014). Associations between medical student empathy and personality: A multi-institutional study. *PLoS One, 9*(3), e89254. doi:10.1371/journal.pone.0089254.

Costa, P., Magalhães, E., & Costa, M. J. (2013). A latent growth model suggests that empathy of medical students does not decline over time. *Advances in Health Sciences Education, 18*, 509–522. doi:10.1007/s10459-012-9390-z. Retrieved from: http://link.springer.com/article/10.1007/s10459-012-9390-z?null.

Costa, P. T., Jr., & McCrea, R. B. (1992). *Revised NEO Personality Inventory (NEO PI-R) and NEO Five Factor Inventory (NEO-FFI): Professional manual.* Odessa, FL: Psychological Assessment Resources.

Coulehan, J. L., & Williams, P. (2001). Vanquishing virtue: The impact of medical education. *Academic Medicine, 76*, 598–605.

Cousins, N. (1985). How patients appraise physicians. *New England Journal of Medicine, 313*, 1422–1424.

Coutts, L. C., & Rogers, J. C. (2000). Humanism: Is its evaluation captured in commonly used performance measures? *Teaching and Learning in Medicine, 12*, 28–32.

Coutts-van Dijk, L. C., Bray, J. H., Moore, S., & Rogers, J. (1997). Prospective study of how students' humanism and psychosocial beliefs relate to specialty matching. *Academic Medicine, 72*, 1106–1108.

Crabb, W. T., Moracco, J. C., & Bender, R. C. (1983). A comparative study of empathy training with programmed instruction for lay helpers. *Journal of Counseling Psychology, 30*, 221–226.

Craig, K. D., & Weiss, S. M. (1971). Vicarious influences on pain-threshold determinations. *Journal of Personality and Social Psychology., 19*, 53–59.

Crandall, S. J., & Marion, G. S. (2009). Commentary: Identifying attitudes towards empathy: An essential feature of professionalism. *Academic Medicine, 84*, 1174–1176.

Cristy, B. L. (2001). Wounded healer: The impact of a therapist's illness on the therapeutic situation. *Journal of the American Academy of Psychoanalysis, 29*, 33–42.

Cronbach, L. J. (1951). Coefficient alpha and the internal structure of tests. *Psychometrika, 16*, 297–334.

Cross, D. G., & Sharpley, C. F. (1982). Measurement of empathy with the Hogan Empathy Scale. *Psychological Reports, 50*, 62.

Crouse, B. B., & Mehrabian, A. (1977). Affiliation of opposite-sex strangers. *Journal of Research in Personality, 11*, 38–47.

Cummings, S. A., Savitz, L. A., & Konrad, T. R. (2001). Reported response rates to mailed physician questionnaires. *Health Sciences Research, 35*, 1347–1355.

Cyphert, F. R., & Gant, W. L. (1970). The Delphi technique: A tool for collecting opinions in teacher education. *The Journal of Teacher Education, 21*, 417–425.

D'Orazio, D. M. (2004). Letter to the editor. *Sexual Abuse: A Journal of Research and Treatment, 16*, 173–174.

Dalton, R., Sunblad, L., & Hylbert, S. (1976). Using principles of social learning in training for communication in empathy. *Journal of Counseling Psychology, 23*, 454–457.

Daly, M., & Wilson, M. (1988). *Homicide*. New York: Aldine de Gruyter.

Damasio, A. (2003). *Looking for Spinoza: Joy, sorrow and the feeling brain*. New York: Harcourt Brace.

Damasio, H., Grabowski, T., Frank, R., Galaburda, A. M., & Damasio, A. R. (1994). The return of Phineas Gage: Clues about the brain from the skull of a famous patient. *Science, 264*, 1102–1105.

Darwin, C. (1965). *The expression of emotion in man and animals*. New York: St. Martin's Press (Originally published in 1872).

Darwin, C. (1981). *The descent of man, and selection in relation to sex*. NJ: Princeton University Press (Originally published in 1871).

DasGupta, S., & Charon, R. (2004). Personal illness narratives: Using reflective writing to teach empathy. *Academic Medicine, 79*, 351–356.

Davies M. F. (2003). Confirmatory bias in the evaluation of personality descriptions: Positive test strategies and output inference. *Journal of Personality and Social Psychology, 85*, 736–744. doi: 10.1037/0022-3514.85.4.736.

Davis, M. S. (1968). Physiological, psychological and demographic factors in patient compliance with doctor's orders. *Medical Care, 6*, 115–122.

Davis, M. H. (1983). Measuring individual differences in empathy: Evidence for a multidimensional approach. *Journal of Personality and Social Psychology, 44*, 113–126.

Davis, M. R. (1985). Perception of affective reverberation component. In A. P. Goldstein & G. Y. Michaels (Eds.), *Empathy: Development, training, and consequences* (pp. 62–108). Hillsdale, NJ: Erlbaum.

Davis, M. H. (1994). *Empathy: A social psychological approach*. Boulder, CO: Westview.

Davis, M. H., & Franzoi, S. L. (1991). Stability and change in adolescent self-consciousness and empathy. *Journal of Research in Personality, 25*, 70–87.

Davis, M. H., Luce, C., & Kraus, S. J. (1994). The heritability of characteristics associated with dispositional empathy. *Journal of Personality, 62*, 369–391.

Davison, A. N., & Peters, A. (1970). *Myelination*. Springfield, IL: Charles C Thomas.

Dawes, R. M. (1999). A message from psychologists to economists: Mere predictability doesn't matter like it should (without a good story appended to it). *Journal of Economic Behavior & Organization, 39*, 20–40.

Dawkins, R. (1999). *The selfish gene*. Oxford, UK: Oxford University Press.

Dawson, G. (1994). Development of emotional expression and emotion regulation in infancy: Contribution of the frontal lobe. In G. Dawson & K. W. Fischer (Eds.), *Human behavior and the developing brain* (pp. 346–379). New York: Guilford.

Day, S. C., Norcini, J. J., Shea, J. A., & Benson, J. A., Jr. (1989). Gender differences in clinical competence of residents in internal medicine. *Journal of General Internal Medicine, 4*, 309–312.

de Quervain, D. J. F., Fischbacher, U., Treyer, V., Schellhammer, M., Schnyder, U., Buck, A., & Fehr, E. (2004). The neutral basis of altruistic punishment. *Science, 305*, 1254–1258.

Deardroff, P. A., Finch, A. J., Jr., Kendall, P. C., Liran, F., & Indrisano, V. (1975). Empathy and socialization in repeat offenders, first offenders, and normals. *Journal of Counseling Psychology, 22*, 453–455.

Deardroff, P. A., Kendall, P. C., Finch, A. J., Jr., & Sitartz, A. M. (1977). Empathy, locus and control and anxiety in college students. *Psychological Reports, 40*, 1236–1238.

DeCasper, A. J., & Fifer, W. P. (1980). Of human bonding: Newborns prefer their mothers' voices. *Science, 208*, 1174–1176.

DeCasper, A. J., & Prescott, P. A. (1984). Human newborn's perception of male voices preference, discrimination, and reinforcing value. *Developmental Psychology, 17*, 481–491.

Decety, J. (2015). The neural pathways, development and functions of empathy. *Current Opinions in Behavioral Sciences, 3*, 1–3. Retrieved from: www.sciencedirect.com.

Decety, J., & Chaminade, T. (2003). Neural correlates of feeling sympathy. *Neuropsychologia, 41*, 127–138.

Decety, J., & Cowell, J. M. (2015). Empathy, justice, and moral behavior. *AJOB Neuroscience, 6*, 1–12. doi:10.1080/21507740.2015.1047055.

Decety, J., & Jackson, P. L. (2004). The functional architecture of human empathy. *Behavior and Cognitive Neuroscience Review, 3*, 71–100.

Decety, J., & Jackson, P. L. (2006). A social-neuroscience perspective on empathy. *Current Directions in Psychological Science, 15*, 54–58.

Decety, J., & Lamm, C. (2006). Human empathy through the lens of social neuroscience. *The Scientific World Journal, 6*, 1146–1163.

Dehning, S., Reiß, E., Krause, D., Gasperi, S., Meyer, S., Dargel, S., …. Siebeck, M. (2014). Empathy in high-tech and high-touch medicine. *Patient Education and Counseling. 95*, 259–264. Retrieved from: http://dx.doi.org/10.1016/j.pec.2014.01.013.

DeKruif. (1926). *Microb hunters*. New York: Harcourt, Brace.

Del Canale, S., Louis, D. Z., Maio, V., Wang, X., Rossi, G., Hojat, M., & Gonnella, J. S. (2012). The relationship between physician empathy and disease complications: An empirical study of primary care physicians and their diabetic patients in Parma, Italy. *Academic Medicine, 87*, 1243–1249. doi:10.1097/ACM.0b013e3182628fbf.

Delgado-Bolton, R., San-Martin, M., Alcorta-Garza, A., & Vivanco, L. (in press). Medical empathy of physicians-in-training who are enrolled in professional training program: A comparative intercultural study in Spain. *Atención Primaria*. Retrieved from: http://dx.doi.org/10.1016/j.aprim.2015.10.005.

Demos, E. (1988). Affect and the development of self: A new frontier. In A. Goldberg (Ed.), *Frontiers in self psychology: Progress in self psychology* (Vol. 3, pp. 27–33). Hillsdale, NJ: Analytic Press.

Derbyshire, S. W. G. (2000). Exploring the pain "neuromatrix". *Current Review of Pain, 4*, 467–477.

Derntl, B., Finkelmeyer, A., Eickhoff, S., Kellermann, T., Falkenberg, D., Schneider, F., & Habel, U. (2010). Multidimensional assessment of empathic abilities: Neural correlates and gender differences. *Psychoneuroendocrinology, 35*, 67–82. doi:10.1016/j.psyneuen.2009.10.006.

DeValck, C., Bensing, J., Bruynooghe, R., & Batenburg, V. (2001). Cure-oriented versus care-oriented attitudes in medicine. *Patient Education and Counseling, 45*, 119–126.

Diaz-Narvaez, V.P., Calzadilla-Nunez, A., Carrasco, D., Bustos, A., Zamorano, A., Silva, H., Lopez Tagle, E., Hubermann, J. (2016). Levels of empathy among dental students in five Chilean universities. *Health, 8*, 32–41. Retrieved from: http://dx.doi.org/10.4236/health.2016.81005.

Diaz-Narvaez, V. P., Coronado, A. M.E., Bilbao, J.L., Gonzalez, F., Padilla, M., Howard, M., Silva, G., Alboleda, J., Bullen, M., Utsman, R., Fajardo, E., Alonso, L.M., & Cervantes, M. (2015). Empathy levels of dental students of Central America and the Caribbean. *Health, 7*, 1678–1686. Retrieved from: http://dx.doi.org/10.4236/health.2015.712182.

Diaz-Narvaez, V. P., Gutierrez-Ventura, F.G., de Villalba, T.V., Salcedo-Rioja, M., Galzadilla-Nunez, A., Hamdan-Rodriguiz, M. (2015). Empathy levels of dentistry students in Peru and Argentina. *Health, 7*, 1268–1274. Retrieved from: http://dx.doi.org/10.4236/health.2015.710141.

Di Blasi, Z., Harkness, E., Ernst, E., Georgiou, A., & Kleijnen, J. (2001). Influence of context effect on health outcomes: A systematic review. *Lancet, 357*, 757–762.

Di Pellegrino, G., Fadiga, L., Fogassi, L., Gallese, V., & Rizzolutti, G. (1992). Understanding motor events: A neurophysiological study. *Experimental Brain Research, 91*, 176–180.

DiLillo, M., Cicchetti, A., Lo Scalzo, A., Taroni, F., & Hojat, M. (2009). The Jefferson Scale of Physician Empathy: Preliminary psychometrics and group comparisons in Italian physicians. *Academic Medicine, 84*, 1198–1202.

Dillard, J. P., & Hunter, J. E. (1989). On the use and interpretation of the Emotional Empathy Scale, the Self-Consciousness Scale, and the Self-Monitoring Scale. *Communication Research, 16*, 104–129.

DiLollo, V., & Berger, S. M. (1965). Effect of apparent pain in others on observers' reaction time. *Journal of Personality and Social Psychology, 2*, 573–575.

DiMascio, A., Boyd, R. W., & Greenblatt, M. (1957). Physiological correlates of tension and antagonism during psychotherapy: A study of "interpersonal physiology.". *Psychosomatic Medicine, 19*, 99–104.

DiMatteo, M. R. (1979). A social-psychological analysis of physician-patient rapport toward a science of the art of medicine. *Journal of Social Issues, 35*, 12–33.

DiMatteo, M. R., Hays, R. D., & Prince, L. M. (1986). Relationship of physicians' nonverbal communication skills to patient satisfaction, appointment noncompliance, and physician workload. *Health Psychology, 5*, 581–594.

DiMatteo, M. R., Prince, I. M., & Taranta, A. (1979). Patients' perceptions of physicians' behavior: Determinants of patient commitment to the therapeutic relationship. *Journal of Community Health, 4*, 280–290.

DiMatteo, M. R., Sherbourne, C. D., Hays, R. D., Ordway, L., Kravitz, R. L., McGlynn, E. A., … Rogers, W. H. (1993). Physicians' characteristics influence patients' adherence to medical treatment: Results from the Medical Outcomes Study. *Health Psychology, 12*, 93–102.

DiMatteo, M. R., Taranta, A., Friedman, H. S., & Prince, L. M. (1980). Predicting patient satisfaction from physicians' nonverbal communication skills. *Medical Care, 17*, 376–387.

Dimberg, U., Thunberg, M., & Elmehed, K. (2000). Unconscious facial reactions to emotional facial expressions. *Psychological Science, 11*, 86–89.

Diseker, R. A., & Michielutte, R. (1981). An analysis of empathy in medical students before and following clinical experience. *Journal of Medical Education, 56*, 1004–1010.

Divinagarcia, R. M., Harkin, T. J., Bonk, S., & Schluger, N. W. (1998). Screening by specialists to reduce unnecessary test ordering in patients evaluated for tuberculosis. *Chest, 114*, 664–666.

Doherty, R. W. (1997). The emotional contagion scale: A measure of individual differences. *Journal of Nonverbal Behavior, 21*, 131–154.

Doidge, N. (2007). *The brain that changes itself: Stories of personal triumph from frontiers of brain science*. New York: Penguin Books.

Domes, G., Heinrichs, M., Michel, A., Berger, C., & Herpertz, S. C. (2007). Oxytocin improves "mind-reading" in humans. *Biological Psychiatry, 61*, 731–733. doi:10.1016/j.biopsych.2006.07.015.

Dovidio, J. F. (1991). The empathy-altruistic hypothesis: Paradigm and promise. *Psychological Inquiry, 2*, 126–128.

Downie, R. S. (1991). Literature and medicine. *Journal of Medical Ethics, 17*, 93–96.

Dubnicki, C. (1977). Relationship among therapist empathy and authoritarianism. *Journal of Counseling and Clinical Psychology, 45*, 958–959.

Duff, P. (2002). Professionalism in medicine: An A–Z primer. *Obstetrics and Gynecology, 99*, 1127–1128.

Duke, P., Grosseman, S., Novack, D. H., & Rosenzweig, S. (2015). Preserving third-year medical students' empathy and enhancing self-reflection using small group "virtual hangout" technology. *Medical Teacher.* Posted online December 2014. doi:10.3109/0142159X.2014.956057.

Dunstone, D. C., & Reames, H. R. J. (2001). Physician satisfaction revisited. *Social Science & Medicine, 52*, 825–837.

Durkheim, E. (1951). *Suicide: A study in sociology, (J.A. Spaulding & G. Simpson, Trans.)*. Glencoe, IL: Free Press.

Dymond, R. F. (1949). A scale for the measurement of empathic ability. *Journal of Consulting Psychology, 13*, 127–133.

Dymond, R. F. (1950). Personality and empathy. *Journal of Counseling Psychology, 14*, 343–350.

Dyrbye, L. N., Eacker, A. M., Harper, W., Power, D. V., Massie Jr, F. S., Satele, D., … Shanafelt, T. D. (2012). Distress and empathy do not drive changes in specialty preference among US medical students. *Medical Teacher, 34*, e116–e122. doi:10.3109/0142159x.2012.644830.

Dziobek, I., Rogers, K., Fleck, S., Bahnemann, M., Heekeren, H. R., Wolf, O. T., & Convit, A. (2008). Dissociation of cognitive and emotional empathy in adults with Asperger Syndrome using multifaceted empathy test (MET). *Journal of Autism and Developmental Disorders, 38*, 464–473.2.

Eagly, A. H. (1987). *Sex differences in social behavior: A social role interpretation.* Hillside, NJ: Erlbaum.

Eagly, A. H. (1995). The science and politics of comparing women and men. *American Psychologist, 50,* 145–158.

Eagly, A. H., & Crowley, M. (1986). Gender and helping behavior: A meta-analytic review of the social psychological literature. *Psychological Bulletin, 100,* 283–308.

Eagly, A. H., & Steffen, V. J. (1986). Gender and aggressive behavior: A meta-analytic review of the social psychological literature. *Psychological Bulletin, 100,* 309–330.

Eagly, A. H., & Wood, W. (1999). The origin of sex differences in human behavior: Evolved dispositions versus social roles. *American Psychologist, 54,* 408–423.

Eagly, A. H., & Wood, W. (2013). The nature-nurture debate: 25 years of challenges in the psychology of gender. *Perspectives on Psychological Science, 8,* 340–357. Retrieved from: http://dx.doi.org/10.1177/1745691613484767.

Eddins-Folensbee, F. F., Harris, T. B., Miller-Wasik, M., & Thompson, B. (2012). Students versus faculty members as admission interviewers: Comparisons of ratings data and admission decisions. *Academic Medicine, 87,* 458–462.

Edmonds, D. (2015). *Would you kill the fat man? The trolley problem and what your answer tells us about right and wrong?* NJ: Princeton University Press.

Edwards, A. L. (1957). *The social desirability variable in personality assessment and research.* New York: Dryden.

Edwards, M. T., & Zimet, C. N. (1976). Problems and concerns among medical students. *Journal of Medical Education, 51,* 619–625.

Edwards-Lee, T. A., & Saul, R. E. (1999). Neuropsychiatry of the right prefrontal lobe. In B. L. Miller & J. L. Cummings (Eds.), *The human prefrontal lobes: Functional and disorders.* New York: Guilford Press.

Egan, G. (1975). *The skilled helper.* Monterey, CA: Brooks/Cole.

Egolf, B., Lasker, J., Wolf, S., & Potvin, L. (1992). Featuring health risks and mortality: The Roseto effect, a 50-year comparison of mortality rates. *American Journal of Public Health, 82,* 1089–1092.

Ehrlich, C. H., & Jaffe, C. (2002). Social support for dying. In J. D. Morgan (Ed.), *Social support: A reflection of humanity* (pp. 17–31). Amityville, NY: Baywood Publishing.

Eibel-Eibesfeldt, I. (1979). *The biology of peace and war.* New York: Viking.

Eisenberg, N. (1983). The relation between empathy and altruism: Conceptual and methodological issues. *Academic Psychology Bulletin, 5,* 195–208.

Eisenberg, N. (1989). *Empathy and related emotional responses* (Vol. 44). San Francisco: Jossey-Bass.

Eisenberg, N., Fabes, R. A., Murphy, B., Karbon, M., Maszk, P., Smith, M., … Suh, K. (1994). The relations of emotionality and regulation to dispositional and situational empathy-related responding. *Journal of Personality and Social Psychology, 66,* 776–797.

Eisenberg, N., & Lennon, R. (1983). Sex differences in empathy and related capacities. *Psychological Bulletin, 94,* 100–131. doi:10.1037/0033-2909.94.1.100.

Eisenberg, N., & Miller, P. A. (1987). The relation of empathy to prosocial and related behaviors. *Psychological Bulletin, 101,* 91–119.

Eisenberg, A., Rosenthal, S., & Schlussel, Y. R. (2015). Medicine as a performing art: What we can learn about empathic communication from theater arts. *Academic Medicine, 90,* 272–276. doi:10.1097/ACM.0000000000000626.

Eisenberg, N., & Strayer, J. (1987a). Critical issues in the study of empathy. In N. Eisenberg & J. Strayer (Eds.), *Empathy and its development* (pp. 3–13). Cambridge: Cambridge University Press.

Eisenberg, N., & Strayer, J. (1987b). *Empathy and its development.* Cambridge: Cambridge University Press.

Eisenberg-Berg, N., & Lennon, R. (1980). Altruism and the assessment of empathy in the preschool years. *Child Development, 51,* 552–557.

Eisenberg-Berg, N., & Mussen, P. (1978). Empathy and moral development in adolescence. *Developmental Psychology, 14*, 185–186.

Eisenberger, N., Leiberman, M., & Williams, K. (2003). Does rejection hurt? An fMRI study of social exclusion. *Science, 302*, 290–292.

Eisenthal, S. E., Emery, R., Lazare, A., & Udin, H. (1979). Adherence and negotiated approach in patienthood. *Archives of General Psychiatry, 36*, 393–398.

Ekman, P. (1992). An argument for basic emotions. *Cognition and Emotion, 6*, 169–200.

Ekman, P., & Friesen, W. V. (1974). Detecting deception from the body or face. *Journal of Personality and Social Psychology, 29*, 288–298.

Elam, C. L., & Johnson, M. M. S. (1992). An analysis of admission committee voting patterns. *Academic Medicine, 67*(10 Suppl.), S72–S75.

Elizur, A., & Rosenheim, E. (1982). Empathy and attitudes among medical students: The effects of group experience. *Journal of Medical Education, 57*, 675–683.

Engel, G. L. (1977). The need for a new medical model: A challenge for biomedicine. *Science, 196*, 129–136.

Engel, G. L. (1990). The essence of the biopsychosocial model: From 17th to 20th century science. In H. Balner (Ed.), *A challenge for biomedicine?* (pp. 13–18). Amsterdam and Rockland, MA: Swets & Zeitlinger, Inc.

Engler, C. M., Saltzman, G. A., Walker, M. L., & Wolf, F. M. (1981). Medical student acquisition and retention of communication and interviewing skills. *Journal of Medical Education, 56*, 572–579.

Englis, B. G., Vaughan, K. B., & Lanzetta, J. T. (1982). Conditioning of counter-empathetic emotional response. *Journal of Experimental and Social Psychology, 18*, 375–391.

Entman, S. S., Glass, C. A., Hickson, G. B., Githens, P. B., Whetten-Goldstein, K., & Sloan, F. A. (1994). The relationship between malpractice claims history and subsequent obstetric care. *Journal of the American Medical Association, 272*, 1588–1591.

Erera, P. I. (1997). Empathy training for helping professionals: Model and evaluation. *Journal of Social Work Education, 33*, 245–260.

Eres, R., Decety, J., Louis, W. R., & Molenberghs, P. (2015). Individual differences in local gray matter density are associated with differences in affective and cognitive empathy. *Neuroimage, 117*, 305–310.

Eron, L. D. (1958). The effect of medical education on attitudes: A follow-up study. *Journal of Medical Education, 33*, 25–33.

Eslinger, P. J. (1998). Neurological and neuropsychological bases of empathy. *European Neurology, 93*, 193–199.

Eslinger, P. J., Satish, U., & Grattan, L. M. (1996). Alterations in cognitive- and affective-based empathy after cerebral damage. *Journal of International Neuropsychological Society, 2*, 15–16.

Evans, B. J., Stanley, R. O., & Burrows, G. D. (1993). Measuring medical students' empathy skills. *British Journal of Medical Psychology, 66*, 121–133.

Eysenck, H. J., & Eysenck, S. B. G. (1975). *Manual of the Eysenck Personality Questionnaire (junior and adult)*. Essex: Hodder & Stoughton.

Fabrega, H., Ulrich, R., & Keshavan, M. (1994). Gender differences in how medical students learn to rate psychopathology. *Journal of Nervous and Mental Disease, 182*, 471–475.

Fahrbach, S. E., Morrell, I. I., & Pfaff, D. W. (1985). Role of oxytocin in the onset of estrogen-facilitated maternal behavior. In J. A. Amico & A. G. Robinson (Eds.), *Oxytocin: Clinical and laboratory studies* (pp. 372–388). Amsterdam: Elsevier.

Falvo, D., & Tippy, P. (1988). Communicating information to patients. Patient satisfaction and adherence as associated with resident skill. *Journal of Family Medicine, 26*, 643–647.

Fan, Y., Duncan, N. W., de Greck, M., & Northoff, G. (2011). Is there a core neural network in empathy? An fMRI based quantitative meta-analysis. *Neuroscience & Biobehavioral Reviews, 35*, 903–911.

Farber, N. J., Novack, D. H., & O'Brien, M. K. (1997). Love, boundaries, and the patient-physician relationship. *Archives of Internal Medicine, 157*, 2291–2294.

Feighny, K. M., Arnold, L., Monaco, M., Munro, S., & Earl, B. (1998). In pursuit of empathy and its relation to physician communication skills: Multidimensional empathy training for medical students. *Annals of Behavioral Science and Medical Education, 5*, 13–21.

Feingold, A. (1990). Gender differences in effect of physical attractiveness on romantic attraction: A comparison across five research paradigms. *Journal of Personality and Social Psychology, 59*, 981–993. doi:10.1037/0022-3514.59.5.981.

Feingold, A. (1992). Gender differences in mate selection preferences: A test of the parental invest-ment model. *Psychological Bulletin, 112*, 125–139. doi:10.1037/0033-2909.112.1.125.

Feingold, A. (1994). Gender differences in personality: A meta-analysis. *Psychological Bulletin, 116*, 429–456.

Feldman, C., & Kornfield, J. (1991). *Stories of the spirit, stories of the heart*. New York: Harper Collins.

Feldman, R., Weller, A., Zagoor-Sharon, O., & Levine, A. (2007). Evidence for a neuroendocrino-logical foundation of human affiliation: Plasma oxytocin levels across pregnancy and the post-partum period predict mother-child bonding. *Psychological Science, 18*, 965–970.

Fenichel, O. (1945). *The psychoanalytic theory of neurosis*. New York: W.W. Norton.

Ferguson, E., James, D., & Madeley, I. (2002). Factors associated with success in medical school: Systematic review of the literature. *British Medical Journal, 324*, 952–957.

Fernandez-Olano, C., Montoya-Fernandez, J., & Salinas-Sanchez, A. S. (2008). Impact of clinical interview training on the empathy level of medical students and medical and residents. *Medical Teacher, 30*, 322–324. doi:10.1080/0142159070180229.

Ferrante, J. M., Chen, P. H., & Kim, S. (2007). The effect of patient navigation on time to diagnosis, anxiety, and satisfaction in urban minority women with abnormal mammograms: A randomized controlled trial. *Journal of Urban Health: Bulletin of the New York Academy of Medicine, 85*, 114–124.

Feshbach, N. D. (1982). Sex differences in empathy and social behavior in children. In N. Eisenberg (Ed.), *The development of prosocial behavior* (pp. 315–338). New York: Academic Press.

Feshbach, N. D. (1989). Empathy training and prosocial behavior. In J. Groebel & R. A. Hinde (Eds.), *Aggression and war: Their biological and social bases* (pp. 101–111). Cambridge: Cambridge University Press.

Feshbach, N. D., & Roe, K. (1968). Empathy in six and seven year olds. *Child Development, 39*, 133–145.

Festinger, L. (1964). *Conflict, decision, and dissonance*. Stanford, CA: Stanford University Press.

Feudtner, C., Christakis, D. A., & Christakis, N. A. (1994). Do clinical clerks suffer ethical ero-sion? Students' perception of their ethical environment and personal development. *Academic Medicine, 69*, 670–679.

Ficklin, F. L., Browne, V. L., Powell, R. C., & Carter, J. E. (1988). Faculty and house staff mem-bers as role models. *Journal of Medical Education, 63*, 392–396.

Field, T. M., Woodson, R., Greenberg, R., & Cohen, D. (1982). Discrimination and imitation of facial expressions by neonates. *Science, 218*, 179–181.

Fields, S. K., Hojat, M., Gonnella, J. S., Mangione, S., Kane, G., & Magee, M. (2004). Comparisons of nurses and physicians on an operational measure of empathy. *Evaluation & the Health Professions, 27*, 80–94. doi:10.1177/0163278703261206.

Fields, S. K., Mahan, P., Hojat, M., Tillman, P., & Maxwell, K. (2011). Measuring empathy in healthcare profession students using the Jefferson Scale of Physician Empathy: Health Provider-Student Version. *Journal of Interprofessional Care, 25*, 287–293. doi:10.3109/13561 820.2011.566648.

Fifer, W. P., & Moon, C. M. (1994). The role of mother's voice in the organization of brain function in the newborn. *Acta Pædiatrica Scandinavica, 397*, 86–93.

Figley, C. R. (1995). *Compassion fatigue: Coping with secondary traumatic stress disorder in those who treat the traumatized*. New York, NY: Brunner/Mazel.

Fine, V. K., & Therrien, M. E. (1977). Empathy in the doctor-patient relationship: Skill training for medical students. *Journal of Medical Education, 52*, 752–757.

Fishbein, R. H. (1999). Scholarship, humanism, and the young physician. *Academic Medicine, 74*, 646–651.

Fishbein, M., & Ajzen, I. (1975). *Belief, attitude, intention, and behavior: An introduction to theory and research.* Reading, MA: Addison-Wesley.

Fjortoft, N., Van Winkle, L. J., & Hojat, M. (2011). Measuring empathy in pharmacy students. *American Journal of Pharmaceutical Education, 75*(6). Article 109. doi:10.5688/ajpe756109.

Flagler, E. (1997). Narrative ethics: A means to enrich medical education. *Annals of the Royal College of Physicians & Surgeons of Canada, 30*, 217–220.

Fleming, A. S., Corter, C., Stallings, J., & Steiner, M. (2002). Testosterone and prolactin are associated with emotional responses to infant cries in new fathers. *Hormones and Behavior, 42*, 399–413.

Fleming, A. S., Ruble, D., Krieger, H., & Wong, P. Y. (1997). Hormonal and experiential correlates of maternal responsiveness during pregnancy and the puerperium in human mothers. *Hormones and Behavior, 31*, 145–158.

Flores, G. (2002). Mad scientists, compassionate healers, and greedy egotists: The portrayal of physicians in the movies. *Journal of the American Medical Association, 94*, 635–658.

Flores, G., Gee, D., & Kastner, B. (2000). The teaching of cultural issues in US and Canadian medical schools. *Academic Medicine, 75*, 451–455.

Fonagy, P. (2001). *Attachment theory and psychoanalysis.* New York: Other Press.

Fonagy, P., & Target, M. (1996). Playing with reality: I. Theory of mind and the normal development of psychic reality. *International Journal of Psychoanalysis, 77*, 217–233.

Forouzan, I., & Hojat, M. (1993). Stability and change of interest in obstetrics and gynecology among medical students: Eighteen years of longitudinal data. *Academic Medicine, 68*, 919–922.

Forstater, A. T., Chauhan, N., Allen, A., Hojat, M., & Lopez, B. L. (2011). An emergency department shadowing experiences for emergency medicine residents: Can it prevent erosion of empathy? (Abstract). *Academic Emergency Medicine, 18*, s2.

Forsythe, M., Calnan, M., & Wall, B. (1999). Doctors as patients: Postal survey examining consultants and general practitioners adherence to guidelines. *British Medical Journal, 319*, 605–608.

Fox, C. M., Harper, A. P., Hyner, G. C., & Lyle, R. M. (1994). Loneliness, emotional expression, marital quality and major life events in women who developed breast cancer. *Journal of Community Health, 19*, 467–482.

Frances, A., First, M. B., & Pincus, H. A. (1995). *DSM-IV guidebook.* Washington, DC: American Psychiatric Association.

Francis, V., & Morris, M. (1969). Gaps in doctor-patient communication: Patients' response to medical advice. *The New England Journal of Medicine, 280*, 535–540.

Frank, E., & Harvey, L. K. (1996). Preventive advice rates of women and men physicians. *Archives of Family Medicine, 5*, 215–219.

Fratiglioni, L., Wang, H. X., Ericsson, K., Maytan, M., & Winblad, B. (2000). Influence of social network on occurrence of dementia: A community-based longitudinal study. *Lancet, 355*, 1315–1319.

Free, N. K., Green, B. L., Grace, M. C., Chernus, L. A., & Whitman, R. M. (1985). Empathy and outcome in brief focal dynamic therapy. *American Journal of Psychiatry, 142*, 917–921.

Freeman, H. P., Muth, B., & Kerner, J. F. (1995). Expanding access to cancer screening and clinical follow-up among the medically underserved. *Cancer Practice, 3*, 19–30.

Freemon, B., Negrete, V. F., Davis, M., & Korsch, B. M. (1971). Gaps in doctor-patient communication: Doctor-patient interaction analysis. *Pediatric Research, 5*, 298–311.

Frenk, J. (1998). Medical care and health improvement: The critical link. *Annals of Internal Medicine, 129*, 419–420.

Fretz, B. R. (1966). Postural movement in a counseling dyad. *Journal of Counseling Psychology, 13*, 343.

Freud, S. (1955). Group psychology and the analysis of the ego. In J. Strachey (Ed. & Trans.), *The standard edition of the complete psychological works of Sigmund Freud* (Vol. 18). London: Hogarth Press and the Institute of Psychoanalysis (original work published in 1921).

Freud, S. (1958a). Recommendation to physicians practicing psychoanalysis. In J. Strachey (Ed. & Trans.), *The standard edition of the complete psychological works of Sigmund Freud* (Vol. 12, pp. 109–120). London: Hogarth Press and the Institute of Psychoanalysis (original work published in 1912).

Freud, S. (1958b). On beginning the treatment. In J. Starchey (Ed. & Trans.), *The standard edition of the complete psychological works of Sigmund Freud* (Vol. 12, pp. 121–144). London: Hogarth Press and the Institute of Psychoanalysis (original work published in 1913).

Freud, S. (1960). Jokes and their relation to the unconscious. In J. Strachey (Ed. & Trans.). *The standard edition of the complete psychological works of Sigmund Freud* (entire Vol. 8). London: Hogarth Press and the Institute of Psychoanalysis (original work published in 1905).

Freud, S. (1964). An outline of psychoanalysis. In J. Strachey (Ed. & Trans.), *The standard edition of the complete psychological works of Sigmund Freud* (Vol. 23, pp. 139–301), London: Hogarth Press and the Institute of Psychoanalysis (original work published in 1938).

Friedman, E. (1990). The perlis of detachment. *Health Care Forum Journal, 33*, 9–10.

Friedman, H. S., Prince, L. M., Riggio, R. E., & DiMatteo, M. R. (1980). Understanding and assessing nonverbal expressiveness: The affective communication test. *Journal of Personality and Social Psychology, 39*, 333–351.

Friedrich, B., Evans-Lacko, S., London, J., Rhydderch, D., & Henderson, C. (2013). Anti-stigma training for medical students: The education not discrimination project. *British Journal of Psychiatry, 202*, s89–s94. doi:10.1192/bjp.bp.112.114017.

Frodi, A., & Macauley, J. (1977). Are women always less aggressive than men? A review of the experimental literature. *Psychological Bulletin, 84*, 634–660.

Fruen, M., Rothman, A., & Steiner, J. (1974). Comparisons of characteristics of male and female medical school applicants. *Journal of Medical Education, 49*, 137–145.

Fuertes, J. N., Boylan, L. S., & Fontanella, J. A. (2008). Behavioral indices in medical care outcomes: The working alliance, adherence, and related factors. *Journal of General Internal Medicine, 24*, 80–85. doi:10.1007/s11606-008-0841-4.

Fussel, F. W., & Bonney, W. C. (1990). A comparative study of childhood experience of psychotherapists and physicists: Implications for clinical practice. *Psychotherapy, 27*, 505–512.

Gabard, D. L., Lowe, D. L., Deusinger, S. S., Stelzner, D. M., & Crandall, S. J. (2013). Analysis of empathy in doctor of physical therapy students: A multi-site study. *Journal of Allied Health, 42*, 10–16.

Gabbard, G. O. (1994). On love and lust in erotic transference. *Journal of the American Psychoanalytic Association, 42*, 385–403.

Gabbard, G. O., & Nadelson, C. (1995). Professional boundaries in the physician-patient relationship. *Journal of the American Medical Association, 273*, 1445–1449.

Galanter, M., Talbott, D., Gallegos, K., & Rubenstone, E. (1990). Combined alcoholics anonymous and professional care for addicted physicians. *American Journal of Psychiatry, 147*, 64–68.

Gallagher, H. L., & Frith, C. D. (2003). Functional imaging of 'theory of mind'. *Trends in Cognitive Sciences, 7*, 77–83.

Gallese, V. (2001). The 'shared manifold' hypothesis: From mirror neurons to empathy. *Journal of Conscious Studies, 8*, 33–50.

Gallese, V. (2003). The roots of empathy: The shared manifold hypothesis and the neural basis of intersubjectivity. *Psychopathology, 36*, 171–180.

Gallese, V., Fadiga, L., Fogassi, L., & Rizzolatti, G. (1996). Action cognition in the premotor cortex. *Brain, 119*, 593–609.

Gallese, V., Keysers, C., & Rizzolatti, G. (2004). A unifying view of the basis of social cognition. *Trends in Cognitive Sciences, 8*, 394–403.

Gartrell, N., Herman, J., Olarte, S., Feldstein, M., & Localio, R. (1986). Psychiatrist-patient sexual contact: Results of a national survey: I. Prevalence. *American Journal of Psychiatry, 143*, 1126–1131.

Gaufberg, E. H., Joseph, R. C., Pels, R. J., Wyshak, G., Wieman, D., & Nadelson, C. C. (2001). Psychosocial training in U.S. internal medicine and family practice residency programs. *Academic Medicine, 76*, 738–742.

Gazzola, V., Rizzolatti, G., Wicker, B., & Keysers, C. (2007). The anthropomorphic brain: The mirror neuron system responds to human and robotic actions. *Neuroimage, 35*, 1674–1684.

Geary, D. D. (1995). Sexual selection and sex differences is spatial cognition. *Learning and Individual Differences, 7*, 289–301. doi:10.1016/1041-6080(95)90003-9.

Geisinger, K. F. (1994). Cross-cultural normative assessment: Translation and adaptation issues influencing the normative interpretation of assessment instruments. *Psychological Assessment, 6*, 304–312.

Geller, G., Tambor, E. S., Chase, G. A., & Holtzman, N. A. (1993). Measuring physicians' tolerance for ambiguity and its relationship to their reported practices regarding genetic testing. *Medical Care, 31*, 989–1001.

Gelmann, E. P., & Stewart, J. P. (1975). Faculty and students as admissions interviewers: Results of a questionnaire given to applicants. *Journal of Medical Education, 50*, 626–628.

Gendreau, P., Burke, D. M., & Grant, B. A. (1980). A second evaluation of the Rideau inmate volunteer program. *Canadian Journal of Criminology, 22*, 66–77.

Ghetti, C., Chang, J., & Gosman, G. (2009). Burnout, psychological skills, and empathy: Balint training in obstetrics and gynecology residents. *Journal of Graduate Medical Education, 1*, 231–235. doi:10.4300/JGME-D-09-00049.1.

Gianakos, D. (1996). Empathy revisited. *Archives of Internal Medicine, 156*, 135–136.

Gibson, E. J., & Walk, R. D. (1960). The visual cliff. *Scientific American, 202*, 64–71.

Gillberg, C. (1992). The Emanuel Miller memorial lecture 1991: Autism and autistic-like conditions: Subclasses among disorders of empathy. *Journal of Child Psychology and Psychiatry, 33*, 813–842.

Gillberg, C. (1996). The long-term outcome of childhood empathy disorders. *European Child, and Adolescent Psychiatry, 5*(Suppl.), 52–56.

Gilligan, C. (1982). *In a different voice: Psychological theory and women's development*. Cambridge, MA: Harvard University Press.

Gilligan, C., & Attanucci, J. (1988). Two moral orientations: Gender differences and similarities. *Merrill-Palmer Quarterly, 34*, 223–237.

Girgis, A., & Sanson-Fisher, R. W. (1995). Breaking bad news: Consensus guidelines for medical practitioners. *Journal of Clinical Oncology, 13*, 2449–2456.

Gladding, S. T. (1978). Empathy, gender, and training as factors in the identification of normal infant cry-signals. *Perceptual & Motor Skills, 47*, 267–270.

Gladstein, G. A. (1977). Empathy and counseling outcome: An empirical and conceptual review. *The Counseling Psychologist, 6*, 70–79.

Gladstein, G. A., and associates. (1987). *Empathy and counseling: Explorations in theory and research*. New York: Springer-Verlag.

Gladstein, G., & Feldstein, J. (1983). Using film to increase counselor empathic experiences. *Counselor Education and Supervision, 23*, 125–131.

Glaser, K., Hojat, M., Veloski, J. J., Blacklow, R. S., & Goepp, C. E. (2004). Science, verbal, or quantitative skills: Which is the most important predictor of physician competence? *Educational and Psychological Measurement, 52*, 395–406.

Glaser, K. M., Markham, F. W., Adler, H. M., McManus, R. P., & Hojat, M. (2007). Relationships between scores on the Jefferson scale of physician empathy, patient perceptions of physician empathy, and humanistic approaches to patient care: A validity study. *Medical Science Monitor, 13*, 291–294.

Gleichgerrcht, E., & Decety, J. (2013). Empathy in clinical practice: How individual dispositions, gender, and experience moderate empathic concern, burnout, and emotional distress in physicians. *PLoS One, 8*(1–12), e61526. doi:10.1371/journal.pone.0061526. Retrieved from: www.plosone.org.

Glynn, L. M., Christenfeld, N., & Gerin, W. (1999). Gender, social support, and cardiovascular response to stress. *Psychosomatic Medicine, 61*, 234–242.

Goldberg, P. E. (2000). The physician-patient relationship: Three psychodynamic concepts that can be applied to primary care. *Archives of Family Medicine, 9*, 1164–1168.

Golden, L. (1992). *Aristotle on tragic and comic mimesis*. Atlanta, GA: Scholars Press.

Golden, T. (2002). Acknowledging the masculine and feminine in offering support. In J. D. Morgan (Ed.), *Social support: A reflection of humanity* (pp. 73–84). Amityville, NY: Baywood Publishing.

Goldstein, A. P., & Michaels, G. Y. (1985). *Empathy: Development, training, and consequences*. Hillsdale, NJ: Erlbaum.

Goleman, D. (1995). *Emotional intelligence: Why it can matter more than I.Q.*. New York: Bantam Books.

Gonçalves-Pereira, M., Trancas, B., Loureiro, J., Papoila, A., & Caldas-De-Almeida, J. M. (2013). Empathy as related to motivations for medicine in a sample of first-year medical students. *Psychological Reports, 11*, 73–88. doi:10.2466/17.13.PR0.112.1.73-88.

Gonnella, J. S., & Hojat, M. (2001). Biotechnology and ethics in medical education of the new millennium: Physician roles and responsibilities. *Medical Teacher, 23*, 371–377.

Gonnella, J. S., Hojat, M., Erdmann, J. B., & Veloski, J. J. (1993a). What have we learned, and where do we go from here? *Academic Medicine, 68*(Suppl.), S79–S87.

Gonnella, J. S., Hojat, M., Erdmann, J. B., & Veloski, J. J. (1993b). What have we learned, and where do we go from here? In J. S. Gonnella, M. Hojat, J. B. Erdmann, & J. J. Veloski (Eds.), *Assessment measures in medical school, residency, and practice: The connections* (pp. 155–173). New York: Springer.

Gonnella, J. S., Hojat, M., & Veloski, J. J. (2011). AM last page: The Jefferson longitudinal study of medical education. *Academic Medicine, 86*, 404.

Gonnella, J. S., Mangione, S., Nasca, T. J., & Hojat, M. (2005). Empathy scores in medical school and ratings of empathic behavior in residency training 3 years later. *The Journal of Social Psychology, 145*, 663–672.

Gonullu, P., & Oztuna, D. (2012). A Turkish adaptation of the student version of the Jefferson Scale of Physician Empathy. *Marmara Medical Journal, 25*, 87–92. doi:10.5472/MMJ.2012.02272.1. Retrieved from: http://www.mmj.dergisi.org/pdf/pdf_MMJ_634.pdf.

Good, R. S. (1972). After office hours: The third ear. *Obstetrics & Gynecology, 40*, 760–762.

Goodchild, C. E., Skinner, T. C., & Parkin, T. (2005). The value of empathy in dietetic consultation: A pilot study to investigate its effect on satisfaction, autonomy and agreement. *Journal of Human Nutrition and Diet, 18*, 181–185.

Goodwin, J. S., Hunt, W. C., Key, C. R., & Samet, J. M. (1987). The effect of marital status on stage, treatment, and survival of cancer patients. *Journal of the American Medical Association, 258*, 3125–3130.

Gorsuch, R. L. (1974). *Factor analysis*. Philadelphia: W.B. Saunders.

Goubert, L., Craig, K. D., Vervoort, T., Morley, S., Sullivan, M. J. L., Williams, A. C. C., … Crombez, G. (2005). Facing others in pain: The effects of empathy. *Pain, 118*, 285–288.

Gough, H. G. (1987). *California Psychological Inventory administrator's guide*. Palo Alto, CA: Consulting Psychologist Press, Inc.

Gough, H. G., & Hall, W. B. (1977). A comparison of physicians who did or did not respond to a postal questionnaire. *Journal of Applied Psychology, 62*, 777–780.

Gould, S. J. (1981). *The mismeasurement of man*. New York: W.W. Norton.

Gouveia, L., Lelorain, S., Brédart, A., Dolbeault, S., Bonnaud-Antignac, A., Cousson-Gélie, F., & Sultan, S. (2015). Oncologists' perception of depressive symptoms in patients with advanced cancer: accuracy and relational correlates. *BMC Psychology, 3*, 6. http://doi.org/10.1186/s40359-015-0063-6.

Grant, J. P. (1991). *The state of the world's children*. Oxford: Oxford University Press.

Grattan, L. M., & Eslinger, P. J. (1989). Higher cognitive and social behavior: Changes in cognitive flexibility and empathy after lesions. *Neuropsychology, 3*, 185.

Gray, J. (1992). *Men are from Mars, women are from Venus: A practical guide for improving communication and getting what you want in a relationship*. New York: Harper & Collins.

Green, J. A., & Gustafson, G. E. (1983). Individual recognition of human infants on the basis of cries alone. *Developmental Psychobiology, 16*, 485–493.

Green, A., Peters, T. J., & Webster, D. J. T. (1991). An assessment of academic performance and personality. *Medical Education, 25*, 343–348.

Greenberg, L. S., Watson, J. C., Elliot, R., & Bohart, A. C. (2001). Empathy. *Psychotherapy, 38*, 380–384.

Greenson, R. R. (1960). Empathy and its vicissitudes. *International Journal of Psychoanalysis, 41*, 418–424.

Greenson, R. (1967). *The techniques and practice of psychoanalysis*. New York: International University Press.

Greif, E. B., & Hogan, R. (1973). The theory and measurement of empathy. *Journal of Counseling Psychology, 20*, 280–284.

Gross, E. B. (1992). Gender difference in physician stress. *Journal of the American Medical Women's Association, 29*, 57–68.

Grosseman, S., Hojat, M., Duke, P. M., Mennin, S., Rosenzweig, S., & Novack, D. (2014). Empathy, self-reflection, and curriculum choice. *The Interdisciplinary Journal of Problem-Based Learning, 8*, 35–41. Retrieved from: http:/dx.doi.org/10.7771/1541-5015.1429.

Grosseman, S., Novack, D. H., Duke, P., Mennin, S., Rosenzweig, S., Davis, T., & Hojat, M. (2014). Residents' and standardized patients' perspectives on empathy: Issues of agreement. *Patient Education and Counseling, 96*, 22–28. Retrieved from: http://dx.doi.org/10.1016/j.pec.2014.04.007.

Grossman, M., & Wood, W. (1993). Sex differences in intensity of emotional experience: A social role interpretation. *Journal of Personality and Social Psychology, 65*, 1010–1022.

Gruen, R. J., & Mendelsohn, G. (1986). Emotional responses to affective displays in others: The distinction between empathy and sympathy. *Journal of Personality and Social Psychology, 51*, 609–614.

Gruin, P., Peng, T., Lopez, G., & Nagda, B. A. (1999). Context, identity, and intergroup relations. In D. A. Prentice & D. T. Miller (Eds.), *Cultural divides: Understanding and overcoming group conflict* (pp. 133–172). New York: Russell Sage Foundation.

Guillemin, F., Bombardier, C., & Beaton, D. (1993). Cross-cultural adaptation of health-related quality of life measures: Literature review and proposed guidelines. *Journal of Clinical Epidemiology, 46*, 1417–1432.

Gulanick, N., & Schmeck, R. (1977). Modeling praise and criticism in teaching empathic responding. *Counselor Education and Supervision, 16*, 284–290.

Gustafson, J. P. (1986). *The complex secret of brief psychotherapy*. New York: W.W. Norton.

Guttman, H., & Laporte, L. (2002). Alexithymia, empathy, and psychological symptoms in family context. *Comprehensive Psychiatry, 43*, 448–455.

Guzzetta, R. A. (1976). Acquisition and transfer of empathy by the parents of early adolescents through structured learning training. *Journal of Community Psychology, 23*, 449–453.

Hafferty, F. W. (1998). Beyond curriculum reform: Confronting medicine's hidden curriculum. *Academic Medicine, 73*, 403–407.

Hall, E. T. (1966). *The hidden dimension*. Garden City, NJ: Doubleday.

Hall, J. A. (1978). Gender effects in decoding nonverbal cues. *Psychological Bulletin, 85*, 845–857.

Hall, J. A. (1984). *Nonverbal sex differences: Communication accuracy and expressive style*. Baltimore: Johns Hopkins University Press.

Hall, J. A. (1990). *Nonverbal sex differences: Accuracy of communication and expressive style*. John Hopkins University Press.

Hall, J. A. (1998). How big are nonverbal sex differences? The case of smiling and sensitivity to nonverbal cues. In D. J. Canary & K. Dindia (Eds.), *Sex differences and similarities in communication: Critical essays and empirical investigations of sex and gender in interaction* (pp. 155–177). Mahwah, NJ: Erlbaum.

Hall, J. A. (2005). The gender similarities hypothesis. *American Psychologist, 60*, 581–592. doi:10.1037/0003-066x.60.6.581.

Hall, J. A., Carter, J. D., & Horgan, T. G. (2000). Gender differences in the nonverbal communication of emotion. In A. H. Fischer (Ed.), *Gender and emotion: Social psychological perspectives* (pp. 97–117). Paris: Cambridge University Press.

Hall, J. A., & Dornan, M. C. (1988). Meta-analysis of satisfaction with medical care: Description of research domain and analysis of overall satisfaction level. *Social Science & Medicine, 27*, 637–644.

Hall, J. A., & Gunnery, S. D. (2013). Gender differences in nonverbal communication. In J. A. Hall & M. L. Knapp (Eds.), Nonverbal communication (Vol. 2, Handbook of communication science, pp. 639–669). Berlin: deGruyterMouton.

Hall, M., Hanna, L.A., Hanna, A., & McDevitt, C. (2015). Empathy in UK pharmacy students: Assessing differences by gender, level in the degree programme, part-time employment and medical status. *Pharmacy Education, 15*, 241–247.

Hall, J. A., Irish, J. T., Roter, D. L., Ehrlic, C. M., & Miller, L. H. (1994). Gender in medical encounters: An analysis of physician and patient communication in a primary care setting. *Health Psychology, 13*, 384–392.

Hall, J. A., Roter, D. L., & Katz, N. R. (1988). Meta-analysis of correlates of provider behavior in medical encounters. *Medical Care, 26*, 657–675.

Halpern, J. (2001). *From detached concern to empathy: Humanizing medical practice.* New York: Oxford University Press.

Halsband, U., Schmitt, J., Weyers, M., Binkofski, F., Grutzner, G., & Freund, H. J. (2001). Recognition and imitation of pantomimed motor acts after unilateral parietal and premotor lesions: A perspective on apraxia. *Neuropsychology, 39*, 200–216.

Hamilton, W. D. (1964). The genetic evolution of social behavior. *Journal of Theoretical Biology, 7*, 1–52.

Hamilton, N. G. (1984). Empathic understanding. In J. Lichtenberg, M. Bornstein, & D. Silver (Eds.), *Empathy II* (pp. 217–222). Hillsdale, NJ: The Analytic Press.

Han, S., Fan, Y., & Mao, L. (2008). Gender difference in empathy for pain: An electrophysiological investigation. *Brain Research, 1196*, 85–93. doi:10.1016/j.brainres.2007.12.062.

Haney, C., Banks, C., & Zimbardo, P. (1973). Interpersonal dynamics in a simulated prison. *International Journal of Criminology and Penology, 1*, 69–97.

Haque, O. S., & Waytz, A. (2012). Dehumanization in medicine: Causes, solutions, and functions. *Perspectives on Psychological Sciences, 7*, 176–186. doi:10.1177/1745691611429706.

Hari, R., Forss, N., Avikainen, S., Kirveskari, E., Salenius, S., & Rizzolatti, G. (1998). Activation of human primary motor cortex during action observation: A neuromagnetic study. *Proceedings of the National Academy of Sciences of the United States of America, 95*, 15061–15065.

Harrigan, J. A., & Rosenthal, R. (1983). Physicians' head and body position as determinants of perceived rapport. *Journal of Applied Social Psychology, 13*, 496–509.

Harsch, H. H. (1989). The role of empathy in medical students' choice of specialty. *Academic Psychiatry, 13*, 96–98.

Hartup, W. W., & Stevens, N. (1999). Friendships and adaptation across the life span. *American Psychological Society, 8*, 76–79.

Hasan, S., Al-Sharqawi, N., Dashti, F., AbdulAziz, M., Abdullah, A., Shukkur, M., … Thalib, L. (2013). Level of empathy among medical students in Kuwait University, Kuwait. *Medical Principles and Practice.* Open Access. doi:10.1159/000348300.

Hasan, S. H., Babar, M. G., Chen, K. K., Ahmed, S. I., & Mitha, S. (2013). An assessment of pharmacy students' empathy levels in Malaysia. *Journal of Advanced Pharmacy Education & Research, 3*, 531–540.

Hass, J. S., Cook, E. F., Puopolo, A. L., Burnstin, H. R., Clearly, P. D., & Brennan, T. A. (2000). Is professional satisfaction of general internists associated with patient satisfaction? *Journal of General Internal Medicine, 15*, 122–128.

Hasse, R. F., & Tepper, D. T., Jr. (1972). Nonverbal components of empathic communication. *Journal of Counseling Psychology, 19*, 417–424.

Hatcher, S. L., Nadeau, M. S., Walsh, L. K., Reynolds, M., Gala, J., & Marz, K. (1994). The teaching of empathy for high school and college students: Testing Rogerian methods with the Interpersonal Reactivity Index. *Adolescence, 29*, 961–974.

Hebb, D. (1946). *The organization of behaviour.* New York: John Wiley & Sons.

Heilman, K. M., Scholes, R., & Watson, R. T. (1975). Auditory affective agnosia: Disturbed comprehension of affective speech. *Journal of Neurology, Neurosurgery and Psychiatry, 38*, 69–72.

Hein, G., Engelmann, J.B., Vollberg, M.C., & Tobler, P.N. (2016). How learning shapes the empathic Pain. *Proceedings of the National Academy of Sciences, 113*, 80–85.

Hein, G., & Singer, T. (2008). I feel how you feel but not always: The empathic brain and its modulation. *Current Opinion in Neurobiology, 18*, 153–158.

Heinrichs, M., & Domes, G. (2008). Neuropeptides and social behavior: Effects of oxytocin and vasopressin in humans. *Progress in Brain Research, 170*, 337–350.

Heinrichs, M., Meinlschmidt, G., Wippich, W., Ehlert, U., & Hemmhammer, D. H. (2004). Selective Amnesic effects of oxytocin on human memory. *Physiology and Behavior, 83*, 31–38.

Hekmat, H., Khajavi, F., & Mehryar, A. H. (1974). Psychoticism, neuroticism, and extraversion: The personality determinants of empathy. *Journal of Clinical Psychology, 30*, 559–561.

Hekmat, H., Khajavi, F., & Mehryar, A. H. (1975). Some personality correlates of empathy. *Journal of Counseling and Clinical Psychology, 43*, 89.

Hemmerdinger, H. M., Stoddart, A. D. R., & Lilford, R. J. (2007). A systematic review of tests of empathy in medicine. *BMC Medical Education, 7*, 24. doi:10.1186/1472-6920-7-24. Retrieved from: http://www.biomedcentral.com/1472-6920/7/24.

Henderson, S. (1974). Care-eliciting behavior in man. *The Journal of Nervous and Mental Disease, 159*, 172–181.

Henderson, J. T., & Weisman, C. S. (2001). Physician gender effects on preventive screening and counseling: An analysis of male and female patients' health care experiences. *Medical Care, 39*, 1281–1292.

Hennen, B. K. (1975). Continuity of care in family practice. *The Journal of Family Practice, 2*, 371–372.

Henry-Tillman, R., Deloney, L. A., Savidge, M., Graham, C. J., & Klimberg, S. (2002). The medical student as patient navigator as an approach to teaching empathy. *The American Journal of Surgery, 183*, 659–662.

Herman, J. (2000). Reading for empathy. *Medical Hypotheses, 54*, 167–168.

Hess, U., Blairy, S., & Phillippot, P. (1999). Facial mimicry. In P. Phillippot, R. Feldman, & E. Coats (Eds.), *The social context of nonverbal behavior* (pp. 213–241). Cambridge: Cambridge University Press.

Hickson, G. B., Clayton, E. W., Entman, S. S., Miller, C. S., Githens, P. B., Whetten-Goldstein, K., & Sloan, F. A. (1994). Obstetricians' prior malpractice experience and patients' satisfaction with care. *Journal of the American Medical Association, 272*, 1583–1587.

Hickson, G. B., Clayton, E. W., Githens, P. B., & Sloan, F. A. (1992). Factors that prompted families to file medical malpractice claims following perinatal injuries. *Journal of the American Medical Association, 267*, 1359–1363.

Hill, E., Berthoz, S., & Frith, U. (2004). Brief report: Cognitive processing of own emotions in individuals with autistic spectrum disorder and in their relatives. *Journal of Autism and Developmental Disorders, 34*, 229–235.

Hinshelwood, R. (1989). *A dictionary of Kleinian thought*. London: Free Association Press.

Hirshberg, C., & Barasch, M. I. (1995). *Remarkable recovery*. New York: Riverside Books.

Hislop, T. G., Waxler, N. E., Coldman, A. J., Elwood, J. M., & Kan, L. (1987). The prognostic significance of psychosocial factors in women with breast cancer. *Journal of Chronic Diseases, 40*, 729–735.

Hittelman, J. H., & Dickes, R. (1979). Sex differences in neonatal eye contact time. *Merrill-Pamler Quarterly, 25*, 171–184.

Hobfolls, S. E., & Benor, D. (1981). Prediction of student clinical performance. *Medical Education, 15*, 231–236.

Hodges, S. D., & Wegner, D. M. (1997). Automatic and controlled empathy. In W. Ickes (Ed.), *Empathic accuracy* (pp. 311–339). New York: Guilford.

Hoffman, M. L. (1977). Sex differences in empathy and related behaviors. *Psychological Bulletin, 84*, 712–722.

Hoffman, M. L. (1978). Psychological and biological perspectives on altruism. *International Journal of Behavioral Development, 1*, 323–339.

Hoffman, M. L. (1981). The development of empathy. In J. Rushton & R. Sorrentino (Eds.), *Altruism and helping behavior: Social personality and developmental perspectives* (pp. 41–63). Hillsdale, NJ: Erlbaum.

Hoffman, M. L. (1982). The measurement of empathy. In C. E. Izard (Ed.), *Measuring emotions in infants and children* (pp. 279–296). Cambridge: Cambridge University Press.

Hoffman, T. L., & Reif, S.D. (1978). *'Intro aging': Simulation game*. Thorofare, NJ: Charles B. Slack Inc.

Hoffman, S. B., Brand, F. R., Beatty, P. G., & Hamill, L. A. (1985). Geriatrix: A role-playing game. *Gerontologist, 25*, 568–572.

Hogan, R. (1969). Development of an empathy scale. *Journal of Consulting and Clinical Psychology, 33*, 307–316.

Hogan, R. (1976). Moral conduct and moral character: A psychological perspective. *Psychological Bulletin, 79*, 217–232.

Hogan, R., & Dickstein, E. (1972). A measure of moral value. *Journal of Consulting and Clinical Psychology, 39*, 210–214.

Hogan, R., & Mankin, D. (1970). Determinants of interpersonal attraction: A clarification. *Psychological Reports, 26*, 235–238.

Hogan, R., & Weiss, D. S. (1974). Personality correlates of superior academic achievement. *Journal of Consulting Psychology, 21*, 144–151.

Hojat, M. (1982a). Loneliness as a function of selected personality variables. *Journal of Clinical Psychology, 38*, 137–141.

Hojat, M. (1982b). Psychometric characteristics of the UCLA Loneliness Scale. *Educational and Psychological Measurement, 42*, 917–925.

Hojat, M. (1983). Comparison of transitory and chronic loners on selected personality variables. *British Journal of Psychology, 74*, 199–202.

Hojat, M. (1992). Social and economic factors in patients with coronary disease. *Journal of the American Medical Association, 268*, 195–196.

Hojat, M. (1993). The world's declaration of the rights of the child: Anticipated challenges. *Psychological Reports, 72*, 1011–1022.

Hojat, M. (1995). Developmental pathways to violence: A psychodynamic paradigm. *Peace Psychology Review, 1*, 177–196.

Hojat, M. (1996). Perception of maternal availability in childhood and selected psychosocial characteristics in adulthood. *Genetic, Social, and General Psychology Monographs, 122*, 425–450.

Hojat, M. (1997). The U.N. Convention: Lost in the clash of adverse opinions. *American Psychologist, 52*, 1384–1385.

Hojat, M. (1998). Satisfaction with early relationships with parents and psychosocial attributes in adulthood: Which parent contributes more? *Journal of General Psychology, 159*, 203–220.

Hojat, M. (2009). Ten approaches for enhancing empathy in health and human services cultures. *Journal of Health and Human Services Association, 31*, 412–450.

Hojat, M. (2014). Assessments of empathy in medical school admissions: What additional evidence is needed? *International Journal of Medical Education, 5*, 7–10. doi:10.5116/ijme.52b7.5294.

Hojat, M., Axelrod, D., Spandorfer, J., & Mangione, S. (2013). Enhancing and sustaining empathy in medical students. *Medical Teacher, 35*, 996–1001. doi:10.3109/0142159X.2013.802300.

Hojat, M., Bianco, J. A., Mann, D., Massello, D., & Calabrese, L. H. (2015). Overlap between empathy, teamwork and integrative approach to patient care. *Medical Teacher, 37*, 755–758. doi:10.3109/0142159x.2014.971722.

Hojat, M., Borenstein, B. D., & Shapurian, R. (1990). Perception of childhood dissatisfaction with parents and selected personality traits in adulthood. *The Journal of Genetic Psychology, 117*, 241–253.

Hojat, M., & Crandall, R. (Eds.). (1989). *Loneliness: Theory, research, and applications*. Newbury, CA: Sage.

Hojat, M., Erdmann, J. B., Veloski, J. J., Nasca, T. J., Callahan, C., Julian, E., & Peck, J. (2000). A validity study of the writing sample section of the Medical College Admission Test. *Academic Medicine, 75*, S25–S27.

Hojat, M., Erdmann, J. B., & Gonnella, J. S. (2014). *Personality assessments and outcomes in medical education and the practice of medicine (AMEE Guide 79)*. Dundee, UK: Association for Medical Education in Europe (AMEE). First published in 2013 in *Medical Teacher, 35*, e1267–e1301.

Hojat, M., Fields, S. K., Rattner, S. L., Griffiths, M., Cohen, M. J. M., & Plumb, J. (1997). Attitudes toward the physician-nurse alliance: Comparisons of medical and nursing students. *Academic Medicine, 72*, 1–3.

Hojat, M., Fields, S. K., & Gonnella, J. S. (2003). Empathy: An NP/MD comparison. *The Nurse Practitioner, 28*, 45–47.

Hojat, M., Glaser, K., Xu, G., Veloski, J. J., & Christian, E. B. (1999). Gender comparisons of medical students' psychosocial profile. *Medical Education, 33*, 342–349.

Hojat, M., Glaser, K. M., & Veloski, J. J. (1996). Associations between selected psychosocial attributes and ratings of physician competence. *Academic Medicine, 71*, S103–S105.

Hojat, M., & Gonnella, J. S. (2015). Eleven years of data on the Jefferson Scale of Empathy-Medical Student Version (JSE-S): Proxy norm data and tentative cutoff scores. *Medical Principles and Practice, 24*, 344–350. doi:10.1159/000381954. Retrieved from: http://www.karger.com/doi/10.1159/000381954.

Hojat, M., Gonnella, J. S., Erdmann, J. B., Rattner, S. L., Veloski, J. J., Glaser, K., & Xu, G. (2000). Gender comparisons of income expectations in the USA at the beginning of medical school during the past twenty-eight years. *Social Science & Medicine, 50*, 1665–1672.

Hojat, M., Gonnella, J. S., Erdmann, J. B., Veloski, J. J., Louis, D. Z., Nasca, T. J., & Rattner, S. L. (2000). Physicians' perceptions of the changing health care system: Comparisons by gender and specialties. *Journal of Community Health, 25*, 455–471.

Hojat, M., Gonnella, J. S., Erdmann, J. B., & Vogel, W. H. (2003). Medical students' cognitive appraisal of stressful life events as related to personality, physical well-being, and academic performance: A longitudinal study. *Personality and Individual Differences, 35*, 219–235.

Hojat, M., Gonnella, J. S., Mangione, S., Nasca, T. J., Veloski, J. J., Erdmann, J. B., … Magee, M. (2002). Empathy in medical students as related to academic performance, clinical competence and gender. *Medical Education, 36*, 522–527. doi:10.1046/j.1365-2923.2002.01234.x.

Hojat, M., Gonnella, J. S., Mangione, S., Nasca, T. J., & Magee, M. (2003). Physician empathy in medical education and practice: Experience with the Jefferson Scale of Physician Empathy. *Seminars in Integrative Medicine, 1*, 25–41.

Hojat, M., Gonnella, J. S., Nasca, T. J., Fields, S. K., Alcorta-Gonzalez, A., Ibarra, D., … Torres-Ruiz, A. (2003). Comparisons of American, Israeli, Italian and Mexican physicians and nurses on four dimensions of the Jefferson Scale of Attitudes toward Physician Nurse Collaboration. *International Journal of Nursing Studies, 40*, 426–435.

Hojat, M., Gonnella, J. S., Nasca, T. J., Mangione, S., Veloski, J. J., & Magee, M. (2002a). The Jefferson Scale of Physician Empathy: Further psychometric data and differences by gender and specialty at item level. *Academic Medicine [Supplement], 77*, S58–S60.

Hojat, M., Gonnella, J. S., Nasca, T. J., Mangione, S., Vergare, M., & Magee, M. (2002b). Physician empathy: Definition, components, measurement, and relationship to gender and specialty. *American Journal of Psychiatry, 159*, 1563–1569.

Hojat, M., Gonnella, J. S., & Veloski, J. (2010). Rebuttals to critics of studies of decline on empathy [Letter to the editor]. *Academic Medicine, 85*, 1812.

Hojat, M., & Herman, M. W. (1985). Developing an instrument to measure attitudes toward nurses: Preliminary psychometric findings. *Psychological Reports, 56*, 571–579.

Hojat, M., & LaNoue, M. (2014). Exploration and confirmation of the latent variable structure of the Jefferson Scale of Empathy. *International Journal of Medical Education, 5*, 73–81. doi:10.5116/ijme.533f.0c41.

Hojat, M., Louis, D. Z., Maio, V., & Gonnella, J. S. (2013). Empathy and health care quality [Editorial]. *American Journal of Medical Quality, 28*, 6–7. doi:10.1177/1062860612464731.

Hojat, M., Louis, D. Z., Markham, F. W., Wender, R., Rabinowitz, C., & Gonnella, J. S. (2011). Physicians' empathy and clinical outcomes in diabetic patients. *Academic Medicine, 86*, 359–364. doi:10.1097/ACM.0b013e3182086fe1.

Hojat, M., Louis, D. Z., Maxwell, K., Markham, F., Wender, R., & Gonnella, J. S. (2010). Patient perceptions of physician empathy, satisfaction with physician, interpersonal trust, and compliance. *International Journal of Medical Education, 1*, 83–87. doi:10.5116/ijme.4d00.b701.

Hojat, M., Louis, D. Z., Maxwell, K., & Gonnella, J. S. (2011). The Jefferson Scale of Empathy (JSE): An update. *Health Policy Newsletter, 24*, 5–6. Retrieved from: http://jdc.jefferson.edu/cgi/viewcontent.cgi?article=1727&context=hpn.

Hojat, M., Mangione, S., Gonnella, J. S., Nasca, T., Veloski, J. J., & Kane, G. (2001). Empathy in medical education and patient care [Letter to the editor]. *Academic Medicine, 76*, 669.

Hojat, M., Mangione, S., Kane, G., & Gonnella, J. S. (2005). Relationships between scores of the Jefferson Scale of Physician Empathy (JSPE) and the Interpersonal Reactivity Index (IRI). *Medical Teacher, 27*, 625–628. doi:10.1080/01421590500069744.

Hojat, M., Mangione, S., Nasca, T. J., Cohen, M. J. M., Gonnella, J. S., Erdmann, J. B., … Magee, M. (2001). The Jefferson Scale of Physician Empathy: Development and preliminary psychometric data. *Educational and Psychological Measurement, 61*, 349–365.

Hojat, M., Mangione, S., Nasca, T. J., Rattner, S. L., Erdmann, J. B., Gonnella, J. S., & Magee, M. (2004). An empirical study of decline of empathy in medical school. *Medical Education, 38*, 934–941. doi:10.1111/j.1365-2929.2004.01911.x.

Hojat, M., Michalec, B., Veloski, J., & Tykocinski, M. L. (2015). Can empathy, other personality attributes, and level of positive social influence in medical school identify potential leaders in medicine? *Academic Medicine, 90*, 505–510. doi:10.1097/ACM.0000000000000652.

Hojat, M., Nasca, T. J., Cohen, M. J. M., Fields, S. K., Rattner, S. L., Griffiths, M., … Garcia, A. (2001). Attitudes toward physician-nurse collaboration: A cross-cultural study of male and female physicians and nurses in the United States and Mexico. *Nursing Research, 50*, 123–128.

Hojat, M., Nasca, T. J., Magee, M., Feeney, K., Pascual, R., Urbano, F., & Gonnella, J. S. (1999). A comparison of the personality profiles of internal medicine residents, physician role models, and the general population. *Academic Medicine, 74*, 54–60.

Hojat, M., Paskin, D. L., Callahan, C. A., Nasca, T. J., Louis, D. Z., Veloski, J. J., … Gonnella, J. S. (2007). Components of postgraduate competence: Analyses of 30 years of longitudinal data. *Medical Education, 41*, 282–289.

Hojat, M., Robeson, M., Damjanov, I., Veloski, J. J., Glaser, K., & Gonnella, J. S. (1993). Students' psychosocial characteristics as predictors of academic performance in medical school. *Academic Medicine, 68*, 635–637.

Hojat, M., Robeson, M., Veloski, J. J., Blacklow, R. S., Xu, G., & Gonnella, J. S. (1994). Gender comparisons prior to, during, and after medical school using two decades of longitudinal data at Jefferson Medical College. *Evaluation and the Health Professions, 17*, 290–306.

Hojat, M., Samuel, S., & Thompson, T. L. (1995). Searching for the lost key under the light of biomedicine: A triangular biopsychosocial paradigm may cast additional light on medical education, research and patient care. In S. K. Majumdar, L. M. Rosenfeld, D. B. Nash, & A. M. Audet (Eds.), *Medicine & health care into the 21st century* (pp. 310–325). Easton, PA: Pennsylvania Academy of Science.

Hojat, M., & Shapurian, R. (1986). Anxiety and its measurement: A study of psychometric characteristics of a short form of the Taylor Manifest Anxiety Scale in Iranian students. *Journal of Social Behavior and Personality, 1*, 621–630.

Hojat, M., Shapurian, R., Foroughi, D., Nayerahmadi, H., Farzaneh, M., Shafieyan, M., & Parsi, M. (2000). Gender differences in traditional attitudes toward marriage and the family: An empirical study of Iranian immigrants in the United States. *Journal of Family Issues, 21*, 419–434.

Hojat, M., Shapurian, R., & Mehryar, A. H. (1986). Dimensionality of the short form of the Beck Depression Inventory. *Psychological Reports, 59*, 1069–1070.

Hojat, M., Shapurian, R., Nayerahmadi, H., Farzaneh, M., Foroughi, D., Parsi, M., & Azizi, M. (1999). Premarital sexual, childrearing, and family attitudes of Iranian men and women in the United States and in Iran. *Journal of Psychology, 133*, 19–31.

Hojat, M., Spandorfer, J., Isenberg, G., Vergare, M., & Fassihi, R. (2012). Psychometrics of the scale of attitudes toward physician-pharmacist collaboration: A study with medical students. *Medical Teacher, 34*, e833–e837.

Hojat, M., Spandorfer, J., Louis, D. Z., & Gonnella, J. S. (2011). Empathic and sympathetic orientations toward patient care: Conceptualization, measurement, and psychometrics. *Academic Medicine, 86*, 989–995. doi:10.1097/ACM.0b013e31822203d8.

Hojat, M., Veloski, J. J., Louis, D. Z., Xu, G., Ibarra, D., Gottlieb, J. E., & Erdmann, J. B. (1999). Perceptions of medical seniors of the current changes in the United States health care system. *Evaluation and the Health Professions, 22*, 169–183.

Hojat, M., Veloski, J. J., & Zeleznik, C. (1985). Predictive validity of the MCAT for students with two sets of scores. *Journal of Medical Education, 60*, 911–918.

Hojat, M., Vergare, M., Isenberg, G., Cohen, M., & Spandorfer, J. (2015). Underlying construct of empathy, optimism, and burnout in medical students. *International Journal of Medical Education, 6*, 12–16. doi:10.5116/ijme.54c3.60cd.

Hojat, M., Vergare, M., Maxwell, K., Brainard, G., Herrine, S. K., Isenberg, G. A., … Gonnella, J. S. (2009). The devil is in the third year: A longitudinal study of erosion of empathy in medical school. *Academic Medicine, 84*, 1182–1191.

Hojat, M., & Vogel, W. H. (1989). Socioemotional bonding and neurobiochemistry. *Journal of Social Behavior and Personality, 2*, 135–144.

Hojat, M., Vogel, W. H., Zeleznik, C., & Borenstein, B. D. (1988). Effects of academic and psychosocial predictors of performance in medical school on coefficients of determination. *Psychological Reports, 63*, 383–394.

Hojat, M., & Xu, G. (2004). A visitor's guide to effect sizes: Statistical versus practical (clinical) importance of research findings. *Advances in Health Sciences Education, 9*, 241–249.

Hojat, M., Zuckerman, M., Gonnella, J. S., Mangione, S., Nasca, T., Vergare, M., & Magee, M. (2005). Empathy in medical students as related to specialty interest, personality, and perception of mother and father. *Personality and Individual Differences, 39*, 1205–1215. doi:10.1016/j.paid.2005.04.007.

Holden, C. (2004). Image studies show how brain thinks about pain. *Science, 303*, 1121.

Holland, J. C. (2001). Improving the human side of cancer care: Psycho-oncology's contribution. *Cancer Journal, 7*, 458–471.

Holland, J. C., Geary, N., Marchini, A., & Tross, S. (1987). An international survey of physician attitudes and practice in regard to revealing the diagnosis of cancer. *Cancer Investigation, 5*, 151–154.

Holleman, W. L. (2000). The play's the thing: Using literature and drama to teach about death and dying. *Family Medicine, 32*, 523–524.

Hollowell, E. E., & De Ville, K. A. (2003). *Physicians: Avoid treating family members*. Retrieved from: http://www.nchealthlaw.com/mla10.html.

Holmes, C. A. (1992). The wounded healer. *International Journal of Communicative Psychoanalysis & Psychotherapy, 6*, 33–36.

Holtzman, J. M., Beck, J. D., & Coggin, P. G. (1978). Geriatric program for medical students: II. Impact of two educational experiences on students attitudes. *Journal of American Geriatric Society, 26*, 355–359.

Holtzman, J. M., Beck, J. D., & Ettinger, R. L. (1981). Cognitive knowledge and attitudes toward the aged dental and medical students. *Educational Gerontology, 6*, 195–207.

Holub, P. G. (2011). The influence of narrative in fostering affective development of medical professionalism in an online class. Doctoral dissertation completed at the Nova Southeastern University, Ft. Lauderdale, FL. ISBN: 978-1-124-43810-8.

Hong, M., Bahn, G. H., Lee, W. H., & Moon, S. J. (2011). Empathy in Korean psychiatric residents. *Asia-Pacific Psychiatry, 3*, 83–90. doi:10.1111/j.1758-5872.2011.00123x.

Hong, M., Lee, W. H., Park, J. H., Yoon, T. Y., Moon, D. S., & Lee, S. M. (2012). Changes of empathy in medical college and medical school students: 1-year follow up study. *BMC Medical Education, 12*, 122. doi:10.1186/1472-6920-12-122. Retrieved from: http://www.biomedcentral.com/1472-6920/12/122.

Hooper, E. M., Comstock, L. M., Goodwin, J. M., & Goodwin, J. S. (1982). Patient characteristics that influence physician behavior. *Medical Care, 20*, 630–638.

Hoover, R. N. (2000). Cancer: Nature, nurture, or both. *The New England Journal of Medicine, 343*, 135–136.

Hornblow, A. R., Kidson, M. A., & Ironside, W. (1988). Empathic processes: Perception by medical students of patients' anxiety and depression. *Medical Education, 22*, 15–18.

Hornblow, A. R., Kidson, M. A., & Jones, K. V. (1977). Measuring medical students' empathy: A validation study. *Medical Education, 11*, 7–12.

Hornstein, H. A. (1978). Promotive tension and prosocial behavior: A Lewinian analysis. In L. Wispe (Ed.), *Altruism, sympathy, and helping: Psychological and sociological principles* (pp. 177–207). New York: Academic Press.

Horton, P. C. (1995). The comforting substrate and the right brain. *Bulletin of the Menninger Clinic, 59*, 480–486.

House, J. S., Landis, K. R., & Umberson, D. (1988). Social relationships and health. *Science, 241*, 540–544.

House, J. S., Robbins, C., & Metzner, H. L. (1982). The association of social relationships and activities with mortality: Prospective evidence from the Tecumseh Community Health Study. *American Journal of Epidemiology, 116*, 123–140.

Houston, W. R. (1938). The doctor himself as a therapeutic agent. *Annals of Internal Medicine, 11*, 1416–1425.

Howell, E. A., Gardiner, B., & Concato, J. (2002). Do women prefer female obstetricians? *Obstetrics and Gynecology, 100*, 827–828.

Hróbjartsson, A., & Gøtzsche, P. C. (2001). Is the placebo powerless? An analysis of clinical trials comparing placebo with no treatment. *The New England Journal of Medicine, 344*, 1594–1632.

Hsiao, C. Y., Tsai, Y. F., & Kao, Y. C. (2012). Psychometric properties of a Chinese version of the Jefferson Scale of Empathy—Health Profession Students. *Journal of Psychiatric and Mental Health Nursing, 12*, 866–873. doi:10.1111/jpm.12024. Retrieved from: http://onlinelibrary.wiley.com/doi/10.1111/jpm.12024/pdf.

Hsieh, N. K., Herzig, K., Gansky, S. A., & Danley, D. (2006). Changing dentists' knowledge, attitudes and behavior regarding domestic violence through an interactive multimedia tutorial. (2006). *Journal of American Dental Association, 137*, 596, 603.

Hu, L., & Bentler, P. M. (1998). Fit indices in covariance structure modeling: Sensitivity to underparameterized model misspecification. *Psychological Methods, 3*, 424–453.

Hubel, D. H. (1967). Effect of distortion of sensory input on the visual system of kittens. *The Physiologist, 10*, 17–54.

Hubel, D. H., & Wiesel, T. N. (1963). Receptive fields of cell in striate cortex of young, visually inexperienced kittens. *Journal of Neurophysiology, 26*, 994–1002.

Hubel, D. H., & Wiesel, T. N. (1970). The period of susceptibility to the physiological effects of unilateral eye closure in kittens. *Journal of Physiology, 206*, 419–436.

Hudson, G. R. (1993). Empathy and technology in the coronary care unit. *Intensive and Critical Care Nursing, 9*, 55–61.

Humphrey, N. (1983). *Consciousness regained*. Oxford: Oxford University Press.

Hunsdahl, J. B. (1967). Concerning Einfühlung (empathy): A concept analysis of its origin and early development. *Journal of History of the Behavioral Sciences, 3*, 180–191.

Hunt, E., & Agnoli, F. (1991). The Whorfian hypothesis: A cognitive psychology perspective. *Psychological Review, 98*, 337–389.

Hurlemann, R., Patin, A., Onur, O. A., Cohen, M. X., Baumgartner, T., Metzler, S., ... Kendrick, K. M. (2010). Oxytocin enhances amygdala-dependent, socially reinforced learning ad emotional empathy in humans. *Journal of Neuroscience, 30*, 4999–5007. doi:10.1523/NEUROSCI.5538-09.2010.

Hurwitz, B. (2000). Narrative and the practice of medicine. *Lancet, 365*, 2086–2089.

Hyde, J. S. (1984). How large are gender differences in aggression? *Developmental Psychology, 20*, 722–736.

Hyde, J. S. (2005). The gender similarities hypothesis. *American Psychologist, 60*, 581–592. Retrieved from: http://dx.doi.org/10.1037/0003-066X.60.6.581.

Hyyppa, M. T., Kronholm, E., & Mattlar, C. (1991). Mental well-being of good sleepers in a random sample population. *British Journal of Medical Psychology, 64*, 25–34.

Iacoboni, M. (2009a). Imitation, empathy, and mirror neurons. *Annual Review of Psychology, 60*, 653–670.

Iacoboni, M. (2009b). *Mirroring people: The science of empathy and how we connect with others.* New York: Farrar, Straus & Giroux.

Iacoboni, M., Molnar-Szakacs, I., Gallese, V., Buccino, G., Mazziotta, J. C., & Rizzolatti, G. (2005). Grasping the intentions of others with one's own mirror neuron system. *PLoS Biology, 3*, e79.

Iacoboni, M., Woods, R. P., Brass, M., Bekkering, H., Mazziotta, J. C., & Rizzolatti, G. (1999). Cortical mechanisms of human imitation. *Science, 286*, 2526–2528.

Ickes, W. (1997). *Empathic accuracy.* New York: Guilford Press.

Ickes, W., Gesn, P. R., & Graham, T. (2000). Gender differences in empathic accuracy: Differential ability of differential motivation? *Personal Relationships, 7*, 95–109. doi:10.1111/j.1475-6811.2000.tb00006.x.

Ingelfinger, F. J. (1980). Arrogance. *The New England Journal of Medicine, 303*, 1507–1511.

Insel, T. R. (2000). Toward a neurology of attachment. *Review of General Psychology, 4*, 176–185.

Isabella, R. A., & Belsky, J. (1991). Interaction synchrony and the origin of infant-mother attachment: A replication study. *Child Development, 62*, 373–384.

Ishikawa, H., Takayama, T., Yamazaki, Y., Skei, Y., & Katsumata, N. (2002). Physician-patient communication and patient satisfaction in Japanese cancer consultation. *Social Science & Medicine, 55*, 301–311.

Ivey, A. (1971). *Microcounseling: Innovations in interviewing training.* Springfield, IL: Charles C Thomas.

Ivey, A. E. (1974). Microcounseling and media therapy: State of the art. *Counselor Education and Supervision, 4*, 173–183.

Jack, D. C. (1993). *Silencing the self: Women and depression.* Cambridge, MA: Harvard University Press.

Jackson, S. W. (1992). The listening healer in the history of psychological healing. *American Journal of Psychiatry, 149*, 1623–1632.

Jackson, S. W. (2001). The wounded healer. *Bulletin of the History of Medicine, 75*, 1–36.

Jackson, P. L., Brunet, E., Meltzoff, A. N., & Decety, J. (2006). Empathy examined through the neural mechanisms involved in imagining how I feel versus how you feel pain. *Neuropsychologia, 44*, 754–761.

Jackson, P. L., & Decety, J. (2004). Motor cognition: A new paradigm to study self-other interactions. *Current Opinion in Neurobiology, 14*, 259–263.

Jackson, P. L., Meltzoff, A. N., & Decety, J. (2005). How do we perceive the pain of others? A window into the neural process involved in empathy. *Neuroimage, 24*, 771–779.

Jackson, P. L., Rainville, P., & Decety, J. (2006). To what extent do we share the pain of others? Insight from the neural bases of pain empathy. *Pain, 125*, 5–9.

Jaffe, D. S. (1986). Empathy, counteridentification, countertransference: A review with some personal perspectives on the "analytic instrument". *Psychoanalytic Quarterly, 15*, 215–243.

Jaffee, S., & Hyde, J. S. (2000). Gender differences in moral orientation: A meta-analysis. *Psychological Bulletin, 126*, 703–726.

James, W. (1890). *Principles of psychology*. New York: Holt.

Jamison, R., & Johnson, J. E. (1975). Empathy and therapeutic orientation in paid and volunteer crisis phone workers, professional therapists, and undergraduate college students. *Journal of Community Psychology, 3*, 269–274.

Janssens, J. M. A. M., & Gerris, J. R. M. (1992). Child rearing, empathy and prosocial develop-ment. In J. M. A. M. Janssens & J. R. M. Gerris (Eds.), *Child rearing: Influence on prosocial development* (pp. 57–75). Amsterdam: Swets & Zeitlinger.

Jarski, R. W., Gjerde, C. L., Bratton, B. D., Brown, D. D., & Matthes, S. S. (1985). A comparison of four empathy instruments in simulated patient-medical student interactions. *Journal of Medical Education, 60*, 545–551.

Jensen, N. (1994). The empathic physician. *Archives of Internal Medicine, 154*, 108.

Jessimer, M., & Markham, R. (1997). Alexithymia: A right hemisphere dysfunctional specific to recognition of certain facial expressions? *Brain and Cognition, 34*, 246–258.

Johnson, J. A., Cheek, J. M., & Smither, R. (1983). The structure of empathy. *Journal of Personality and Social Psychology, 45*, 1299–1312.

Johnston, M. A. C. (1992). A model program to address insensitive behaviors toward medical students. *Academic Medicine, 67*, 236–237.

Jones, A. H. (1987). Reflections, projections, and the future of literature-and-medicine. In D. Wear, M. Kohn, & S. Stocker (Eds.), *Literature and medicine: A claim for a discipline* (pp. 29–40). McLean, VA: Society for Health and Human Values.

Jones, A. H. (1997). Literature and medicine: Narrative ethics. *Lancet, 349*, 1243–1246.

Joreskog, K. G. (1993). Testing structural equation models. In K. A. Bollen & J. S. Long (Eds.), *Testing structural equation models*. Newbury Park, CA: Sage.

Jose, P. E. (1989). The role of gender and gender role similarity in readers' identification with story characters. *Sex Roles, 21*, 697–713.

Jumroonrojana, K., & Zartrungpak, S. (2012). Development of the Jefferson Scale of Physician Empathy-student version (Thai version). *Journal of the Psychiatric Association of Thailand, 57*, 213–224.

Jung, C. G. (1964). *Man and his symbols*. Garden City, NY: Doubleday.

Kaiser, H. (1960). The application of electronic computer factor analysis. *Educational and Psychological Measurement, 20*, 141–151.

Kalisch, B. J. (1971). An experiment in the development of empathy in nursing students. *Nursing Research, 20*, 202–211.

Kalisch, B. J. (1973). What is empathy? *American Journal of Nursing, 73*, 1548–1552.

Kalliopuska, M. (1992a). Attitudes towards health, health behavior, and personality factors among school students very high on empathy. *Psychological Reports, 70*, 1119–1122.

Kalliopuska, M. (1992b). Self-esteem and narcissism among the most and least empathetic Finnish baseball players. *Perceptual & Motor Skills, 75*, 945–946.

Kalliopuska, M. (1994). Empathy related to living in towns versus the countryside. *Psychological Reports, 74*, 896–898.

Kandel, E. R. (1998). A new intellectual framework for psychiatry. *American Journal of Psychiatry, 155*, 457–469.

Kane, G. C., Gotto, J. L., Mangione, S., West, S., & Hojat, M. (2007). Jefferson Scale of Patient's Perceptions of Physician Empathy: Preliminary psychometric data. *Croatian Medicine Journal, 48*, 81–86.

Kanter, S. L. (2012). What are the most revealing interview questions? *Academic Medicine, 87*, 387–388.

Kaplan, N. B., & Bloom, S. W. (1960). The use of sociological and social psychological concepts in physiological research. *Journal of Nervous and Mental Disease, 131*, 128–134.

Kaplan, G. A., Salonem, J. T., & Cohen, R. D. (1988). Social connections and mortality from all causes and from cardiovascular disease: Prospective evidence from eastern Finland. *American Journal of Epidemiology, 128*, 370–380.

Kaplan, R. M., Satterfield, J. M., & Kington, R. S. (2012). Building a better physician: The case for the new MCAT. *The New England Journal of Medicine, 366*, 1265–1268.

Kaplan, R. M., & Simon, H. J. (1990). Compliance in medical care: Reconsideration of self-predictions. *Annals of Behavioral Medicine, 12*, 66–71.

Karen, R. (1994). *Becoming attached*. New York: Warner Books.

Karniol, R., Gabay, R., Ochion, Y., & Harari, Y. (1998). Is gender or gender-role orientation a better predictor of empathy in adolescence? *Sex Roles, 39*, 45–59.

Kassebaum, D. G., & Szenas, P. L. (1994). Factors influencing the specialty choice of 1993 medical school graduates. *Academic Medicine, 69*, 164–170.

Kassirer, J. P. (1998). Doctor discontent. *New England Journal of Medicine, 339*, 1543–1545.

Kataoka, H. U., Koide, N., Hojat, M., & Gonnella, J. S. (2012). Measurement and correlates of empathy among female Japanese physicians. *BMC Medical Education, 12*, 48. doi:10.1186/1472-6920-12-48. Retrieved from: http://www.biomedcentral.com/1472-6920/12/48.

Kataoka, H., Koide, N., Ochi, K., Hojat, M., & Gonnella, J. S. (2009). Measurement of empathy among Japanese medical students: Psychometrics and score differences by gender and level of medical education. *Academic Medicine, 84*, 1192–1197.

Katz, R. L. (1963). *Empathy: Its nature and uses*. New York: Free Press.

Katz, J. (1984). *The silent world of doctor and patient*. New York: Free Press.

Kause, D. R., Robbins, A., Heidrich, R., Abrassi, I. B., & Anderson, L. A. (1980). The long-term effectiveness of interpersonal skills training in medical school. *Journal of Medical Education, 55*, 595–601.

Kay, J. (1990). Traumatic deidealization and the future of medicine. *Journal of the American Medical Association, 263*, 572–573.

Kazanowski, M., Perrin, K., Potter, M., & Sheehan, C. (2007). The silence of suffering: Breaking the sound barriers. *Journal of Holistic Nursing, 25*, 195–203. doi:10.1177/0898010107305501.

Keller, S., Shiflett, S. C., Schleifer, S. J., & Bartlett, J. A. (1994). *Human stress and immunity*. San Diego, CA: Academic Press.

Kelman, H. C. (1958). Compliance, identification, and internalization: Three processes of attitude change. *Conflict Resolution, 2*, 51–60.

Kendall, P. C., & Wilcox, C. E. (1980). Cognitive behavioral treatment for impulsivity: Concrete versus conceptual training in non-self-controlled problem children. *Journal of Counseling and Clinical Psychology, 48*, 80–91.

Kennedy, S., Kiecolt-Glaser, J. K., & Glaser, R. (1988). Immunological consequences of acute and chronic stressors: Mediating role of interpersonal relationships. *British Journal of Medical Psychology, 61*, 77–85.

Kenny, D. T. (1995). Determinants of patient satisfaction with the medical consultation. *Psychology and Health, 10*, 427–437.

Kerr, W. A. (1947). *The empathy test: Form A*. Chicago: Psychometric Affiliates.

Kerr, R. F., & Speroff, B. J. (1954). Validation and evaluation of the Empathy Test. *Journal of General Psychology, 50*, 269–276.

Kestenbaum, R., Farber, E. A., & Sroufe, L. A. (1989). Individual differences in empathy among preschoolers: Relation to attachment history. In N. Eisenberg (Ed.), *Empathy and related emotional responses* (pp. 51–64). San Francisco: Jossey-Bass.

Ketterer, M. W., & Buckholtz, C. D. (1989). Somatization disorder. *Journal of the American Osteopathic Association, 89*, 489–490.

Keverne, E. B., Nevison, C. M., & Martel, F. L. (1997). Early learning and social bond. *Annals of the New York Academy of Sciences, 807*, 329–339.

Keysers, C. (2011). *The empathic brain: How discovery of mirror neuron changes our understanding of human nature*. First published as a Kindle e-book, subsequently published by Social Brain Press in the U.S.

Keysers, C., Kohler, E., Umilta, M. A., Nanetti, L., Fogassi, L., & Gallese, V. (2003). Audiovisual mirror neurons and action recognition. *Experimental Brain Research, 153*, 628–636.

Keysers, C., & Perrett, D. I. (2004). Demystifying social cognition: A Hebbian perspective. *Trends in Cognitive Sciences, 8*, 501–507.

Keysers, C., Wicker, B., Gazzola, V., Anton, J. L., Fogassi, L., & Gallese, V. (2004). A touching sight: SII/VP activation during the observation and experience of touch. *Neuron, 42*, 335–346.

Khademalhosseini, M., Khademalhosseini, Z., & Mahmoodian, F. (2014). Comparison of empathy score among medical students in both basic and clinical levels. *Journal of Advances in Medical Education & Professionalism, 2*, 88–91.

Kiecolt-Glaser, J. K., Garner, W., Speicher, C. E., Penn, G. M., Holiday, J. E., & Glaser, R. (1984). Psychosocial modifiers of immunocompetence in medical students. *Psychosomatic Medicine, 46*, 7–14.

Kiersma, M. E., Chen, A. M. H., Yehle, K. S., & Plake, K. S. (2013). Validation of an empathy scale in pharmacy and nursing students. *American Journal of Pharmaceutical Education, 77*, Article 94. doi:10.5688/ajpe77594.

Kim, S. S., Kaplowitz, S., & Johnston, M. V. (2004). The effects of physician empathy on patient satisfaction and compliance. *Evaluation and the Health Professions, 27*, 237–251.

Kimmelman, M., Giacobbe, J., Faden, J., Kumar, G., Pinckney, C. C., & Steer, R. (2012). Empathy in osteopathic medical students: A cross-sectional analysis. *Journal of the American Osteopathic Association, 112*, 347–355.

Kimura, D. (1999). Sex differences in the brain. *Scientific American,* May 13 issue.

King, S., & Holosko, M. J. (2012). The development and initial validation of the empathy scale for social workers. *Research on Social Work Practice, 22*, 174–185. doi:10.1177/1049731511417136.

Kipper, D. A., & Ben-Ely, Z. (1979). The effectiveness of the psychodramatic double method, the reflection method, and lecturing in the training of empathy. *Journal of Clinical Psychology, 35*, 370–375.

Klaus, M. H., Jerauld, R., Kreger, N. S., McAlpine, W., Steffa, M., & Kennell, J. H. (1972). Maternal attachment: Importance of the first post-partum days. *New England Journal of Medicine, 286*, 460–463.

Klaus, M., & Kennell, J. H. (1970). Mothers separated from their newborn infants. *Pediatric Clinics of North America, 17*, 1015–1037.

Kleinman, A. (1988). *The illness narratives: Suffering, healing, and the human condition.* New York: Basic Books.

Kleinman, A. (1995). *Writing at the margin: Discourse between anthropology and medicine.* Berkeley, CA: University of California Press.

Kleinman, A., Eisenberg, L., & Good, B. (1978). Culture, illness, and care: Clinical lessons from anthropologic and cross-cultural research. *Annals of Internal Medicine, 88*, 251–258.

Kline, R. B. (1998). *Principles and practice of structural equation modeling.* New York: Guilford Press.

Kliszcz, J., Hebanowski, M., & Rembowski, J. (1998). Emotional and cognitive empathy in medical schools. *Academic Medicine, 73*, 541.

Kliszcz, J., Nowicka-Sauer, K., Trzeciak, B., Nowak, P., & Sadowska, A. (2006). Empathy in health care providers–validation study of the Polish version of the Jefferson Scale of Empathy. *Advances in Medical Sciences, 51*, 219–225. Retrieved from: http://www.advms.pl/ms_2006/Kliszcz_J_et%20al_Empathy%20in%20health%20care%20providers.pdf.

Knafo, A., Zahn-Waxler, C., Van Hule, C., Robinson, J. L., & Rhee, S. H. (2008). The developmental origins of disposition toward empathy: Genetic and environmental contributions. *Emotion, 8*, 737–752. Retrieved from: http://dx.doi.org/10.1037/a0014179.

Knapp, B. L. (1984). *A Jungian approach to literature.* Carbondale, IL: Southern Illinois University.

Knight, J. A. (1981). *Doctor-to-be: Coping with trials and triumphs of medical school.* New York: Appleton-Century.

Koenig, H. G. (2002). *Spirituality in patient care.* Philadelphia: Templeton Foundation Press.

Kohler, E., Keysers, C., Umilta, M. A., Fogassi, L., Gallese, V., & Rizzolatti, G. (2002). Hearing sounds, understanding actions: Action representation in mirror neurons. *Science, 297*, 846–848.

Kohn, L. T., Corrigan, J. M., & Donaldson, M. S. (2000). *To err is human: Building a safe health system.* Washington, DC: National Academy Press.

Kohut, H. (1959). Introspection, empathy and psychoanalysis. *Journal of American Psychoanalysis, 7*, 459–483.

Kohut, H. (1971). *Analysis of the self: A systematic approach to the psychoanalytic treatment of narcissistic personality disorders.* New York: International Universities Press.

Kohut, H. (1984). Introspection, empathy, and the semicircle of mental health. In J. Lichtenberg, M. Bornstein, & D. Silver (Eds.), *Empathy* (Vol. 1, pp. 81–100). Hillsdale, NJ: Erlbaum.

Kolb, B., & Taylor, L. (1981). Affective behavior in patients with localized cortical excisions: Role of lesion site and side. *Science, 214*, 81–89.

Kolenikov, S., & Bollen, K. A. (2012). Testing negative error variances: Is a Heywood case a symptom of misspecification? *Sociological Methods & Research, 41*, 124–167.

Konner, M. (2004). The ties that bind [Comment]. *Nature, 429*, 705.

Konrath, S. H., O'Brien, E. H., & Hsing, C. (2011). Changes in dispositional empathy in American college students over time: A meta-analysis. *Personality and Social Psychology Review, 15*, 180–189.

Korsch, B. M., Gozzi, E. K., & Francis, V. (1968a). Gaps in doctor-patient interaction and patient satisfaction. *Pediatrics, 42*, 855–871.

Korsch, B. M., Gozzi, E. K., & Francis, V. (1968b). Gaps in doctor-patient communication: I. Doctor-patient interaction and patient satisfaction. *Pediatrics, 42*, 855–871.

Kosfeld, M., Heinrichs, M., Zak, P., Fischbacher, U., & Fehr, E. (2005). Oxytocin increases trust in humans. *Nature, 435*, 673–676. doi:10.1038/nature03701.

Koženy, J., Tišanská, L., & Hoschl, C. (2013). Assessing empathy among Czech medical students: A cross-sectional study. *Československá Psychologie, 57*, 246–254.

Kramer, C. (1974). Folk linguistics. *Psychology Today, 8*, 82–85.

Kramer, D., Ber, R., & Moore, M. (1987). Impact of workshop on students' and physicians' rejecting behaviors in patient interviews. *Journal of Medical Education, 62*, 904–910.

Kramer, D., Ber, R., & Moore, M. (1989). Increasing empathy among medical students. *Medical Education, 23*, 168–173.

Krasner, M. S., Epstein, R. M., Beckman, H., Suchman, A. L., Chapman, B., Mooney, C. J., & Quill, T. E. (2009). Association of an educational program in mindful communication with burnout, empathy, and attitudes among primary care physicians. *Journal of the American Medical Association, 302*, 1284–1293. doi:10.1001/jama.2009.1384.

Krebs, D. (1975). Empathy and altruism. *Journal of Personality and Social Psychology, 32*, 1134–1146.

Kremer, J. F., & Dietzen, L. L. (1991). Two approaches to teaching accurate empathy to undergraduates: Teacher-intensive and self-directed. *Journal of College Student Development, 32*, 69–75.

Krevans, J., & Gibbs, J. C. (1996). Parents' use of inductive discipline: Relations to children's empathy and prosocial behavior. *Child Development, 67*, 3263–3277.

Kring, A. M., & Gordon, A. L. (1998). Sex differences in emotion. *Journal of Personality and Social Psychology, 74*, 686–703.

Kugiumutzakis, G. (1998). Neonatal imitation in the intersubjective companion space. In S. Braten (Ed.), *Intersubjective communication and emotion in early ontogeny* (pp. 63–88). Cambridge: Cambridge University Press.

Kumagai, A. K. (2008). A conceptual framework for the use of illness narratives in medical education. *Academic Medicine, 83*, 653–658.

Kunyk, D., & Olson, J. K. (2001). Clarification of conceptualizations of empathy. *Journal of Advanced Nursing, 35*, 317–325.

Kupfer, D. J., Drew, F. L., Curtis, E. K., & Rubinstein, D. N. (1978). Personality style and empathy in medical students. *Journal of Medical Education, 53*, 507–509.

Kurtines, W., & Hogan, R. (1972). Sources of conformity in unspecialized college students. *Journal of Abnormal Psychology, 80*, 49–51.

Kurtz, R. R., & Grummon, D. L. (1972). Different approaches to the measurement of therapist empathy and their relationship to therapy outcomes. *Journal of Consulting and Clinical Psychology, 39*, 106–115.

La France, M. (1979). Nonverbal synchrony and rapport: Analysis by the cross-lag panel technique. *Social Psychology Quarterly, 42*, 66–70.

La France, M. (1982). Posturre mirroring and rapport. In M. Davis (Ed.), *Interaction rhythms: Periodicity in communication behavior* (pp. 279–298). New York: Human Sciences Press.

LaFrance, M., Hecht, M. A., & Paluck, E. L. (2003). The contingent smile: A meta-analysis of sex differences in smiling. *Psychological Bulletin, 129*, 305–334.

Lakin, J. L., Jefferis, V. E., Cheng, C. M., & Chartland, T. L. (2003). The chameleon effect as social glue: Evidence for the evolutionary significance of nonconscious mimicry. *Journal of Nonverbal Behavior, 27*, 145–162.

Lamm, C., Batson, D., & Decety, J. (2007). The neural substrate of human empathy: Effects of perspective-taking and cognitive appraisal. *Journal of Cognitive Neuroscience, 19*, 42–58.

LaMonica, E. L. (1981). Construct validity of an empathy instrument. *Research in Nursing & Health, 4*, 389–400.

LaMonica, E. L., Carew, D. K., Winder, A. E., Haase, A. M., & Blanchard, K. H. (1976). Empathy training as the major thrust of a staff development program. *Nursing Research, 25*, 447–451.

Lamont, L. M., & Lundstrom, W. J. (1977). Identifying successful industrial salesmen by personality and personal characteristics. *Journal of Marketing Research, 14*, 517–529.

Lamothe, M., Boujut, E., Zenasni, F., & Sultan, S. (2014). To be or not to be empathic: The combined role of empathic concern and perspective taking in understanding burnout in general practice. *BMC Family Practice, 15*, 15. doi:10.1186/1471-2296-15-15. Retrieved from: http://www.biomedcentral.com/1471-2296/15/15.

Lancaster, T., Hart, R., & Gardner, S. (2002). Literature and medicine: Evaluating a special study module using the nominal group technique. *Medical Education, 36*, 1071–1076.

Lane, F. E. (1986). Utilizing physician empathy with violent patients. *American Journal of Psychotherapy, 40*, 448–456.

Lanzetta, J. T., & Englis, B. G. (1989). Expectation of cooperation and competition and their effects on observers' vicarious emotional response. *Journal of Personality and Social Psychology, 56*, 543–554.

Lanzetta, J. T., & Kleck, R. E. (1970). Encoding and decoding nonverbal affect in humans. *Journal of Personality and Social Psychology, 16*, 12–19.

LaRocco, J. M., House, J. S., & French, J. R. P. (1980). Social support, occupational stress, and health. *Journal of Health and Social Behavior, 21*, 202–218.

Larson, D. (1993). *The helper's journey: Working with people facing grief, loss, and life-threatening illness*. Champaign, IL: Research Press.

Larson, E. B., & Yao, X. (2005). Clinical empathy as emotional labor in the patient-physician relationship. *Journal of the American Medical Association, 293*, 1100–1106.

Laskowski, C., & Pellicore, K. (2002). The wounded healer archetype: Applications to palliative care practice. *American Journal of Hospice & Palliative Care, 19*, 403–407.

Lawrence, E. J., Shaw, P., Baker, D., Baron-Cohen, S., & David, A. S. (2004). Measuring empathy: Reliability and validity of the Empathy Quotient. *Psychological Medicine, 34*, 911–924.

Layton, J. M. (1979). The use of modeling to teach empathy to nursing students. *Research in Nursing & Health, 2*, 163–176.

Layton, J. M., & Wykle, M. H. (1990). A validity study of four empathy instruments. *Research in Nursing & Health, 13*, 319–325.

Lazarus, R. S. (1982). Thoughts on the relations between emotion and cognition. *American Psychologist, 37*, 1019–1024.

Lee, B. K., Bahn, G. H., Lee, W. H., Park, J. H., Yoon, T. Y., & Baek, S. B. (2009). The relationship between empathy and medical education system, grades, and personality in medical college students and medical school students. *Korean Journal of Medical Education, 21*, 117–124. doi:10.3946/kjme.2009.21.2.117.

Leiper, R., & Casares, P. (2000). An investigation of the attachment organization of clinical psychologists and its relationship to clinical practice. *British Journal of Medical Psychology, 73*, 449–464.

Lelorain, S., Brédart, A., Dolbeault, S., Cano, A., Bonnaud-Antignac, A., Cousson-Gélie, F., & Sultan, S. (2014). How can we explain physician accuracy in assessing patient distress? A multilevel analysis in patients with advanced cancer. *Patient Education and Counseling, 94*, 322–327. doi:10.1016/j.pec.2013.10.029.

Lelorain, S., Brédart, A., Dolbeault, S., Cano, A., Bonnaud-Antignac, A., Cousson-Gélie, F., & Sultan, S. (2015). How does a physician's accurate understanding of a cancer patient's unmet needs contribute to patient perception of physician empathy? *Patient Education and Counseling, 98*, 734–741. http://doi.org/10.1016/j.pec.2015.03.00.

Lelorain, S., Sultan, S., Zenasni, F., Catu-Pinault, A., Juar, P., Boujut, E., & Rigal, L. (2013). Empathic concern and professional characteristics associated with clinical empathy in French general practitioners. *European Journal of General Practice, 19*, 23–28. doi:10.3109/1381478 8.2012.709842.

Leombruni, P., Di Lillo, M., Miniotti, M., Picardi, A., Alessandri, G., Sica, C., ... Torta, R. (2014). Measurement properties and confirmatory factor analysis of the Jefferson Scale of Empathy in Italian medical students. *Perspectives on Medical Education*. Published online: 08 Aug 2014. doi:10.1007/s40037-014-0137-9.

Lerner, A. (1978). *Poetry in the therapeutic experience*. Elmsford, NY: Pergamon Press.

Lerner, A. (2001). Poetry therapy. In R. J. Corsini (Ed.), *Handbook of innovative therapies* (pp. 472–479). New York: John Wiley & Sons.

Lerner, M. J., & Meindl, J. R. (1981). Justice and altruism. In J. P. Rushton & J. R. Sorrentino (Eds.), *Altruism and helping behavior: Social, personality, and developmental perspectives* (pp. 213–232). Hillsdale, NJ: Erlbaum.

Letourneau, C. (1981). Empathy and stress: How they affect parental aggression. *Social Work, 26*, 383–389.

Levasseur, J., & Vance, A. R. (1993). Doctors, nurses, and empathy. In H. M. Spiro, M. G. Mccrea Curnen, E. Peschel, & D. S. James (Eds.), *Empathy and practice of medicine* (pp. 76–84). New Haven: Yale University Press.

Levenson, R. W., & Ruef, A. M. (1992). Empathy, a physiological substrate. *Journal of Personality and Social Psychology, 63*, 234–246.

Levine, L. E., & Hoffman, M. L. (1975). Empathy and cooperation in 4-year olds. *Developmental Psychology, 4*, 533–534.

Levinson, W. (1994). Physician-patient communication: A key to malpractice prevention. *Journal of the American Medical Association, 272*, 1619–1620.

Levinson, W., Gorawara-Bhat, R., & Lamb, J. (2000). A study of patient clues and physician responses in primary care and surgical settings. *Journal of the American Medical Association, 284*, 1021–1027.

Levinson, W., Roter, D., Mullooly, J. P., Dull, V. T., & Frankel, R. (1997). Physician-patient communication: The relationship with malpractice claims among primary care physicians and surgeons. *Journal of the American Medical Association, 277*, 553–559.

Levy, J. (1997). A note on empathy. *New Ideas in Psychology, 15*, 179–184.

Levy, D. (Ed.). (1999). *Medical milestones from the National Heart, Lung, and Blood Institute's Framingham Heart Study*. Center for Bio-Medical Communication.

Lewin, K. (1936). *A dynamic theory of personality*. New York: McGraw-Hill.

Lewinsohn, R. (1998). Medical theories, science, and the practice of medicine. *Social Science & Medicine, 46*, 1261–1270.

Lewis, J. M. (1998). For better or worse: Interpersonal relationships and individual outcome. *American Journal of Psychiatry, 155*, 582–589.

Lewis, T., Amini, F., & Lannon, R. (2000). *A general theory of love*. New York: Vintage Books.

Li, L., Wang, J., Hu, X., & Xu, C. (2015). Empathy in Chinese pharmacy undergraduates: Implication for integrating humanities into professional pharmacy education. *Indian Journal of Pharmaceutical Education and Research, 49*, 31–39. doi: 10.5530/ijper.49.1.5.

Lichtenstein, P., Holm, N. V., Verkasalo, P. K., Iliadou, A., Kaprio, J., Koskenvuo, M., ... Hemminki, K. (2000). Environmental and heritable factors in the causation of cancer: Analyses of cohort twins from Sweden, Denmark, and Finland. *New England Journal of Medicine, 343*, 78–85.

Lieberman, M. D. (2007). Social cognitive neuroscience: A review of core processes. *Annual Review of Psychology, 58,* 259–289.

Lieberman, Matthew D. (2007) Social Cognitive Neuroscience: A Review of Core Processes. *Annual Review of Psychology; 58,* 259–289.

Lief, H. I., & Fox, R. C. (1963). Training for "detached concerns" in medical students. In H. I. Lief, V. F. Lief, & N. R. Lief (Eds.), *The psychological basis of medical practice* (pp. 12–35). New York: Harper & Row.

Lief, H. I., Lief, V. F., & Lief, N. R. (Eds.). (1963). *The psychological basis of medical practice.* New York: Harper & Row.

Lieu, T. A., Schroeder, S. A., & Altman, D. F. (1989). Specialty choice at one medical school: Recent trends and analysis of predictive factors. *Academic Medicine, 64,* 622–629.

Likert, R. (1932). A technique for the measurement of attitudes. *Archives of Psychology, 140,* 5–35.

Lilienfeld, R. (1978). *The rise of systems theory: An ideological analysis.* New York: John Wiley & Sons.

Lim, B. T., Moriarty, H., Huthwaite, M., Gray, L., Pullon, S., & Gallagher, P. (2013). How well do medical students rate and communicate clinical empathy? *Medical Teacher, 35,* e946–e951. doi:10.3109/0142159X.2012.715783.

Lim, B. T., Moriarty, H., & Huthwaite, M. (2011). "Being-in-role": A teaching innovation to enhance empathy communication skills in medical students. *Medical Teacher, 33,* e663–e669. doi:10.3109/0142159X2011.611193.

Lin, C., Li, L., Wan, D., Wu, Z., & Yan, Z. (2012). Empathy and avoidance in treating patients living with HIV/AIDS (PLWHA) among service providers in China. *AIDS Care, 24,* 1341–1348. doi:10.1080/09540121.2011.648602.

Linley, P. A., & Joseph, S. (2007). Therapy work and therapists' positive and negative well-being. *Journal of Social and Clinical Psychology, 26,* 385–403.

Linn, L. S. (1974). Care vs. cure: How the nurse practitioner views the patient. *Nursing Outlook, 22,* 641–644.

Linn, L. S. (1975). A survey of the "care-cure" attitudes of physicians, nurses, and their students. *Nursing Forum, 14,* 145–161.

Linn, L. S., Cope, D. W., & Leake, B. (1984). The effect of gender and training of residents on satisfaction ratings by patients. *Journal of Medical Education, 59,* 964–966.

Linn, L. S., DiMatteo, M. R., Cope, D. W., & Robbins, A. (1987). Measuring physicians' humanistic attitudes, values, and behaviors. *Medical Care, 25,* 504–515.

Linn, L. S., Yager, J., Cope, D., & Leake, B. (1985). Health status, job satisfaction, job stress, and life satisfaction among academic and clinical faculty. *Journal of the American Medical Association, 254,* 2775–2782.

Lipner, R. S., Blank, L. L., Leas, B. F., & Fortna, G. S. (2002). The value of patient and peer ratings in recertification. *Academic Medicine, 77,* S64–S66.

Litvack-Miller, W., McDougall, D., & Romney, D. M. (1997). The structure of empathy during middle childhood and its relationship to prosocial behavior. *Genetic, Social, and General Psychology Monographs, 123,* 303–324.

Loggia, M. L., Mogil, J. S., & Bushnell, C. M. (2008). Empathy hurts: Compassion for another increases both sensory and affective components of pain perception. *Pain, 136,* 68–176.

Lopez, G. E., Gurin, P., & Nagda, B. A. (1998). Education and understanding structural causes for group inequalities. *Political Psychology, 19,* 305–329.

Lott, D. A. (1998). Brain development, attachment and impact on psychic vulnerability. *Psychiatric Times, 15.* Retrieved 20 Dec 2004 from: http://www.psychiatrictimes.com.

Lounsburg, M. L., & Bates, J. E. (1982). The cries of infants of differing levels of perceived temperamental difficultness: Acoustic properties and effects on listeners. *Child Development, 53,* 677–686.

Lu, M. C. (1995). Why it was hard for me to learn compassion as a third-year medical student. *Cambridge Quarterly of Healthcare Ethics, 4,* 454–458.

Luborsky, L., Chandler, M., Auerbach, A. H., Cohen, J., & Bacharach, H. M. (1971). Factors influencing the outcome of psychotherapy: A review of quantitative research. *Psychological Bulletin, 75*, 145–185.

Ludmerer, K. M. (1999). *Time to heal. American medical education from the turn of the century to the era of managed care*. New York: Oxford University Press.

Luscher, T. F., & Vetter, W. (1990). Adherence to medication. *Journal of Human Hypertension, 4*(Suppl. 1), 43–46.

Lutchmaya, S., Baron-Cohen, S., & Raggatt, P. (2002). Foetal testosterone and vocabulary size in 18 and 24-month old infants. *Infant Behavior & Development, 24*, 418–424.

Lynch, J. J. (1977). *The broken heart: The consequences of loneliness*. New York: Basic books.

Maccoby, E. E., & Jacklin, C. N. (1974). *The psychology of sex differences*. Stanford, CA: Stanford University Press.

MacKay, R., Hughes, J. R., & Carver, E. J. (Eds.). (1990). *Empathy in the helping relationship*. New York: Springer.

MacLean, P. D. (1967). The brain in relation to empathy and medical education. *Journal of Nervous and Mental Disease, 144*, 374–382.

MacLean, P. D. (1990). *The triune brain evolution*. New York: Plenum Press.

Macmillan, M. B. (2000). Restoring Phineas Gage: A 150th retrospective. *Journal of History of Neurosciences, 9*, 42–62.

MacPherson, H., Mercer, S. W., Scullion, T., & Thomas, K. J. (2003). Empathy, enablement, and outcome: An exploratory study on acupuncture patient's perceptions. *Journal of Alternative & Complementary Medicine, 9*, 869–876.

Magalhães, E., Costa, P., & Costa, M. (2012). Empathy of medical students and personality: Evidence from the Five-Factor Model. *Medical Teacher, 34*, 807–812.

Magalhães, E., Salgueira, A. P., Costa, P., & Costa, M. J. (2011). Empathy in senior year and first year medical students: A cross-sectional study. *BMC Medical Education, 11*, 52. doi:10.1186/1472-6920-11-52. Retrieved from: http://www.biomedcentral.com/1472-6920/11/52.

Magee, M., & Hojat, M. (1998). Personality profiles of male and female positive role models in medicine. *Psychological Reports, 82*, 547–559.

Magee, M., & Hojat, M. (2001). Impact of health care system on physicians' discontent. *Journal of Community Health, 26*, 357–365.

Magee, M., & Hojat, M. (2010). Rocking chair and empathy: A pilot study [Letter to the editor]. *Family Medicine, 42*, 467.

Maheux, B., Beaudoin, C., Berkson, L. C. L., Des Marchais, J., & Jean, P. (2000). Medical faculty as humanistic physicians and teachers: The perceptions of students at innovative and traditional medical schools. *Medical Education, 34*, 630–634.

Maheux, B., & Beland, F. (1989). Students' perceptions of values emphasized in three medical schools. *Journal of Medical Education, 61*, 308–316.

Maheux, B., Duford, F., Beland, F., Jacques, A., & Levesque, A. (1990). Female medical practitioners: More preventive and patient oriented? *Medical Care, 28*, 87–92.

Main, M., & Solomon, J. (1990). Procedures for identifying infants as disorganized/disoriented during the Ainsworth strange situation. In M. Greenberg, D. Cicchetti, & E. M. Cummings (Eds.), *Attachment in the preschool years: Theory, research and intervention* (pp. 121–160). Chicago: University of Chicago Press.

Makoul, G. (1998). Perpetuating passivity: Reliance and reciprocal determinism in physician-patient interaction. *Journal of Health Communication, 3*, 233–259.

Makoul, G. (2001). Essential elements of communication in medical encounters: The Kalamazoo consensus statement. *Academic Medicine, 76*, 390–393.

Makoul, G., & Strauss, A. (2003). Building therapeutic relationships during patient visits. *Journal of General Internal Medicine, 18*(Suppl. 1), 275.

Malno, R. B., Boag, T. J., & Smith, A. A. (1957). Physiological study of personal interaction. *Psychosomatic Medicine, 19*, 105–119.

Mandel, E. D., & Schweinle, W. E. (2012). A study of empathy decline in physician assistant students at completion of first didactic year. *The Journal of Physician Assistant Education, 23*, 16–24.

Mandell, H., & Spiro, H. (1987). *When doctors get sick*. New York: Plenum.

Mangione, S., Kane, G. C., Caruso, J. W., Gonnella, J. S., Nasca, T. J., & Hojat, M. (2002). Assessment of empathy in different years of internal medicine training. *Medical Teacher, 24*, 370–373.

Mann, L., Wise, T. N., Trinidad, A., & Kohanski, R. (1994). Alexithymia, affect recognition, and the five-factor model of personality in normal subjects. *Psychological Reports, 74*, 563–567.

Manning, R., Levine, M., & Collins, A. (2007). The Kitty Genovese murder and social psychology of helping: The parable of the 38 witnesses. *American Psychologist, 62*, 555–562.

Mansen, T. J. (1993). Role-taking abilities of nursing education administrators and their perceived leadership effectiveness. *Journal of Professional Nursing, 9*, 347–357.

Marcus, E. R. (1999). Empathy, humanism, and the professionalization process of medical education. *Academic Medicine, 74*, 1211–1215.

Markham, B. (1979). Can a behavioral science course change medical students' attitudes? *Journal of Psychiatric Education, 3*, 44–54.

Markus, H. R., & Kitayama, S. (1991). Culture and the self: Implications for cognition, emotion, and motivation. *Psychological Review, 98*, 224–253.

Marmot, M. G., & Syme, S. L. (1976). Acculturation and coronary heart disease in Japanese-Americans. *American Journal of Epidemiology, 104*, 225–247.

Marshall, W. L., & Maric, A. (1996). Cognitive and emotional components of generalized empathy deficits in child molesters. *Journal of Child Sexual Abuse, 5*, 101–111.

Marshall, P. A., & O'Keefe, J. P. (1994). Medical students' first person narrative of a patient's story of AIDS. *Social Science & Medicine, 40*, 67–76.

Marte, A. L. (1988). How does it feel to be old? Simulation game provides "into aging" experience. *Journal of Continuing Education in Nursing, 19*, 166–168. doi:10.3928/0022-0124-19880701-06.

Martin, R. (2007). *The psychology of humor: An integrative approach*. San Diego, CA: Elsevier Academic Press.

Martin, G. B., & Clark, R. D. (1982). Distress crying in neonates: Species and peer specificity. *Developmental Psychology, 18*, 3–9.

Martin, R. A., & Lefcourt, H. M. (1983). Sense of humor as a moderator of the relation between stress and mood. *Journal of Personality and Social Psychology, 45*, 1313–1324.

Marx, B. P., Heidt, J. M., & Gold, S. D. (2005). Perceived uncontrollability and unpredictability, self-regulation, and sexual revictimization. *Review of General Psychology, 9*, 67–90.

Maslach, C. (1993). Burnout: A multidimensional perspective. In W. B. Schaufeli, C. Maslach, & F. T. Marek (Eds.), *Professional burnout: Recent developments in theory and research*. Washington, DC: Taylor & Francis.

Matravers, D. (2014). Empathy as a route to knowledge. In A. Coplan & P. Goldie (Eds.), *Empathy: Philosophical and psychological perspectives* (pp. 19–30). New York: Oxford University Press.

Matthews, K. A., Batson, C. D., Horn, J., & Rosenman, R. H. (1981). Principles in his nature which interest him in the fortune of others: The heritability of empathic concern for others. *Journal of Personality, 49*, 237–247.

Matthews, D. A., & Feinstein, A. R. (1989). A new instrument for patients' rating of physician performance in the hospital setting. *Journal of General Internal Medicine, 4*, 14–22.

Matthews, D. A., Suchman, A. L., & Branch, W. T. (1993). Making "connexions": Enhancing the therapeutic potential of patient-clinician relationships. *Annals of Internal Medicine, 118*, 973–977.

Maurer, R. E., & Tindall, J. H. (1983). Effect of postural congruence on client's perception of counselor empathy. *Journal of Counseling Psychology, 30*, 158–163.

Mayerson, E. W. (1976). *Putting the ill at ease*. New York: Harper & Row.

Mays, L. C., Carter, A. S., Eggar, H. L., & Pajer, K. A. (1991). Reflection on stillness: Mother's reaction to the still-face situation. *Journal of Academy of Child and Adolescent Psychiatry, 30*, 22–28.

McClintock, M. K. (1971). Menstrual synchrony and suppression. *Nature, 229*, 244–245.

McEwen, B. S. (1998). Protective and damaging effects of stress mediators. *New England Journal of Medicine, 338*, 171–179.

McKellar, P. (1957). *Imagining and thinking: A psychological analysis*. New York: Basic Books.

McKenna, L., Boyle, M., Brown, T., Williams, B., Molloy, A., Lewis, B., & Molloy, L. (2011). Levels of empathy in undergraduate midwifery students: An Australian cross-sectional study. *Women and Birth: Journal of the Australian College of Midwives, 24*, 80–84. doi:10.1016/j.wombi.2011.02.003.

McKenna, L., Boyle, M., Brown, T., Williams, B., Molloy, A., Lewis, B., & Molloy, L. (2012). Levels of empathy in undergraduate nursing students. *International Journal of Nursing Practice, 18*, 246–251. doi:10.1111/j.1440-172X.2012.02035.x.

McKinlay, J. B., & McKinlay, S. M. (1981). Medical measures and the decline of mortality. In P. Conrad & R. Kern (Eds.), *The sociology of health and illness: Critical perspectives* (pp. 12–30). New York: St. Martin's Press.

Mclean, M. (2004). The choice of role models by students at a culturally diverse South African medical school. *Medical Teacher, 26*, 133–141.

McLellan, M. F., & Husdon Jones, A. (1996). Why literature and medicine? *Lancet, 348*, 109–111.

McLellan, J. D., Jansen-McWilliams, L., Comer, D. M., Gardner, W. P., & Kelleher, K. J. (1999). The Physician Belief Scale and psychosocial problems in children: A report from the pediatric research in office settings and the ambulatory sentinel practice network. *Journal of Developmental & Behavioral Pediatrics, 20*, 24–30.

McManus, I. C. (1995). Humanity and the medical humanities. *Lancet, 346*, 1143–1145.

McMillan, J. R., Clifton, A. K., McGrath, D., & Gale, W. S. (1977). Women's language: Uncertainty or interpersonal sensitivity and emotionality. *Sex Roles, 3*, 545–559.

McMillan, L. R., & Shannon, D. M. (2011). Psychometric analysis of the JSPE nursing student version R: Comparison of senior BSN students and medical students' attitudes toward empathy in patient care. *International Scholarly Research Network Nursing*, Article ID 726063. doi:10.5402/2011/726063. Retrieved from: http://dx.doi.org/10.5402/2011/726063.

McTighe, A. (2014). *Effects of medical education on empathy in osteopathic medical students*. Doctoral dissertation completed at Department of Psychology, Philadelphia College of Osteopathic Medicine, Philadelphia, Pennsylvania, USA.

McVey, L. J., Davis, D. E., & Cohen, H. J. (1989). The aging game: An approach to education in geriatrics. *Journal of the American Medical Association, 262*, 1507–1509.

Mead, G. H. (1934). *Mind, self and society*. Chicago: University of Chicago Press.

Means, J. J. (2002). Mighty prophet/wounded healer. *Journal of Pastoral Care, 56*, 41–49.

Meeuwesen, L., Schaap, C., & Van der Staak, C. (1991). Verbal analysis of doctor-patient communication. *Social Science & Medicine, 32*, 1143–1150.

Mehrabian, A. (1969). Significance of posture and position in the communication of attitude and status relationships. *Psychological Bulletin, 71*, 359–372.

Mehrabian, A. (1972). *Nonverbal communication*. Chicago: Aldine-Atherton.

Mehrabian, A. (1996). The Balanced Emotional Empathy Scale (BEES). Unpublished document. Information Retrieved from: www.kaaj.com/psych/scales/emp.html.

Mehrabian, A. (1997). Relations among personality scales of aggression, violence, and empathy: Validational evidence bearing on the Risk of Eruptive Violence Scale. *Aggressive Behavior, 23*, 433–445.

Mehrabian, A., & Epstein, N. A. (1972). A measure of emotional empathy. *Journal of Personality, 40*, 525–543.

Mehrabian, A., & O'Reilly, E. (1980). Analysis of personality measures in terms of basic dimensions of temperament. *Journal of Personality and Social Psychology, 38*, 492–503.

Mehrabian, A., Young, A. L., & Sato, S. (1988). Emotional empathy and associated individual differences. *Current Psychology: Research & Reviews, 7*, 221–240.

Mello, M. M., Studdert, D. M., DesRoches, C. M., Peugh, J., Zapert, K., Brennan, T. A., & Sage, W. M. (2004). Caring for patients in a malpractice crisis: Physician satisfaction and quality of care. *Health Affairs, 23*, 42–53.

Meltzoff, J., & Kornreich, M. (1970). *Research in psychotherapy*. New York: Atherton.

Meltzoff, A. N., & Moore, M. K. (1977). Imitation of facial and manual gestures by human neonates. *Science, 198*, 75–78.

Meltzoff, A. N., & Moore, M. K. (1983). Newborn infants imitate adult facial gestures. *Child Development, 54*, 702–709.

Meltzoff, A. N., & Prinz, W. (2002). *The imitative mind: Development, evolution, and brain bases.* Cambridge: Cambridge University Press.

Melzack, R. (1990). Phantom limb and the concept of neuromatrix. *Trends in Neurosciences, 13*, 88–92.

Mengel, M. B. (1987). Physician ineffectiveness due to family-of-origin issues. *Family Systems Medicine, 5*, 176–190.

Menks, F. (1983). The use of a board game to simulate the experience of old age. *Gerontologist, 23*, 565–568.

Mercer, S. W., Maxwell, M., Heaney, D., & Watt, G. C. M. (2004). The consultation and rational empathy (CARE) measure: Development and preliminary validation and reliability of an empathy-based consultation process measure. *Family Practice, 21*, 699–705. doi:10.1093/fampra/cmh621.

Mercer, S. W., McConnachie, A., Maxwell, M., Heaney, D., & Watt, G. C. (2005). Relevance and practical use of the Consultation and Relational Empathy (CARE) measure in general practice. *Family Practice, 22*, 328–334.

Mercer, S. W., & Reynolds, W. J. (2002). Empathy and quality of care. *British Journal of General Practice, 52*, S9–S12.

Mercer, S. W., Watt, G. C. M., & Reilly, D. (2001). Empathy is important for enablement. *British Medical Journal, 322*, 865.

Merlyn, S. (1998). Improving doctor-patient communication: Not an option, but a necessity. *British Medical Journal, 316*, 1922.

Mestre, M. V., Samper, P., Frias, M. D., & Tur, A. M. (2009). Are women more empathic than men? A longitudinal study in adolescence. *The Spanish Journal of Psychology, 12*, 76–83. doi:10.1017/S1138741600001499.

Metcalfe, J., & Mischel, W. (1999). A hot/cool system analysis of delay of gratification: Dynamics of willpower. *Psychological Review, 106*, 3–19.

Meyers, A. R. (1987). Lumping it: The hidden denomination of the medical malpractice crisis. *American Journal of Public Health, 77*, 1544–1548.

Michalec, B. (2010). As assessment of medical student school stressors on preclinical students' level of clinical empathy. *Current Psychology, 29*, 210–221.

Michalec, B., Veloski, J. J., Hojat, M., & Tykocinski, M. L. (2015). Identifying potential engaging leaders within medical education: The role of positive influence on peers. *Medical Teacher, 37*, 677–683. doi:10.3109/0142159X.2014.947933.

Michalska, M. J., Kinzler, K. D., & Decety, J. (2013). Age-related sex differences in explicit measures of empathy do not predict brain responses across childhood and adolescence. *Developmental Cognitive Neuroscience, 3*, 22–32.

Milgram, S. (1963). Behavioral study of obedience. *Journal of Abnormal and Social Psychology, 67*, 371–378.

Milgram, S. (1968). Some conditions of obedience and disobedience to authority. *Human Relations, 6*, 259–276.

Miller, K. (2002). *Communication theories: Perspective, processes, and context.* Boston: McGraw-Hill.

Miller, P. A., & Eisenberg, N. (1988). The relation of empathy to aggressive and externalizing/antisocial behavior. *Psychological Bulletin, 103*, 324–344.

Miller, M. N., & McGowen, K. R. (2000). The Painful truth: Physicians are not invincible. *Southern Medical Journal, 91*, 966–972.

Milner, K., Squire, L. R., & Kanel, E. R. (1998). Cognitive neuroscience and the study of memory. *Neuron, 20*, 445–468.

Misra-Hebert, A. D., Isaacson, J. H., Kohn, M., Hull, A. L., Hojat, M., Papp, K. K., & Calabrese, L. (2012). Improving empathy of physicians through guided reflective writing. *International Journal of Medical Education, 3*, 71–77. doi:10.5116/ijme.4f7e.e332.

Montanari, P. (2012). Psychometric analysis of the Jefferson Scale of Empathy (JSE) health professional students (HPS) version: An Italian validation study with undergraduate nursing students. Nursing graduation dissertation completed at Universita degli Studi dell'Aquila, Italy.

Montgomery Hunter, K., Charon, R., & Coulehan, J. L. (1995). The study of literature in medical education. *Academic Medicine, 70*, 787–794.

Moore, D. B. (1996). Illegal action-official reaction: Affect theory, criminology, and the criminal justice system. In D. L. Nathanson (Ed.), *Knowing feeling: Affect, script, and psychotherapy* (pp. 346–378). New York: W.W. Norton.

Moore, P. J., Adler, N. E., & Robertson, P. A. (2000). Medical malpractice: The effect of doctor-patient relations on medical patient perceptions and malpractice intentions. *Western Journal of Medicine, 173*, 244–250.

Moore, B. E., & Fine, B. D. (1968). *A glossary of psychoanalytic terms and concepts*. New York: American Psychoanalytic Association.

Morelli, S. A., Rameson, L. T., & Lieberman, M. D. (2014). The neural components of empathy: Predicting daily prosocial behavior. *Social Cognitive and Affective Neuroscience, 9*, 39–47. doi:10.1093/SCAN/nss088.

Moreno, J. L. (1934). *Who shall survive?* Washington, DC: Nervous and Mental Disease Publishing Co.

Moreto, G. (2015). Evaluating empathy in undergraduate medical students at São Paulo University using two instruments. Doctoral dissertation, São Paulo University, Brazil.

Morgan, J. D. (Ed.). (2002). *Social support: A reflection of humanity*. Amityville, NY: Baywood Publishing Company.

Mori, M. S., Vigh, A., Miayata, T., & Yoshihara, S. (1990). Oxytocin is the major prolactin releasing factor in the posterior pituitary. *Endocrinology, 125*, 1009–1013.

Morrison, I., Lloyd, D., di Pellegrino, G., & Roberts, N. (2004). Vicarious responses to pain in anterior cingulated cortex: Is empathy a multisensory issue? *Cognitive & Affective Behavioral Neuroscience, 4*, 270–278.

Morse, J. M., Anderson, G., Bottorff, J. L., Yonge, O., O'Brien, B., Solberg, S. M., & McIlveen, K. H. (1992). Exploring empathy: A conceptual fit for nursing practice? *Image: Journal of Nursing Scholarship, 24*, 273–280.

Morse, D. S., Edwardsen, E. A., & Gordon, H. S. (2008). Missed opportunities for interval empathy in long cancer communication. *Archives of Internal Medicine, 168*, 1853–1858.

Morse, J. M., & Mitcham, C. (1997). Coempathy: The contagion of physical distress. *Journal of Advanced Nursing, 26*, 649–657.

Moser, R. S. (1984). Perceived role-taking behavior and course grades in junior year college nursing students. *Journal of Nursing Education, 23*, 294–297.

Moss, H. A. (1967). Sex, age, and state as determinants of mother-infant interaction. *Merrill-Palmer Quarterly, 13*, 19–36.

Mostafa, A., Hoque, R., Mosrafa, M., Rana M., & Mostafa, F. (2014). Empathy in undergraduate medical students of Bangladesh: Psychometric analysis and differences by gender, academic year, and specialty preference. *International Scholarly Research Notices Psychiatry*, Article ID 375439. Retrieved from: http://dx.doi.org/10.1155/2014/375439.

Moyers, T. B., & Miller, W. (2013). Is low therapist empathy toxic? *Psychology of Addictive Behaviors, 27*, 878–884.

Mullins-Nelson, J. L., Salekin, R. T., & Leistico, A. R. (2006). Psychopathy, empathy, and perspective-taking ability in a community sample: Implications for the successful psychotherapy concept. *International Journal of Forensic Mental Health, 5*, 133–149.

Mumford, L. (1967). *The myth of the machine*. New York: Harcourt, Brace & World.

Murray, H. A. (1938). *Explorations in personality*. Englewood Cliffs, NJ: Prentice-Hall.

Mussen, P., & Eisenberg-Berg, N. (1977). *Roots of caring, sharing, and helping: The development of prosocial behavior in children*. San Francisco: W.H. Freeman.

Musson, D. M. (2009). Personality and medical education. *Medical Education, 43*, 395–397.

Naftulin, D. H., Ware, J. E., Jr., & Donnelly, F. A. (1973). The Doctor Fox lecture: A paradigm of educational seduction. *Journal of Medical Education, 48*, 630–635.

Narváez, V. P. D., Palacio, L. M. A., Caro, S. E., Silva, M. G., Castillo, J. A., … Acosta, J. I. (2014). Empathic orientation among medical students from three universities in Barranquilla, Colombia and one university in the Dominican Republic. *Archivos Argentinos de Pediatria, 112*, 41–49. Retrieved from: http://dx.doi.org/10.5546/aap.2014.eng.41.

Nasr Esfahani, M., Behzadipour, M., Jalili Nadoushan, A., & Shariat, S. V. (2014). A pilot randomized controlled trial on the effectiveness of inclusion of a distant learning component into empathy training. *Medical Journal of the Islamic Republic of Iran, 28*(65), 1–6.

Nathanson, D. L. (Ed.). (1996). *Knowing feeling: Affect, script, and psychotherapy.* New York: W.W. Norton.

Nauta, W. J. H., & Feirtag, M. (1986). *Fundamental neuroanatomy.* New York: W.H. Freeman.

Nelson, D. W., & Baumgarte, R. (2004). Cross-cultural misunderstandings reduce empathic responding. *Journal of Applied Social Psychology, 34*, 391–401.

Neubauer, R. B., & Neubauer, A. (1990). *Nature's thumbprint: The new genetics of personality.* Reading, MA: Addison-Wesley.

Neumann, M., Edehäuser, F., Tauschel, D., Fischer M. R., Wirtz, M., Woopen, C., … Scheffer, C. (2011). Empathy decline and its reasons: A systematic review of studies with medical students and residents. *Academic Medicine, 86*, 996–1009.

Neumann, M., Scheffer, C., Tauschel, D., Lutz, G., Wirtz, M., & Edelhäuser, F. (2012). Physician empathy: Definition, outcome-relevance and its measurement in patient care and medical education. *GMS Zeitschrift Für Medizinische Ausbildung, 29*, 11–21. Retrieved from: http://www.ncbi.nlm.nih.gov/pmc/articles/PMC3296095/.

Neuwirth, Z. E. (1997). Physician empathy—Should we care? *Lancet, 350*, 606.

Newberg, A., & Waldman, R. (2010). Yawn, it's one of the best things you can do for your brain. In *How god changes your brain?* New York: Ballantine books/Random House.

Newman, T. B. (2003). The power of stories over statistics. *British Medical Journal, 327*, 1224–1427.

Newton, B. W. (2010). Rebuttals to critics of studies of decline on empathy [Letter to the editor]. *Academic Medicine, 85*, 1812–1813.

Newton, N., Feeler, D., & Rawlins, C. (1968). Effect of lactation on maternal behavior in mice with comparative data on humans. *Lying-in: Journal of Reproductive Medicine, 1*, 257–262.

Newton, N., & Newton, M. (1967). Psychologic aspects of lactation. *New England Journal of Medicine, 277*, 1179–1188.

Newton, B. W., Savidge, M. A., Barber, L., Cleveland, E., Clardy, J., Beeman, G., & Hart, T. (2000). Differences in medical students' empathy. *Academic Medicine, 75*, 1215.

Nicholas, D. (2002). Social support of the bereaved: Some practical suggestions. In J. D. Morgan (Ed.), *Social support: A reflection of humanity* (pp. 33–43). Amityville, NY: Baywood Publishing.

Nightingale, S. D., Yarnold, P. R., & Greenberg, M. S. (1991). Sympathy, empathy, and physician resource utilization. *Journal of General Internal Medicine, 6*, 420–423.

Nolte, J. (1993). *The human brain: An introduction to its functional anatomy* (3rd ed.). St. Louis: Mosby.

Norsica, I., Demuru, E., & Palagi, E. (2016). She more than he: Gender bias supports the empathic nature of yawn contagion in *homo sapiens. Royal Society Open Science, 3*, 150459. Retrieved from: http://dx.doi.org/10.1098/rsos.150459.

Novack, D. H. (1987). Therapeutic aspects of the clinical encounter. *Journal of General Internal Medicine, 2*, 346–355.

Novack, D. H., Epstein, R. M., & Paulsen, R. H. (1999). Toward creating physician-healers: Fostering medical students' self-awareness, personal growth, and well-being. *Academic Medicine, 74*, 516–520.

Nummenmaa, L., Hirvonen, J., Parkkola, R., & Hietanen, J. (2008). Is emotional contagion special? An fMRI study on neural system for affective and cognitive empathy. *Neuroimage, 43*, 571–580.

Nunes, P., Williams, S., Sa, B., & Stevenson, K. (2011). A study of empathy decline in students from five health disciplines during their first year of training. *International Journal of Medical Education, 2*, 12–17. doi:10.5116/ijme.4d47.ddb0.

O'Conner, J. P., Nash, D. B., Buehler, M. L., & Bard, M. (2002). Satisfaction higher for physician executives who treat patients, survey finds. *Physician Executive, 28*, 16–21.

O'Sullivan, J., & Whelan, T. A. (2011). Adversarial growth in telephone counsellors: Psychological and environmental influences. *British Journal of Guidance & Counselling, 39*, 307–323. doi:1 0.1080/03069885.2011.567326.

Oatley, K. (2004). Scripts, transformation, and suggestiveness of emotions in Shakespeare and Chekhov. *Review of General Psychology, 8*, 323–340.

Ochsner, K. N., Zaki, J., Hanelin, J., Ludlow, D. H., Knierim, K., Ramchandram, T., … Mackey, S. C. (2008). Your pain or mine? Common and distinct neural systems supporting the perception of pain in self and others. *Social Cognitive and Affective Neuroscience, 3*, 144–160.

Ogle, J., Bushnell, J., & Caputi, P. (2013). Empathy is related to clinical competence in medical care. *Medical Education, 47*, 824–831. doi:10.1111/medu.12232.

Olinick, S. L. (1984). A critique of empathy and sympathy. In J. Lichtenbergh, M. Borenstein, & D. Silver (Eds.), *Empathy I* (pp. 137–166). Hillsdale, NJ: Analytic Press.

Oliver, J. (1939). An ancient poem on the duties of a physician, Part 1. *Bulletin of the History of Medicine, 7*, 315.

Olson, J., & Hanchett, E. (1997). Nurse-expressed empathy, patient outcomes, and development of a middle-range theory. *Image—The Journal of Nursing Scholarship, 29*, 71–76.

Ong, L. M., DeHaes, J. M., Hoos, A. M., & Lammies, F. B. (1995). Doctor-patient communication: A review of the literature. *Social Science & Medicine, 40*, 903–918.

Oppenheim, A. (1992). *Questionnaire design: Interviewing and attitude measurement*. London: Printer Publishing.

Orlando, I. (1961). *The dynamic nurse-patient relationship*. New York: Putman.

Orlando, I. (1972). *The discipline and teaching of nursing process*. New York: Putman.

Ornish, D. (1998). *Love and survival: The scientific basis for the healing power of intimacy*. New York: Harper Collins.

Orth-Gomer, K., & Johnson, J. V. (1987). Social network integration and mortality: A six-year follow-up study of random sample of the Swedish population. *Journal of Chronic Diseases, 40*, 949–957.

Ortmeyer, C. F. (1974). Variations in mortality, morbidity, and health care by marital status. In L. L. Erhardt & J. E. Beln (Eds.), *Mortality and morbidity in the United States* (pp. 159–184). Cambridge, MA: Harvard University Press.

Osler, W. (1932). *Aequanimitas with other addresses to medical schools, nurses, and practitioners of medicine*. Philadelphia, PA: Blakiston.

Osofsky, J. D., & O'Connell, E. J. (1977). Patterning of newborn behavior in an urban population. *Child Development, 48*, 532–536.

Ouzouni, C., & Nakakis, K. (2012). An exploratory study of student nurses' empathy. *Health Science Journal, 6*, 534–552.

Pacala, J. T., Boult, C., Bland, C., & O'Brien, J. (1995). Aging game improves medical students' attitudes toward caring for elderly. *Gerontology and Geriatrics Education, 15*, 45–57.

Pacala, J. T., Boult, C., & Hepburn, K. (2006). Ten years' experience conducting the Aging game workshop: was it worth it? *Journal of American Geriatric Society, 54*, 144–149.

Page, K. M., & Novak, M. A. (2002). Empathy leads to fairness. *Bulletin of Mathematical Biology, 64*, 1101–1116.

Papadakis, M. A., Teherani, A., Banach, M. A., Knettler, T. R., Rattner, S. L., Stern, D. T., … Hodgson, C. S. (2005). Disciplinary action by ethical boards and prior behavior in medical school. *New England Journal of Medicine, 353*, 2673–2682.

Papousek, M., Papousek, H., & Symmes, D. (1991). The meanings of melodies in motherese in tone and stress languages. *Infant Behavior & Development, 14*, 415–440.

Park, K. H., Roh, H., Suh, D. H., & Hojat, M. (2015). Empathy in Korean medical students: Findings from a nationwide survey. *Medical Teacher, 37*, 943–948. doi:10.3109/01421 59X.2014.956058.

Parlow, J., & Rothman, A. (1974). Attitudes toward social issues in medicine of five health science facilities. *Social Science & Medicine, 8*, 351–358.

Paro, H., Daud-Gallotti, R. M., Tiberio, I. C., Pinto, R. M. C., & Martins, M. A. (2012). Brazilian version of the Jefferson Scale of Empathy: Psychometric properties and factor analysis. *BMC Medical Education, 12*, 73.

Pascalis, O., DeSchonen, S., Morton, J., Deruella, C., & Fabre-Grenet, M. (1995). Mother's face recognition by neonates: A replication and extension. *Infant Behavior & Development, 18*, 79–85.

Patterson, C. H. (1984). Empathy, warmth, and genuineness in psychotherapy: A review of reviews. *Psychotherapy, 21*, 431–438.

Paulhus, D. L. (1991). Measurement and control of response bias. In J. P. Robinson, P.R. Shaver, & L. S. Wrightsman (Eds.). *Measures of personality and social psychological attitudes* (pp. 17–59). San Diego, CA: Academic Press.

Peabody, F. W. (1984). The care of the patient. *Journal of the American Medical Association, 252*, 813–818.

Pecukonis, E. V. (1990). A cognitive/affective empathy training program as a function of ego development in aggressive adolescent females. *Adolescence, 25*, 59–76.

Pedersen, R. (2009). Empirical research on empathy in medicine: A critical review. *Patient Education and Counseling, 76*, 307–322. doi:10.1016/j.pec.2009.06.012.

Pedersen, C. A., Ascher, J. A., Monroe, Y. L., & Prange, A. J. J. (1982). Oxytocin induces maternal behavior in virgin female rats. *Science, 216*, 648–649.

Pedersen, C. A., & Prange, A. J. J. (1979). Induction of maternal behavior in virgin rats after intra-cerebroventicular administration of oxytocin. *Proceedings of the National Academy of Sciences of the United States of America, 76*, 6661–6665.

Pellegrino, E. (1979). *Humanism and the physician.* Knoxville, TN: University of Tennessee Press.

Pennebaker, J. W. (1990). *Opening up: The healing power of confining in others.* New York: William Morrow.

Pennebaker, J. W., Kiecolt-Glaser, J. K., & Glaser, K. (1988). Disclosure of traumas and immune function: Health implications for psychotherapy. *Journal of Consulting and Clinical Psychology, 56*, 239–245.

Pennington, R. E., & Pierce, W. L. (1985). Observations of empathy of nursing-home staff: A predictive study. *International Journal of Aging and Human Development, 21*, 281–291.

Penninx, B. W., van Tilburg, T., & Kriegsman, D. M. (1997). Effects of social support and personal coping resources on mortality in older age: The Longitudinal Aging Study, Amsterdam. *American Journal of Epidemiology, 146*, 510–519.

Perls, F. S. (1969/1992). *Gestalt therapy verbatim.* Gouldsboro, ME: The Gestalt Journal Press, Inc.

Perry, R. J., Rosen, H. R., Kramer, J. H., Beer, J. S., Levenson, R. L., & Miller, B. L. (2001). Hemispheric dominance for emotions, empathy and social behaviour: Evidence from right and left handers with frontotemporal dementia. *Neurocase, 7*, 145–160.

Peschel, E. R. (1980). *Medicine and literature.* New York: Neale Watson.

Peter, E., & Gallop, R. (1994). The ethic of care: A comparison of nursing and medical students. *Image—The Journal of Nursing Scholarship, 26*, 47–50.

Piaget, J. (1967). *Six psychological studies.* New York: Random House.

Pigman, G. W. (1995). Freud and the history of empathy. *International Journal of Psychoanalysis, 76*, 237–256.

Platek, S. M., Critton, S. R., Myers, T. E., & Gallup, G. G. (2003). Contagious yawning: The role of self awareness and mental state attribution. *Cognitive Brain Research, 17*, 223–227.

Platek, S. M., Keenan, J. P., Gallup, G. G., & Mohamed, F. B. (2004). Where am I? The neurological correlates of self and other. *Cognitive Brain Research, 19*, 114–122.

Platek, S. M., Mohamed, F. B., & Gallup, G. G. (2005). Contagious yawning and the brain. *Cognitive Brain Research, 23*, 448–452.

Platt, F. W., & Keller, V. F. (1994). Empathic communication: A teachable and learnable skill. *Journal of General Internal Medicine, 9*, 222–226.

Plutchik, R. (1987). Evolutionary bases of empathy. In N. Eisenberg & J. Strayer (Eds.), *Empathy and its development* (pp. 38–46). New York: Cambridge University Press.

Pohl, C. A., Hojat, M., & Arnold, L. (2011). Peer nominations as related to academic attainment, empathy, and specialty interest. *Academic Medicine, 86,* 747–751. doi:10.1097/ACM.0b013e318217e464.

Polgar, C., & Thomas, S. (1988). *Introduction to research in health sciences.* Edinburgh: Churchill Livingston.

Pollak, O. (1976). *Human behavior and the helping professions.* New York: Spectrum Publications.

Pollak, I. K., Arnold, R. M., Jeffrey, A. S., Alexander, S. C., Olsen, M. K., Abernethy, A. P., … Tulsky, J. A. (2007). Oncologist communication about emotions during visits with patients with advanced cancer. *Journal of Clinical Oncology, 25*, 5748–5752.

Poole, A. D., & Sanson-Fisher, R. W. (1980). Long-term effects of empathy training on the interview skills of medical students. *Patient Counseling and Health Education, 2*, 125–127.

Potash, J. S., Chen, J. Y., Lam, C. L., & Chau, V. T. (2014). Art-making in a family medicine clerkship: How does it affect medical student empathy? *BMC Medical Education, 14*, 247. doi:10.1186/s12909-014-0247-4. Retrieved from: www.biomedcentral.com/1472-6920/14/247.

Powell, A. S., Boakes, J. P., & Slater, P. (1988). Hostility and the medical student: How a trait measure influences perception of medical specialties. *Medical Education, 22*, 222–230.

Preston, S. D., & deWaal, F. B. M. (2002). Empathy: It's ultimate and proximate bases. *Behavioral and Brain Sciences, 25*, 1–20.

Preusche, I., & Wagner-Menghin, M. (2013). Rising to the challenge: Cross-cultural adaptation and psychometric evaluation of the adapted German version of the Jefferson Scale of Physician Empathy for students (JSPE-S). *Advances in Health Science Education: Theory and Practice, 18*, 573–587. doi:10.1007/s10459-012-9393-9.

Price, B. H., Daffner, K. R., Stowe, R. M., & Mesulam, M. (1990). The compartmental learning disabilities of early frontal lobe damage. *Brain, 113*, 1383–1393.

Prinz, W. (1997). Perception and action planning. *European Journal of Cognitive Psychology, 9*, 129–154.

Pumilia, C. V. (2002). Psychological impact of the physician-patient relationship on compliance: A case study and clinical strategies. *Progress in Transplantation, 12*, 10–16.

Puryear, J. B., & Lewis, L. A. (1981). Description of the interview process in selecting students for admission to U.S. medical school. *Journal of Medical Education, 56*, 881–885.

Quill, T. E. (1987). Medical resident education: A cross-sectional study of the influence of the ambulatory preceptor as a role model. *Archives of Internal Medicine, 147*, 971–973.

Radley, C. (1992). Imagining ethics: Literature and practice of ethics. *Journal of Clinical Ethics, 3*, 38–45.

Rahimi-Madiseh, M., Tavakol, M., Dennick, R., & Nasiri, J. (2010). Empathy in Iranian medical students: A preliminary psychometric analysis and differences by gender and year of medical school. *Medical Teacher, 32*, e471–e478 (web paper).

Rahm, E. T. (2006). Tracking the subprocesses of decision-based action in the human frontal lobes. *Neuroimage, 30*, 656–667. doi:10.1016/j.neuroimage.2005.09.045.

Rakel, D. P., Hoeft, T. J., Barrett, B. P., Chewning, B. A., Craig, B. M., & Niu, M. (2009). Practitioner empathy and the duration of the common cold. *Family Medicine, 41*, 494–501.

Rankin, K. P., Gorno-Tempini, M. L., Allison, S. C., Stanley, C. M., Glenn, S., & Weiner, M. W. (2006). Structural anatomy of empathy in neurodegenerative disease. *Brain, 129*, 2945–2956.

Rankin, K. P., Kramer, J. H., & Miller, B. L. (2005). Patterns of cognitive and emotional empathy in frontotemporal lobar degeneration. *Cognitive Behavioral Neurology, 18*, 28–36.

Raudonis, B. M. (1993). The meaning and impact of empathic relationships in hospice nursing. *Cancer Nursing, 16*, 304–309.

Ray, O. (2004). How the mind hurts and heals the body. *American Psychologist, 59*, 29–40.

Raynolds, P., Boyd, P. T., & Blacklow, R. S. (1994). The relationships between social ties and survival among black and white breast cancer patients: National Cancer Institute, Cancer Survival Study Group. *Cancer Epidemiology, Biomarkers & Prevention, 3*, 253–259.

Reed, V. A., Jernstedt, C., & Reber, E. S. (2001). Understanding and improving medical student specialty choice: Synthesis of the literature using decision theory as a referent. *Teaching and Learning in Medicine, 13*, 117–129.

Reik, T. (1948). *Listening with the third ear: The inner experience of a psychoanalyst*. New York: Farrar, Straus.

Reiser, M. F., Reeves, R. B., & Armington, J. (1955). Effects of variation in laboratory procedure and experimenter upon the ballistoeargram, blood pressure, and heart rate in healthy young men. *Psychosomatic Medicine, 17*, 185–199.

Reisetter, B. C. (2003). Relationship between psychosocial physician characteristic and physician price awareness. Doctoral dissertation, University of Mississippi, Dissertation Abstracts International, 63(10-B), p. 4620.

Reisetter, B. C., Bently, J. P., & Wilkin, N. E. (2005). Relationship between psychosocial physician characteristics and physician price awareness. *Journal of Pharmaceutical Marketing & Management, 17*, 51–76. doi:10.1300/j058v17n01_05.

Reiter-Palmon, R., & Connelly, M. S. (2000). Item selection counts: A comparison of empirical key and rational scale validities in theory-based and non-theory-based item pools. *Journal of Applied Psychology, 85*, 143–151.

Rempel, J. K., Holmes, J. G., & Zanna, M. P. (1985). Trust in close relationships. *Journal of Personality and Social Psychology, 49*, 95–112.

Reverby, S. (1987). A caring dilemma: Womanhood and nursing in historical perspective. *Nursing Research, 36*, 1–5.

Reynolds, W. J. (2000). *The measurement and development of empathy in nursing*. Burlington, VT: Ashgate.

Richard, F. D., Bond, C. F., Jr., & Stokes-Zoota, J. J. (2003). One hundred years of social psychology quantitatively described. *Review of General Psychology, 7*, 331–363.

Richard, G. V., Nakamoto, D. M., & Lockwood, J. H. (2001). Medical career choices: Traditional and new possibilities. *Journal of the American Medical Association, 285*, 2249–2250.

Richards, H. L., Fortune, D. G., Weildmann, A., Sweeney, S. K. T., & Griffiths, C. E. M. (2004). Detection of psychological distress in patients with psoriasis: Low consensus between dermatologist and patient. *British Journal of Dermatology, 151*, 1227–1233. doi:10.1111/j.1365-2133.2004.06221.x.

Richter, C. P. (1957). On the phenomenon of sudden death in animals and man. *Psychosomatic Medicine, 19*, 191–198.

Ridley, M., & Dawkins, R. (1981). The natural selection of altruism. In J. P. Rushton & R. M. Sorrentino (Eds.), *Altruism and helping behavior: Social, personality, and developmental perspectives* (pp. 19–39). Hillsdale, NJ: Erlbaum.

Riess, H., Kelley, J., Bailey, R., Dunn, E., & Phillips, M. (2012). Empathy training for resident physicians: A randomized controlled trial of a neuroscience-informed curriculum. *Journal of General Internal Medicine, 27*, 1280–1286. doi:10.1007/s11606-012.2063-z.

Riess, H., Kelley, J. M., Bailey, R., Konowitz, P. M., & Gray, S. T. (2011). Improving empathy and relational skills in otolaryngology residents: A pilot study. *Otolaryngology-Head and Neck Surgery, 144*, 120–122. doi:10.1177/0194599810390897.

Riggio, R. E., Tucker, J., & Coffaro, D. (1989). Social skills and empathy. *Personality and Individual Differences, 10*, 93–99.

Rizzolatti, G., & Arbibi, M. A. (1998). Language within our grasp. *Trends in Neuroscience, 21*, 188–194.

Rizzolatti, G., & Craighero, L. (2004). The mirror-neuron system. *Annual Review of Neuroscience, 27*, 169–192.

Rizzolatti, G., Fadiga, L., Gallese, V., & Fogassi, L. (1996). Premotor cortex and the recognition of motor action. *Cognitive Brain Research, 3*, 131–141.

Roberts, B. W., & DelVecchio, W. F. (2000). The rank-order consistency of personality traits from childhood to old age: A quantitative review of longitudinal studies. *Psychological Bulletin, 126*, 3–25.

Robinson, J. P. (1978). General attitudes toward people. In J. P. Robinson & P. R. Shaver (Eds.), *Measures of social psychological attitudes* (pp. 587–627). Ann Arbor, MI: Institute for Social Research.

Robinson, J. L., Zahn-Waxler, C., & Emde, R. N. (1994). Patterns of development in early empathic behavior: Environmental and child constitutional influences. *Social Development, 3*, 125–145.

Rodriguez, M. S., & Cohen, S. (1998). Social support. In H. S. Friedman (Ed.), *Encyclopedia of mental health* (pp. 535–544). San Diego, CA: Academic Press.

Roe, A. (1957). Early determinants of vocational choice. *Journal of Consulting Psychology, 4*, 212–217.

Roe, K. V. (1977). A study of empathy in young Greek and U.S. children. *Journal of Cross-Cultural Psychology, 8*, 493–502.

Rogers, C. R. (1959). A theory of therapy: Personality and interpersonal relationships as developed in the client-centered framework. In S. Koch (Ed.), *Psychology, a study of science: Foundations of the person and the social context* (pp. 184–256). New York: McGraw-Hill.

Rogers, C. R. (1975). Empathic: An unappreciated way of being. *Counseling Psychologist, 5*, 2–11.

Rogers, C. R., Gendlin, E., Kiesler, D., & Truax, C. B. (1967). *The therapeutic relationship and its impact*. Madison: University of Wisconsin Press.

Roghmann, K. J., Hengst, A., & Zastowny, T. R. (1979). Satisfaction with medical care: Its measurement and relation to utilization. *Medical Care, 17*, 461–479.

Roh, M. S., Hahm, B. J., Lee, D. H., & Suh, D. H. (2010). Evaluation of empathy among Korean medical students: A cross-sectional study using Korean version of the Jefferson Scale of Physician Empathy. *Teaching and Learning in Medicine: An International Journal, 22*, 167–171. doi:10.1080/10401334.2010.488191. Retrieved from: http://dx.doi.org/10.1080/1040133 4.2010.488191.

Rokeach, M. (1973). *The nature of human values*. New York: Free Press.

Romano, J. M., Jensen, M. P., Turner, J. A., Good, A. B., & Hops, H. (2000). Chronic pain patient-partner interactions: Further support for a behavioral model of chronic pain. *Behavior Therapy, 31*, 415–440.

Rosenberg, M. (1957). *Occupation and values*. Glencoe, IL: Free Press.

Rosenberg, M. (1965). *Society and adolescent self-image*. Princeton, NJ: Princeton University Press.

Rosenberg, M. J., & Hovland, C. I. (1960). Cognitive, affective, and behavioral components of attitudes. In M. J. Hovland & M. J. Rosenberg (Eds.), *Attitude organization and change* (pp. 1–14). New Haven, CT: Yale University Press.

Rosenberg, D. A., & Silver, H. K. (1984). Medical student abuse—An unnecessary and preventable cause of stress. *Journal of the American Medical Association, 251*, 739–742.

Rosenfeld, H. M. (1965). Effect of an approval-seeking induction on interpersonal proximity. *Psychological Reports, 17*, 120–122.

Rosenhan, D. L. (1973). On being sane in insane places. *Science, 179*, 250–258.

Rosenow, E. C. (1999). The challenge of becoming a distinguished clinician. *Mayo Clinic Proceedings, 74*, 635–637.

Rosenthal, R., Hall, J. A., DiMatteo, M. R., Rogers, P. L., & Archer, D. (1979). *Sensitivity to non-verbal communication: The PONS test*. Baltimore, MD: Johns Hopkins University Press.

Rosenthal, S., Howard, B., Schlussel, Y. R., Herrigel, D., Smolarz, B. G., Gable, B., … Kaufman, M. (2011). Humanism at heart: Preserving empathy in third-year medical students. *Academic Medicine, 86*, 350–358.

Ross, J. B., & McLaughlin, M. M. (1949). *The portable medieval reader*. New York: Penguin Books USA Inc.

Ross, E. D., & Mesulam, M. M. (1979). Dominant language functions of the right hemisphere? Prosody and emotional gesturing. *Archives of Neurology, 36*, 144–148.

Roter, D. L., & Hall, J. A. (1997). Gender differences in patient-physician communication. In S. J. Gallant, G. P. Keita, & R. Royak-Schater (Eds.), *Health care for women: Psychological, social, and behavioral influences* (pp. 57–71). Washington, DC: American Psychological Association.

Roter, D. L., Hall, J. A., Kern, D. E., Baker, L. R., Cole, K. A., & Roca, R. P. (1995). Improving physicians' interviewing skills and reduction in patients' emotional distress: A randomized clinical trial. *Archives of Internal Medicine, 155*, 1877–1884.

Roter, D. L., Hall, J. A., Merisca, R., Nordstrom, B., Cretin, D., & Svarstad, B. (1998). Effectiveness of interventions to improve patient compliance: A meta-analysis. *Medical Care, 36*, 1138–1161.

Roter, D. L., Hall, J. A., & Aoki, Y. (2002). Physician gender effects in medical communication. *Journal of the American Medical Association, 288*, 756–764.

Roter, D., Lipkin, M., & Korsgaard, A. (1991). Sex differences in patients' and physicians' communication during primary care medical visits. *Medical Care, 29*, 1088–1093.

Rovezzi-Carroll, S., & Fitz, P. A. (1984). Predicting allied health major fields of study with selected personality characteristics. *College Student Journal, 18*, 43–51.

Ruby, P., & Decety, J. (2004). How would you feel versus how would you think she would feel? A neuroimaging study of perspective taking with social emotions. *Journal of Cognitive Neuroscience, 16*, 988–999.

Rueckert, L., & Naybar, N. (2008). Gender differences in empathy: The role of the right hemisphere. *Brain and Cognition, 67*, 162–167. doi:10.1016/j.bandc.2008.01.002.

Rushton, J. P. (1981). The altruistic personality. In P. J. Rushton & R. M. Sorrentino (Eds.), *Altruism and helping behavior: Social, personality, and developmental perspectives* (pp. 251–266). Hillsdale, NJ: Erlbaum.

Rushton, J. P. (2004). Genetic and environmental contributions to pro-social attitudes: A twin study of social responsibility. *Proceedings of the Royal Society of Biological Sciences, 271*, 2583–2585. doi:10.1098/rspb.2004.2941.

Rushton, J. P., Chrisjohn, R. D., & Fekker, G. C. (1981). The altruistic personality and the self-report Altruism Scale. *Personality and Individual Differences, 2*, 293–302.

Rushton, J. P., Fulker, D. W., Neale, M. C., Nias, D. K. B., & Eysenck, H. J. (1986). Altruism and aggression: The heritability of individual differences. *Journal of Personality and Social Psychology, 50*, 1192–1198.

Russek, L. G., & Schwartz, G. E. (1997). Perceptions of parental caring predict health status in midlife: A 35-year follow up of the Harvard Mastery of Stress study. *Psychosomatic Medicine, 59*, 144–149.

Russell, D., Peplau, L. A., & Cutrona, C. B. (1980). The revised UCLA Loneliness Scale: Concurrent and discriminant validity evidence. *Journal of Personality and Social Psychology, 39*, 472–480.

Rutgen, M., Seidel, E. M., Riecansky, I., & Lamm, C. (2015). Reduction of empathy for pain by placebo analgesia suggests functional equivalence of empathy and first-hand emotion experience. *The journal of Neuroscience, 35*, 8938–8947. doi:10.1523/JNEUROSCI.3936-14.2015.

Rutter, M., Caspi, A., Fergusson, D., Horwood, L. J., Goodman, R., Maughan, B., … Carroll, J. (2005). Sex differences in developmental reading ability: New findings from 4 epidemiological studies. *Journal of the American Medical Association, 291*, 2007–2012.

Sackett, D. H., & Haynes, R. B. (1976). *Compliance with therapeutic regimens*. Baltimore, MD: Johns Hopkins University Press.

Safdar, B., Heins, A., Homel, P., Miner, J., Neighbor, M., De Sandre, P., & Todd, K. (2009). Impact of physician and patient gender on pain management in the emergency department—A multicenter study. *Pain Medicine, 10*, 364–372.

Sage, W. M. (2002). Putting the patient in patient safety: Linking patient complaints and malpractice risk. *Journal of the American Medical Association, 287*, 3003–3005.

Sagi, A., & Hoffman, M. L. (1976). Empathic distress in newborns. *Developmental Psychology, 12*, 175–176.

Salk, L. (1960). The effects of normal heartbeat sound on the behavior of the newborn infant: Implications for mental health. *World Mental Health, 12*, 168–175.

Salovey, P., & Mayer, J. D. (1990). Emotional intelligence. *Imagination, Cognition, and Personality, 9*, 185–211.

Sandler, G. (1980). The importance of the history in the medical clinic and the cost of unnecessary tests. *American Heart Journal, 100*, 928–931.

Sandoval, A. M., Hancock, D., Poythress, N., Edens, J. F., & Lilienfeld, S. (2000). Construct validity of the Psychopathic Personality Inventory in a correctional sample. *Journal of Personality
Assessment, 74*, 262–281.

Sanson-Fisher, R., & Maguire, P. (1980). Should skills in communication with patients be taught
in medical schools? *Lancet, 2*, 523–526.

Sanson-Fisher, R. W., & Poole, A. D. (1978). Training medical students to empathize: An experimental study. *Medical Journal of Australia, 1*, 473–476.

Sapolsky, R. M. (2004). *Why zebras don't get ulcers* (3rd ed.). New York: Times Books.

Schachter, S. (1959). *The psychology of affiliation*. Stanford, CA: Stanford University Press.

Schafer, R. (1959). Generative empathy in the treatment situation. *Psychoanalytic Quarterly, 28*,
342–373.

Schaflen, A. E. (1964). The significance of posture in communication systems. *Psychiatry, 27*,
316–331.

Schlesinger, M. (2002). A loss of faith: The sources of reduced political legitimacy for the
American medical profession. *Milbank Quarterly, 80*, 185–235.

Schmidt, C. W., & Baker, L. R. (1986). Psychotherapy in ambulatory practice. In L. R. Barker,
J. R. Burton, & P. D. Zieve (Eds.), *Principles of ambulatory medicine* (pp. 133–139). Baltimore:
Williams & Wilkins.

Schmitt, D. P. (2012). When the difference is in the detail: A critique of Zentner and Mitura (2012)
"Stepping out of the caveman's shadow: Nations' gender gap predicts degree of sex differentiation in mate preferences". *Evolutionary Psychology, 10*, 720–726.

Schneiderman, L. J. (2002). Empathy and the literary imagination. *Annals of Internal Medicine,
137*, 627–629.

Schoenbach, V., Kaplan, B. H., Fredman, L., & Kleinbaum, D. G. (1986). Social ties and mortality
in Evans County, Georgia. *American Journal of Epidemiology, 123*, 577–591.

Schore, A. N. (1996). *Affect regulation and the origin of the self: The neurobiology of emotional
development*. Hillsdale, NJ: Erlbaum.

Schroeder, T. (1925). The psycho-analytic method of observation. *International Journal of
Psychoanalysis, 6*, 155–170.

Schulte-Ruther, M., Markowitsch, H., Fink, G., & Piefke, M. (2007). Mirror neuron and theory of
mind mechanisms involved in face-to-face interactions: A functional magnetic resonance
imaging approach to empathy. *Journal of Cognitive Neuroscience, 19*, 1354–1372.

Schutle-Ruther, M., Markowitsch, H. J., Shah, N. J., Fink, G. R., & Piefke, M. (2008). Gender
differences in brain networks supporting empathy. *Neuroimage, 42*, 393–403. doi:10.1016/j.
neuroimage.2008.04.180.

Schutte, N. S., Malouff, J. M., Bobik, C., Coston, T. D., Greeson, C., Jedulicka, C., … Wendorf,
G. (2001). Emotional intelligence and interpersonal relations. *Journal of Social Psychology,
141*, 523–536.

Schwaber, E. (1981). Empathy: A mode of analytic listening. *Psychoanalytic Inquiry, 1*,
357–392.

Schwartz, B., & Bohay, R. (2012). Can patient help teach professionalism and empathy to dental
students? Adding patient video to lecture course. *Journal of Dental Education, 76*, 174–184.

Schweller, M., Costa, F. O., Antônio, M. Â., Amaral, E. M., & de Carvalho-Filho, M. A. (2014).
The impact of simulated medical consultations on the empathy levels of students at one medical school. *Academic Medicine, 89*, 632–637.

Scourfield, J., Martin, N., Lewis, G., & McGuffin, P. (1999). Heritability of social cognitive skills
in children and adolescents. *British Journal of Psychiatry, 175*, 564.

Seaberg, D. C., Godwin, S. A., & Perry, S. J. (1999). Teaching empathy in an emergency medicine
residency. *Academic Emergency Medicine, 6*, 485.

Seaberg, D. C., Godwin, S. A., & Perry, S. J. (2000). Teaching patient empathy: The ED visit
program. *Academic Emergency Medicine, 7*, 1433–1436.

Seeman, T. E., Berkman, L. F., & Kohout, F. (1993). Intercommunity variation in the association
between social ties and mortality in elderly: A comparative analysis of three communities.
Annals of Epidemiology, 3, 325–335.

Seeman, T. E., & Syme, L. (1987). Social network and coronary artery disease: A comparison of the structure and function of social relations and predictors of disease. *Psychosomatic Medicine, 49*, 341–354.

Seifritz, E., Esposito, F., Neuhoff, J. G., Luthi, A., Mustovic, H., Dammann, G., … Di Salle, F. (2003). Differential sex-independent amygdala response to infant crying and laughing in parents versus nonparents. *Biological Psychiatry, 54*, 1367–1375.

Self, D. J., Schrader, D. E., Baldwin, D. C., Jr., & Wolinsky, F. D. (1993). The moral development of medical students: A pilot study of the possible influence of medical education. *Medical Education, 27*, 26–34.

Shallice, T. (2001). "Theory of Mind" and the prefrontal cortex. *Brain, 124*, 247–248.

Shamasundar, M. R. C. (1999). Reflections: Understanding empathy and related phenomena. *American Journal of Psychotherapy, 53*, 232–245.

Shamay-Tsoory, S. G., Tomer, R., Berger, B. D., & Aharon-Peretz, J. (2003). Characterization of empathy deficit following prefrontal brain damage: The role of the right ventromedial prefrontal cortex. *Cognitive Neuroscience, 15*, 324–337.

Shamay-Tsoory, S. G., Tomer, R., Goldsher, D., Berger, B. D., & Aharon-Peretz, J. (2004). Impairment in cognitive and affective empathy in patients with brain lesions: Anatomical and cognitive correlates. *Journal of Clinical and Experimental Neuropsychology, 26*, 1113–1127.

Shapiro, T. (1974). The development and distortions of empathy. *Psychoanalytic Quarterly, 43*, 4–25.

Shapiro, J. (2002). How do physicians teach empathy in the primary care setting? *Academic Medicine, 77*, 323–328.

Shapiro, D. E., Boggs, S. R., Melamed, B. G., & Graham-Pole, J. (1992). The effect of varied physician affect on recall, anxiety, and perceptions in women at risk of breast cancer: An analogue study. *Health Psychology, 11*, 61–66.

Shapiro, J., & Hunt, L. (2003). All the world's a stage: The use of theatrical performance in medical education. *Medical Education, 37*, 922–927.

Shapiro, J., Morrison, E., & Boker, J. (2004). Teaching empathy to first year medical students: Evaluation of an elective literature and medical course. *Education for Health, 17*, 73–84.

Shapiro, A. K., & Shapiro, E. (1984). Patient-provider relationships and the placebo effect. In J. D. Matarazzo, S. M. Weiss, J. A. Herd, N. E. Miller, & S. M. Weiss (Eds.), *Behavioral health: A handbook of health enhancement and disease prevention* (pp. 371–383). New York: Wiley-Interscience.

Shapiro, R. S., Simpson, D. E., & Lawrence, S. L. (1989). Survey of sued and non-sued physicians and suing patients. *Annals of Internal Medicine, 149*, 2190–2196.

Shapurian, R., & Hojat, M. (1985). Psychometric characteristics of a Persian version of the Eysenck Personality Questionnaire. *Psychological Reports, 57*, 631–639.

Shariat, S. V., Eshtad, E., & Ansari, S. (2010). Empathy and its correlates in Iranian physicians: A preliminary psychometric study of the Jefferson Scale of Physician Empathy. *Medical Teacher, 32*, e417–e421. doi:10.3109/0142159X.2010.498488 (web paper).

Shariat, S. V., & Habibi, M. (2013). Empathy in Iranian medical students: Measurement model of the Jefferson Scale of Empathy. *Medical Teacher, 35*, e913–e918. doi:10.3109/01421 59x.2012.714881.

Shariat, S. V., & Kaykhavoni, A. (2010). Empathy in medical residents at Iran University of Medical Sciences. *Iranian Journal of Psychiatry and Clinical Psychology, 16*, 248–256.

Shaver, P., & Hazan, C. (1989). Being lonely, falling in love: Perspectives from attachment theory. In M. Hojat & R. Crandall (Eds.), *Loneliness: Theory, research, and applications* (pp. 105–124). Newbury, CA: Sage.

Sheehan, C. A., Perrin, K. O., Potter, M. L., Kazanowski, M. K., & Bennett, L. A. (2013). Engendering empathy in baccalaureate nursing students. *International Journal of Caring Sciences, 6*, 456–464.

Sheehan, K. H., Sheehan, D. V., White, K., Leibowitz, A., & Baldwin, D. C., Jr. (1990). A pilot study of medical student 'abuse': Student perceptions of mistreatment and misconduct in medical school. *Journal of the American Medical Association, 263*, 533–537.

Shelton, W. (1999). Can virtue be taught? *Academic Medicine, 74*, 671–674.

Sherif, C. W., Sherif, M., & Nebergall, R. E. (1965). *Attitudes and attitude change: The social judgment-involvement approach*. Philadelphia: W.B. Saunders.

Sherman, J. J., & Cramer, A. (2005). Measurement of changes in empathy during dental school. *Journal of Dental Education, 69*, 338–345.

Sherman, J. J., & Cramer, A. (2010). Rebuttals to critics of studies of decline on empathy [Letter to the editor]. *Academic Medicine, 85*, 1813.

Shorey, H. S., & Snyder, C. R. (2006). The role of adult attachment styles in psychopathology and psychotherapy outcomes. *Review of General Psychology, 10*, 1–20.

Shorter, E. (1986). *Bedside manners: The troubled history of doctors and patients*. Harmondsworth, UK: Viking.

Siegel, D. J. (1999). *The developing mind: How relationships and the brain interact to shape who we are*. New York: Guilford.

Sieratzki, J. S., & Woll, B. (1996). Why do mothers cradle babies on their left? *Lancet, 347*, 1746–1748.

Sierles, F. S., Vergare, M., Hojat, M., & Gonnella, J. S. (2004). Academic performance of psychiatrists compared other specialists before, during, and after medical school. *American Journal of Psychiatry, 161*, 1477–1482.

Silver, H. K. (1982). Medical students and medical school. *Journal of the American Medical Association, 247*, 309–310.

Silver, H. K., & Glicken, A. D. (1990). Medical student abuse: Incidence, severity, and significance. *Journal of the American Medical Association, 263*, 527–532.

Simmons, J. M. P., Robie, P. W., Kendrick, S. B., Schumacher, S., & Roberge, L. P. (1992). Residents' use of humanistic skills and content of resident discussions in a support group. *American Journal of the Medical Sciences, 303*, 227–232.

Simner, M. L. (1971). Newborn response to the cry of another infant. *Developmental Psychology, 5*, 136–140.

Simpson, M., Buckman, R., Stewart, M., Maguire, P., Kipkin, M., Novack, D., & Till, J. (1991). Doctor-patient communication: The Toronto consensus statement. *British Medical Journal, 303*, 1385–1387.

Sims, A. (1988). *Symptoms in the mind: An introduction to descriptive psychotherapy*. London: Baillier, Tindall, W.B. Saunders.

Singer, T., & Frith, C. (2005). The painful side of empathy. *Nature Neuroscience, 8*, 845–846.

Singer, T., Seymour, B., O'Doherty, J., Kaube, H., Dolan, R. J., & Frith, C. D. (2004). Empathy for pain involves the affective but not sensory components of pain. *Science, 303*, 1157–1162. doi:10.1126/science.1093535.

Singer, T., Seymour, B., O'Doherty, J., Stephan, K. E., Dolan, R. J., & Frith, C. (2006). Empathic neural responses are modulated by the perceived fairness of others. *Nature, 439*(7075), 466–469. doi:10.1038/nature04271.

Skeff, K. M., & Mutha, S. (1998). Role models: Guiding the future of medicine. *New England Journal of Medicine, 339*, 2015–2017.

Skelton, J. R., Macleod, J. A. A., & Thomas, C. P. (2000). Teaching literature and medicine to medical students: Part II. Why literature and medicine? *Lancet, 356*, 2001–2003.

Slipp, S. (2000). Subliminal stimulation research and its implications for psychoanalytic theory and treatment. *Journal of the American Academy of Psychoanalysis, 28*, 305–320.

Sloan, F. A., Mergenhagen, P. M., Burfield, W. B., Bovjerg, R. R., & Hassan, M. (1989). Medical malpractice experience of physicians: Predictable or haphazard? *Journal of the American Medical Association, 262*, 3291–3297.

Smith, B. H. (1981). Narrative versions, narrative theories. In W. J. T. Mitchell (Ed.), *On narrative* (pp. 209–232). Chicago: University of Chicago Press.

Smith, R. C. (1984). Teaching interviewing skills to medical students: The issue of countertransference. *Journal of Medical Education, 59*, 582–588.

Smith, G. R. (1991). *Somatization disorder in the medical setting*. Washington, DC: American Psychiatric Press.

Smolarz, B. G. (2005). Determining the relationship between medical student empathy and undergraduate college major. Master's degree thesis completed at the Albany Medical College, The Graduate College of Union University, Schenectady, New York.

Smotherman, W. P., & Robinson, S. R. (1994). Milk as the proximal mechanism for behavioral change in the newborn. *Acta Pædiatrica Scandinavica, 397*, 64–70.

Smyth, J., Stone, A., Hurewitz, A., & Kaell, A. (1999). Effects of writing about stressful experiences on symptom reduction in patients with asthma or rheumatoid arthritis: A randomized trial. *Journal of the American Medical Association, 281*, 1304–1309.

Sochting, I., Skoe, E. E., & Marcia, J. E. (1994). Care-oriented moral reasoning and prosocial behavior: A question of gender role orientation. *Sex Roles, 31*, 131–147.

Soenens, B., Duriez, B., Vansteenkiste, M., & Goossens, L. (2007). The intergeneration transmission of empathy-related responding in adolescence: The role of maternal support. *Personality and Social Psychology Bulletin, 33*, 200–311. doi:10.1177/0146167206296300.

Solomon, R. C. (1976). *The passion.* New York: Anchor/Doubleday.

Sommer, R. (1969). *Personal space.* Englewood Cliffs, NJ: Prentice-Hall.

Soncini, F., Silvestrini, G., Poscia, A., Clorba. V., Conti, A., Murru, C., ... Ziglio, A. (2013). Public health physicians and empathy: Are we really empathic? The Jefferson Scale applied to Italian resident doctors in public health. *European Journal of Public Health, 23*(Suppl. 1), 264–265. doi:10.1093/eurpub/ckt124.068.

Sorce, J. F., Emde, R. N., Campos, J., & Klinnert, M. D. (1985). Maternal emotional signaling: Its effect on the visual cliff behavior of 1-year-olds. *Developmental Psychology, 21*, 195–200.

Sotile, W. M., & Sotile, M. O. (1996). *The medical marriage: A couple's survival manual.* New York: Carol Publication.

Southard, E. E. (1918). The empathic index in the diagnosis of mental diseases. *Journal of Abnormal Psychology, 13*, 199–214.

Sox, H. C. (2002). Medical professionalism in the new millennium: A physician charter. *Annals of Internal Medicine, 136*, 243–246.

Speedling, E. J., & Rose, D. N. (1985). Building an effective doctor-patient relationship: From patient satisfaction to patient participation. *Social Science & Medicine, 21*, 115–120.

Spelke, E. S. (2005). Sex differences in intrinsic aptitude for mathematics and science? A critical review. *American Psychologist, 60*, 950–958.

Spiegel, D. (1990). Can psychotherapy prolong cancer survival? *Psychosomatics, 31*, 361–366.

Spiegel, D. (1993). *Living beyond limits: New hope and help for facing life-threatening illness.* New York: Times Books.

Spiegel, D. (1994). Health caring: Psychological support for patients with cancer. *Cancer, 74*, 1453–1457.

Spiegel, D. (2004). Mind matters—Group therapy and survival in breast cancer. *The New England Journal of Medicine, 345*, 1–3.

Spiegel, D., & Bloom, J. R. (1983). Group therapy and hypnosis reduce metastatic breast carcinoma pain. *Psychosomatic Medicine, 45*, 333–339.

Spiegel, D., Bloom, J. R., Kraemer, H. C., & Gottheil, E. (1989). Effect of psychosocial treatment on survival of patients with metastatic breast cancer. *Lancet, 2*, 888–891.

Spiegel, D., Bloom, J. R., & Yalom, I. D. (1981). Group support for patients with metastatic breast cancer. *Archives of General Psychiatry, 38*, 527–533.

Spinella, M. (2002). A relationship between smell identification and empathy. *International Journal of Neuroscience, 112*, 605–612.

Spiro, H. M. (1986). *Doctors, patients and placebos.* New Haven: Yale University Press.

Spiro, H. (1992). What is empathy and can it be taught? *Annals of Internal Medicine, 116*, 843–846.

Spiro, H. (1998). *The power of hope: A doctor's perspective.* New Haven: Yale University Press.

Spiro, H. (2009). Commentary: The practice of empathy. *Academic Medicine, 84*, 1177–1179.

Spiro, H. M., McCrea Curnen, M. G. M., Peschel, E., & St. James, D. (1993). *Empathy and the practice of medicine: Beyond pills and the scalpel.* New Haven: Yale University Press.

Spreng, R. N., McKinnon, M. C., Mar, R. A., & Levine, B. (1999). The Toronto Empathy Questionnaire: Scale development and initial validation of a factor analytic solution to multiple empathy measures. *Journal of Personality Assessment, 91*, 62–71. doi:10.1080/00223890802484381.

Spreng, R. N., McKinnon, M. C., Mar, R. A., & Levine, B. (2009). The Toronto Empathy Questionnaire: Scale development and initial validation of a factor analytic solution to multiple empathy measures. *Journal of Personality Assessment, 91*, 62–71. doi:10.1080/00223890802484381.

Squier, R. W. (1990). A model of empathic understanding and adherence to treatment regimens in practitioner-patient relationships. *Social Science & Medicine, 30*, 325–339.

Stamps, P. L., & Boley Cruz, N. T. (1994). *Issues in physician satisfaction: New perspectives*. Ann Arbor, MI: Health Administration Press.

Stansfield, R. B., Schwartz, A., O'Brien, C. L., Dekhtyar, M., Dunham, L., & Quirk, M. (2016). Development of a metacognitive effort construct of empathy during clinical training: A longitudinal study of the factor structure of the Jefferson Scale of Empathy. *Advances in Health Sciences Education : Theory and Practice, 21*, 5–17. http://doi.org/10.1007/s10459-015-9605-1.

Starcevic, V., & Piontek, C. M. (1997). Empathic understanding revisited: Conceptualization, controversies, and limitations. *American Journal of Psychotherapy, 51*, 317–328.

Starfield, B., Wray, C., Hess, K., Gross, R., Birk, P., & D'Lugoff, B. (1981). The influence of patient-practitioner agreement on outcome of care. *American Journal of Public Health, 71*, 127–131.

Starr, P. (1982). *Social transformation of American medicine*. New York: Basic Books.

Staub, E. (1978). *Positive social behavior and morality: Social and personal influences* (Vol. 1). New York: Academic Press.

Staudenmayer, H., & Lefkowitz, M. S. (1981). Physician-patient psychological characteristics influencing medical decision-making. *Social Science & Medicine, 15*, 77–81.

Stebbins, C. A. (2005). Enhancing empathy in medical students using Flex Care™ communication training. Doctoral dissertation completed at Iowa State University. Dissertation Abstracts International, 66(4-B), p. 1962.

Stein, M. D., Fleisman, J., Mor, V., & Dresser, M. (1993). Factors associated with patient satisfaction among HIV-infected persons. *Medical Care, 31*, 182–188.

Steinbrook, R. (2002). Nursing in the crossfire. *New England Journal of Medicine, 346*, 1757–1766.

Steiner, J. F. (2005). The use of stories in clinical research and health policy. *Journal of the American Medical Association, 294*, 2901–2904.

Stephan, W. G., & Finlay, K. (1999). The role of empathy in improving inter-group relations. *Journal of Social Issues, 55*, 729–743.

Stepien, K. A., & Baernstien, A. (2006). Educating for empathy: A review. *Journal of General Internal Medicine, 21*, 524–530.

Ster, M. P., Ster, B., Petek, D., & Gorup, E. C. (2014). Validation of Slovenian version of Jefferson Scale of Empathy for students. *Slovenian Journal of Public Health, 53*, 89–100. doi:10.2478/sjph-2014-0010.

Stern, D. (1985). *The interpersonal world of the infant: A view from psychoanalysis and developmental psychology*. New York: Basic Books.

Stern, D. T., Frohna, A. Z., & Gruppen, L. A. (2005). The prediction of professional behaviour. *Medical Education, 39*, 75–82.

Sternberg, R. J. (2004). Culture and intelligence. *American Psychologist, 59*, 325–338.

Stewart, M. A. (1996). Effective physician-patient communication and health outcomes: A review. *Canadian Medical Association Journal, 152*, 1423–1433.

Stewart-Williams, S., & Thomas, A. G. (2013). The ape that thought it was a peacock: Does evolutionary psychology exaggerate human sex differences? *Psychological Inquiry, 24*, 137–168. Retrieved from: http://dx.doi.org/10.1080/1047840X.2013.804899.

Stiles, W., Putman, S., Wolfe, M., & James, S. (1979). Interaction exchange structure and patient satisfaction with medical interview. *Medical Care, 17*, 667–679.

Stokes, J. (1980). Grief and the performing arts: A brief experiment in humanistic medical education. *Journal of Medical Education, 55*, 215.

Stotland, E. (1969). Exploratory investigation of empathy. In L. Berkowitz (Ed.), *Advances in experimental social psychology* (pp. 271–314). New York: Academic Press.

Stotland, E. (1978). Fantasy-empathy research: An integration. In E. Stotland, K. E. Matthews Jr., S. E. Sherman, R. O. Hansson, & B. Z. Richardson (Eds.), *Empathy, fantasy, and helping* (pp. 103–122). Beverly Hills, CA: Sage.

Stotland, E., Mathews, K. E., Jr., Sherman, S. E., Hansson, R. O., & Richardson, B. Z. (1978). *Empathy, fantasy and helping* (Vol. 65). Beverly Hills: Sage.

Strauss, M. B. (1968). *Familiar medical quotations*. Boston: Little, Brown.

Street, R. L., Makoul, G., Arora, N. K., & Epstein, R. M. (2009). How does communication heal? Pathways linking clinician-patient communication to health outcomes. *Patient Education and Counseling, 74*, 295–301.

Streit, U. (1980). Attitudes toward psycho-social factors in medicine: An appraisal of the ATSIM scale. *Medical Education, 14*, 259–266.

Streit-Forest, U. (1982). Differences in empathy: A preliminary analysis. *Journal of Medical Education, 57*, 65–67.

Stuss, D. T. (2001). The right frontal lobes are necessary for theory of mind. *Brain, 124*, 279–286.

Su, R., Rounds, J., & Armstrong, P. I. (2009). Men and things, women and people: A meta-analysis of sex differences in interests. *Psychological Bulletin, 135*, 859–884. Retrieved from: http://dx.doi.org/10.1037/a0017364.

Suchman, A. L., Markakis, K., Beckman, H. B., & Frankel, R. (1997). A model of empathic communication in the medical interview. *Journal of the American Medical Association, 277*, 678–682.

Suh, D. H., Hong, J. S., Lee, D. H., Gonnella, J. S., & Hojat, M. (2012). The Jefferson Scale of Physician Empathy: A preliminary psychometric study and group comparisons in Korean physicians. *Medical Teacher, 34*, e464–e468. doi:10.3109/0142159x.2012.668632 (web paper).

Sullivan, P. (1990). Pay more attention to your own health, physicians warned. *Canadian Medical Association Journal, 142*, 1309–1310.

Sultan, S., Attali, C., Gilberg, S., Zenasni, F., & Hartemann, A. (2011). Physicians' understanding of patients' personal representations of their diabetes: Accuracy and association with self-care. *Psychology and Health, 18*, 1–17.

Surbone, A. (1992). Truth telling to the patient. *Journal of American Medical Association, 268*, 1661–1662.

Surrey, J. L., & Bergman, S. J. (1994). Gender differences in rational development: Implications for empathy in the doctor-patient relationship. In L. S. More & M. A. Milligan (Eds.), *The empathic practitioner: Empathy, gender, and medicine* (pp. 113–131). New Brunswick, NJ: Rutgers University Press.

Sutherland, J. A. (1993). The nature and evolution of phenomenological empathy in nursing: An historical treatment. *Archives of Psychiatric Nursing, 7*, 369–376.

Swain, J. E., Lorberlaum, J. P., Kose, S., & Strathearn, L. (2007). Brain basis of early parent-infant interactions: Psychology, physiology, and in vivo functional neuroimaging studies. *Journal of Child Psychology and Psychiatry, 48*, 262–287.

Szalita, A. B. (1976). Some thoughts on empathy. The eighteenth annual Frieda Fromm-Reichmann memorial lecture. *Psychiatry, 39*, 142–152.

Tai, Y. F., Scherfler, C., Brooks, D. J., Sawamoto, N., & Castiello, U. (2004). The human premotor cortex is 'mirror' only for biological actions. *Current Biology, 14*, 117–120. doi:10.1016/j.cub.2004.01.005.

Takooshian, H. (2014). Fifty years later: What have we learnt from the 1964 Kitty Genovese tragedy? *The General Psychologist, 49*(1–2), 34.

Tannen. (1990). *You just don't understand: Women and men in conversation*. New York: Ballantine.

Taragin, M. I., Sonnenberg, F. A., Karns, M. E., Trout, R., Shapiro, S., & Carson, J. L. (1994). Does physician performance explain interspecialty differences in malpractice claim rates? *Medical Care, 32*, 661–667.

Tausch, R. (1988). The relationship between emotions and cognitions: Implications for therapist empathy. *Person-Centered Review, 3*, 277–291.

Tavakol, S., Dennick, R., & Tavakol, M. (2011a). Empathy in UK medical students: Differences by gender, medical year and specialty interest. *Education for Primary Care, 22*, 297–303.

Tavakol, S., Dennick, R., & Tavakol, M. (2011b). Psychometric properties and confirmatory factor analysis of the Jefferson Scale of Physician Empathy. *BMC Medical Education, 11*, 54. doi:10.1186/1472-6920-11-54. Retrieved from: http://www.biomedcentral.com/1472-6920/11/54.

Taylor, S. E., Klein, L. C., Gruenewald, T. L., Gurung, R. A. R., & Fernandes-Taylor, S. (2003). Affiliation, social support and biobehavioral response to stress. In J. Suls & K. A. Wallston (Eds.), *Social psychological foundations of health and illness* (pp. 314–331). Malden, MA: Blackwell.

Taylor, S. E., Klein, L. C., Lewis, B. P., Gruenewald, T. L., Gurung, R. A., Regan, A. R., & Updegraff, J. (2000). Biobehavioral responses to stress in females: Tend-and-befriend, not fight-or-flight. *Psychological Review, 107*, 411–429. doi:10.1037/0037/0033-295X.107.3.411.

Therrien, M. E. (1979). Evaluating empathy skills training for parents. *Social Work, 24*, 417–419.

Thom, D. H., Hall, M. A., & Pawlson, L. G. (2004). Measuring patients' trust in physicians when assessing quality of care. *Health Affairs, 23*, 124–132.

Thomas, L. (1985). *The youngest science*. Oxford: Oxford University Press.

Thompson, B. M., Hearn, G. N., & Collins, M. J. (1992). Patient perceptions of health professional interpersonal skills. *Australian Psychologist, 27*, 91–95.

Thorndike, E. L. (1926). *The measurement of intelligence*. New York: Teacher's College, Columbia University.

Titchener, E. B. (1909). *Lectures on the experimental psychology of the thought-processes*. New York: Macmillan.

Titchener, E. B. (1915). *A beginner's psychology*. New York: Macmillan.

Tomkins, S. S. (1962). *Affect, imagery, consciousness: I. The positive effects*. New York: Springer.

Tomkins, S. S. (1963). *Affect, imagery, consciousness: II. The negative effects*. New York: Springer.

Tomkins, S. S. (1987). Script theory. In J. Aronoff, A. J. Rubin, & R. A. Zucker (Eds.), *The emergence of personality* (pp. 147–216). New York: Springer.

Tooby, J., & Cosmides, L. (1990). On the universality of human nature and the uniqueness of the individual: The role of genetic and adaptation. *Journal of Personality, 58*, 17–67.

Tranel, D., Bechara, A., & Denburg, N. L. (2002). Asymmetric functional roles of right and left ventromedial prefrontal cortices in social conduct, decision-making, and emotional processing. *Cortex, 38*, 589–612.

Trautmann Banks, J. (2002). The story inside. In R. Charon & M. Montello (Eds.), *Stories matter: The role of narrative in medical ethics* (pp. 219–226). New York: Routledge.

Triandis, H. C. (1995). *Individualism & collectivism*. Boulder, CO: Westview Press.

Trivers, R. L. (1972). Parental investment and sexual selection. In B. Campbell (Ed.), *Sexual selection and the descent of man* (pp. 136–179). Chicago, IL: Aldine.

Trommsdorff, G. (1991). Child-rearing and children's empathy. *Perceptual & Motor Skills, 72*, 387–390.

Trommsdorff, G. (1995). Person-context relations as developmental conditions for empathy and prosocial action: A cross-cultural analysis. In T. A. Kindermann & J. Valsiner (Eds.), *Development of person-context relations* (pp. 189–208). Hillsdale, NJ: Erlbaum.

Tronick, E., Als, H., Adamson, L., Wise, S., & Brazelton, T. B. (1978). The infant's response to entrapment between contradictory messages in face-to-face interaction. *Journal of the American Academy of Child Psychiatry, 17*, 1–13.

Trout, D. L., & Rosenfeld, H. M. (1980). The effect of postural lean and body congruence on the judgment of psychotherapeutic rapport. *Journal of Nonverbal Behavior, 4*, 176–190.

Truax, C. B., Altmann, H., & Millis, W. A. (1974). Therapeutic relationships provided by various professionals. *Journal of Community Psychology, 2*, 33–36.

Truax, C. B., & Carkhuff, R. (1967). *Towards effective counseling and psychotherapy: Training and practice.* Chicago: Aldine.

Tucker, D., Luu, P., & Derryberry, D. (2005). Love hurts: The evolution of empathic concern through the encephalization of nociceptive capacity. *Development and Psychopathology, 17,* 699–713.

Turner, J. A., Deyo, R. A., Loeser, J. D., von Korff, M., & Fordyce, W. E. (1994). The importance of placebo effect on pain treatment and research. *Journal of the American Medical Association, 271,* 1609–1614.

Twenge, J. M. (1997). Changes in masculine and feminine traits over time: A meta-analysis. *Sex Roles, 36,* 305–325. Retrieved from: http://dx.doi.org/10.1007/BF02766650.

Uchino, B. N., Cacioppo, J. T., & Kiecolt-Glaser, J. K. (1996). The relationship between social support system and physiological processes: A review with emphasis on underlying mechanisms and implications for health. *Psychological Bulletin, 119,* 488–531.

Umilta, M. A., Kohler, E., Gallese, V., Fogassi, L., Fadiga, L., Keysers, C., & Rizzolatti, G. (2001). I know what you are doing: A neurophysiological study. *Neuron, 31,* 155–165.

Underwood, B., & Moore, B. (1982). Perspective-taking and altruism. *Psychological Bulletin, 91,* 143–173.

Uvnas-Moberg, K. (1997). Physiological and endocrine effects of social contact. *Annals of the New York Academy of Sciences, 807,* 146–163.

Valeriani, M., Betti, V., Le Pera, D., De Armas, L., Miliucci, R., Restuccia, D., … Aglioti, S. M. (2008). Seeing the pain of others while being in pain. A laser-evoked potential study. *Neuroimage, 40,* 1419–1428.

Vallabh, K. (2011). Psychometrics of the student version of the Jefferson Scale of Physician Empathy (JSPE-S) in final-year medical students in Johannesburg in 2008. *South African Journal of Bioethics and Law, 4,* 63–68. Retrieved from: http://www.sajbl.org.za/index.php/sajbl/article/view/164/140.

Valliant, G. E. (1977). *Adaptation to life.* Boston: Little, Brown.

Van Honk, J., Schutter, D., Bos, P., Kruijt, A., Lentjes, E., & Baron-Cohen, S. (2011). Testosterone administration impairs cognitive empathy in women depending on second-to-fourth digit ratio. *National Academy of Sciences, 108,* 3448–3452.

Van Orum, W., Foley, J. M., Burns, P. R., DeWolfe, A. S., & Kennedy, E. C. (1981). Empathy, altruism, and self-interest in college students. *Adolescence, 16,* 799–808.

Van Winkel, L. J., Fjortoft, N., & Hojat, M. (2011). Validation of an instrument to measure pharmacy and medical students' attitudes toward physician-pharmacist collaboration. *American Journal of Pharmaceutical Education, 75*(9), Article 178.

Van Winkle, L. J., Bjork, B. C., Chandar, N., Cornell, S., Fjortoft, N., Green, J. M., … Burdick, P. (2012). Interprofessional workshop to improve mutual understanding between pharmacy and medical students. *American Journal of Pharmaceutical Education, 76*(8), Article 150. Retrieved from: http://www.ncbi.nlm.nih.gov/pmc/articles/PMC3475779/.

Van Winkle, L. J., Burdick, P., Bjork, B. C., Chandar, N., Green, J. M., Lynch, S. M., … Robson, C. (2014). Critical thinking and reflection on community service for a medical biochemistry course raise students' empathy, patient-centered orientation, and examination scores. *Medical Science Educator, 24,* 279–290. doi:10.1007/s40670-014-0049-7.

Van Winkle, L. J., Fjortoft, N., & Hojat, M. (2012). Impact of a workshop about aging on the empathy scores of pharmacy and medical students. *American Journal of Pharmaceutical Education, 76*(1), Article 9. doi:10.5688/ajpe7619. Retrieved from: http://www.ncbi.nlm.nih.gov/pmc/articles/PMC3298407/.

Van Winkle, L. J., La Salle, S., Richardson, L., Bjork, B. C., Burdick, P., Chandar, N., … Viselli, S. M. (2013). Challenging medical students to confront their biases: A case study simulation approach. *Medical Science Educator, 23,* 217–224.

Van Zanten, M., Boulet, J. R., Norcini, J., & McKinley, D. (2005). Using standardised patient assessment to measure professional attributes. *Medical Education, 39,* 20–29. doi:10.1111/j.1365-2929.2004.02029.x.

Varkey, P., Chutka, D. S., & Lesnick, T. G. (2006). The aging game: Improving medical students' attitudes toward caring for the elderly. *Journal of the American Medical Directors Association, 7*, 224–229.

Vaughan, K. B., & Lanzetta, J. T. (1981). The effect of modification of expressive displays on vicarious emotional arousal. *Journal of Experimental Social Psychology, 17*, 16–30.

Velicer, W. F., & Fava, J. L. (1998). Effects of variables and subject sampling on factor pattern recovery. *Psychological Methods, 3*, 231–251.

Veloski, J., & Hojat, M. (2006). Measuring specific elements of professionalism: Empathy, teamwork, and lifelong learning. In D. T. Stern (Ed.), *Measuring Medical Professionalism* (pp. 117–145). Oxford: Oxford University Press.

Verbrugge, L. M. (1979). Marital status and health. *Journal of Marriage and the Family, 41*, 267–285.

Viviani, P. (2002). Motor competence in the perception of dynamic events: A tutorial. In W. Prinz & B. Hommel (Eds.), *Common mechanisms in perception and action* (pp. 406–442). New York: Oxford University Press.

Voinescu, B. I., Szentagotai, A., & Coogan, A. (2009). Residents' clinical empathy: Gender and specialty comparisons—A Romanian study. *Acta Medica Academica, 38*, 11–15. doi:10.5644/ama.v38i1.50.

Voyer, D., Voyer, S., & Bryden, M. P. (1995). Magnitude of sex differences in spatial abilities: A meta-analysis and consideration of critical variables. *Psychological Bulletin, 117*, 250–270. doi:10.1037/0033-2909.117.2.250.

Wagner, H. L., Buck, R., & Winterbotham, M. (1993). Communication of specific emotions: Gender differences in sending accuracy and communication measures. *Journal of Nonverbal Behavior, 17*, 29–53.

Wagoner, N. E., Suriano, J. R., & Stoner, J. A. (1986). Factors used by program directors to select residents. *Journal of Medical Education, 61*, 10–21.

Waisman, M. (1966). Listening with the third ear in eczematous eruptions. *Medical Times, 94*, 1108–1113.

Wallace, D. S., Paulson, R. M., Lord, C. G., & Bond, C. F., Jr. (2005). Which behaviors do attitudes predict? Meta-analyzing the effects of social pressure and perceived difficulty. *Review of General Psychology, 9*, 214–227.

Walton, H. J. (1987). Personality assessment of future doctors. *Journal of the Royal Society of Medicine, 80*, 27–30.

Ward, J., Cody, J., Schaal, M., & Hojat, M. (2012). The empathy enigma: An empirical study of decline in empathy among undergraduate nursing students. *Journal of Professional Nursing, 28*, 34–40. doi:10.1016/j.profnurs.2011.10.007.

Ward, J., Schaal, M., Sullivan, J., Bowen, M. E., Erdmann, J. B., & Hojat, M. (2008). The Jefferson Scale of Attitudes toward Physician-Nurse Collaboration: A study with undergraduate nursing students. *Journal of Interprofessional Care, 22*, 375–386.

Ward, J., Schaal, M., Sullivan, J., Bowen, M. E., Erdmann, J. B., & Hojat, M. (2009). Reliability and validity of the Jefferson Scale of Empathy in undergraduate nursing students. *Journal of Nursing Measurement, 17*, 73–88. doi:10.1891/1061-3749.17.1.73.

Wasserman, R. C., Inui, T. S., Barriatua, R. D., Carter, W. B., & Lippincott, P. (1984). Pediatric clinicians' support for patients makes a difference: An outcome-based analysis of clinician-parent interaction. *Pediatrics, 74*, 1047–1053.

Watson, J. B. (1924). *Behaviorism*. New York: W.W. Norton.

Watson, J. C. (2002). Re-visioning empathy. In D. Cain & J. Seeman (Eds.), *Humanistic psychotherapies: Handbook of research and practice* (pp. 445–471). Washington, DC: American Psychological Association.

Watson, P. J., Grisham, S. O., Trotter, M. V., & Biderman, M. D. (1984). Narcissism and empathy: Validity evidence for the Narcissistic Personality Inventory. *Journal of Personality Assessment, 48*, 301–305.

Watts, D. (2012). Cure for the common cold. *New England Journal of Medicine, 367*, 1184–1185.

Waxler-Morrison, N., Anderson, J. M., & Richardson, E. (1990). *Cross-cultural caring: A handbook for health professionals in Western Canada*. Vancouver: University of British Columbia Press.

Wear, D., & Aultman, J. M. (2005). The limits of narrative: Medical student resistance to confronting inequality and oppression in literature and beyond. *Medical Education, 39*, 1056–1065.

Wear, D., Nixon, L.L. (2002). Literary inquiry and professional development in medicine: Against abstraction. *Perspectives in Biology and Medicine, 45*, 104–124.

Weaver, M. J., Ow, C. L., Walker, D. J., & Degenhardt, E. F. (1993). A questionnaire for patients' evaluations of their physicians' humanistic behaviors. *Journal of General Internal Medicine, 8*, 135–139.

Webb, C. (1996). Caring, curing, coping: Toward an integrated model. *Journal of Advanced Nursing, 23*, 960.

Weijters, B., Baumgartner, H., & Schillewaert N. (2013). Reversed item bias: An integrated model. *Psychological Methods, 18*, 320–334.

Weinberg, M. K., Tronick, E. Z., & Cohn, J. F. (1999). Gender differences in emotional expressivity and self-regulation during early infancy. *Developmental Psychology, 35*, 175–188.

Weinberg, M. K., & Tronik, E. Z. (1996). Infant affective reaction to the resumption of maternal interaction after the still-face. *Child Development, 67*, 905–914.

Weisman, J. S., Betancourt, J., Campbell, E. G., Park, E. R., Kim, M., Clarridge, B., ... Maina, A. W. (2005). Resident physicians' preparedness to provide cross-cultural care. *Journal of the American Medical Association, 294*, 1058–1067.

Weisman, C. S., & Teitelbaum, M. A. (1985). Physician gender and the physician-patient relationship: Recent evidence and relevant questions. *Social Science & Medicine, 20*, 1119–1127.

Weiss, R. F., Boyer, J. L., Lombardo, J. P., & Stich, M. H. (1973). Altruistic drive and altruistic reinforcement. *Journal of Personality and Social Psychology, 25*, 390–400.

Weissman, S. H., Haynes, R. A., Killan, C. D., & Robinowitz, C. (1994). A model to determine the influence of medical school on students' career choices. *Academic Medicine, 69*, 58–59.

Wellman, H. (1991). *The child's theory of mind*. Cambridge, MA: Bradford Books/MIT Press.

Wellman, B. (1998). Social network. In H. S. Friedman (Ed.), *Encyclopedia of mental health* (pp. 525–544). San Diego, CA: Academic Press.

Wen, D., Ma, X., Li, H., Liu, Z., Xian, B., & Liu, Y. (2013). Empathy in Chinese medical students: Psychometric characteristics and differences by gender and year of medical education. *BMC Medical Education, 13*, 130. doi:10.1186/1472-6920-13-130.

Wen, D., Ma, X., Li, H., & Xian, B. (2013). Empathy in Chinese physicians: Preliminary psychometrics of the Jefferson Scale of Physician Empathy (JSE) [Letter to the editor]. *Medical Teacher, 35*, 609–610.

Weng, H. C., Steed, J. F., Yu, S. W., Liu, Y. T., Hsu, C. C., Yu, T. J., & Chen, W. (2011). The effect of surgeon empathy and emotional intelligence on patient satisfaction. *Advances in Health Sciences Education, 16*, 591–600. doi:10.1007/s10459-011-9278-3.

Werner, A., & Schneider, J. M. (1974). Teaching medical students interactional skills: A research-based course in doctor-patient relationship. *New England Journal of Medicine, 290*, 1232–1237.

West, C. P., Dyrbye, L. N., Rabatin, J. T., Call, T. G., Davidson, J. H., Multari, A., ... Shanafelt, T. D. (2014). Intervention to promote physician well-being, job satisfaction, and professionalism: A randomized clinical trial. *JAMA Internal Medicine, 174*, 527–533. doi:10.1001/jamainternmed.2013.14387.

West, C. P., Huschka, M. M., Novotny, P. J., Sloan, J. A., Kolars, J. C., Habermann, T. M., & Shanafelt, T. D. (2006). Association of perceived medical errors with resident distress and empathy. *Journal of American Medical Association, 269*, 1071–1078.

West, C. P., Tan, A. D., Habermann, T. M., Sloan, J. A., & Shanafelt, T. D. (2009). Association of resident fatigue and distress with perceived medical errors. *Journal of American Medical Association, 302*, 1294–1300.

Wester, W. C., & Smith, A. H. J. (1984). *Clinical hypnosis: A multidisciplinary approach.* Philadelphia: Lippincott.

Westerman, M. A. (2005). What is interpersonal behavior? Post-cartesian approach to problematic interpersonal pattern and psychotherapy process. *Review of General Psychology, 9,* 16–34.

White, K. L. (1991). *Healing the schism: Epidemiology, medicine, and the public's health.* New York: Springer-Verlag.

Whittemore, P. B., Burstein, A. G., Loucks, S., & Schoenfeld, L. S. (1985). A longitudinal study of personality changes in medical students. *Journal of Medical Education, 60,* 404–405.

Whorf, B. L. (1956). *Language, thought, and reality: Selected writings of Benjamin Lee Whorf.* New York: John Wiley & Sons.

Wicker, B., Keysers, C., Plailly, J., Royet, J. P., Gallese, V., & Rizzolatti, G. (2003). Both of us disgusted in my insula: The common neural basis of seeing and feeling disgust. *Neuron, 40,* 655–664.

Wickramasekera, I. E., & Szylk, J. P. (2003). Could empathy be a predictor of hypnotic ability? *International Journal of Clinical & Experimental Hypnosis, 51,* 390–399.

Wiehe, V. R. (2003). Empathy and narcissism in a sample of child abuse perpetrators and a comparison sample of foster parents. *Child Abuse & Neglect, 27,* 541–555.

Wiesenfeld, A. R., Whitman, P. B., & Malatesta, C. Z. (1984). Individual differences among adult women in sensitivity to infants: Evidence in support of an empathy concept. *Journal of Personality and Social Psychology, 46,* 118–124.

Wiklund, I., Oden, A., & Sanne, H. (1988). Prognostic importance of somatic and psychosocial variables after a first myocardial infarction. *American Journal of Epidemiology, 128,* 786–795.

Wilkes, M., Milgrom, E., & Hoffman, J. R. (2002). Toward more empathic medical students: A medical student hospitalization experience. *Medical Education, 36,* 528–533.

Williams, C. A. (1989). Empathy and burnout in male and female helping professionals. *Research in Nursing & Health, 12,* 169–178.

Williams, R. B., Barefoot, J. C., Califf, R. M., Haney, T. L., Saunders, W. B., & Pryor, D. B. (1992). Prognostic importance of social and economic resources among medically treated patients with angiographically documented coronary artery disease. *Journal of the American Medical Association, 267,* 524.

Williams, B., Boyle, M., Brightwell, R., Devenish, S., Hartley, P., McCall, M., … Webb, V. (2012). Paramedic empathy levels: Results from seven Australian universities. *International Journal of Emergency Services, 1,* 111–121. Retrieved from: www.emeraldinsight.com/doi/abs/10.1108/20470891211275902.

Williams, B., Boyle, M., Tozer-Jones, J., Devenish, S., Hartley, P., McCall, M., … O'Meara, P. (2015). Undergraduate paramedic students' empathy levels: A two-year longitudinal study. *Journal of Nursing Education and Practice, 5,* 58–64. doi:10.5430/jnep.v5n1p58. Retrieved from: http://dx.doi.org/10.5430/jnep.v5n1p58.

Williams, B., Boyle, M., & Earl, T. (2013). Measurement of empathy levels in undergraduate parametric students. *Prehospital and Disaster Medicine, 28,* 145–149. doi:10.1017/S1049023X1300006X.

Williams, B., Brown, T., Boyle, M., McKenna, L., Palermo, C., & Etherington, J. (2014). Levels of empathy in undergraduate emergency health, nursing, and midwifery students: A longitudinal study. *Advances in Medical Education and Practice, 5,* 299–306. Retrieved from: http://dx.doi.org/10.2147/AMEP.S66681.

Williams, B., Brown, T., Boyle, M., & Dousek, S. (2013). Psychometric testing of the Jefferson Scale of Empathy Health Profession Students' version with Australian paramedic students. *Nursing and Health Sciences, 15,* 45–50. doi:10.1111/j.1442-2018.2012.00719.x.

Williams, B., Brown, T., McKenna, L., Boyle, M. J., Palermo, C., Nestel, D., … Russo, V. (2014). Empathy levels among health professional students: A cross-sectional study at two universities in Australia. *Advances in Medical Education and Practice, 5,* 107–113. doi:10.2147/AMEP.S57569. Retrieved from: http://dx.doi.org/10.2147/AMEP.S57569.

Williams, B., Brown, T., & McKenna, L. (2013). DVD empathy simulations: An interventional study. *Medical Education, 47*, 1142–1143.

Williams, B., Sadasivan, S., Kadirvelu, A., & Olaussen, A. (2014). Empathy level among first year Malaysian medical students: An observational study. *Advances in Medical Education and Practice, 5*, 149–156. doi:10.2147/AMEP.S58094.

Willingham, W. W., & Cole, N. S. (1997). *Gender and fair assessment*. Hillsdale, NJ: Erlbaum.

Wilmer, H. A. (1968). The doctor-patient relationship and issues of pity, sympathy and empathy. *British Journal of Medical Psychology, 41*, 243–248.

Wilson, S. E., Prescott, J., & Becket, G. (2012). Empathy levels in first- and third-year students in health and non-Health disciplines. *American Journal of Pharmaceutical Education, 76*(2), Article 24. Retrieved from: http://www.ncbi.nlm.nih.gov/pmc/articles/PMC3305933/.

Windholz, M. J., Marmar, C. R., & Horowitz, M. J. (1985). A review of research in conjugal bereavement: Impact on health and efficacy of intervention. *Comprehensive Psychiatry, 26*, 433–447.

Winefield, H. R., & Chur-Hansen, A. (2000). Evaluating the outcome of communication skill teaching for entry-level medical students: Does knowledge of empathy increase? *Medical Education, 34*, 90–94.

Winnicott, D. W. (1987). *Babies and their mothers*. Reading, MA: Addison-Wesley.

Wispe, L. (1978). *Altruism, sympathy, and helping: Psychological and sociological principles*. New York: Academic Press.

Wispe, L. (1986). The distinction between sympathy and empathy: To call forth a concept, a word is needed. *Journal of Personality and Social Psychology, 50*, 314–321.

Wittstein, I. S., Thiemann, D. R., Lima, J. A. C., Baughman, K. L., Schulman, S. P., … Chapman, H. C. (2005). Neurohormunal features of myocardial stunning due to sudden emotional stress. *New England Journal of Medicine, 352*, 539–548.

Wolf, E. S. (1980). The dutiful physician: The central role of empathy in psychoanalysis, psychotherapy, and medical practice. *Hillside Journal of Clinical Psychiatry, 2*, 41–56.

Wolf, S. (1992). Prediction of myocardial infarction over a span of 30 years in Roseto, Pennsylvania. *Integrative Physiological & Behavioral Science, 27*, 246–257.

Wolf, T. M., Balson, P. M., Faucett, J. M., & Randall, H. M. (1989). A retrospective study of attitude change during medical education. *Medical Education, 23*, 19–23.

Wolfgang, A. (1979). *Nonverbal behavior: Applications and cultural implications*. New York: Academic Press.

Wood, W., & Eagly, A. H. (2002). A cross-cultural analysis of the behavior of women and men: Implications for the origin of sex differences. *Psychological Bulletin, 128*, 699–727.

Wood, W., & Eagly, A. H. (2010). Gender. In S. T. Fiske, D. T. Gilbert, & G. Lindzey (Eds.), *The handbook of social psychology* (Vol. 1, 5th ed., pp. 629–667). New York: McGraw-Hill.

World Health Organization. (1948). *World Health Organization Constitution: Basic documents*. Geneva: Author.

Worly, B. (2013). Professionalism education of OB/GYN resident physicians: What makes a difference? *Open Journal of Obstetrics and Gynecology, 3*, 137–141. doi:10.4236/ojog.2013.31A026.

Wright, S. (1996). Examining what residents look for in their role models. *Academic Medicine, 71*, 290–292.

Xia, L., Hongyu, S., & Xinwei, F. (2011). Study on correlation between empathy ability and personality characteristics of undergraduate nursing students. *Chinese Nursing Research, 32*, 2933–2935.

Yaghmaei, M., Monajemi, A., & Soltani-Arabshahi, K. (2014). The effect of storytelling course on medical students' empathy toward patients. *International Journal of Body, Mind & Culture, 1*, 127–134.

Yang, K. T., & Yang, J. H. (2013). A study of the effect of a visual arts-based program on the scores of Jefferson Scale of Physician Empathy. *BMC Medical Education, 13*, 142. Retrieved from: http://www.biomedcentral.com/1472-6920/13/142.

Yarnold, P. R., Bryant, F. B., Nightingale, S. D., & Martin, G. J. (1996). Assessing physician empathy using the Interpersonal Reactivity Index: A measurement model and cross-sectional analysis. *Psychology, Health & Medicine, 1*, 207–221.

Yarnold, P. R., Greenberg, M. S., & Nightingale, S. D. (1991). Comparing resource use of sympathetic and empathetic physicians. *Academic Medicine, 66*, 709–710.

Yarnold, P. R., Martin, G. J., & Soltysik, R. C. (1993). Androgyny predicts empathy for trainees in medicine. *Perceptual & Motor Skills, 77*, 576–578.

Yates, S. (2001). Finding your funny bone: Incorporating humour into medical practice. *Australian Family Physician, 30*, 22–24.

Yedidia, M. J., Gillespie, C. C., Kachur, E., Schwartz, M. D., Ockene, J., Chepaitis, A. E., … Lipkin, M. (2003). Effect of communications training on medical student performance. *Journal of the American Medical Association, 290*, 1157–1165.

Younger, J. B. (1990). Literary works as a mode of knowing. *Journal of Nursing Scholarship, 22*, 39–43.

Youssef, F. F., Nunes, P., Sa, B., & Williams, S. (2014). An exploration of changes in cognitive and emotional empathy among medical students in the Caribbean. *International Journal of Medical Education, 5*, 185–192. doi:10.5116/ijme.5412.e641.

Yu, J., & Kirk, M. (2009). Evaluation of empathy measurement tools in nursing: Systematic review. *Journal of Advanced Nursing, 65*, 1790–1806. doi:10.1111/j.1365-2648.2009.05071.x.

Zachariae, R., Pedersen, C. G., Jensen, A. B., Ehrnrooth, E., Rossen, P. B., & von der Maase, H. (2003). Association of perceived physician communication style with patient satisfaction, distress, cancer-related self-efficacy, and perceived control over the disease. *British Journal of Cancer, 88*, 658–665.

Zahedi, F. (2011). The challenge of truth telling across cultures: A case study. *Journal of Medical Ethics and History of Medicine, 4*, 11–19.

Zahn-Waxler, C., & Radke-Yarrow, M. (1990). The origin of empathic concern. *Motivation and Emotion, 14*, 107–130.

Zahn-Waxler, C., Radke-Yarrow, M., & King, R. A. (1979). Child rearing and children's prosocial initiations toward victims of distress. *Child Development, 50*, 319–330.

Zahn-Waxler, C., Robinson, J. L., & Emde, R. N. (1992). The development of empathy in twins. *Developmental Psychology, 28*, 1038–1047.

Zeldow, P. B., & Daugherty, S. R. (1987). The stability and attitudinal correlates of warmth and caring in medical students. *Medical Education, 21*, 353–357.

Zeleznik, C., Hojat, M., Goepp, C. E., Amadio, P., Kowlessar, O. D., & Borenstein, B. D. (1988). Measurement of certainty in medical school examination: A pilot study on non-cognitive dimensions of test-taking behavior. *Journal of Medical Education, 63*, 881–891.

Zeleznik, C., Hojat, M., & Veloski, J. J. (1983). Levels of recommendation for students and academic performance in medical school. *Psychological Reports, 52*, 851–858.

Zell, E., Krizan, Z., & Teener, S. R. (2015). Evaluating similarities and differences using metasynthesis. *American Psychologist, 70*, 10–20. Retrieved from: http://dx.doi.org/10.1037/a0038208.

Zenasni, F., Boujut, E., de Vaure, C. B., Catu-Pinault, A., Tavani, J. L., Rigal, L., … Sultan, S. (2012). Development of a French-language version of the Jefferson Scale of Physician Empathy and association with practice characteristics and burnout in a sample of general practitioners. *The International Journal of Person Centered Medicine, 2*, 759–766. Retrieved from: http://www.ijpcm.org/index.php/IJPCM/article/view/295.

Zentner, M., & Mitura, K. (2012). Stepping out of the caveman's shadow: Nations' gender gap predicts degree of sex differentiation in mate preferences. *Psychological Science, 23*, 1176–1185. doi:10.1177/0956797612441004.

Zhou, Q., Eisenberg, N., Losoya, S. H., Fabes, R. A., Reiser, M., Guthrie, I. K., … Shepard, S. A. (2002). The relations of parental warmth and positive expressiveness to children's empathy-related responding and social functioning: A longitudinal study. *Child Development, 73*, 893–915.

Zhou, Q., Valiente, C., & Eisenberg, N. (2003). Empathy and its measurement. In S. J. Lopez & C. R. Snyder (Eds.), *Positive psychological assessment: A handbook of models and measures* (pp. 269–284). Washington, DC: American Psychological Association.

Zimbardo, P. (2007). *Lucifer effect: Understanding how good people turn evil.* New York: Random House.

Zinn, W. (1990). Transference phenomenon in medical practice: Being whom the patient needs. *Annals of Internal Medicine, 113,* 298.

Zuckerman, M. (2002). Zuckerman-Kuhlman Personality Questionnaire (ZKPQ): An alternative five-factor model. In B. DeRaad & M. Perugini (Eds.), *Big five assessment* (pp. 377–396). Seattle, WA: Hogrefe & Huber.

Zuckerman, M., DePauls, B. M., & Rosenthal, R. (1981). Verbal and nonverbal communication of deception. In L. Berkowitz (Ed.), *Advances in experimental social psychology* (Vol. 14). New York: Academic Press.

Zuger, A. (2004). Dissatisfaction with medical practice. *New England Journal of Medicine, 350,* 69–75.

About the Author

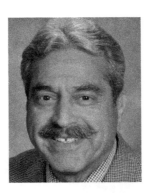

Mohammadreza Hojat, Ph.D. is a Research Professor of Psychiatry and Human Behavior, and Director of the Jefferson Longitudinal Study of Medical Education at Sidney Kimmel (formerly Jefferson) Medical College at Thomas Jefferson University in Philadelphia, PA, USA. He was born in Mashhad, Iran, received his bachelor's degree in educational psychology from Pahlavi University (currently University of Shiraz), his master's degree in psychology from the University of Tehran in Iran, and his doctoral degree in psychological services from the University of Pennsylvania. Dr. Hojat is a licensed psychologist in the Commonwealth of Pennsylvania, and has published more than 200 articles in peer-reviewed journals and 13 book chapters on educational, psychological, and social issues. Dr. Hojat has led the development of 10 psychometrically sound instruments (including the Jefferson Scale of Empathy) for the assessment of health professions education and patient outcomes, and professional development of health professionals-in-training and in-practice. Dr. Hojat's research on measurement, development, erosion, enhancement, and correlates of empathy in health professions education and patient care has received broad media coverage, featured in the *New York Times, Wall Street*

© Springer International Publishing Switzerland 2016
M. Hojat, *Empathy in Health Professions Education and Patient Care*,
DOI 10.1007/978-3-319-27625-0

Journal, Philadelphia Inquirer, the *National Public Radio* and television program segments. Dr. Hojat is a manuscript referee for several American and European professional journals, and has served as a co-editor of two books: *Loneliness: Theory, Research, and Applications* (Sage Publications, 1987), and *Assessment Measures in Medical School, Residency, and Practice: The Connections* (Springer, 1993). The original edition of his book *"Empathy in Patient care: Antecedents, Development, Measurement, and Outcomes"* was published in 2007 by Springer, which was expanded and updated in 2016 under a new title *"Empathy in Health Professions Education and Patient Care"* (Springer Intertnational Publishing).

Index

© Springer International Publishing Switzerland 2016
M. Hojat, *Empathy in Health Professions Education and Patient Care*,
DOI 10.1007/978-3-319-27625-0

Sotile, M.O., 131
Sotile, W.M., 131
Southard, E.E., 5
Sox, H.C., 209
Spandorfer, J., 10, 74, 79, 80, 115, 156, 158,
    210, 257, 292, 314
Speedling, E.J., 192
Spelke, E.S., 186
Speroff, B.J., 63, 153, 164
Spiegel, D., 23, 26
Spiro, H., 73, 75, 132, 133, 214, 226, 328
Spiro, H.M., 28, 90, 96, 130, 132, 133, 143, 205
Spreng, R.N., 65
Squier, R.W., 130, 132, 192, 193
Squire, L.R., 237
Sroufe, L.A., 4, 50
St. James, D., 90, 130
Stallings, J., 180
Stamps, P.L., 172
Stanley, R.O., 84, 207
Stansfield, R.B., 284
Starcevic, V., 13, 14, 75, 227
Starfield, B., 133
Starr, P., 207
Staub, E., 152
Staudenmayer, H., 191, 196
Stebbins, C.A., 232
Steed, J.F., 297
Steele, J., 115, 304
Steer, R., 308
Stefanis, C.N., 159
Steffen, V.J., 184
Steiger, J.H., 211
Stein, M.D., 192
Steinbrook, R., 208
Steiner, J., 185
Steiner, J.F., 227, 228
Steiner, M., 180
Stelzner, D.M., 306
Stephan, W., 129
Stephan, W.G., 29, 216
Stepien, K.A., 212, 233
Ster, B., 284
Ster, M.P., 284
Stern, D., 55
Stern, D.T., 268
Stern, J., 8
Sternberg, C., 55
Sternberg, R.J., 146
Stevens, N., 21
Stevenson, K., 173, 309
Stewart, J.P., 266
Stewart, M.A., 191–193, 195
Stewart-Williams, S., 186

Stich, M.H., 215
Stiles, W., 192
Stoddart, A.D.R., 66, 324
Stokes, J., 230
Stokes-Zoota, J.J., 125
Stone, A., 229
Stoner, J.A., 266
Stotland, E., 5, 64–66, 156, 216, 217, 252
Strathearn, L., 245
Straus, A., 43
Strauss, A., 141
Strauss, M.B., 151
Strayer, J., 4, 5, 43, 181
Street, R.L., 192
Streit, U., 156
Streit-Forest, U., 11, 155, 160, 267
Stuss, D.T., 243
Su, R., 178, 186
Suchman, A.L., 77, 78, 130, 194, 220, 221, 294
Suh, D.H., 106, 159, 173, 174, 283, 284, 302
Sullivan, J., 285
Sullivan, P., 131
Sultan, S., 115, 156, 195, 196, 294, 295, 298
Sunblad, L., 215
Surbone, A., 147
Suriano, J.R., 266
Sutherland, J.A., 77
Svrakic, D.M., 157
Swain, J.E., 245
Swan, J.E., 197
Swartz, M.H., 165, 196
Sweeney, B., 227
Sweeney, S.K.T., 297
Syme, L., 23, 24
Syme, S., 19, 22
Syme, S.L., 22
Symmes, D., 47
Szalita, A.B., 38, 139, 226
Szenas, P.L., 159
Szentagotai, A., 114, 174, 303
Szylk, J.P., 155

T

Tai, Y.F., 241
Takayama, T., 147
Takooshian, H., 139
Talbott, D., 26
Tambor, E.S., 163
Tannen, 178
Tanner, J., 174
Taragin, M.I., 164, 194
Taranta, A., 144, 192
Target, M., 53

Subject Index

© Springer International Publishing Switzerland 2016

M. Hojat, *Empathy in Health Professions Education and Patient Care*,

DOI 10.1007/978-3-319-27625-0

CPSIA information can be obtained
at www.ICGtesting.com
Printed in the USA
BVHW040155270819
556921BV00004B/9/P